Developmental Psychopathology

Developmental Psychopathology
Epidemiology, Diagnostics and Treatment

Edited by

Cecilia Ahmoi Essau and Franz Petermann

University of Bremen, Germany

harwood academic publishers

Australia • Canada • China • France • Germany • India • Japan
Luxembourg • Malaysia • The Netherlands • Russia • Singapore
Switzerland • Thailand • United Kingdom

Amsteldijk 166
1st Floor
1079 LH Amsterdam
The Netherlands

British Library Cataloguing in Publication Data

Developmental psychopathology: epidemiology, diagnostics
and treatment
1. Child psychopathology
I. Essau, Cecilia Ahmoi   II. Petermann, Franz
618.9'2'89

ISBN 90-5702-190-0

Table of Contents

Foreword

No one knows for certain when the field of developmental psychopathology was born, but we know it is still quite young. About twenty years ago, Thomas Achenbach began the first chapter of his new textbook, *Developmental Psychopathology*, with the words, "This book is about a field that hardly exists yet." At the time, Achenbach and several contemporaries were concerned that much of the literature on child psychological dysfunction was little more than a downward extension of theory and research on adults. This small group worked to counter that adultocentric trend, nurturing the embryonic field into a healthy childhood, and perhaps by now, adolescence.

From these efforts, an increasingly rich body of research has been built, one that may serve as a model for adult psychopathology research in several important respects. For example, developmental psychopathology, much more than adult psychopathology, construes dysfunction in two quite complementary ways: a categorical approach, reflected in the DSM and ICD systems; and a dimensional approach, reflected in the empirically-derived taxonomies, most notably those derived from principal components analyses of the Child Behavior Checklist. A strong research base is being built within both approaches, and many researchers rely on both concurrently to enrich their research efforts.

As another example of its ascendency, and distinctive features, developmental psychopathology is built on the notion that the patterning and expression of psychopathology are influenced by developmental period and by social and cultural context. The biological, cognitive and social transformations that occur with development can produce marked discontinuities in the kinds of problem behaviour and psychopathology individuals show. Moreover, because children and adolescents are much less free to select and structure their own environments than are adults, special attention needs to be paid to the impact of such involuntary environments as schools and families on young people, and the impact of the youngsters on those environments.

To make matters more complex, such developmental theorists as Stephen Hinshaw and Jerome Kagan have cautioned us to recognize heterotypic continuity — a consistency across time in an underlying problem or disorder that is masked by developmental variations in the outward display, as when the core problem of aggression is manifest as pushiness in early childhood, threatening and bullying in preadolescence, and confrontational crime involving weapons in late adolescence. The challenge for researchers is to clearly delineate the ways in which psychopathology is continuous and discontinuous, across the developmental trajectory. Such complexity illustrates that, although developmental psychopathologists do not have all the answers, we do have some of the most fascinating questions.

As befits a young and vital field, developmental psychopathology has begun to generate some implicit basic principles. One of the most important of these is that the union of a developmental perspective with the study of child and adolescent psychopathology can enrich the study of the origins, course and outcome of various forms of child and adolescent dysfunction, and inform efforts to prevent and intervene. This core idea is reflected in the various chapters of this beautifully organized volume.

The chapters collectively provide an introduction to some of the most important basics of the field. The heart of the book is a series of thoughtful reviews, structured in parallel fashion, summarizing the state of knowledge on major syndromes of childhood and adolescence — conduct disorder, opposition, defiant disorder, attention — deficit/hyperactivity disorder pervasive developmental disorder, anxiety disorders, mood disorders, substance in disorders, feeding and eating disorders, and elimination disorders. The chapters devote special attention to such developmentally sensitive issues as course and outcome, family factors, peer relations, etiological models and evidence of their validity, and interventions that are particularly relevant to young people. The uniform coverage of such topics, across syndromes, makes the volume equally valuable as a researcher's resource book and as a text for an advanced course in the field.

The quality of this book reflects both the scholarship and energy of its two editors — Cecilia Ahmoi Essau, the prolific emerging leader in the field of European developmental psychopathology, and Franz

Petermann, the senior scholar whose important contributions in the area span many years. The editors offer especially thoughtful introductory chapters, summarizing key issues faced by researchers in developmental psychopathology, and noting how these issues have been addressed thus far; topics include the question of how patterns of child and adolescent dysfunction should be organized and classified, how assessment of dysfunction should be carried out, what kinds of research designs are used to answer various questions, and what forms of data and analytic strategies may be appropriate for the assessment of frequency, risk and change.

A final chapter, by Joseph Sergeant and Pier Prins, highlights enduring issues in the field — for example, how 'abnormality' should be defined, the relative importance of person versus situation factors, comorbidity among syndromes, and the issue of continuity/discontinuity noted above. This intriguing chapter is a particularly useful finale; it presents a picture of the 'big questions' that have driven and shaped the field of developmental psychopathology and that are likely to remain with us for the duration.

The contributors to this book have captured much of the spirit that energizes developmental psychopathology in the 1990s; the reviews, critiques and proposals advanced herein can serve to guide new investigators who want to venture in, and to update experienced workers on recent developments. Although we cannot yet know the ultimate shape of this young discipline known as developmental psychopathology, we can be confident that many of the shapers are here, in the list of contributors to this volume.

John R. Weisz

Preface

Developmental psychopathology has emerged as a new discipline, the presence of which has been manifested through the growing number of theoretical, review and empirical papers that reflect this orientation, and through its influence in prevention and intervention of disorders (Cicchetti and Cohen, 1995). Additionally, there have been various journals devoted to the discipline of developmental psychopathology. The substantial increase of interest and research attention in developmental psychopathology has been spurred by the findings that between 17 to 22% of adolescents below 18 years of age have had some type of psychiatric disorder (Kazdin and Kagan, 1994). Furthermore, some disorders such as conduct disorder which occur in childhood not only often continue into adulthood, but they also have a lifelong consequence (Feehan et al., 1994; Kazdin and Kagan, 1994; McGee et al., 1994). As reported by Feehan and colleagues (1993), about two-thirds of the adolescents with a disorder at age 15 still have a disorder at age 18.

Given these findings, literature regarding developmental psychopathology is accumulating at a rapid pace. Yet, when mental health professionals need information which is scientifically (e.g., prevalence rates and risk factors of specific psychiatric disorders) and clinically relevant (e.g., choice of treatment and treatment guidelines), their search often results in frustration. With this in mind, the aim of this book is to provide a comprehensive coverage of the most common psychiatric disorders reported in children and adolescents.

This volume is divided into three parts. Part 1 covers a brief introduction to the field of developmental psychopathology, general issues on the current classification systems, assessment strategies, and on research methods and designs. Part 2 contains eight chapters that provide a comprehensive summary of the most recent empirical findings for specific psychiatric disorders. The disorders covered are those which seem to increase in frequency during childhood and adolescence, including conduct disorder and oppositional defiant disorder, attention-deficit/hyperactivity disorder, pervasive developmental disorders, anxiety disorders, mood disorders, substance use disorders, feeding and eating disorders, and elimination disorders. These disorders not only rise or peak in frequency in these age groups, but they also seem to cause long-term psychosocial impairment in adulthood. Where information is available, the topics covered in each chapter include: definition and classification, epidemiology, risk factors, comorbidity, course and outcome, assessment, treatment and concluding remarks. Part 3 contains a chapter on progress and unresolved issues in developmental psychopathology and provides some recommendations for future studies in this field.

This book was written for professionals, advanced students and researchers who are interested in developmental psychopathology. It will be most useful to psychologists, psychiatrists, social workers, pediatricians, counselors and other mental health professionals. It is hoped that this volume will not only serve to illustrate our current knowledge of psychopathology, but also serve as a springboard to a better understanding of how and where we have to further enhance our knowledge. Thus, by reviewing recent literature on assessment strategies and research designs, as well as the prevalence and nature of common disorders, and some unresolved issues, this volume may stimulate and facilitate further progress in this field. This in turn may contribute to an improved understanding of the nature, course, outcome and treatment of psychiatric disorders in children and adolescents.

In a project such as this, many people need to be acknowledged. Among the foremost are the contributors, whose expertise and dedication to the project have been outstanding, and for being so patient with our requests to clarify, expand, or shorten sections of their work. Without them, a comprehensive scholarly coverage of the various topics would not have been so easily achieved. Finally, we thank the editorial staff at Harwood Academic Publishers for their support and patience.

REFERENCES

Cicchetti, D., and Cohen, D.J. (1995). Perspectives on developmental psychopathology. In D. Cicchetti and D.J. Cohen (Eds.), *Developmental psychopathology. Volume 1: Theory and methods* (pp. 3–20). New York: Wiley.

Feehan, M., McGee, R. and Williams, S.M. (1993). Mental health disorders from age 15 to age 18 years. *Journal of the American Academy of Child and Adolescent Psychiatry*, **32**, 1118–1126.

Feehan, M., McGee, R., Nada-Raja, S. and Williams, S.M. (1994). DSM-III-R disorders in New Zealand 18-year-olds. *Australian and New Zealand Journal of Psychiatry*, **28**, 87–99.

Kazdin, A.E. and Kagan, J. (1994). Models of dysfunction in developmental psychopathology. *Clinical Psychology: Science and practice, Summer*, 35–52.

McGee, R., Williams, S. and Feehan, M. (1994). Behavior problems in New Zealand children. In P.R. Joyce, R.T. Mulder, M.A. Oakley-Browne, J.D. Sellman and W.G.A. Watkins (Eds.), *Development, personality and psychopathology* (pp. 15–22). Christchurch: Christchurch School of Medicine.

McGee, R., Feehan, M. and Williams, S. (1995). Long-term follow-up of a birth cohort. In F.C. Verhulst and H.M. Koot (Eds.), *The epidemiology of child and adolescent psychopathology* (pp. 366–384). Oxford: Oxford University Press.

List of Contributors

Richard J. Butler
Department of Clinical Psychology
Leeds Community and Mental
    Health Services
High Royds Hospital
Menston, Ilkley
W. Yorks LS29 6AQ
UK

Wendy M. Craig
Department of Psychology
Queen's University
Kingston, Ontario
Canada K7L 3N6

Lisa Dierker
Genetic Epidemiology Research
    Unit
School of Medicine
40 Temple Street
New Haven
Connecticut 06510–3223
USA

Paul M. G. Emmelkamp
Klinische Psychologie
Academisch Ziekenhuis
Oostersingel 59
9713 EZ Groningen
The Netherlands

Cecilia Ahmoi Essau
Klinische Psychologie
Universität Bremen
Grazer Straße 2
28359 Bremen
Germany

Michael Feehan
Faculty Research Centre
Faculty of Health Studies,
    Rm AF 205
Auckland Institute of
    Technology
Private Bag 92006
Auckland 1020
New Zealand

Julie Hakim-Larson
Department of Psychology
University of Windsor
401 Sunset
Windsor, Ontario
Canada N9B 3P4

Michael Kusch
Zentrum für Kinderheilkunde der
    Universität Bonn
Adenauerallee 119
53113 Bonn
Germany

Rob McGee
University of Otago
Department of Preventive and
    Social Medicine
Otago Medical School
P.O. Box 913, Dunedin
New Zealand

Kathleen R. Merikangas
Genetic Epidemiology Research
    Unit   .
School of Medicine
40 Temple Street
New Haven
Connecticut 06510–3223
USA

Debra J. Pepler
York University
Department of Psychology
    (Clinical-Developmental)
Faculty of Arts
Behavioral Sciences Building
4700 Keele St.
North York, Ontario
Canada M3J 1P3

Franz Petermann
Klinische Psychologie
Universität Bremen
Grazer Straße 2
28359 Bremen
Germany

Ulrike Petermann
Sondererziehung und
    Rehabilitation der Universität
    Dortmund
Emil-Figge-Str. 50
44221 Dortmund
Germany

Pier J.M. Prins
Vakgroep Klinische Psychologie
Universiteit van Amsterdam
Roetersstraat 15
1018 WB Amsterdam
The Netherlands

Linda Reinstein
Department of Psychology
University of Windsor
401 Sunset
Windsor, Ontario
Canada N9B 3P4

Agnes Scholing
Klinische Psychologie
Academisch Ziekenhuis
Oostersingel 59
9713 EZ Groningen
The Netherlands

Joseph A. Sergeant
Vakgroep Klinische Psychologie
Universiteit van Amsterdam
Roetersstraat 15
1018 WB Amsterdam
The Netherlands

Cheryl Thomas
Department of Psychology
University of Windsor
401 Sunset
Windsor, Ontario
Canada N9B 3P4

Bedirhan Üstun
Mental Health Divison
World Health Organization
Avenue Appia
CH-1211 Geneva
Switzerland

Sylvia Voelker
Department of Psychology
University of Windsor
401 Sunset
Windsor, Ontario
Canada N9B 3P4

John R. Weisz
Department of Psychology
University of California at
    Los Angeles
405 Hilgard Avenue
Los Angeles
California 90024–1563
USA

CHAPTER **1**

INTRODUCTION AND GENERAL ISSUES

Cecilia Ahmoi Essau and Franz Petermann

The patterns and processes of change in psychopathology form the basis of an emergent scientific discipline termed "Developmental psychopathology" (Cicchetti, 1984; Kazdin, 1989). This discipline has been variously defined as "... the study of the origins and course of individual patterns of behavioral maladaptation ..." (Sroufe and Rutter, 1984, p. 18), "... the study of the prediction of development of maladaptive behaviors and processes" (Lewis and Miller, 1990, p. xiii), and "... the study of how and why psychopathology develops and ceases ..." (Loeber, 1991, p. 97). In these definitions the key concept is temporality (Powers *et al.*, 1989); the recognition that the expression of "abnormal behaviour" is dynamic and changes across the lifespan of the individual. Research in the area is concerned with the "... origins and time course of a given disorder, its varying manifestations with development, its precursors and sequelae, and its relation to nondisordered patterns of behavior" (Sroufe and Rutter, 1984, p. 18). This suggests that the study at mental ill-health need to occur against a backdrop of normal development and developmental deviations across the life span.

Also, central to the developmental perspective of psychopathology is the consideration of continuity. That is, the degree to which psychopathology may alter or remain constant over time in terms of its behavioural indicators, and its covariance with "normal" developmental change. This perspective reflects a shift from an initial research focus on the description of psychiatric disorder to answering questions concerning "what leads to what?" (McGee *et al.*, 1995, p. 366). Generally, this involves a process of identifying individuals with psychiatric disorder, studying what happens to them over a period of time, and identifying factors which place them at risk of, or protect them from, developing persistent psychiatric problems (McGee *et al.*, 1995; Werry, 1992). Calls have been made for a greater application of research and clinical resources to child and adolescent mental health services in

order to reduce longer-term distress and disability. As proposed by
Werry (1992) "… we need to know much more accurately who will get
better without treatment, who is heading towards more durable disorder, who will get real benefit from treatment, and what are risk and protective factors" (p. 478).

COMPONENTS AND TASKS OF DEVELOPMENTAL PSYCHOPATHOLOGY

Developmental psychopathology needs to be conceptualized in terms
of what Achenbach (1990) called a "macroparadigm" which coordinate
relevant theoretical models such as social learning theory, attachment
theory, cognitive-developmental theory and family system. In viewing
developmental psychopathology within the framework of macroparadigm, collaborative, multidisciplinary, and multidomain studies on
various types of population are needed (Cicchetti, 1990); this enables
studying psychopathology in the context of maturational and developmental processes (Achenbach, 1990) for better understanding, predicting, and management of normal and abnormal behaviour. As shown by
chapters in this volume, the topics covered in the area of developmental psychopathology are both broad and diversified, indicating the need
to have an overaching perspective to view their relationships. Also, as
we can see in the second section of this book, psychiatric disorders,
despite the presence of some common characteristics, have diverse and
complex etiologies that involve biological, familial, and psychosocial
factors.

Cicchetti and Cohen (1995) have recently identified some related
aspects of developmental psychopathology, including: (i) investigating
population with high risk factors and population with a disorder by
applying knowledge of normal development; (ii) studying individuals
who despite the presence of risk factors do not have the disorder, and
trying to understand pathways that lead to competent adaptation;
(iii) identifying mechanisms and processes that moderate the outcome
of risk factor by assessing level of functioning using different assessment
strategies; (iv) studying the interactions between constitutional and psychosocial factors over the course of life; (vi) evaluating the influence
of biological, psychological, and sociological factors to determine
individual differences, the continuity of adaptive or maladaptive behavioural patterns, and the different pathways by which the same develop-

mental outcomes may be achieved; and (vii) identifying factors and mechanisms which may divert an individual from a certain pathway into an adaptive course.

Knowledge of developmental psychopathology is critical for the prevention of psychiatric disorders (Cicchetti and Cohen, 1995). Information with respect to the timing, persistence, correlates or risk factors, and precursors of the disorder at different developmental stages may provide useful information for prevention. It is also important to target prevention and intervention efforts for the individual's period of developmental transition and "sensitive periods" (Cicchetti and Cohen, 1995). For example, information about early developmental deviations and their link with subsequent psychopathology may prevent the occurrence of full-blown psychopathology. Thus, in order to increase its effectiveness, prevention and intervention strategies for psychiatric disorders need to be sensitive to the individual's developmental stage.

In this respect, Achenbach (1990) has proposed that research in the domain of developmental psychopathology should include studies which: (i) estimate the prevalence of specific problems in the general population at each developmental stage; (ii) identify variables that could distinguish individuals who are normal from those who are deviant for their age; (iii) identify syndrome patterns of problems that require help; and (iv) explore the associations between characteristics of particular developmental periods and the outcomes of these characteristics longitudinally. Such studies help identify the characteristics and patterns of problems at different ages, and identify developmental continuities and discontinuities in functioning (Achenbach, 1990). Sroufe and Rutter (1984) similarly emphasized the importance of a developmental perspective for understanding psychopathology. They argued: "Only by understanding the nature of the developmental process — with progressive transformation and reorganization of behavior as the developing organism continuously transact with the environment — is it possible to understand the complex links between early adaption and later disorder" (p. 20).

NORMAL DEVELOPMENT

To enhance our knowledge of maladaptive behaviour, it is crucial to know what may be expected at different developmental stages. Normative studies may provide information on typical ages at which children acquire particular skills such as cognitive performance and academic achievement. As proposed by several theorists (Erikson, 1980; Piaget, 1983), children develop through various stages of cognitive, social, moral, and social-emotional development. Within each developmental stage, the children are confronted with new challenges to which they must adapt, and that a failure to adapt successfully is often linked to poor psychosocial well-being (Kellam *et al.*, 1975; Kellam, 1990). In 1948, Havighurst introduced the concept of developmental tasks, defined as tasks that individuals have to solve at different stages in their lives to feel well and to be successful in solving subsequent tasks.

Three transitional periods have been identified as crucial: (i) between the ages of 18 to 24 months, during which the children become mobile and begin mastering language; (ii) around age 5, which is associated with major advancement in cognitive performance; (iii) puberty, which is characterized with a large increase of sex hormone and dramatic physical changes, major changes of educational and social status, and the need to prepare for adult roles (Achenbach, 1990; Piaget, 1983; Tanner, 1989). Perhaps, because of all these dramatic changes, pubertal timing has been reported to affect the person's psychological well-being. Numerous studies have for example shown that early maturing girls tend to have a more negative body image, more emotional and psychosomatic problems (Buchanan *et al.*, 1992; Stattin and Magnusson, 1990), and show more norm-breaking behaviour as compared with later maturing girls (Aro and Taipale, 1987; Caspi and Moffitt, 1991; Caspi *et al.*, 1993; Dorn *et al.*, 1988; Petersen, 1988; Stattin and Magnusson, 1990). Although these developmental stages are relatively arbitrary, they neithertheless serve as a guideline for the typical sequences of development in various domains of functioning (Erikson, 1980; Piaget, 1983).

Various factors such as dispositional (e.g., temperament) (Hetherington, 1989; Zahn-Waxler *et al.*, 1990), familial (e.g., parental stress, parenting and discipline styles, child maltreatment) (Cicchetti and Lynch, 1995; Garmezy and Rutter, 1983; Patterson, 1982) or contextual factors (e.g., school, peers) have been considered to increase or hinder normal developmental process during early childhood. However, the role that many of these factors especially that of familial factors have on child's development have been questioned (Pike and Plomin, 1996). First, these factors may have different affect in children although they are in the same family. For example, the occurrence of a specific life events such as a death of a family member, although shared by all the children in the family may be experienced differently by each child.

Second, it could be that the relationship between such factors and the children's developmental outcome may be mediated by genetic factors. In this respect, Plomin and his colleagues (Pike and Plomin, 1996) have suggested the use of behaviour genetic methods in studying psychopathology. By means of the behavioural genetic methods, molecular genetic tools are used to identify specific genes involved in behavioural dimensions and disorders (Pike and Plomin, 1996).

RESEARCH FINDINGS IN DEVELOPMENTAL PSYCHOPATHOLOGY

The last few years have shown a substantial increase of developmental psychopathology research. This increase has been spurred by findings of recent epidemiological studies which estimate that between 17 to 22% of adolescents below the age of 18 years have suffered some types of psychiatric disorders (see review by Kazdin and Kagan, 1994). Importantly, the chronological patterns of the major disorders is apparently changing, with an increased tendency towards an earlier age of onset. Using the Epidemiologic Catchment Area Study (ECA) data, Burke *et al.* (1991, p. 789) found a "... gradual shift to increased rates for major depression between the ages of 15 and 19 years ... " among the more recent birth cohorts. Similar shifts, though not as large, were found for substance use disorders. Using data from nine epidemiologic surveys and three family studies, the Cross-National Collaborative Group (1992) has similarly found an increased risk and lower age of onset for major depression among those in more recent birth cohorts. Declining age of onset estimates are particularly significant as disorders with an earlier reported onset tend to follow a more chronic course and are associated with the most subsequent disability during the productive years (Rey, 1992). However, according to Werry (1992), the view that early onset portends a worse prognosis still remains open to question. Major challenges involve describing the psychopathological consequences of children's failure to make age-appropriate responses to environmental demands, and predicting children who will be at a high risk of psychopathology, and at what developmental stages (Costello *et al.*, 1993).

According to numerous studies, children have an increased risk for psychiatric disorders if they have specific conditions or problems such as having difficult temperament, have academic problems, have parent(s) with psychopathology, and inconsistent parent-child interaction. The list of risk factors, as shown in chapters 4 to 11 are broad. This makes it difficult to identify the contribution of each factor on the onset of the disorder. Other problems are related to (Kazdin, 1995): (i) the co-occurrence of factors such as low income being related to poor housing and marital accord; (ii) interaction of factors with each other and with other variables. For example, family size may have the greatest influence on risk in lower compared to higher family income; (iii) Accumulation of factors (e.g., academic impairment may lead to truancy and drop out of school). As reported by recent studies high risk children can be characterized as having an accumulation of difficulties and adversities (Blanz *et al.*, 1991; Fergusson and Lynskey, 1996; Shaw *et al.*, 1994).

On the other hand, not all children raised in adverse circumstances or have risk factors end up in having psychiatric disorders (Fergusson and Lynskey, 1996). Factors that may protect against or mitigate the effects of risk factors and confer resilience to those with high risk environments include the presence of: (i) high intelligence or problem solving skills (Herrenkohl *et al.*, 1994; Seifer *et al.*, 1992); (ii) strong interests outside the family or the presence of a confiding adult outside their family (Jenkins and Smith, 1990; Werner, 1989); (iii) warm, nurturant or supportive relationships with at least one parent (Bradley *et al.*, 1994; Seifer *et al.*, 1992; Herrenkohl *et al.*, 1994); and (iv) have an easy temperament during childhood (Werner, 1989; Wyman *et al.*, 1991).

Psychopathology in children and adolescents has a negative impact on school work (i.e., school functioning difficulties, low grade point averages) or social life. Most disorders have a life long consequence. Taking conduct disorder as an example, numerous studies have shown the presence of this disorder in childhood or adolescence to predict multiple problems in adulthood such as having poor school attainment, social dysfunction, suffer various types of psychiatric symptoms, criminal behavior, and poor occupational adjustment (Kazdin, 1995; Robins, 1966). These findings lend support to the view of some authors (Weiner, 1982) for the continuity between early and later disorder, considering that adolescents with signs of behavioural disorders rarely outgrow them. On the other hand, Sroufe and Rutter (1984) proposed that although the actual degree of continuity may vary, an underlying coherence to the individual's course of development would still remain. This expectation of coherence is distinct from an expectation of behavioural stability, which Sroufe and Rutter (1984) considered to be rare. In support of this contention, they cited the conclusion of Kohlberg *et al.* (1972). Despite finding a lack of stability for particular emotional symptoms (perhaps due to dependence on situational factors), Kohlberg *et al.* (1972) argued that the child's general pattern of adaptation would better predict later pathology. Researchers should not look for continuity in behaviour *per se*, but rather, causal connections between experiences at one age and their subsequent psychological or behavioural outcomes. Similarly, Kazdin (1989, p. 181) used the term "developmental symptom substitution" to describe the observation that abnormal behaviours may be replaced at later ages by different (and perhaps more age-appropriate) behaviour, whilst the underlying pathology may remain constant.

The continuity of disorder could be attributable to common risk factors such as socio-economic disadvantage, rather than the presence of disorder in an earlier developmental period leading directly to the experience of disorder in a later period. According to Sroufe and Rutter (1984), continuity lies not in isomorphic behaviours over time but in lawful relations to later behaviour. Their thesis is that disordered behaviour does not arise without changing environmental supports or altered environmental challenges: "Even where qualitative change in functioning occurs, as when a well functioning individual later shows severely disordered behavior ... it is presumed that the particular form of maladaptation will be related to the adaptational history" (p. 22). In this they referred to the individual's history of functioning relative to what may be expected given their age or developmental level, as opposed to a history of disorder *per se*. They concluded that there was little connection between adult disorder and the same disordered behaviour in childhood. However, there was a very real likelihood that early patterns of maladaptation may leave individuals differentially vulnerable to adult disorders. Venables (1989, p. 348), in discussing test-retest reliability in longitudinal studies, made the observation that what may be most important is: "... the extent to which a measure has long term predictive value, that is, behavior "A" is a good predictor of behavior "B" rather than necessarily a predictor of the behavior "A" which is shown by the subject at a later stage in development." Thus, a particular adolescent disorder (e.g., depression) may not necessarily predict the same disorder in adulthood but it may well elevate the risk of disorder in general or some other disorder (e.g., substance dependence).

Children and adolescents with one disorder generally have at least one other disorders as well (i.e., comorbidity). Some of the most frequent comorbidity patterns are that of anxiety disorders and depression (see Chapters 5, 7, 8 of this volume) and between attention deficit/hyperactivity disorder and conduct and oppositional defiant disorders (see Chapter 4).

Comorbidity rates however differ across studies, with values ranging from 20 to 70%. According to Wittchen's review (1996), these variations in rates may have been influenced by numerous factors, including: (i) the extent to which diagnostic exclusions and hierarchies are used, as proposed in the revised version of the third edition of the Diagnostic and Statistical Manual of Mental Disorders (DSM-III-R; American Psychiatric Association, APA, 1987), the fourth edition of the DSM (DSM-IV; APA, 1994), and the tenth revision of the International Classification of Diseases (ICD-10; World Health Organization, 1993); (ii) the type and number of diagnostic classes included. For example, it is useful to indicate which specific sub-types of anxiety disorders are included in studies that examine the comorbidity of anxiety disorders with other disorders; (iii) the time frame of assessment for each disorder; (iv) the assessment method (structured, standardized, and semi-structured diagnostic interview). For example, among adults, the use of standardized instruments has produced about twice higher diagnoses as clinicians would assign (Wittchen, 1995). Also the sequence in which disorders are assessed and the use of stem questions and memory probes significantly influence the types of symptom reported (Kessler *et al.*, 1994); and (v) the use of different research designs (cross-sectional, longitudinal designs) and statistical analyses.

In a review of the possible causes of comorbidity, Caron and Rutter (1991), suggested that the co-occurrence of two or more disorders (i) could have resulted from shared and overlapping risk factors; or (ii) that the co-occurring of conditions could have consisted of a single condition with multiple manifestations; or (iii) that one disorder causes or lowers the threshold for the expression of the other; or (iv) one disorder represents an early manifestation of the other; or (v) the comorbidity could be due to overlapping diagnostic criteria.

MODELS OF DEVELOPMENTAL PSYCHOPATHOLOGY

A number of models have been developed to help understand the etiology of psychopathology: The *environmental model* considers behaviour as a function of the environmental forces that act on the individual. Of importance for this model is the role of critical periods wherein certain environmental influences will have a greater effect in other periods (Lewis, 1988). In the *goodness-of-fit model*, psychopathology appears as the consequence of the mismatch between an individual's characteristics and environmental demand (Thomas and Chess, 1977).

In the *transactional model*, children's development is considered as a product of a continous dynamic interaction between the children and the experiences provided by the family and social contexts (Sameroff, 1995); experience may affect development by causing a developmental change that will not appear unless the experience occurred, and by sustaining an already-achieved state of development (Gottlieb, 1991).

Kazdin and Kagan (1994) have recently questioned the strategies used to develop models of developmental psychopathology. The first common assumption is that of single causal pathways of dysfunction. That is, individuals suffering from certain psychopathology are assumed to have the same characteristics. Yet we know from the literature and clinical practice about the limitation of this "one size fits all" model (Kazdin and Kagan, 1994, p. 36) in that a particular risk factor do not necessarily generate the same outcome in most people, suggesting the presence of several different pathway which could lead to a particular psychopathology (Tremblay *et al.*, 1992; Werner and Smith, 1992). Furthermore, risk factors not only co-occur and interact with each other, but the types of risk factors, the strength of association among the factors and their impact vary with the person's developmental stages (Kazdin, 1995; Rutter and Giller, 1983; Rutter *et al.*, 1975).

Second, being indifferent to the sources of information for assessing major constructs. As discussed in chapter 2 of this volume, it is recommended that multiple sources of information and assessment methods be used because of problems inherent in each method and because the frequency and quality of behaviour tend to vary across situation. The latter reflects the interaction between the child's characteristics and reinforcement contingencies associated with different settings (Mash and Krahn, 1995). The choice of informant is also important since informant may influence the reporting of the presence and the severity of a disorder (Rutter *et al.*, 1970). As reported by several authors (Achenbach *et al.*, 1987; Offord *et al.*, 1991; Verhulst and Koot, 1992), the rates of agreement between different informants are poor to moderate.

Third, there is a lack of attention to the "package" of influences and outcomes, and to their relations. Not only do factors come in package, so are its outcome (Kazdin and Kagan, 1994). As discussed earlier, the co-occurrence of disorders is common (see also chapters 4–11). Thus, future studies need to explore the extend to which "packages of factors" may lead to package of outcome (i.e., comorbidity), and also to examine factors that could distinguish between these with one disorder from those with comorbid disorders.

To advance our understanding of dysfunction, several strategies need to be considered. First, there is a need to expand the sources of assessment (Kazdin and Kagan, 1994). The assessment methods should include a broad range of symptoms to ensure that other symptoms which may have important implications for managing and treating the case are not overlooked (Kazdin, 1995). Also, the fact that the children's problem (e.g., conduct disorder) varies across situations (e.g., home, school), suggest the importance to assess parent and teacher evaluations of child dysfunction and performance at home and in school, respectively (Kazdin, 1995; Verhulst and Koot, 1992). In this respect, Achenbach (1990) has introduced the multiaxial model of assessment by using parent and teacher reports, cognitive and physical assessment, and direct assessment of the child. The model uses the normative-developmental approach to determine the extend and the degree to which a child's behaviour deviate from those in the same age group can be determined. This approach futhermore allows the identification of various areas in which help is needed. In addition to the individual's personal characteristics, there is a need to include a broad domain and social context such as family and peers. In other words, there is a need to study children's behaviour and development in relationship to the child's social context. Children with attention deficit/hyperactivity disorder, for example, may not show any problems doing non-demanding and unstructured task, but may display problems in doing a structured task in the classroom.

Culture is also an important determinant of the child's behaviour; the physical and social settings, the customs of child care and rearing may all play a role in the child's behaviour. Culturally mediated values and expectation such as child-rearing and socialization practices may help shape the children's problems (Weisz, 1989) and the kinds of problems parents perceive as distressing (Weisz et al., 1988). As suggested by Dragun (1973), psychopathology in a particular culture may reflect an exaggeration of frequent adaptive behaviour that are socially shared. The "problem suppression-facilitation model", proposed by Weisz and Eastman (1995), views that cultural forces may influence the incidence of child psychopathology by suppressing culturally unacceptable behaviour and facilitating desirable one. To test this model, Weisz et al. (1993) compared the prevalence of over- and undercontrolled problems among the 12–16 year old adolescents using the Child Behavior Checklist (Achenbach, 1983). As hypothesized, the Thai adolescents reported more overcontrolled problems than American adolescents. These findings were interpreted as being consistent with the hypothesis that over-controlled problems are being fostered by cultural pressures (which is parallel with the Buddhist-influence in Thai tradition and child rearing practices) for self-control, emotional restraint, and social inhibition of strong emotions. Traditional Thai also emphasis on quiteness, inhibition, introspection, and deference (Weisz *et al.*, 1988). The Thais are known to be intolerable of aggressive and disrespectful behaviour, and children are taught to be polite and deference. All these have been interpreted as discouraging the development of undercontrolled behaviour problems and to foster the development of overcontrolled behaviour problems.

In the "adult-distress threshold model", cultural factors are presumed to influence adults' expectancies and beliefs about the children, which in turn influence how distressing the child behaviour will be, and the type of actions that will take in response (Weisz and Eastman, 1995). This model was tested by comparing adults perception of the seriousness of over- and undercontrolled problems by using different vignettes. The Thai compared to American adults rated the children's behavioural and emotional problem as less serious, unusual, and less likely to worry (Weisz *et al.*, 1988). Adults in these 2 cultures also differ in the way in which they referred their children to clinics. The main reason for clinic referral among Americans were that of externalizing problems, whereas among Thais this was related to internalizing problems (Weisz *et al.*, 1987). Mash and Krahn (1995) similarly argued that "children's dependency on significant adults and the central role that adults play in defining childhood disorders necessitate that the role of social context be considered in conceptualizing research and in deciding how samples of children are recruited, how data are collected, and how findings are interpreted" (p. 112). The nature of the children's problems in terms of the severity of the problems and the associated features may differ among children who are referred by adults. The likelihood that parents seek help for their children may be influenced by the extend to which the child's behaviour is noticeable and bothersome, as well as by parent's mental health status and treatment history, and perceived benefits of treatment (Mash and Krahn, 1995).

Second, there is a need to identify and aggregate risk factors since many factors tend to aggregate over time and contribute to an outcome (Kazdin and Kagan, 1994). However, as discussed earlier, a particular risk factor may not necessarily produce the same outcome in most people. Rather a risk factor may interact with the person's characteristics such as sex, ethnicity, and age. Taking conduct disorder as an example, early aggressive behaviour predicted later antisocial behaviour among boys but not among girls (Kazdin, 1995). A major challenge for future research is to identify the contribution of each factors, and as to how they may co-occur to produce specific outcomes. Futhermore, some factors may act in a direct and/or indirect way (Mash and Krahn, 1995). For example, marital discord may directly affect the children through exposure or experiencing of adversive situation at home, or indirectly through interference of the parent's ability to provide consistent discipline or adversely influence parental attitudes and satisfaction in the parent-child interaction.

Third, a large number of samples and multiple areas of child functioning (e.g., physical, intellectual, psychosocial) are necessary to study the association between risk factors and developmental psychopathology (Mash and Krahn, 1995). This is important because only a small number of those with high risk factors will end up in developing the disorder, and also because it is impossible to foresee as to which of the person's areas of functioning will be affected and how they are affected.

Fourth, there is a need to do both the within-group and within-individual analysis (Kazdin and Kagan, 1994). Within-group analysis allows the examination of factors that are common among individuals in the group, whereas within-individual analysis expands this focus beyond that of the usual level of analysis which views certain variables as the basis of group membership. The need for both of these analyses can best be illustrated with findings of family studies. Specifically, family studies have reported (Hammen, 1991; Keller *et al.*, 1986; Lee and Gotlib, 1991; Weissman *et al.*, 1987), that children whose parents have psychiatric disorders showed an increased rate for having the disorders compared to those whose parents are not psychiatrically ill. Yet, not all children of psychiatrically ill parents have psychiatric disorders, nor do children who have problems show the same kind of disorder or the same course and outcome of their disorder. Explanation for these differences include: parental differential treatment (Dunn *et al.*, 1990; McHale and Pawletko, 1992; Pike *et al.*, 1996; Plomin and Daniels, 1987), child characteristics such as physical disability or beauty, and position in the family (e.g., birth order) (Block, 1983; Elder *et al.*, 1986). For example, the results of Tarullo *et al.*'s (1995) longitudinal study showed maternal depression as predictor of the older sibling's symptoms, whereas that of low maternal engagement and high maternal critical-irritable behaviour predicted younger sibling's symptoms. Using data from the Nonshared Environment and Adolescent Development Project, Pike and colleagues

(1996) reported differences of parent's negativity within identical twins correlated significantly with the twin differences in antisocial behaviour.

These findings stressed the importance of evaluating the family system as a whole, and examine feelings related to equity and fairness within the family (McHale and Pawletko, 1992). Experiences outside the family such as peers and teachers may even have a stronger effects on psychopathology as adolescent siblings begin to make their own ways outside the family. As stated by Pike and Plomin (1996, p. 569): "The news once was that genetic influences are important in the development of psychopathology. This is now not only old news, but well-accepted news. Although often of moderate if not substantial importance, genetics is not the only key to understanding psychiatric disorders. The environment is also important ...".

Fifth, factors that are related to and generate a particular outcome for testing mechanisms or processes through which these factors operate should be identified (Kazdin and Kagan, 1994). Research need to go beyond identifying factors that produce an outcome, but also to examine the process involved. As argued by Kazdin and Kagan (1994), understanding the notion of process forces us to be involved with the dynamic, reciprocal, and interactive characteristics of human functioning.

SUMMARY

Developmental psychopathology is an emerging discipline that can be used to study the origins and course of maladaptive behaviour. The conceptualization of developmental psychopathology in terms of macroparadigm allows studying psychiatric disorders in the context of maturational and developmental processes using relevant theoretical models. In studying developmental psychopathopology, one needs a solid general knowledge of research and theory on development in order to know the typical ages at which certain skills are acquired.

There has been an accumulative number of research in the area of developmental psychopathology. This increase has been spurred by recent findings that between 17 to 22% of adolescents have had some types of psychiatric disorders. Several factors (e.g., dispositional, familial and contextual factors) have been identified to be associated with an increased risk for psychiatric disorders. However, recent studies have also shown that individual raised in adverse circumstances or with certain risk factors do not necessarily develop psychiatric disorders. Factors such as high intelligence level, having strong interest outside the family, having warm relationship with one parent may protect against the effects of risk. Recent studies have also indicated that the presence of psychopathology is often associated with the presence of at least one additional disorders, and with psychosocial impairment in various areas such as in academic or social life. Numerous models have been developed to enhance our understanding of the etiology of psychopathology, however, they have been critized because of the limitation inherent in the strategies used to develop them. Finally, in this chapter we have made a number of proposal to expand our assumption on the contribution of factors in the development of psychopathology. We believed that our understanding of psychopathology can be enhanced through the expansion of sources of assessment, identification and aggregation of risk factors, inclusion of large sample size and assessment of multiple areas of functioning.

REFERENCES

Achenbach, T.M. (1990). Conceptualization of developmental psychopathology. In M. Lewis and S.M. Miller (Eds.), *Handbook of developmental psychopathology* (pp. 3–14). New York: Plenum Press.

Achenbach, T.M., McConaughy, S.H., and Howell, C.T. (1987). Child/adolescent behavioral and emotional problems: Implications of cross-informant correlations for situational specificity. *Psychological Bulletin,* **101**, 213–232.

American Psychiatric Association (1987). *Diagnostic and Statistical Manual of Mental Disorders* (3rd ed., rev.). Washington, DC: American Psychiatric Association.

American Psychiatric Association (1994). *Diagnostic and Statistical Manual of Mental Disorders* (4th ed.). Washington, DC: American Psychiatric Association.

Aro, H., and Taipale, V. (1987). The impact of timing of puberty on psychosomatic symptoms among fourteen- to sixteen-year old Finnish girls. *Child Development,* **58**, 261–268.

Blanz, B., Schmidt, M.H., and Esser, G. (1991). Familial adversities and child psychiatric disorders. *Journal of Child Psychology and Psychiatry,* **32**, 939–950.

Block, J.H. (1983). Differential premises arising from differential socialization of the sexes: Some conjectures. *Child Development,* **54**, 1335–1354.

Buchanan, C.M., Eccles, J.S., and Becker, J.B. (1992). Are adolescents the victims of raging hormones: Evidence of activational effects of hormones on moods and behavior at adolescence. *Psychological Bulletin,* **111**, 62–107.

Burke, K.C., Burke, J.D., Rae, D.S., and Regier, D.A. (1991). Comparing age of onset of major depression and other psychiatric disorders by birth cohorts in five US community populations. *Archives of General Psychiatry,* **48**, 789–795.

Bradley, R.H., Whiteside, L., Mundfrom, D.J., Casey, P.H., Kelleher, K.J., and Pope, S.K. (1994). Early indicators of resilience and their relation to experiences in the home environments of low birthweight, premature children living in poverty. *Child Development,* **65**, 346–360.

Caron, C., and Rutter, M. (1991). Comorbidity in child psychopathology: Concepts, issues, and research strategies. *Journal of Child Psychology and Psychiatry,* **32**, 1063–1080.

Carlson, E.A., and Sroufe, L.A. (1995). Contribution of attachment theory to developmental psychopathology. In D. Cicchetti and D.J. Cohen (Eds.), *Developmental psychopathology. Volume 1: Theory and methods* (pp. 581–617). New York: Wiley.

Caspi, A., and Moffitt, T.E. (1991). Individual differences are accentuated during periods of social change: The sample case of girls at puberty. *Journal of Personality and Social Psychology,* **61**, 157–168.

Caspi, A., Lynam, D., Moffitt, T.E., and Silva, P.A. (1993). Unraveling girls' delinquency: Biological, dispositional, and contextual contributions to adolescent misbehavior. *Developmental Psychology,* **29**, 19–30.

Cicchetti, D. (1984). The emergence of developmental psychopathology. *Child Development,* **55**, 1–7.

Cicchetti, D., and Cohen, D.J. (1995). Perspectives on developmental psychopathology. In D. Cicchetti and D.J. Cohen (Eds.), *Developmental psychopathology. Volume 1: Theory and methods* (pp. 3–20). New York: Wiley.

Cicchetti, D., and Lynch, M. (1995).Failures in the expectable environment and their impact on individual development: The case of child maltreatment. In D. Cicchetti and D.J. Cohen (Eds.), *Developmental psychopathology. Volume 2: Risk, disorder, and adaptation* (pp. 32–72). New York: Wiley.

Costello, E.J., Burns, B.J., Angold, A., and Leaf, P.J. (1993). How can epidemiology improve mental health services for children and adolescents? *Journal of the Academy of Child and Adolescent Psychiatry,* **32**, 1106–1113.

Cross-National Collaborative Group (1992). The changing rate of major depression: Cross- national comparison. *JAMA,* **268**, 3098–3105.

Dorn, L.D., Crockett, LJ., and Petersen, A.C. (1988). The relations of pubertal status to intrapersonal changes in young adolescents. *Journal of Early Adolescence,* **8**, 405–419.

Dunn, J., Stocker, C., and Plomin, R. (1990). Nonshared experiences within the family: Correlates of behavioral problems in middle childhood. *Developmental Psychopathology,* **2**, 113–126.

Elder, G.H., Caspi, A., and Van Nguyen, T. (1986). Resourceful and vulnerable children: Family influences in hard times. In R.K. Silbereisen, K. Eyferth, and G. Rudinger (Eds.), *Development as action in context: Problem behavior and normal youth development* (pp. 167–186). New York: Springer.

Erikson, E.H. (1980). Elements of a psychoanalytic theory of psychosocial development. In S.I. Greenspan and G.H. Pollock (Eds.), *The course of life: Psychoanalytic contributions toward understanding personality development: Vol. 1. Infancy and early childhood* (pp. 11–61). Adelphi, MD: NIMH Mental Health Study Center.

Feehan, M., McGee, R., and Williams, S.M. (1993). Mental health disorders from age 15 to age 18 years. *Journal of the American Academy of Child and Adolescent Psychiatry, 32*, 1118–1126.

Feehan, M., McGee, R., Nada-Raja, S., and Williams, S.M. (1994). DSM-III-R disorders in New Zealand 18-year-olds. *Australian and New Zealand Journal of Psychiatry,* **28**, 87–99.

Fergusson, D.M., and Lynskey, M.T. (1996). Adolescent resiliency to family adversity. *Journal of Child Psychology and Psychiatry, 37*, 281–292.

Garmezy, N., and Rutter, M. (1983). Acute reaction to stress. In M. Rutter and L. Herzov (Eds.), *Child psychiatry: A modern approach* (2nd ed.), (pp. 152–177). Oxford, England: Blackwell.

Hammen, C. (1991). *Depression runs in families: The social context of risk and resilience in children of depressed mothers.* New York: Springer.

Havighurst, R.J. (1948). *Developmental tasks and education.* New York: McKay.

Hay, D.F., and Angold, A. (1993). Introduction: Precursors and causes in development and pathogenesis. In D.F. Hay and A. Angold (Eds.), *Precursors and causes in development and psychopathology* (pp. 1–21). Chichester: Wiley.

Herrenkohl, E.C., Herrenkohl, R.C., and Egolf, B. (1994). Resilient early school-age children from maltreating homes: Outcomes in late adolescence. *American Journal of Orthopsychiatry,* **64**, 301–309.

Hetherington, E.M. (1989). Coping with family transitions: Winners, losers and survivors. *Child Development,* **60**, 1–14.

Hill, P. (1989). Adolescent psychiatry. Edinburgh: Churchhill, Livingstone.

Jenkins, J.N., and Smith, M.A. (1990). Factors protecting children living in disharmonious homes: Maternal reports. *Journal of the Academy of Child and Adolescent Psychiatry,* **29**, 60–69.

Kazdin, A.E. (1995). Conduct disorder. In F.C. Verhulst and H.M. Koot (Eds.), *The epidemiology of child and adolescent psychopathology* (pp. 258–291). Oxford: Oxford University Press.

Kazdin, A.E. (1989). Identifying depression in children: A comparison of alternative selection criteria. *Journal of Abnormal Child Psychology,* **17**, 437–455.

Kazdin, A.E., and Kagan, J. (1994). Models of dysfunction in developmental psychopathology. *Clinical Psychology: Science and practice, Summer,* 35–52.

Kellam, S.G. (1990). Developmental epidemiologic framework for family research on depression and aggression. In G.R. Patterson (Ed.), *Depression and aggression in family interaction* (pp. 11–48). Hillsdale, NJ: Lawrence Erlbaum.

Kellam, S.G., Branch, J.D., Agrawal, K.C., and Ensminger, M.E. (1975). *Mental health and going to school: The Woodlawn program of assessment, early intervention, and evaluation.* Chicago: University of Chicago Press.

Keller, M.B., Beardslee, W.R., Dorer, D.J., Lavori, P.W., Samuelson, H., and Klerman, G.L. (1986). Impact of severity and chronicity of parental affective illness on adaptive functioning and psychopathology in children. *Archives of General Psychiatry,* **43**, 930–937.

Kessler, R.C., McGonagle, K.A., Zhao, S., Nelson, C.B., Hughes, M., Eshleman, S., Wittchen, H.-U., and Kendler, K.S. (1994). Lifetime and 12-month prevalence of DSM-III-R psychiatric disorders in the United States: Results from the National Comorbidity Survey. *Archives of General Psychiatry,* **51**, 8–19.

Kohlberg, L., LaCrosse, J., and Ricks, D. (1972). The predictability of adult mental health from childhood behavior. In B. Wolman (Ed.), *Manual of child psychopathology* (pp. 1217–1284). New York: McGraw-Hill.

Lee, C.M., and Gotlib, I.H. (1991). Clinical status and emotional adjustment of children of depressed mothers. *American Journal of Psychiatry,* **40**, 1055–1060.

Lewis, M. (1988). Models of developmental psychopathology. In M. Lewis and S.M. Miller (Eds.), *Handbook of developmental psychopathology* (pp. 15–27). New York: Plenum Press.

Lewis, M., and Miller, S.M. (Eds.) (1990). *Handbook of developmental psychopathology.* New York: Plenum Press.

Loeber, R. (1991). Questions and advances in the study of developmental pathways. In D. Cicchetti and S. Toth (Eds.), *Rochester symposium on developmental psychopathology, Volume 3: Models and integrations* (pp. 97–116). Rochester: University of Rochester Press.

Mash, E.J., and Krahn, G.L. (1995). Research strategies in child psychopathology. In M. Hersen and R.T. Hammerman (Eds.), *Advanced abnormal child psychology* (pp. 105–133). Hillsdale, NJ: Lawrence Erlbaum.

McGee, R., Williams, S., and Feehan, M. (1994). Behavior problems in New Zealand children. In P.R. Joyce, R.T. Mulder, M.A. Oakley-Browne, J.D. Sellman, and W.G.A. Watkins (Eds.), *Development, personality and psychopathology* (pp. 15–22). Christchurch: Christchurch School of Medicine.

McGee, R., Feehan, M., and Williams, S. (1995). Long-term follow-up of a birth cohort. In F.C. Verhulst and H.M. Koot (Eds.), *The epidemiology of child and adolescent psychopathology* (pp. 366–384). Oxford: Oxford University Press.

McHale, S.M., and Pawletko, T.M. (1992). Differential treatment in two family contexts. *Child Development, 63,* 68–81.

Offord, D.R., Boyle, M.H., and Racine, Y.A. (1991). The epidemiology of antisocial behavior. In D.J. Pepler and K.H. Rubin (Eds.), *The development and treatment of childhood aggression* (pp. 31–54). Hillsdale, NJ: Erlbaum.

Patterson, G. (1982). *Coercive family process.* Eugene, OR: Castalia.

Petersen, A.C. (1988). Adolescent development. *Annual Review of Psychology, 39,* 583–607.

Piaget, J. (1983). Piaget's theory. In P.H. Mussen (Ed.), *Handbook of child psychology: Vol. 1. History, theory, and methods* (4th ed., pp. 1–25). New York: Wiley.

Pike, A., and Plomin, R. (1996). Importance of nonshared environmental factors for childhood and adolescent psychopathology. *Journal of the American Academy of Child and Adolescent Psychiatry, 35,* 560–570.

Pike, A., Reiss, D., Hetherington, E.M., and Plomin, R. (1996). Using MZ differences in the search for nonshared environmental effects. *Journal of Child Psychology and Psychiatry, 37,* 695–704.

Plomin, R., and Daniels, D. (1987). Why are children in the same family so different from each other? *Behavoral and Brain Science, 10,* 1–16.

Powers, S.L., Hauser, S.T., and Kilner, L.A. (1989). *Adolescent mental health. American Psychologist, 44,* 200–208.

Rey, J.M. (1992). The Epidemiologic Catchment Area (ECA) study: Implications for Australia. *Medical Journal of Australia, 156,* 200–203.

Robins, L.N. (1966). *Deviant children grow up: A sociological and psychiatric study of sociopathic personality.* Baltimore: Williams and Wilkens.

Rutter, M (1987). Psychosocial resilience and protective mechanisms. *American Journal of Orthopsychiatry, 57,* 316–331.

Rutter, M. (1990). Psychosocial resilience and protective mechanisms. In J. Rolf, A.S. Masten, D. Cicchetti, K.H. Neuechterlain, and S. Weintraub (Eds.), *Risk and protective factors in the development of psychopathology* (pp. 181–214). New York: Cambridge University Press.

Rutter, M., and Giller, H. (1983). *Juvenile delinquency: Trends and perspectives.* Harmondsworth: Penguin.

Rutter, M., Yule, B., Quinton, D., Rowlands, O., Yule, W., and Berger, M. (1975). Attainment and adjustment in two geographical areas. III. Some factors accounting for area differences. *British Journal of Psychiatry, 126,* 520–533.

Rutter, M., Tizard, J., and Whitmore, K. (1970). *Education, health and behavior.* London: Longmans.

Sameroff, A.J. (1995). General systems theories and developmental psychopathology. In D. Cicchetti and D.J. Cohen (Eds.), *Developmental psychopathology. Volume 1: Theory and methods* (pp. 659–695). New York: Wiley.

Seifer, R., Sameroff, A.J., Baldwin, C.P., and Baldwin, A. (1992). Child and family factors that ameliorate risk between 4 and 13 years of age. *Journal of the American Academy of Child and Adolescent Psychiatry, 31,* 893–903.

Shaw, D.S., Vondra, J.I., Hommerding, K.D., Keenan, K., and Dunn, M. (1994). Chronic family adversity and early child behavior problems: A longitudinal study of low income families. *Journal of Child Psychology and Psychiatry, 35,* 1109–1122.

Sroufe, L.A., and Rutter, M. (1984). The domain of developmental psychopathology. *Child Development, 55,* 17–29.

Stattin, H., and Magnusson, D. (1990). *Paths through life — Volume 2: Pubertal maturation in female development.* Hillsdale, NJ: Erlbaum.

Tanner, J.M. (1989). *Foetus into man: Physical growth from conception to maturity* (2nd Ed.). Wale: Castlemead Publications.

Tarullo, L.B., DeMulder, E.K., Ronsaville, D.S., Brown, E., and Radke-Yarrow, M. (1995). Maternal depression and maternal treatment of siblings as predictors of child psychopathology. *Developmental Psychopathology, 31*, 395–405.

Thomas, A., and Chess, S. (1977). *Temperament and development.* New York: Brunner/Mazel.

Tremblay, R.E., Masse, B., Perron, D., Leblanc, M., Schwartzman, E., and Ledingham, J.E. (1992). Early disruptive behavior, poor school achievement, delinquent behavior, and delinquent personality: Longitudinal analyses. *Journal of Consulting and Clinical Psychology, 60*, 64–72.

Venables, P.H. (1989). The Emanuel Miller memorial lecture. Childhood markers for adult disorders. *Journal of Child Psychology and Psychiatry, 30*, 347–364.

Verhulst, F.C., and Koot, H.M. (1992). *Child psychiatric epidemiology: Concepts, methods, and findings.* Newbury Park, CA: Saga.

Weiner, I.B. (1982). *Child and adolescent psychopathology.* New York: Wiley.

Weissman, M.M., Gammon, G.D., John, K., Merikangas, K.R., Prusoff, B.A., and Scholomskas, D. (1987). Children of depressed parents: Increased psychopathology and early onset of major depression. *Archives of General Psychiatry, 44*, 847–853.

Weisz, J.R. (1989). Culture and the development of child psychopathology: Lessons from Thailand. In D. Cicchetti (Ed.), *Rochester symposium on developmental psychopathology, Volume 1: The emergence of a discipline* (pp. 89–117). Hillsdale, NJ: Erlbaum.

Weisz, J.R., and Eastman, K.L. (1995). Cross-cultural research on child and adolescent psychopathology. In F.C. Verhulst and H.M. Koot (Eds.), *The epidemiology of child and adolescent psychopathology* (pp. 42–65). Oxford: Oxford University Press.

Weisz, J.R., Suwanlert, S., Chaiyasit, W., Weiss, B., Walter, B.R., and Anderson, W.W. (1988). Thai and American perspectives on over- and undercontrolled child behavior problems: Exploring the threshold model among parents, teachers, and psychologists. *Journal of Consulting and Clinical Psychology, 56*, 601–609.

Werner, E. (1989). High risk children in young adulthood: A longitudinal study from birth to 32 years. *American Journal of Orthopsychiatry, 59*, 72–81.

Werner, E.E., and Smith, R.S. (1992). *Overcoming the odds: High risk children from birth to adulthood.* Ithaca, NY: Cornell University Press.

Werry, J.S. (1992). Child and adolescent (early onset) schizophrenia: A review in light of DSM-III-R. *Journal of Autism and Developmental Disorders, 22*, 601–624.

Wittchen, H.-U. (1995). Comorbidity of mood disorders — diagnosis and treatment. *Depression, 3*, 131–133.

Wittchen, H.-U. (1996). Critical issues in the evaluation of comorbidity of psychiatric disorders. *British Journal of Psychiatry, 168*, 9–16.

World Health Organization (1993). *International Classification of Mental and Behavioral Disorders.* Geneva: World Health Organization.

Wyman, P.A., Cowen, E.L., Work, W.C., and Parker, G.R. (1991). Developmental and family correlates of resilience in urban children who have experienced major life stress. *American Journal of Community Psychology, 19*, 405–426.

Zahn-Waxler, C., Iannotti, R., Cunnings, E.M., and Denham, S. (1990). Antecedents of problem behaviors in children of depressed mothers. *Development and Psychopathology, 2*, 271–291.

CHAPTER 2

CLASSIFICATION AND ASSESSMENT STRATEGIES

Cecilia Ahmoi Essau, Michael Feehan, and Bedirhan Üstun

A sound classification system is a prerequisite for any scientific and clinical work (Achenbach, 1995). With regard to psychiatric disorders in children and adolescents, a robust classification system should: be reliable and valid; have a comprehensive coverage of important disorders; take into account developmental perspectives; be based on principles and rules which are clearly defined; contain information which are clinically important; and finally result in assessment technologies (Remschmidt, 1995; Rutter, 1977).

Classification systems that meet these requirements: (i) provide researchers with a common framework for theory formation about the nature of psychiatric disorders; (ii) provide clinicians with a nomenclature for effective communication that furnishes a basis for description and information retrieval, gives information for making predictions of clinical course and treatment selection, and facilitates understanding and treatment of psychiatric disorders; and (iii) provide administrators with a rationale for planning and resource allocation (Blashfield, 1984; Remschmidt, 1995).

In this chapter, current classification systems and assessment methods commonly used in studying psychiatric disorders in children and adolescents are described.

CLASSIFICATION SYSTEMS

"Clinically" Derived Classification System

Diagnostic and Statistical Manual of Mental Disorders

The Diagnostic and Statistical Manual of Mental Disorders (DSM) developed in the United States is a classification system widely used around the world. In the first version of the DSM (American Psychiatric

Association; APA, 1952), two categories of childhood disorders (Adjustment reaction and childhood schizophrenia) were included, and in the subsequent DSM-II (APA, 1968), the category of behavioural disorder of childhood and adolescence was added. The later versions (DSM-III, APA, 1980; DSM-III-R, APA, 1987; DSM-IV, APA, 1994) have included an expanded number of diagnostic categories specific to children and adolescents. Several other diagnostic classifications such as the depressive disorders can also be applied to adults, children, and adolescents.

The most recent edition, DSM-IV (APA, 1994), categorizes psychiatric disorders into 16 major diagnostic classes (Table 2.1), with the first section being devoted to "Disorders usually first diagnosed in infancy, childhood, or adolescence". Each disorder is described along the following headings: diagnostic features; subtypes and/or specifiers; recording procedures; associated features and disorders, which is further subdivided into "associated descriptive features and mental disorders", "associated laboratory findings", and "associated physical examination findings and general medical conditions"; specific culture, age, and gender features; prevalence; course; familial pattern; and differential diagnosis. In the case that the disorder described has no information on a particular section, that section is excluded.

Table 2.1   Clinical disorders and conditions in DSM-IV

Disorders usually first diagnosed in infancy, childhood, or adolescence
Delirium, dementia, and amnestic and other cognitive disorders
Mental disorders due to a general medical condition not elsewhere classified
Substance-related disorders
Schizophrenia and other psychotic disorders
Mood disorders
Anxiety disorders
Somatoform disorders
Factitious disorders
Dissociative disorders
Sexual and gender identity disorders
Eating disorders
Sleep disorders
Impulse-control disorders not elsewhere classified
Adjustment disorders
Personality disorders
Other conditions that may be a focus of clinical attention

The developers of DSM-IV specifically acknowledge the manual is based on categories of disorder — a limited approach. No assumption is made that each category is discrete. "A categorical approach to classification works best when all members of a diagnostic class are homogeneous, when there are clear boundaries between classes, and when the different classes are mutually exclusive" (APA, 1994, p. xxii). DSM-IV differs from previous versions by giving greater weight to published literature, that is, "more than any other nomenclature of mental disorders, DSM-IV is grounded in empirical evidence" (APA, 1994, p. xvi). Further, DSM-IV employs the concept of diagnostic hierarchies, whereby diagnoses higher in the hierarchy often include symptoms of diagnoses lower in the hierarchy. In this case, individuals who meet the criteria for the diagnoses lower in the hierarchy are not generally given that lower diagnosis. Hierarchies are used in three areas: first, the presence of a psychiatric disorder due to a general medical condition or a substance-induced disorder preempts other diagnoses with the same symptoms. Second, the application of hierarchies require that more pervasive disorder (e.g., schizophrenia) preempts less pervasive disorder (e.g., dysthymic disorder). Third, they are useful when differential diagnostic decisions are not straightforward to make, and when there is a need to have an immediate clinical plan.

DSM-IV continues to apply the multiaxial system introduced in DSM-III, with minor modifications. The use of a multiaxial system ensures that attention be given to certain types of disorder, aspects of environment, and areas of functioning that may be overlooked when the focus is based on a single presenting problem. The multiaxial system in DSM-IV includes 5 axes, which each patient can be evaluated on:

Axis I   Clinical disorders
          Other conditions that may be a focus of clinical attention
Axis II   Personality disorders
          Mental retardation
Axis III General medical conditions
Axis IV   Psychosocial and environmental problems
Axis V   Global assessment of functioning

Axis I includes various types of disorders or conditions other than personality disorders and mental retardation. Axis II includes personality disorders and mental retardation. It also contains prominent maladaptive personality features which fail to meet the threshold for a personality disorder. Axis III is used to report general medical conditions that are relevant for the understanding and management of the individual. Axis IV assesses psychosocial and environmental factors which may be important in the initiation or exacerbation of the disorder. These relate to the availability of primary support groups, the social environment, education level, occupational status, housing, and economic situation, involvement with legal system, and problems with access to health care services. Axis V measures the individual's current psychological, social, and occupational functioning by using a Global Assessment of Functioning Scale.

International Classification of Diseases

The other major classification system widely used world wide is the International Statistical Classification of Diseases and Related Health Problems (ICD; World Health Organization; WHO, 1993), of which Chapter V (F) is devoted to psychiatric disorders (Table 2.2).The chapter is divided into 10 groups, with each category denoted by the letter F followed by a number for the main group. In the latest version of the ICD (ICD-10; WHO, 1993), the disorders with an onset in childhood or adolescence have been expanded and classified into three groups: those comprising mental retardation (F7), developmental disorders (F8), and those comprising behavioural and emotional disorders with onset specific to childhood and adolescence (F9). Other major changes from ICD-9 include the exclusion of the differentiation between psychosis and neurosis as a basic principle for sub-classification. The terms psychosis and neurosis have been replaced with the term "disorders". Disorders which are symptomatically relevant have been grouped together. For example, depressive syndromes are no longer separately classified as psychotic and neurotic depression, but are grouped together under "affective disorders". The clinical description and diagnostic guidelines are described in more detail in ICD-10 than in ICD-9.

Each category in the chapter is accompanied by a brief glossary definition (Sartorius, 1994). Other material produced together with the glossary includes (1) the clinical guidelines of the disorders which appeared in Chapter V; (2) the ICD-10 Diagnostic Criteria for Research on Mental Disorder; (3) diagnostic guidelines for use in primary health care settings; (4) crosswalks between the various revisions of the ICD and reference materials for comparing classifications produced by other systems (e.g., DSM-III) or other associations with a special interest (e.g., classifi-

Table 2.2   Mental and behavioral disorders in ICD-10

F0	Organic, including symptomatic, mental disorders
F1	Mental and behavioral disorders due to psychoactive substance use
F2	Schizophrenia, schizotypal and delusional disorders
F3	Mood (affective) disorders
F4	Neurotic, stress-related and somatoform disorders
F5	Behavioral syndromes associated with physiological disturbances and physical factors
F6	Disorders of adult personality and behaviour
F7	Mental retardation
F8	Disorders of psychological development
F9	Behavioural and emotional disorders with onset usually occurring in childhood and adolescence
F99	Unspecific mental disorder

cation of pain, sleeping disorders); (5) several related classifications such as the reason for encounter, etc; (6) standardized diagnostic instruments for clinical (e.g., SCAN) and epidemiological studies (e.g., CIDI), and a diagnostic computer program for analysizing data obtained using these instruments; (7) standard case histories and videotaped material to train and to assess the reliability of interviewers who make their diagnosis using ICD-10 categories; and (8) the use of multiaxial schema. The ICD-10 multiaxial system may be a useful tool for efficient stimultaneous assessment of the various aspects of the patient's illness. It also allows more thorough, uniform, and consistent collection of data, as well as to generate a database useful in both clinical care and research (Janca *et al.*, 1996).

The multiaxial schema in ICD-10 consists two versions. One version is for children and adolescents (6 axes), and the other for adults (3 axes). The multiaxial classifications of child and adolescent psychiatric disorder are:

Axis I	Clinical psychiatric syndromes
Axis II	Specific disorders of psychological development
Axis III	Intellectual level
Axis IV	Medical conditions
Axis V	Associated abnormal psychological situations
Axis VI	Global assessment of psychosocial functioning

Axis I includes coding for disorders that are of little relevance for children, although these disorders can apply in childhood and adolescence.

Some examples of disorders included in the first axis are schizophrenia, schizotypal and delusional disorders (F20–F29), and disorders of adult personality and behaviour (F60–F69). Specific delays in disorders of psychological development are coded in Axis II independent of their origin, except when delays are solely due to poor schooling. Specific developmental disorders of speech and language (F80) and specific developmental disorders of scholastic skills are some examples of disorders listed under Axis II. Axis III is used to describe a person's current levels of general intellectual functioning. The person can be described as having "intellectual level within the normal range" to "profound mental retardation". Axis IV provides coding of non-psychiatric medical conditions. Axis V provides coding of abnormal psychosocial situations which may be relevant for the precipitating psychiatric disorders or for therapeutic planning. Examples of such situations include abnormal intrafamilial relationships, abnormal qualities of upbringing, acute life events, and societal stressors. Axis VI reflects the patient's psychological, social, and occupational functioning at the time of examination. It deals with disability in functioning that result from psychiatric disorders, specific disorders of psychological development or mental retardation. The levels of disability used ranged from "superior/ good social functioning" to "profound and pervasive social disability".

Comparison of ICD and DSM

In categorization, both ICD-10 Chapter V and DSM-IV are largely similar. Due to the fact that natural classifications should be compatible with international classifications, groups drafting ICD and DSM have worked in close collaboration to establish a good level of similarity and congruence. ICD-10 and DSM-IV are over ninety percent similar in categorization. However, differences remain in style and terms relating to cross-cultural applicability issues.

The ICD-10 lists the codes and names of the disorders with a glossary describing each disorder. Each disorder in DSM-IV has information which can be divided under different categories such as diagnostic features, onset and course. Guidelines and criteria used in the ICD-10 do not take social consequences of the disorder into consideration. In DSM-IV the diagnostic criteria include significant distress and impairment in social, occupational, or other important areas of functioning.

Another difference is related to the multiaxial system. ICD-10 places all the diagnoses included in the DSM-IV Axes I, II, and III on one axis.

In formulating criteria, ICD-10 has depended on expert consensus and has tested these with field trials in various countries world wide, whereas DSM-IV depended more on empirical review (Frances *et al.*, 1994). The final differences are related to definitions of some disorders, which could be attributed to the fact that: ICD has separate clinical and research criteria; different purposes served by the ICD and DSM systems; DSM-IV's greater reliance on empirical evidence (for US or anglosaxon psychiatry) and ICD-10s transcultural applicability.

Critiques of the DSM and ICD Systems

Although both the DSM-IV and ICD-10 represent major advances on previous systems, they have been open to criticism. Except for few disorders, there is little information given about etiological influences on the development of psychiatric disorder, which limit the value of classification systems in both research and clinical practice (Graham and Skuse, 1992). Both systems make little attempt to define criteria of abnormal behaviour in children from different cultural background (Graham and Skuse, 1992). For example, in most Asian countries, children are expected to submit and conform to parental and teacher authority, which would have implications for deciding on a threshold for "oppositional defiant disorder" (Graham and Skuse, 1992).

DSM-IV does not adequately address developmental perspectives on psychiatric disorders. Only brief references are given to developmental factors in diagnostic decision making in children and adolescents. For example, in order to make the diagnosis of Attention-Deficit/Hyperactivity Disorder (ADHD), some hyperactive-impulsive or inattentive symptoms which cause impairment have to be present before age 7 years, however, there is no indication as to why this age is used. Another related issue is its emphasis on a "single, development free set of criteria" (Graham and Skuse, 1992). For example, the diagnostic criteria for DSM-IV major depressive episode can be applied to children, adolescents and adults. The only differences are those related to "depressed mood" and "significant weight loss or weight gain" in that the symptom can be substituted with irritable mood, and with a "failure to make expected weight gains" (p. 327), respectively. There lacks an empirical basis for both the difference and similarities in the manifestation of depressive symptoms at different ages (Angold and Worthman, 1993; Cicchetti and Schneider-Rosen, 1986).

DSM-IV only lists symptoms (e.g., conduct disorders) for a particular diagnosis and does not specify the sources of information to be used as a basis for judging whether a child meets the criteria (e.g., direct observation, interviewing the child or parents or teachers). Although these sources of information are not equivalent to each other, the DSM-IV does indicate which sources of information to use or the relative weight to give to each source. Another related issue is the influence of situational factors on the children's behaviour. Since children's behaviour varies over time and in different settings, the contexts in which children are examined need to be considered. Taking ADHD as an example, DSM-IV acknowledges that although ADHD symptoms appear in multiple contexts (e.g., home, school, work, social situations) it would be unusual for the child to display the same level of dysfunction in all settings or within the same setting at all times. Additionally, DSM-IV states that some environments may stimulate the child's disorganized behaviour. Yet, no explicit guidelines are given as to how many symptoms, in how many settings, are needed to make a ADHD diagnosis. Though both DSM-IV and ICD-10 mention comorbidity, no mention is made as to how children's cognitive, social, and bodily development may influence their ability to experience different symptoms (Costello and Angold, 1995).

For the DSM-IV disorder criteria, generally, once one or two cardinal symptoms are evident (e.g., depressed mood for major depressive episode), all subsequent symptoms (e.g., loss of appetite, suicidal ideation) are given equal weight in making a diagnosis. That is, on a simple count, a child may be classified as having a disorder. To a certain extent this notion of unidimensionality, and symptom equivalency can defy common sense. For example, why should "suicide attempt" and "fatigue" be given the same weight in a diagnosis of major depressive disorder? To make the diagnosis, some symptoms must have caused impairment, however, which symptoms are not specified, nor are criteria of impairment defined. Although there is a general consensus as to the types of symptoms used to define psychiatric disorders (Quay, 1986), major questions exist with regard to defining the boundaries or thresholds for classifying disorder as either present or absent.

The thresholds of symptomatology in the DSM-IV used to differentiate between presence or absence of a disorder have historically been made arbitrarily, and not generally based on empirical data as highlighted by changes made from DSM-III to DSM-IV (Achenbach, 1995). For example, in order to meet the criteria for oppositional defiant disorder, DSM-III lists 5 criteria for which 2 are required, DSM-III-R lists 9 criteria for which 5 are required, and in DSM-IV 8 for which 4 are needed. DSM-IV recognizes this problem when it states that "there is no assumption that each category of mental disorder is a completely discrete entity with absolute boundaries dividing it from other mental disorders or from no mental disorders" (APA, 1994, p. xxii).

Since thresholds for classifying psychiatric disorder have immense impacts for research, some authors (Boyle *et al.*, submitted) have recommended that attention be focused on developing empirical criteria that take into account prevalence, reliability, correlates, and comorbidity for evaluating the extent to which decision rules for classifying children and adolescents with psychiatric disorders are sensible. Also, since the current classification systems involve some arbitrariness it is important to look for convergence of results using different decision rules and approaches. In order to evaluate classification systems, attempts should be made to obtain data from the population of interest since information from clinic samples may not be applicable to general population samples and the reverse. That is, although the conceptual and empirical issues related to thresholds for classifying disorder are similar in both groups, underlying differences in the response patterns of the two groups may make it difficult to generalizing findings from one population to the other.

"Empirical" Approaches to Classification

An empirical approach uses standardized tests and statistical techniques (e.g., factor or cluster analysis) to identify sets of items that are interrelated, with each cluster of behaviours constituting a syndrome. One of the most widely used standardized tests has been the Child Behavior Checklist (CBCL; Achenbach and Edelbrock, 1986).

The main advantage of the empirical approach to classification is that dimensions of the constellations of behaviour are obtained through empirical data. However, there has been some concern about the use of empirical approach in the development of classification systems (Yule, 1981), since certain clusters of behaviour are labelled differently across studies, and in some cases certain dimensions may not even emerge (Gettinger and Kratochwill, 1987). Additionally, the results obtained seem to be dependent on the type of statistical procedures, the scoring format, the number and content of items, and the number of participants used in the analyses. Finally, the exclusion of rarely endorsed symptoms (e.g., autistic behaviour) may limit the instrument for assessing uncommon but severe problems.

ASSESSMENT METHODS

Assessment refers to the collection of information about the individual's repertoire of behaviour (Achenbach, 1995). The general goals of assessment have always been associated with the need to both plan and implement successful intervention strategies for remediating psychiatric disorder. Assessment has several specific functions including allowing the assignment of problems to a diagnostic category; evaluating the presence, absence, or level of specific behaviours, abilities, or skills; specify the severity of symptoms; transforming vague complaints into specific behavioural excesses or deficits and predicting future behaviour under given conditions; for designing research to enhance our knowledge of the nature of psychopathology; and to monitor the impact of treatment or previous efforts (Kanfer and Nay, 1982).

An important consideration when choosing an assessment approach is the reliability and validity of the instruments. Furthermore, assessment methods should also be adequate to test the hypothesis under consideration. Major sources of unreliability that arise from variability in obtaining clinical information and diagnostic formulation have greatly been reduced by using structured diagnostic interviews and the use of explicit diagnostic criteria (Mezzich, 1988; Mezzich and Mezzich, 1987).

Decisions as to which instruments to use generally rely on the research questions and the study design. As a general outline, Achenbach (1995) recommended that the instrument used be standardised; contains multiple items to assess each level of functioning; and have normed score to compare the individual with a relevant reference group. Also, in the assessment of children and adolescents, there is a need to consider measures appropriate to their age and level of development.

Depending on whether it is a clinical or research work, the data should be obtained from multiple sources (e.g., parent, teacher) to help decrease bias that may result from only one informant. Achenbach (1995) recommended five sources of data relevant for assessing children and adolescents. These sources include:

- parent reports (standardized ratings, developmental history, parent interview);
- teacher report (standardized rating, school records, teacher interview);
- cognitive assessment (ability tests, achievement tests, perceptual-motor tests, language tests);
- physical assessment (height, weight, medical examination, neurological examination);

- assessment of the child or adolescent (direct observation, clinical interview, standardized self-ratings by child or adolescent).

The need to assess the multiple aspects of children's functioning (cognitive, educational, emotional, physical) in various situations (home, school) also precludes the use of single methods (Achenbach, 1988). Kazdin and Kagan (1994) have similarly suggested that assessment not be limited to the characteristics of the individual, but also include broad domains and context outside the individuals such as the characteristics of the parents, family, and culture; they also recommended the use of repeated assessments which can be used to identify the child's stable characteristics and the context in which these characteristics appear. Assessment should be based on multiple methods, multiple modalities, and multiple informants. Furthermore, the prevalence, severity, and correlates of certain disorders tend to be dependent on the informant source (Achenbach *et al.*, 1987; Kazdin, 1989; Rutter *et al.*, 1970). As indicated by Rutter *et al.* (1970), quantification of the presence and severity of behaviour vary depending on whether the informant is a parent, teacher, or the child/adolescent. A meta-analysis of cross-informant correlations by Achenbach *et al.* (1987) showed a mean correlation of 0.60 between informants with similar roles to the child, and between informants with different roles in relation to the child it was 0.28; the mean correlation between children's self-reports and reports by parents, teachers, and mental health professionals was 0.22. Based on these findings, it has been recommended that the diagnosis of certain disorders (e.g., conduct disorder) be delineated based on parent-identified versus teacher- or adolescent-identified symptoms (Offord *et al.*, 1991). It is also important to examine how the child's significant others behave toward the child, and how their behaviours may contribute to the child's problem. A major challenge for assessment and taxonomy of psychiatric disorder is the lack of a "gold standard" against which to validate multisource data, and for dealing with the variations among different sources (Achenbach, 1995).

The child's behaviour should be evaluated from a developmental perspective. However, designing age-appropriate methods is difficult as it is closely linked with defining age-appropriate diagnostic systems. In order to correctly identify and to better understand problems in children and adolescents, it is important to evaluate them on the basis of developmental norms or age-appropriate functioning (La Greca and Stone, 1992). For example, nocturnal enuresis is considered to be normal in the 3-year old, but not in the 10-year old.

Achenbach (1988) differentiated between 5 principle types of assessment methods: rating scales, clinical interviews, direct observations, family assessment, and neuropsychological methods.

Rating Scales and Self-report Questionnaires

Many rating scales and self-report questionnaires have been developed to assess children's functioning. They can be used as screening instruments (e.g., the Child Behavior Checklist) to select subjects prior to second-stage interviews, or for defining a case (e.g., the revised Ontario Child Health Study scales; Boyle *et al.*, 1993). Rating scales not only vary in length, but also in the kinds of behaviours covered, the specificity of settings in which behaviours occur, and the age range of children for whom the checklist applies. Some checklists have a comprehensive coverage of a wide spectrum of psychiatric symptoms and disorders, while others cover a single disorder such as depression (Table 2.3). In evaluating rating scales it is necessary to consider the type of disorder plus the nature of the informant. The most commonly used informants are parents and teachers, basically because they are the ones who have the most frequent contact with the child (Achenbach, 1988). It should be recognized that these principal informants will tend to observe behaviours that are situation specific.

Rating scales elicit information through a question-and-answer format; the information elicited can then be used to indicate the presence and absence of moods, feelings, and behaviour constituting an episode of a psychiatric disorder. Subjects respond to the questions or statements by marking one of a given set of responses (Table 2.4). It has been suggested that the instruments which use more than two response alternatives tend to be more reliable and valid, and give more information than those with a dichotomous response (Barkley, 1981).

There are several advantages of using rating scales and questionnaires to assess symptoms of psychiatric disorders. Depending on the wording of questions, they can often be administered and assessed by nonprofessional personnel with a minimum of specialized training or clinical experience. They can be administered quickly to a large group of people at low financial cost, and thus may be used economically as screening devices to determine those potentially in need of psychiatric help and for an early identification of psychiatric problems. The scales can be tested for internal consistency and reliability (Achenbach, 1988). Rating scales when used by themselves have the disadvantage in that

Table 2.3 Rating scales and self-report questionnaires for specific problems

Name (Author)	No. of items	Characteristics
Anxiety		
Fear Survey Schedule for Children — Revised (Ollendick, 1983)	80	Each item to be rated on a 3-point scale (none, some, a lot) Factor analysis produced 5 subscales: fear of failure and criticism, fear of the unknown, fear of injury and small animals, fear of danger and death, fear of medical fear.
Revised Children's Manifest Anxiety Scale (Reynolds & Richmond, 1978)	37	Each item is to be responded "yes" or "no". Contains 3 subscales: physiological symptoms, worry and oversensitivity, and concentration.
Leyton Obsessional Compulsive Scale — Child version (Berg, Rapoport, & Flament, 1986)	44	Child responds to each item "yes" or "no". All items which are positively answered are rated on resistance and interference.
Stait-trait Anxiety Inventory for Children (Spielberger, 1973)	40	The A-trait scale measures an enduring tendency to experience anxiety. The A-state scale measures temporal and situational variations in levels of perceived anxiety.
Depression		
Children's Depression Inventory (Kovacs, 1979)	27	Items use a 3-alternative, forced-choice response format, the child chooses the symptom level that best describes how he/she is feeling.

Table 2.3 *continued*

Name (Author)	No. of items	Characteristics
Reynolds Child Depression Scale (Reynolds, 1989)	30	29 items measure depressive symptoms which the child (age 8–13 years) experienced during the past 2 weeks, and are to be responded on a 4-point scale ("almost never" to "all the time"). The last item is a global dysphoric mood-state rating that consists of 5 "smiley-type" faces ranging from sad to happy. The child places an X over the face which indicates how he/she feels.
Reynolds Adolescent Depression Scale (Reynolds, 1987)	30	Each item is to be rated on a 4-point scale ("almost never" to "most of the time").
Center for Epidemiological Studies — Depression Scale (Radloff, 1977)	20	Items are to be rated on the basis of frequency over the past week.
Attention-deficit hyperactivity		
Werry-Weiss Peters Activity Rating Scale (Werry, 1968)	31	Parents rate specific behaviours within 7 different settings: mealtime, watching TV, doing homework, playing, sleeping, public places, and school. Each item is to be rated as: 0 (none), 1 (a little bit), 2 (very much).

Table 2.4 Examples of questions in the selected rating scales

Instruments (Authors)	Examples of questions	Rating options
Child Behavior Checklist (Achenbach & Edelbrock, 1983)	– has difficulty making friends with others – is afraid or worried too much – likes to be alone – easily tired	0 = not at all true, 1 = a little bit true, 2 = very much true, or very frequent
Revised Ontario Child Health Study scales (Boyle *et al.*, 1993)	– I can't concentrate and can't pay attention for long – I feel hopeless – I have nightmares about being abandoned	0 = never or not true, 1 = sometimes true 2 = somewhat true 3 = often or very true
Beck Depression Inventory (Beck *et al.*, 1962)	Mood: 0 I do not feel sad 1 I feel sad 2 I am sad all the time and I can't snap out of it 3 I am so sad or unhappy that I can't stand it	

they tend to overestimate the prevalence of psychiatric problems. Social desirability may also affect how informants respond to scales; the degree of social desirability may vary among specific items and/or among different informants (Haynes, 1978). Several scales for the assessment of childhood and adolescent mental health and behavioural problems have appeared which have been used in epidemiological studies, studies of clinical populations, and in the clinical or treatment settings. The more common scales include the Child Behavior Checklist, the Revised Behavior Problem Checklist (Quay and Peterson, 1987), the Conners Parent Symptom Questionnaire and Conners Teacher Rating Scale (Goyette *et al.*, 1978), the Revised Ontario Child Health Study Scales (Boyle *et al.*, 1993), and the Symptom Checklist-90-R (Derogatis, 1977).

Child Behavior Checklist (CBCL)

The CBCL is usually used to assess social competence and behaviour problems in children between the ages of 4 and 16 years (Achenbach and Edelbrock, 1986).The social competence items consist of an activities scale (i.e., to measure the child's participation in sports, nonsports hobbies, activities, games, jobs and chores), the social functioning scale (i.e., to measure the children's membership and participation in organizations, the number of friends and contacts with them, and behavior with others and alone), and the school functioning scale (i.e., to measure performance in academic subjects, placement in a regular or a special class, being promoted regularly or held back, and the presence or absence of school problems).

The CBCL is designed in different formats for obtaining information from parents, teachers, and adolescents. It is inexpensive to administer, can be used to collect information about the children's competencies and problems within a short period of time, and has excellent psychometric properies (Bird and Gould, 1995). It has been used not only in a large representative population in the United States, but also in different cultural settings (Achenbach, 1990; Verhulst, 1995; Weisz *et al.*, 1987; Weisz *et al.*, 1989; see Weisz and Eastman, 1995 for review).

Separate norms are available for girls and boys at ages 4–5, 6–11, and 12–16 since it is believed that children make important transitions in their cognitive, physical, educational, and/or social-emotional development during these age periods. Studies that used the CBCL have shown the existence of two broad-band syndromes: Externalizing (undercontrolled) and internationalizing (overcontrolled) (Achenbach and Edelbrock, 1978, 1979). Some characteristics associated with the externalizing syndrome include temper tantrums, aggression, and destructiveness. The internalizing syndrome includes specific cluster of behaviours such as anxious, shy, withdrawn, and depressed. Specific narrow-band syndromes (e.g., schizoid, aggressive, delinquent, socially withdrawn) have been found within the two broad-band syndromes of internalizing and externalizing. Some syndromes which do not fall within one of the two broad-band categories are listed under the "mixed" syndromes.

While internalizing and externalizing categories do exist in both boys and girls, specific problems within these syndromes differ depending on the child's age and gender. For example, the factors for 6–11 year old girls include depressed, social-withdrawal, somatic complaints, schizoid-obsessive, hyperactive, sex problems, delinquent, aggressive, and cruel. The factors for the 12–16 year old boys include somatic complaints, schizoid, uncommunicative, immature, obsessive-compulsive, hostile-withdrawn, delinquent, aggressive and hyperactive (Achenbach and Edelbrock, 1979).

Revised Behavior Problem Checklist (RBPC)

The RBPC (Quay and Peterson, 1987) contains 89 items designed to assess behavioral/emotional disturbance which can be used with respondents as young as 5 years and as old as 20. Factor analysis of the RBPC revealed four major scales (i.e., Conduct Disorder, Socialized Aggression, Attention Problem Immaturity, Anxiety-Withdrawal) and two minor scales (Psychotic Behavior and Motor Excess). The Conduct Disorder scale comprises items that represent the dimension of aggressive, noncompliant, quarrelsome, interpersonally aliented, and acting-out behavior. Socialized Aggression represents a dimension of acting-out, externalizing behavior. The Attention Problem-Immaturity scale reflects problems related to concentration, perseverance, impulsivity, and in following directions at home and in school. The Anxiety-Withdrawal scale contains items relating to anxiety, depression, fear of failure, social inferiority, and social concern. The Psychotic Behavior scale is comprised of items related to overt psychoses (e.g., delusion) and language dysfunction.

Conners Parent Symptom Questionnaire and Conners Teacher Rating Scale

The Conners Parent Symptoms Questionnaire is a 48-item paper-pencil inventory designed for assessing behaviour problems of children aged 3–17 years as observed by their parents in the home setting. Factor analysis of the questionnaire yields six factor scales: conduct problems, learning problems, psychosomatic problems, impulsivity-hyperactivity, and anxiety (Goyette *et al.*, 1978).

The Conners Teacher Rating Scale assesses 28 problem behaviours of children from preschool to grade 12 that are encountered in the classroom by teachers. It yields 4 factors scores: conduct problems, hyperactivity, inattention-passivity, and a hyperactivity index.

The Revised Ontario Child Health Study Scales (OCHS)

The OCHS were developed to measure conduct disorder, oppositional disorder, attention-deficit hyperactivity, overanxious disorder, separation anxiety, and depression according to DSM-III-R criteria. The questionnaire is available in three forms, one for parents, one for teachers, and the other for adolescents aged 12–16 years. The frame for assessment was the past six months. Each item can be scored as "never or not true" (0), "sometimes or somewhat true" (1), and "often or very true" (2).

Some DSM-III-R symptoms are operationalized using 2 or more items. This is especially the case for overanxious disorder and depression. For example, the DSM-III-R symptom of "significant weight loss or weight gain when not dieting" was operationalized using 2 items "significant weight loss" and "weight gain when not dieting", each of which was given a value of 0, 1, or 2. The higher rating obtained by the 2 items indicates symptom presence.

Symptom Checklist-90-R (SCL-90-R)

The SCL-90-R (Derogatis, 1977) is a self-report inventory designed to measure psychological distress, which though actually developed for adults has been widely used among adolescents. The 90 items conform to nine symptom dimensions: somatization, obsessive-compulsive, interpersonal sensivity, depression, anxiety, hostility, phobic anxiety, paranoid ideation, and psychoticism. Three severity indexes are derived: a global severity index which reflects both the intensity of distress and number of reported symptoms; a positive symptom total which is simply the number of symptoms reported; and a positive symptom distress index, which is a measure of intensity, adjusted for the number of symptoms present.

Diagnostic Interviews

A number of structured diagnostic interviews have been designed in recent years. Efforts in the development of structured diagnostic interviews for children and adolescents have been spurred by pioneering work of Rutter and Graham, along with the development of structured interview schedules for adults which has greatly improved diagnostic reliability (Robins *et al.*, 1981). The development of more differentiated taxonomies of childhood disorders and more explicit diagnostic criteria has also required, and consequently led to, a more standardized approach for the assessment of psychiatric symptoms. Unlike rating scales, diagnostic interviews are based on stricter formalizations of the diagnostic process by using specific symptoms and probe questions, detailed coding rules, and diagnostic algorithms. The questions in each diagnostic category are formulated to evaluate the symptoms of the disorder, their duration, and potential exclusion (Table 2.5).

Diagnostic interviews with children or adolescents are needed to obtain information regarding their current functioning, behavioural or

Table 2.5 Examples of questions in the standardized clinical interviews

Instruments	Examples of questions	Rating options
DICA-R (Reich and Welner, 1988)	Was there ever a time during the past 6 months when you found yourself being snappish, irritable (crabby or cranky) a *lot* more than usual?	1 = Yes 2 = Sometimes 4 = No 9 = Don't know
DISC (Costello et al., 1987)	In the past 6 months, were there times when you were **grouchy or irritable, often in a bad mood**, so that even little things would make you mad? IF YES, a) When you are grouchy like this, does it last most of the day? b) Would you say you have been grouchy *a lot of* the time for as long as a year? IF YES, c) Would you say you were like that *most of the time*? IF YES, d) Were you grouchy most of the time for as long as 2 years? e) Now thinking about just the last 6 months ... Was there a time when you were grouchy almost every day? IF YES, f) Did this go on for 2 weeks or more?	0 = No 1 = Sometimes / somewhat 2 = Yes 9 = Don't know

Table 2.5   *continued*

Instruments	Examples of questions	Rating options
K-SADS-P (Puig-Antich and Chambers, 1978)	Do you get annoyed and irritated, or cranky at little things? What kinds of things? Have you been feeling mad or angry also (even if you don't show it)? How angry? More than before? What kinds of things make you feel angry? Do you sometimes feel angry, irritable, or cranky and don't know why? Does this happen often? Do you lose your temper? With your family? Your friends? Who else? At school? What happens? Has anybody said anything about it? How much of the time do you feel angry, irritable, or cranky? When you get mad, what do you think about? Do you think about killing others? Or about hurting them or torturing them? Whom? Do you have a plan? How?	0 = No information 1 = Not at all 2 = Slight 3 = Mild 4 = Moderate 5 = Severe 6 = Extreme 7 = Number 6 plus homicidal plan

Note: DICA-R = Diagnostic Interview for Children and Adolescents —revised version; DISC = Diagnostic Interview Schedule for Children; K-SADS-P = Schedule for Affective Disorders and Schizophrenia for School-age Children (present episode version) psychiatric problems, and their attributions about their current status especially in assessing symptoms which no other informants are aware of. Interviews with parents are used to obtain descriptions and course of the problems, developmental history, family background, and information about the parent's role in the child's problems (Achenbach, 1988).

All structured interviews contain lists of target behaviours, symptoms, and guidelines for conducting the interview and recording responses; they allow a direct derivation of diagnoses so that a second stage investigation is not needed. However, the nature of the target behaviours or diagnostic coverage that are to be assessed, the time frames (e.g., lifetime, 6-month), and the degree of structure imposed on the interview can differ markedly across interviews. Interviews also differ in the classification systems they serve, the expertise needed to administer them, their operational cost, and their product (Robins, 1994). In choosing which interview schedule to use, it is important to specify the goals of the study, and the available resources (Robins, 1994).

A diagnostic interview must be comprehensive in scope and provide the means for determining the presence or absence of psychiatric disorders likely to be encountered in the population (Bird and Gould, 1995). Additionally, it must be feasible in terms of its length and ease of administration, be inexpensive to administer and ideally be equipped with algorithms which can be scored by computer (Bird and Gould, 1995).

There are two types of structured interviews: highly structured and semi-structured. Highly structured interviews specify exact wording and sequence of questions, well-defined rules for recording, and rating of the respondents' answers. Their highly structured forms encourage administration by lay interviewers who have undergone an intensive training in the instruments use. Interviews such as the Diagnostic Interview for Children and Adolescents (Herjanic and Campbell, 1977) and the Diagnostic Interview Schedule for Children (Costello *et al.*, 1987) have been designed for used in large epidemiologic studies. Semi-structured interviews such as the Child Assessment Schedule (Hodges *et al.*, 1982) and the Child Version of the Schedule of Affective Disorders and Schizophrenia (Puig-Antich and Chambers, 1978) contain more general and flexible guidelines for conducting the interview and recording information. That is, the interviewer is allowed some flexibility in what is asked, how questions are phrased, and how responses are recorded. As such, they are primarily designed for use by trained clinicians. However, since the interview may be conducted in a slightly different way by each clinician, close attention needs to be paid to reliability.

The main advantage of diagnostic interviews is that they allow the exploration of the informant's responses together with the direct observation of behaviour. As such they allow interviewers to clarify misunderstandings and resolving ambiguous responses. Structured interviews attempt to reduce variability in obtaining information by specifying the items to be investigated and providing definition for these items, and providing instructions for rating the presence and severity of the items involved. Furthermore, structured interviews can be time consuming, and need to be carried out by trained interviewers. Although structured interviews provide diagnostic classifications they very often can also provide symptom scales. However embedded problem with some symptom scales derived from structured interviews is that items are often "gated" which lead to large number of no (0) responses and non-normally distributed frequency distributions of items.

Diagnostic Interview Schedule for Children (DISC)

The National Institute of Mental Health (NIMH) Diagnostic Interview Schedule for Children (DISC) is a highly structured psychiatric interview developed for used by trained lay interviewers (Piacentini *et al.*, 1993; Schwab-Stone *et al.*, 1993). The first version of the DISC appeared in 1983. Since then it has undergone several revisions, and another major revision (DSC-IV) is currently taking place (Fischer, 1996). The newest version will address DSM-IV and ICD-10 criteria, include a 6-month timeframe, an elective module for lifetime diagnosis, and include a more precise probing for episode onset. The interview has 2 parallel forms, DISC-C which is administered to children, and the DISC-P for administration to the parents or caregivers.

The DISC was designed to be used in epidemiological studies of children aged 9–17 to assess for the presence of major psychiatric disorders found in children and adolescents, including: major affective disorder, attention-deficit disorder, conduct disorder, separation anxiety, avoidant disorder, anorexia nervosa, bulimia, functional enuresis, functional encopresis, alcohol abuse/dependence, cannabis abuse/dependence, tobacco dependence, schizophrenia, cyclothymic disorder, agoraphobia, social phobia, simple phobia, panic disorder, obsessive-compulsive disorder, and substance abuse. Additionally the parent version covers infantile autism, elective mutism, psychogenic fugue, hypochondriasis, Tourette's syndrome, pervasive developmental disorder, psychogenic amnesia, conversion disorder, and tic disorder.

The DISC requires the interviewer to read each question exactly as written, with little freedom allowed to interpret replies. Most response options are limited to "yes", "no", and "sometimes" or "somewhat". DISC questions can be grouped into two categories: (i) "stem" questions which ask about the presence of behaviours. A "No" response to the "stem question" means that the interview has to move forward past more specific prompts of that general question; (ii) "contingent" questions inquire only if a stem question is answered positively to determine whether the elicited behaviour meets a diagnostic criterion. The contingent questions help reduce the false positive responses, and are used to determine whether the symptom meets the specifications for a diagnostic criteria. A third category of questions has been added in the later versions of the DISC, which are asked at the end of each diagnostic section when certain numbers of symptoms have been posivitely answered. These questions assess age at which the first "episode" appeared, impairment associated with the current episode, the context in which the current symptoms may have arisen or been exacerbated, and the need for or receipt of any treatment intervention for the specific conditions.

Computerized versions of the DISC are available such as the PC-DISC which was programmed at Emory University, and the C-DISC developed at the University of Ottawa. The C-DISC is available in two versions: the computer-assist and the computer-administered versions. In the computer-assist version, the computer is used by the interviewer as an aide to asking questions and who then enters subject's responses. In the computer-administered version, the respondents read the questions directly from the screen and enters their own responses directly.

Diagnostic Interview for Children and Adolescents (DICA)

The DICA is a structured interview designed to assess the major psychiatric disorders of childhood adolescence according to DSM-III criteria. The later version, the DICA-R, has been streamlined and expanded to include diagnoses using DSM-III-R criteria, together with onset, duration, severity, and associated impairments of the symptoms (Herjanic and Reich, 1982).The DICA is available in three versions, one for children (ages 6–12), one for adolescents (13–17 years), and another for parents.

The diagnostic categories and areas covered in the child interview are: attention-deficit disorder, oppositional disorder, socialization, conduct disorder, alcohol use, cigarette smoking, drug use, mood disorders, separation anxiety disorder, overanxious disorder, simple phobia, obsessive-compulsive disorder, compulsions, anorexia nervosa, bulimia, somatization disorder, enuresis, encopresis, menstruation, gender identity disorder, sexual experience, psychotic symptoms, and psychosocial stressors. Questions are also available for the interviewer to evaluate the child's general appearance, affect, motor behaviour, speech, attention, flow of thought, general responses to interview, and subjective clinical impressions of the interview. Information relating to the child's developmental and medical history can be obtained through a joint interview of parent and the child, or only in the parent interview.

The Kiddie-Schedule for Affective Disorders and Schizophrenia (K-SADS)

The K-SADS is a semi-structured diagnostic interview designed to be administered by clinicians who are familiar with diagnostic criteria and who are experienced in the assessment of children aged 6 to 18 years (Puig-Antich and Chambers, 1978). It assesses for current psychopathology scored according to DSM-III and Research Diagnostic Criteria for major affective disorder and the disorders of childhood. The semi-structured nature of the instrument allows the clinician to freely reformulate questions to meet immediate contingencies and to introduce additional questions when necessary. The K-SADS is available in two versions: the K-SADS-P and the K-SADS-E. The K-SADS-P is used for evaluating current state or present episode and involves making judgements as to symptom severity. The K-SADS-E has been designed for epidemiological research and is used to measure the presence or absence of lifetime psychopathology.The interview begins with an unstructured interview to establish rapport, to gain a sense of the child's social environment and social functioning (e.g., family composition and relations, friendship patterns and peer relations, favorite activities), and to obtain a history of the present illness, as well as to determine current symptoms, their severity, and chronicity. This phase also help to soften the transition from the unstructured to structured phase of the interview, and to further preserve a sense of rapport. The structured section of the K-SADS focus on specific symptoms.

The K-SADS is administered by first interviewing the parent(s), then the child alone, and by obtaining summary ratings through various informants and sources (parent, child, school, chart and other). The six point severity ratings are scaled from: "no information" to "extreme". The latest version of the instrument, K-SADS-III-R, has 6 sections: major depression, mania, eating disorders, anxiety disorders, behavioural disorders, and psychoses. The interview contains a skip structure which reduce interviewing time for children with only few symptoms. The "essential symptoms" (i.e., screening or gating question) of a disorder are first asked to evaluate the presence of an episode of illness before evaluating additional "qualifying symptoms". If the response to the screening question is negative, the clinician then skips to the next diagnostic category as in the DISC.

Child Assessment Schedule (CAS)

The CAS is a semi-structured interview to assess psychological and behavioral problems in children aged 7–12 (Hodges *et al.*, 1982). Interviewers need to have some clinical experience since some clinical judgement is needed to administer and rate CAS items. It provides information relevant to diagnosis according to DSM-III. The interview is made up of two parts. The first part consists of questions related to school, friends, activities, hobbies, family, fears, worries, self-image, mood, somatic concerns, expression of anger and thought disorder symptomatology. The responses are coded as yes, no, ambiguous, no response, and not applicable. The second part contains questions related to the child's affective, verbal, nonverbal, and interactional style, and performance during the interview.

Interview Schedule for Children (ISC)

The ISC is a semi-structured interview designed to yield symptom ratings and to make diagnosis based on DSM-III criteria (Kovacs, 1985). The main focus of the ISC is on current depressive symptomatology, although symptoms related to overanxious disorder and attention deficit disorder have been added. The ISC additionally covers several broad areas including: (i) major psychopathologic symptoms and subsidiary items; (ii) mental status (e.g., delusions); (iii) signs of psychopathology seen during the interview such as impaired concentration, psychomotor agitation; (iv) developmental milestones like dating and sexual behavior; (v) clinician's impression on presentation (e.g., grooming, social maturity); (vi) severity of the current problems.

It is appropriate for children aged 8 to 17 years. The interview is available in two forms: Form C which is used during an intake interview, and Follow-up form for re-evaluation purposes. The interviewers needs to have clinical experience and be trained in using the interview. The time frame covered for symptoms concerning mood, affective behaviour, cognition, and vegetative functions is the immediate two weeks before the interview. Behaviours related to "acting-out" are evaluated for the past six months. Assessing children with the ISC begins with an unstructured interview by getting information about the nature, history, and duration of the child's problems, which is then followed by the standardized enquiries.

Diagnostic Interview Schedules for Adults

A number of diagnostic interviews designed for adults have also been used with adolescents. These include the Diagnostic Interview Schedule (Robins *et al.*, 1981), the Composite International Diagnostic Interview (Essau and Wittchen, 1993; Wittchen *et al.*, 1991), the Structured Clinical Interview for DSM-III-R (Spitzer *et al.*, 1988), and the Schedules for Clinical Assessment in Neuropsychiatry (SCAN; WHO, 1994).

Diagnostic Interview Schedule (DIS)

The DIS is a fully structured diagnostic interview that permits, through the use of a diagnostic algorithm, the derivation of current and lifetime diagnoses according to three different diagnostic systems (the Feighner Criteria, the Research Diagnostic Criteria, and the DSM-III-R). The DIS diagnoses major psychiatric syndromes such as somatization, anxiety disorder, affective disorders, eating disorders, drug and alcohol disorders, organic brain syndrome, and the subtypes of these disorders (Robins *et al.*, 1981). The DIS inquires about respondent's symptoms or problems that are currently experienced and periods ranging from the past two weeks, the past month, the past six months, and the past year or over a lifetime.

There have been several revisions of the DIS since its development. The newest version (DIS-IV) which has just been completed has profited from experience with the field trials and from studies that use the Composite International Diagnostic Interview and the DISC (Robins *et al.*, 1996). In addition to disorders available in the earlier versions of the DIS, the following disorders have been included: Disorders arising in childhood (ADHD, separation anxiety disorder, oppositional defiant disorder, and conduct disorder), chronic and acute pain disorder, specific phobia (animal type, natural environment type, blood-injection-injury type), and depressive episode due to medical condition, substance induced, and with post-partum onset. The DIS contains both the age of onset and recency questions related to the symptom of each disorder, and determines whether these symptoms have been continuous between those ages. It also contains questions as to time periods of being symptom-free for at least a year long. "Standard impairment questions" ask the extend to which respondent report that the symptoms caused problems in various life areas (family, friends, job, school, etc) and indicate the duration of problems (lasted for at least one month) and their severity. Respondents are also asked whether they ever talked to a doctor or other health professional about the symptoms of the disorder.

Composite International Diagnostic Interview (CIDI)

The CIDI is a fully standardized interview designed to be administered by well-trained lay interviewers (Wittchen *et al.*, 1991). It provides adult diagnoses according to both the ICD-10 and the DSM-IV. It is primarily intended for use in epidemiological studies of psychiatric disorders, but it can be used for other clinical and research purposes. The CIDI was produced in the framework of a major project undertaken by the World Health Organization and the U.S. National Institute of Health (NIH). Its development is the result of many years of close collaboration with many experts and reflects the input from at least five major sources: the DIS, the Present State Examination, findings of the cross-cultural CIDI Field Trials, the Diagnostic Criteria for Research of the ICD-10, and the Schedules for Clinical Assessment in Neuropsychiatry (Essau and Wittchen, 1993).

The CIDI has been designed for use in a variety of cultures and settings (Essau and Wittchen, 1993; Wittchen *et al.*, 1991). It is available in 14 languages and has been tested in a series of WHO field trials in 21 sites. The interview questions are fully spelled out which must be read exactly as written, and are "closed-ended" (i.e., answerable with a number or by choosing among predetermined alternatives).

The CIDI package consists of the CIDI interview, the user and training manual, and computer programs. (i) The *core CIDI interview* contains 15 sections: demographics, disorders resulting from the use of tobacco, somatoform and dissociative disorders, phobic and other anxiety disorders, depressive disorders and dysthymic disorder, manic and bipolar affective disorder, schizophrenia and other psychotic disorders, eating disorders, disorders resulting from the use of alcohol, obsessive-compulsive disorder, disorders resulting from the use of psychoactive substances, organic mental disorders, sexual dysfunction, interview observations, and interview ratings; (ii) The *user manual* includes an introduction to the CIDI and question-by-question specifications, guidelines on how to use the probe flow chart and to handle critical situations; (iii) The *training manual* describes the 5-day training programme required for CIDI users; (iv) *Computer programs* which to facilitate data entry and to check for correct codes and consistency of the data entered, and the diagnostic program which allows the computation of ICD-10 and DSM-IV diagnoses.

In addition, several optional modules are also available in conjunction with the core CIDI, including modules for antisocial personality, posttraumatic stress disorders, pathological gambling, transsexualism, comorbidity, and an expanded substance abuse module (Cottler *et al.*, 1991; Wittchen *et al.*, 1991).

The CIDI incorporates two types of questions: symptom questions and time-related questions: (i) "Symptom questions" ask about problems or experiences that the respondents have had (Table 2.6). Positive answers to these questions are explored further with fully specified probes to determine the clinical significance of the symptom and whether it could have been entirely explained by physical causes or ingesting substances. (ii) "Time-related questions" allow for making diagnoses on a lifetime and a cross-sectional basis. The first CIDI question concerning a symptom asks whether it has ever occurred in the respondent's lifetime. If the symptoms have ever occurred, the respondents are asked as to how recently they occurred, and when the first of the symptoms of the disorder occurred. If the last occurrence was more than a year ago, the respondent is asked the age at which the symptom first appeared (i.e., How old were you the first time you had the symptom?) The CIDI is also available in computerized form. The computer-assisted version is used by the interviewer, who reads the questions out loud to the respondents and enters the respondents' answers directly to the computer. The computer-administered version allows the respondents to read the question directly on the screen and enter their responses on the computer.

Structured Clinical Interview for DSM-III-R (SCID)

The SCID is a semi-structured interview designed to assess DSM-III-R diagnoses of bipolar disorder (mania and hypomania), cyclothymia, major depression, dysthymia, and mood disorders not otherwise specified (Spitzer *et al.*, 1988). It follows the decision-making rules of the DSM-III-R and examines the extent to which diagnostic criteria are fulfilled. Questions are grouped by diagnosis and criteria: If the criterion

Table 2.6 Examples of CIDI question format

1.

Examples for questions with probes

C34 Have you ever had problems with *double vision?*

     MD:. . . . . OTHER:. . . . .   PRB: 1 2 3 4 5

C36 Has your *heart ever beat so hard* that you could feel it pound in your chest?

    IF NO, CODE PRB 1, IF YES, ASK A

    A: Has that happened only when you were exerting yourself or at other times too?

    IF ONLY ON EXERTION, CODE PRB 1, IF OTHER TIMES CONTINUE PROBING

     MD:. OTHER:. . . . .   PRB: 1 2 3 4 5

2.

Example of NO/YES question without probes

D14 Were you worrying a great deal over things that were not really serious?

                             NO. 1

                               YES. 5

IF NOT CODED "5" SKIP TO E14

A. Did you ever have a period of two weeks or more, when nearly
every morning you would [Did you] *wake up at least two hours
before you wanted to?*

                               NO 1

                               YES. 5

Table 2.6 *continued*

3.
Example for time-related question

E13   Have you ever had two weeks or more when nearly every night you had [Did you have] *trouble with waking up too early?*

MD: . . . .   OTHER: . . . .

PRB: 1   3   4   5

4.
Example for age of onset and recency

C14   When was the (first/last) time you were bothered a lot by these pain(s)?

ONS: 1   2   3   4   5   6
AGE ONS:
REC: 1   2   3   4   5   6
AGE REC:

Source: Composite International Diagnostic Interview (Core version 1.0 — November 1990), WHO

is not met, the remaining questions for that diagnosis is skipped. In this respect, SCID is a time-saving interview (Üstün and Tien, 1995). On the other hand, this characteristic could result in a loss of information and incomplete data sets.

The SCID assesses for these problems that occur within the past month (current) and over the lifetime. Responses are coded as: ? = inadequate information, 1 = absent or false, 2 = subthreshold, and 3 = threshold. The SCID also documents information about the onset, course of illness, partial or full remission, impairment or Global Assessment of Functioning, and the differentiation of symptoms from organic causes. The interview is designed for administration by clinicians who are familiar with psychopathology and experienced in making differential diagnosis. Since the SCID is modularized, the interviewers can tailor their interview with their preferred diagnostic coverage. There are standard editions for "patients" (SCID-P) that can be used with psychiatric patients, and for "non-patients" (SCID-NP) to be used in community surveys.

The Schedule for Clinical Assessment in Neuropsychiatry (SCAN)

The SCAN (WHO, 1994) is a set of instruments used to assess and clarify psychopathology and psychiatric disorders in adults, although it has been used among adolescents. It resembles a clinical examination, in that it can be used to discover whether a symptom or sign is present during a specified period of time, and if so, with what severity. Individual items of psychopathology and other clinical information are defined with operationalized rating scales in the SCAN Glossary. The SCAN system additionally has a Manual, an Item Group Checklist to code past episodes, and a Clinical History Schedule to outline the course and history of a disorder (Üstun and Tien, 1995).

The SCAN has computer programs which automate processing of the rating information. Data from the paper version of the SCAN can be entered in a specific computer program. The output is presented as a series of options such as a range of profiles of symptoms and item group scores, an index of definition for probability of caseness, and application of ICD-10 and DSM-IV rules for specific categories (Üstün and Tien, 1995).

Direct Observation

Direct observation involves observing and recording children's overt motor and/or verbal behaviour using operationalized definitions (Remschmidt, 1995). The main emphasis is to examine the relationship between environmental contingencies and behavioural responses (Mash and Terdal, 1981). Direct observation may be conducted in naturalistic environments or in analogue settings. Systematic naturalistic observation consists of directly observing individuals in their natural environments such as at the home, classroom, and playground.

In analogue situations, the children's behaviour is directly observed in settings that are structured to occasion target behaviour (e.g., structured playroom). Since situational or task variables are standardized, analogue observation allows a comparison of the child's performance with that of children in various reference groups in the same setting and under the same conditions. Also, the environment together with relevant situational, contextual or social interactional factors can be controlled or variations held to a minimum.

Major recording techniques used in direct observation include (i) frequency recording, which records the number of times a behaviour occurs within a temporal interval; (ii) duration recording, which is a direct measurement of the amount of time which a child engages in a behaviour; and (iii) interval recording, which involves recording the occurrence or non-occurrence of a behaviour at equal intervals (see Barton and Ascione, 1984; Gettinger and Kratochwill, 1987 for review). Observed behaviour may be recorded using pencil and paper checklists, or audio- and video-recording. Taping of behaviour is advantageous because it allows the scene to be observed repeatedly and a consensus in coding reached.

Direct observation makes it possible to record actual behaviour, identification of environmental contingencies and direct assessment of behavioural change points (Achenbach, 1988). Besides the costs, much time is needed to prepare coding systems for defining, recognizing, and recording the behaviour. Furthermore, data may be affected by the observational techniques used and observer characteristics. Expectancies, experiences, and prior training may influence the reliability of the data collected (Gettinger and Kratochwill, 1987).

Family Assessment

Family assessment methods in developmental psychopathology can be grouped under observational and self-report measures, as well as diagnostic interviews (Jacob and Tennenbaum, 1988). Each assessment technique generally focused on a variety of constructs including affective bonds between family members, interpersonal control, and communication. The interest in exploring these constructs is based on research findings that consistently show greater risk for psychiatric disorders among children and adolescents coming from disrupted, as opposed to stable, family environments. Such studies have focused on parental discord, divorce or separation, conflictful parent-child relationship, and parental psychopathology.

Observational measures provide information on the dyadic interaction of family members either in natural or laboratory settings. Naturalistic observation involves the observation and assessment of family interaction at home, whereas laboratory-based procedures involve studying family interaction in performing defined tasks and problems. Rating of behaviour can be done either by means of detailed coding systems or general rating and through permanent records using audio- or video-tapes (Jacob and Tennenbaum, 1988). Another family assessment method is through the use of self-report questionnaires. Such measures include the assessment of parent-child relationships, sibling relationships, and whole families (Table 2.7). Another approach is through structured interviews, for example, the Expressed Emotion procedure (EE), that can be used to assess the number of critical comments, hostility, and emotional over involvement of parents (Brown and Rutter, 1966).

Another line of research is to assess the presence of parental psychopathology by interviewing parents with standardized diagnostic interviews. This research area is spurred by the findings that children of parents with psychiatric disorders are at a higher risk of having psychiatric disorders than children of parents without disorder. Diagnostic interviews commonly used to assess parental psychopathology (see Wittchen and Essau, 1990 for review) include the Structured Clinical Interview for DSM-III-R (SCID; Spitzer and Williams, 1985), the Diagnostic Interview Schedule (DIS; Robins *et al.*, 1981), the Composite International Diagnostic Interview (CIDI; Wittchen *et al.*, 1991), and the Schedule for Clinical Assessment in Neuropsychiatry (SCAN; WHO, 1994).

Biochemical and Neuropsychological Methods

A number of methods have been used to evaluate the role of biochemical factors in the etiology and maintenance of psychiatric disorders (Ciaranello *et al.*, 1995 for review; Zeichner, 1987). Most assessment techniques are based on the analyses of central nervous system metabolites (e.g., 3-methoxy-4-hydroxyphenylglycol, dopamine-ß-hydroxylase, phenylethylamine, platelet 5-hydroxyptryptamine); neuroendocrine

Table 2.7 Self-report questionnaires for the assessment of family functioning

Questionnaires/Authors	No. of items	Characteristics
Parent-Child Relationships		
1. Child Report of Parental Behavior Inventory (Margolies and Weintraub, 1977)	56	Measures children's perceptions of parental behaviour. The 3 dimensions assessed are: acceptance versus rejection, psychological autonomy versus psychological control, and firm control versus lax control.
2. Parental-Adolescent Communication Scale (Barnes and Olson, 1985)	20	Measures adolescents' and their parents' perceptions and experiences of communicating with each other. The scale is based on the hypothesis that effective communication allows families to achieve and maintain a desired balance on the dimensions of family cohesion and adaptability.
3. Parent-Child Areas of Change Questionnaire (Weiss *et al.*, 1973)	32	Provides information about parent-child problem areas and about the congruence in perceptions of these relationships.
Sibling Relationships		
4. Sibling Relationship Questionnaire (Furman and Buhrmester, 1985)	51	Measures children's view of their relationship with their sibling. The dimensions covered are warmth/closeness, relative status/power, conflict and rivalry.

Table 2.7 *continued*

Questionnaires/Authors	No. of items	Characteristics
Whole Families		
5. Family Adaptability and Cohesion Evaluation Scales (Olson et al., 1979)	30	Measures family cohesion and adaptability. The scale is based on the hypothesis that effective family functioning occurs in families with balanced level of cohesion and adaptability, and maintenance of the balanced levels of these 2 dimensions is facilitated by family communication.
6. Family Environment Scale (Moos and Moos, 1981)	90	Measures family member's perceptions of their family life along the dimensions of interpersonal relationships (cohesion, expressiveness, conflict), personal growth (independence, achievement orientation, intellectual-cultural orientation, active recreational orientation, moral-religious emphasis), and system maintenance (organization, control).
7. Family Assessment Measure (Steinhauer and Tisdall, 1984)	134	Measures family characteristics in the area of task values and norms, accomplishment, role performance, communication, affective expression, affective involvement and control.
8 Family Assessment Devise (Epstein et al., 1983)	53	Designed to measure family functioning along 7 dimensions: problem solving, communication, roles, affective responsiveness, affective involvement, behaviour control, and general functioning.

responses (e.g., dexamethasone suppression test, growth-hormone-releasing products); and allergic reactions and food toxicity (e.g., toxic trace elements).

Neuropsychological methods include several tests designed to indirectly assess brain dysfunctions which may be related to observed or suspected behavioural deficits (see Pennington and Welsh, 1995 for review; Wittling *et al.*, 1995). Tests which contain learning, sensorimotor, perceptual, verbal, and memory tasks are evaluated on the level and pattern of performance, as well as specific abnormal responses. Commonly used neuropsychological test batteries include the Reitan-Indiana Battery (Reitan, 1969), the Halstead Neuropsychological Test Battery for children (Reitan and Davison, 1974), and the Bender Visual-Motor Gestalt Test (Bender, 1946). Another type of neuropsychological assessment deals with general tests of performance and intellectual function. A number of intelligence tests such as the Stanford-Binet Intelligence Scale (Thorndike *et al.*, 1986), the Wechsler Preschool and Primary Scale of Intelligence (Wechsler, 1967), and the Wechsler Intelligence Scale for Children-Revised (Wechsler, 1974) can be used for this purpose.

Psychosocial Impairment

Due to lack of acceptable "gold standards" in validating "caseness", psychosocial impairment has been used as an external validator for psychiatric disorders. The use of functional impairment or dysfunctionality in defining "caseness" is especially important in studies where disorders tend to appear or lie slightly above the diagnostic threshold and when individuals who meet diagnostic criteria do not receive or seek treatment (Bird and Gould, 1995; Bird *et al.*, 1990). The estimates of the prevalence of disorder are considered to be more meaningful when they are related to severity, to need for services, and to personal distress (Bird *et al.*, 1990). Therefore, in some epidemiological studies, the classification of disorder is only made when the individual meets the required symptoms according to a specific diagnostic criteria, and shows some degree of functional impairment (Bird *et al.*, 1988; Feehan *et al.*, 1994; Verhulst *et al.*, 1985).

A number of instruments have been developed to measure psychosocial impairment among those with psychiatric disorders. Examples of instruments are: the Children's Global Assessment (CGAS; Shaffer *et al.*, 1983), the Columbia Impairment Scale (CIS; Bird *et al.*, 1993), and the Social Adjustment Inventory for Children and Adolescents (SAICA;

Table 2.8   The Children's Global Assessment Scale

100–91   *Superior functioning* in all areas (at home, at school, and with peers), involved in a range of activities and has many interests (e.g., has hobbies or participates in extracurricular activities or belongs to an organized group such as Scouts, etc). Likeable, confident, "everyday" worries never get out of hand. Doing well in school. No symptoms.

90–81   *Good functioning in all areas*. Secure in family, school, and with peers. There may be transient difficulties and "everyday" worries that occasionally get out of hand (e.g., mild anxiety associated with an important exam, occasionally "blow-ups" with siblings, parents, or peers).

80–71   *No more than a slight impairment in functioning* at home, at school or with peers. Some disturbance of behaviour or emotional distress may be present in response to life stresses (e.g., parental separations, deaths, birth of a sib) but these are brief and interference with functioning is transient. Such children are only minimally disturbing to others and are not considered deviant by those who know them.

70–61   *Some difficulty in a single area, but generally functioning pretty well* (e.g., sporadic or isolated antisocial acts, such as occasionally playing hooky or petty theft; consistent minor difficulties with school work, mood changes of brief duration; fears and anxieties which do not lead to gross avoidance behavior; self-doubts). Has some meaningful interpersonal relationships. Most people who do not know the child well would not consider him/her deviant but those who do know him/her well might express concern.

65–51   *Variable functioning with sporadic difficulties or symptoms in several but not all social areas*. Disturbance would be apparent to those who encounter the child in a dysfunctional setting or time but not to those who see the child in other settings.

50–41   *Moderate degree of interference in functioning in most social areas or serve impairment of functioning in one area*, such as might result from, for example, suicidal preoccupations and ruminations, school refusal and other forms of anxiety, obsessive rituals, major conversion symptoms, frequent anxiety attacks, frequent episodes of aggressive or other antisocial behaviour with some preservation of meaningful social relationships.

40–31   *Major impairment in functioning in several areas and unable to function in one of these areas*, i.e., disturbed at home, at school, with peers, or in society at large, e.g., persistent aggression without clear instigation; markedly withdrawn and isolated behaviour due to either mood or thought disturbance, suicidal attempts with clear lethal intent. Such children are likely to require special schooling and/or hospitalization or withdrawal from school (but this is not a sufficient criterion for inclusion in this category).

Table 2.8 *continued*

30–21   *Unable to function in almost all areas*, e.g., stays at home, in ward or in bed all day without taking part in social activities OR severe impairment in communication (e.g., sometimes incoherent or inappropriate).

20–11   *Needs considerable supervision* to prevent hurting others or self, e.g., frequently violent, repeated suicide attempts OR to maintain personal hygiene OR gross impairment in all forms of communication, e.g., severe abnormalities in verbal and gestural communication, marked social aloofness, stupor, etc.

10–01   *Needs constant supervision* (24-hour care) due to severely aggressive or self-destructive behavior or gross impairment in reality testing, communication, cognition, affect, or personal hygiene.

Note: From "Shaffer, D., Gould, M.S., Brasic, J., Ambrosini, P., Fischer, P., Bird, H., and Aluwahlia, S. (1983). A Children's Global Assessment Scale (CGAS). *Archives General Psychiatry*, **40**, 1228–1231."

Reprinted with permission from the Diagnostic and Statistical Manual of Mental Disorders, Fourth Edition. Copyright 1983 American Medical Association.

John *et al.*, 1987). (i) The CGAS has been designed for 4–16-year-old children to measure their psychological and social functioning at home, at school, and with peers. Scores range from 1 which indicates that the child is most impaired and is in need of constant supervision, to 100 which indicates children who are at the highest level of adaptive functioning (Table 2.8). A score below 61 is supposed to represent a "definite case", scores between 61 to 70 a "probable case", and a score of 71 or above to represent a "non-case" (Bird *et al.*, 1990); (ii) The CIS has been designed for children aged 9 to 17 years old to measure functioning in interpersonal relations, psychopathology, at school or work, and use of leisure time; (iii) The SAICA is a semi-structured instrument for assessing adaptive functioning in school, peer relations, home life, and spare time activities. The total score may range from 0 ("no problem") to 52 ("very big problem").

CONCLUDING REMARKS

A number of factors need to be considered when assessing children and adolescents such as the type of disorder, level of comorbidity, expected frequency in the population, type of samples (clinical or non-clinical sample), informant choice, and the type of scales/categories used. An over-arching consideration is a recognition that children are undergoing developmental changes which are both rapid and uneven and which may complicate any judgement or interpretation that may be made. Assessment of children implicitly involves comparisons with norms and developmental milestones. The developmental perspective applies to physical factors (e.g., growth, height and weights) at different stages of development, cognitive and emotional development, and difference in development rates.

So, at the minimum the clinician or researcher has chosen measures that reliably and validly indicate the presence or absence of a discrete psychiatric disorder (or a continuous measure indicating the extent of psychiatric dysfunction), has access to data by which to evaluate the information obtained (e.g., norms); has considered the necessity of gathering impairment data; has determined the most appropriate informant or informants; and has chosen instruments that are developmentally, gender, and culture appropriate. Perhaps above all this, remain questions not discussed in this chapter which we will leave to the reader. Why this assessment, with these people, at this time? A consideration of the ethics and philosophies underpinning the proposed assessment is critical. Information does not exist in a vacuum, it has a social meaning and value. Ultimately we need to consider who will benefit from the assessment, who can be harmed or disenpowered, who has initiated the assessment, who owns and has access to the data obtained, and to what extent does the information obtained serve social and political ends.

REFERENCES

Achenbach, T.M. (1995). Developmental issues in assessment, taxonomy, and diagnosis of child and adolescent psychopathology. In D. Cicchetti and D.J. Cohen (Eds.), *Developmental psychopathology. Volume 1: Theory and methods* (pp. 57–80). New York: Wiley.

Achenbach, T.M. (1990). Conceptualization of developmental psychopathology. In M. Lewis and S.M. Miller (Eds.), *Handbook of developmental psychopathology* (pp. 3–14). New York: Plenum Press.

Achenbach, T.M. (1988). Integrating assessment and taxonomy. In M. Rutter, A.H. Tuma, and I.S. Lann (Eds.), *Assessment and diagnosis in child psychopathology* (pp. 300–343). London: David Fulton Publishers.

Achenbach, T.M. and Edelbrock, C. (1983). *Manual for the Child Behavior Checklist and Revised Child Behavior Profile.* Burlington: University of Vermont Department of Psychiatry.

Achenbach, T.M. and Edelbrock, C. (1978). The classification of child psychopathology: A review and analysis of empirical efforts. *Psychological Bulletin,* **85**, 1275–1301.

Achenbach, T.M. and Edelbrock, C. (1979). The Child Behavior Checklist Profile: II. Boys aged 12–16 and girls aged 6–11 and 12–15. *Journal of Consulting and Clinical Psychology,* **47**, 223–233.

Achenbach, T.M. and Edelbrock, C. (1986). *Manual for the Teacher's Report Form and teacher version of the Child Behavior Profile.* Burlington: University of Vermont Department of Psychiatry.

Achenbach, T.M., Verhulst, F.C., Edelbrock, C., Baron, G.D., and Akkerhuis, G.W. (1987). Epidemiological comparisons of American and Dutch children: II. Behavioral/emotional problems reported by teachers for ages 6 to 11. *Journal of the American Academy of Child and Adolescent Psychiatry,* **26**, 326–332.

American Psychiatric Association (1952). *Diagnostic and statistical manual of mental disorders (1st ed.).* Washington, DC: American Psychiatric Association.

American Psychiatric Association (1968). *Diagnostic and statistical manual of mental disorders (2nd ed.).* Washington, DC: American Psychiatric Association.

American Psychiatric Association (1980). *Diagnostic and statistical manual of mental disorders (3rd ed.).* Washington, DC: American Psychiatric Association.

American Psychiatric Association (1987). *Diagnostic and statistical manual of mental disorders (3rd ed. rev.).* Washington, DC: American Psychiatric Association.

American Psychiatric Association (1994). *Diagnostic and statistical manual of mental disorders (4th ed.).* Washington, DC: American Psychiatric Association.

Angold, A. and Worthman, C.M. (1993). Puberty onset of gender differences in rates of depression: A developmental, epidemiologic and neuroendocrine perspective. *Journal of Affective Disorders,* **29**, 145–158.

Barkley, R.A. (1981). *Hyperactive children: A handbook for diagnosis and treatment.* New York: Guilford Press.

Barnes, H.L. and Olson, D.H. (1985). Parent-adolescent communication and the circumflex model. *Child Development,* **56**, 438–447.

Barton, E.J. and Ascione, F.R. (1984). Direct observation. In T.H. Ollendick and M. Hersen (Eds.), *Child behavioral assessment: Principles and procedures* (pp. 166–194). New York: Pergamon Press.

Beck, A.T., Ward, C.H., Mendelson, M., Mock, J.E., and Erbaugh, J.K. (1962). Reliability of psychiatric diagnosis: II. A study of consistency of clinical judgements and ratings. *American Journal of Psychiatry,* **119**, 351–357.

Bender, L. (1946). *Instructions for the use of the visual motor gestalt test.* New York: American Orthopsychiatric Association.

Berg, I., Rapoport, J.L., and Flament, M. (1986). The Leyton Obsessional Inventory-Child version. *Journal of the American Academy of Child Psychiatry,* **25**, 84–91.

Bird, H., Canino, G., Rubio-Stipec, M., Gould, M.S., Ribera, J., Sesman, M., Woodbury, M., Huertas-Goldman, S., Pagan, A., Sanchez-Lacay, A., and Moscoso, M. (1988). Estimates of the prevalence of childhood maladjustment in a community survey in Puerto Rico. *Archives of General Psychiatry,* **45**, 1120–1126.

Bird, H.R. and Gould, M.S. (1995). The use of diagnostic instruments and global measures of functioning in child psychiatry epidemiological studies. In F.C. Verhulst and H.M. Koot (Eds.), *The epidemiology of child and adolescent psychopathology* (pp. 86–103). Oxford: Oxford University Press.

Bird, H.R., Shaffer, D., Fisher, P., Gould, M.S. *et al.* (1993). The Columbia Impairment Scale (CIS): Pilot findings on a measure of global impairment for children and adolescents. *International Journal of Methods in Psychiatric Research,* **3**, 167–176.

Bird, H.R., Yager, T., Staghezza, B., Gould, M., Canino, G., and Rubio-Stipec, M. (1990). Impairment in the epidemiological measurement of childhood psychopathology in the community. *Journal of the American Academy of Child and Adolescent Psychiatry,* **29**, 796–803.

Blashfield, R.K. (1984). *The classification of psychopathology.* New York: Plenum Press.

Boyle, M.H., Offord, D.R., Racine, Y., Fleming, J.E., Szatmari, P., and Sanford, M. (1993). Evaluation of the Revised Ontario Health Study Scales. *Journal of Child Psychology and Psychiatry,* **32**, 189–213.

Boyle, M.H., Offord, D.R., Racine, Y., Szatmari, P., Fleming, J.E., and Sanford, M. (submitted). Identifying thresholds for classifying childhood psychiatric disorders: Issues and prospects.

Brown, G.W. and Rutter, M. (1966). The measurement of family activities and relationships: A methodological study. *Human Relations*, **19**, 241–263.

Ciaranello, R.D., Aimi, J., Dean, R.R., Morilak, D.A., Porteus, M.H., and Cicchetti, D. (1995). Fundamentals of molecular neurobiology. In D. Cicchetti and D.J. Cohen (Eds.), *Developmental psychopathology. Volume 1: Theory and methods* (pp. 109–160). New York: Wiley.

Cicchetti, D. and Schneider-Rosen, K. (1986). An organizational approach to childhood depression. In M. Rutter, C. Izard, and P. Read (Eds.), Depression in young people: Clinical and developmental perspectives. New York: Guilford.

Cottler, L., Robins, L.N., Grant, B.F., Blaine, J., Towle, L., Wittchen, H.-U., and Sartorius, N. (1991). The CIDI-core substance abuse and dependence questions: Cross-cultural and nosological issues. *British Journal of Psychiatry*, **159**, 653–658.

Costello, E.J. and Angold, A. (1995). Developmental epidemiology. In D. Cicchetti and D.J. Cohen (Eds.), *Developmental psychopathology. Volume 1: Theory and methods* (pp. 23–56). New York: Wiley.

Costello, A.J., Edelbrock, C., Dulcan, M.K., Kalas, R., and Klaric, S. (1987). *The Diagnostic Interview Schedule for Children (DISC)*. Pittsburgh: University of Pittsburgh.

Derogatis, L.R. (1977). *The SCL-90 Manual*. Baltimore: John Hopkins University School of Medicine.

Edelbrock, C. and Achenbach, T.M. (1984). The teacher version of the child behavior profile. I. Boys aged 6–11. *Journal of Consulting and Clinical Psychology*, **52**, 207–217.

Epstein, N.B., Baldwin, L.M., and Bishop, D.S. (1983). The McMaster Family Assessment Device. *Journal of Marital and Family Therapy*, **9**, 171–180.

Essau, C.A. and Wittchen, H-U. (1993). An overview of the Composite International Diagnostic Interview (CIDI). *International Journal of Methods in Psychiatric Research*, **3**, 79–85.

Feehan, M., McGee, R., Nada-Raja, S., and Williams, S.M. (1994). DSM-III-R disorders in New Zealand 18-year-olds. *Australian and New Zealand Journal of Psychiatry*, **28**, 87–99.

Fischer, P. (1996). *The NIMH Diagnostic Interview Schedule for Children*. Unpublished manuscript. New York: New York State Psychiatric Institute.

Frances, A., Pincus, H., Widiger, T., First, M., Davis, W., Hall, W., McKinney, K., and Stayna, H. (1994). DSM-IV and International communication in psychiatric diagnosis. In J.E. Mezzich, Y. Honda, and M.C. Kastrup (eds.), *Psychiatric diagnosis: A world perspective* (pp. 11–22). New York: Springer.

Furman, W. and Buhrmester, D. (1985). Children's perceptions of the qualities of sibling relationships. *Child Development*, **56**, 448–461.

Gettinger, M. and Kratochwill, T.R. (1987). Behavioral assessment. In C.L. Frame and J.L. Matson (Eds.), *Handbook of assessment in childhood psychopathology: Applied issues in differential diagnosis and treatment evaluation* (pp. 131–161). New York: Plenum Press.

Goyette, C.H., Conners, C.K., and Ulrich, R.F. (1978). Normative data on revised Conners parent and teacher rating scales. *Journal of Abnormal Child Psychology*, **6**, 221–236.

Graham, P. and Skuse, D. (1992). The developmental perspective in classification. In H. Remschmidt and M.H. Schmidt (Eds.), *Developmental psychopathology* (pp.1–6). Göttingen: Hogrefe and Huber Publisher.

Haynes, S.N. (1978). *Principles of behavioral assessment*. New York: Gardner Press.

Herjanic, B. and Campbell, W. (1977). Differentiating psychiatrically disturbed children on the basis of a structured interview. *Journal of Abnormal Child Psychology*, **5**, 127–134.

Herjanic, B. and Reich, W. (1982). Development of a structured psychiatric interview for children: Agreement between child and parent on individual symptoms. *Journal of Abnormal Child Psychology*, **10**, 307–324.

Hodges, K., McKnew, D., Cytryn, L., and Kline, J. (1982). The Child Assessment Schedule (CAS) diagnostic interview: A report on reliability and validity. *Journal of the American Academy of Child and Adolescent Psychiatry*, **21**, 468–473.

Jacob, T. and Tennenbaum, D.L. (1988). Family assessment methods. In M. Rutter, A.H. Tuma, and I.S. Lann (Eds.), *Assessment and diagnosis in child psychopathology* (pp. 196–231). London: David Fulton Publishers.

Janca, A., Kastrup, M.C., Katschnig, H., López-Ibor, J.J., Mezzich, J.E., and Sartorius, N. (1996). The ICD-10 multiaxial system for use in adult psychiatry: Structure and applications. *Journal of Nervous and Mental Disease,* **184**, 191–192.

John, K., Gammon, G.D., Prusoff, B.A., and Warner, V. (1987). The social adjustment inventory for children and adolescents (SAICA): Testing of a new semistructured interview. *Journal of the American Academy of Child and Adolescent Psychiatry,* **26**, 898–911.

Kanfer, F.H. and Nay, W.R. (1982). Behavioral assessment. In G.T. Wilson and C.M. Franks (Eds), *Contemporary behavior therapy: Conceptual and empirical foundations.* New York: Guildford Press.

Kazdin, A.E. (1989). Identifying depression in children: A comparison of alternative selection criteria. *Journal of Abnormal Child Psychology,* **17**, 437–455.

Kazdin, A.E. and Kagan, J. (1994). Models of dysfunction in developmental psychopathology. *Clinical Pychological: Science and Practice, 1 (summer),* 35–52.

Kovacs, M. (1985). The Interview Schedule for Children. *Psychopharmacology Bulletin,* **21**, 991–994.

Kovacs, M. (1979). *Children's Depression Inventory.* Unpublished test. Pittsburgh: University of Pittsburgh School of Medicine.

La Greca, A.M. and Stone, W.L. (1992). Assessing children through interviews and behavioral observations. In C.E. Walker and M.C. Roberts (Eds.), *Handbook of clinical child psychology* (pp. 63–83). New York: Wiley.

Margolies, P.J. and Weintraub, S. (1977). The revised 56-item CRPBI as a research instrument: Reliability and factor structure. *Journal of Clinical Psychology,* **33**, 472–476.

Mash, E.J. and Terdal, L.G. (1981). Behavioral assessment of childhood disturbance. In E.J. Mash and L.G. Terdal (Eds.), *Behavioral assessment of childhood disorders* (pp. 3–37). New York: Guildford.

Mezzich, J.E. (1988). On developing a psychiatric multiaxial schema for ICD-10. *British Journal of Psychiatry,* **152**, 38–43.

Mezzich, J.E. and Mezzich, A.C. (1987). Diagnostic classification systems in child psychopathology. In C.L. Frame and J.L. Matson (Eds.), *Handbook of assessment in childhood psychopathology: Applied issues in differential diagnosis and treatment evaluation* (pp. 33–60). New York: Plenum Press.

Miller, L.E. (1967). Dimensions of psychopathology in middle childhood. *Psychological Reports,* **21**, 897–903.

Moos, R. and Moos, B.S. (1981). *Family environment scale: Manual.* Palo Alto: Consulting Psychologists Press.

Offord, D.R., Boyle, M.H., and Racine, Y.A. (1991). The epidemiology of antisocial behavior. In D.J. Pepler and K.H. Rubins (Eds.), *The developmental and treatment of childhood aggression* (pp. 31–45). Hillsdale, NJ: Erlbaum.

Ollendick, T.C. (1983). Reliability and validity of the revised Fear Survey Schedule for Children (FSSC-R). *Behaviour Research and Therapy,* **21**, 685–692.

Olson, D.H., Sprenkle, D.H., and Russell, C.S. (1979). Circumflex model of marital and family systems: I. Cohesion and adaptability dimensions, family types, and clinical applications. *Family Process,* **18**, 3–28.

Piacentini, J., Shaffer, D., and Fischer, P.W. (1993). The Diagnostic Interview Schedule for Children — Revised version (DISC-R): II. Concurrent criterion validity. *Journal of the American Academy of Child and Adolescent Psychiatry,* **32**, 658–665.

Pennington, B.F. and Welsh, M. (1995). Neuropsychology and developmental psychopathology. In D. Cicchetti and D.J. Cohen (Eds.), *Developmental psychopathology. Volume 1: Theory and methods* (pp. 254–290). New York: Wiley.

Puig-Antich, J. and Chambers, W. (1978). *The Schedule for Affective Disorders and Schizophrenia for school-aged children.* New York: State Psychiatric Institute, New York.

Quay, H.C. (1986). Classification. In H.C. Quay and J.S. Werry (Eds.), *Psychopathological disorders in childhood* (3rd ed., pp. 1–34). New York: Wiley.

Quay, H.C. and Peterson, D.R. (1987). *Manual for the Revised Behavior Problem Checklist.* Authors: Miami, FL.

Radloff, L.S. (1977). The CES-D scale: A self-report scale for research in the general population. *Applied Psychological Measurement,* **1**, 385–401.

Reich, W. and Welner, Z (1988). *Revised version of the Diagnostic Interview for Children and Adolescents (DICA-R).* St. Louis, MO: Department of Psychiatry.

Reitan, R.M. (1969). *Manual for administration of neuropsychological test batteries for adults and children.* Indianapolis, IN: Reitan.

Reitan, R.M. and Davison, L.W. (1974). *Clinical neuropsychology: Current status and applications.* New York: Winston.

Remschmidt, H. (1995). Grundlagen psychiatrischer Klassifikation und Psychodiagnostik. In F. Petermann (Ed.), *Lehrbuch der Klinischen Kinderpsychologie* (pp. 3–52). Göttingen: Hogrefe.

Reynolds, W.M. (1987). *Reynolds Adolescent Depression Scale.* Odessa, FL: Psychological Assessment Resources.

Reynolds, W.M. (1989). *Reynolds Child Depression Scale.* Odessa, FL: Psychological Assessment Resources.

Reynolds, C.R. and Richmond, B.O. (1978). What I think and feel: A revised measure of children's manifest anxiety. *Journal of Abnormal Child Psychology,* **6**, 271–280.

Robins, L.N. (1994). How to choose among the riches: Selecting a diagnostic instrument. *International Review of Psychiatry,* **6**, 265–271.

Robins, L.N., Cottler, L., Bucholz, K., and Compton, W. (1996). *The Diagnostic Interview Schedule, Version IV.* St. Louis: Washington University.

Robins, L.N., Helzer, J.E., Croughan, J., and Ratcliff, K.F. (1981). National Institute of Mental Health Diagnostic Interview Schedule: Its history, characteristics and validity. *Archives of General Psychiatry,* **38**, 381–389.

Rutter, M. (1977). Classification. In M. Rutter and L. Hersov (Eds.), *Child psychiatry. Modern approaches* (pp. 359–384). Oxford: Blackwell.

Rutter, M., Tizard, J., and Whitmore, K. (1970). *Education, health and behavior.* London: Longmans.

Sartorius, N. (1994). Progress in the development of the classification of mental disorders in the ICD-10. In J.E. Mezzich, Y. Honda, and M.C. Kastrup (eds.), *Psychiatric diagnosis: A world perspective* (pp. 115–124). New York: Springer-Verlag.

Schwab-Stone, M., Fisher, P., Shaffer, D., Piacentini, J., Davies, M., and Gioia, P. (1993). The Diagnostic Interview Schedule for Children — revised version (DISC-R). II. Test-retest reliability. *Journal of the American Academy of Child and Adolescent Psychiatry,* **32**, 643–650.

Shaffer, D., Gould, M.S., Brasic, J., Ambrosini, P., Fisher, P., Bird, H., and Aluwahlia, S. (1983). A children's global assessment scale (CGAS). *Archives of General Psychiatry,* **40**, 1228–1231.

Spielberger, C.D. (1973). *Manual for the state-trait anxiety Inventory for children.* Palo Alto, CA: Consulting Psychologists Press.

Spitzer, R.L., Williams, J.B.W., and Gibbon, M. (1988). *Structured Clinical Interview for DSM-III-R.* New York: New York State Psychiatric Institute, Biometrics Research Department.

Spitzer, R.L. and Williams, J. (1985). *Instruction manual for the Structured Clinical Interview for DSM-III (SCID).* New York: New York State Psychiatric Institute.

Steinhauer, P.D. and Tisdall, G.W. (1984). The integrated use of individual and family psychotherapy. *Canadian Journal of Psychiatry,* **29**, 89–97.

Thorndike, R.L., Hagen, E.P., and Sattler, J.M. (1986). *Stanford-Binet Intelligence Scale: Fourth edition.* Chicago: Riverside.

Üstün, T.B. and Tien, A.Y. (1995). recent developments for diagnostic measures in psychiatry. *Epidemiologic Reviews,* **17**, 210–220.

Verhulst, F.C. (1995). The epidemiology of child and adolescent psychopathology: Strengths and limitations. In F.C. Verhulst and H.M. Koot (Eds.), *The epidemiology of child and adolescent psychopathology* (pp. 1–21). Oxford: Oxford University Press.

Verhulst, F.C., Berden, G.F.M., and Sanders-Woudstra, J.A.R. (1985). Mental health in Dutch children: II. The prevalence of psychiatric disorder and relationship between measures. *Acta Psychiatrica Scandinavica (Suppl. 324)*, 1–45.

Wechsler, D.I. (1967). *Manual for the Wechsler Preschool and Primary Scale of Intelligence (WPPSI)*. New York: Psychological Corporation.

Wechsler, D.I. (1974). *Manual for the Wechsler Intelligence Scale for Children-revised (WISC-R)*. New York: Psychological Corporation.

Weiss, R.L., Hops, H., and Patterson, G.R. (1973). A framework for conceptualizing marital conflict: A technology for altering it, some data for evaluating it. In R.W. Clark and L.A. Hamerlynck (Eds.), *Critical issues in research and practice: Proceedings of the Fourth Banff International Conference*. Champaign, IL: Research Press.

Weisz, J.R., and Eastman, K.L. (1995). Cross-cultural research on child and adolescent psychopathology. In F.C. Verhulst and H.M. Koot (Eds.), *The epidemiology of child and adolescent psychopathology* (pp. 42–65). Oxford: Oxford University Press.

Weisz, J.R., Sigman, M., Weiss, B., and Mosk, J. (1993). Parent reports of behavioral and emotional problems among children in Kenya, Thailand and the United States. *Child Development, 64*, 98–109.

Weisz, J.R., Suwanlert, S., Chaiyasit, W., Weiss, B., Achenbach, T.M., and Trevathan, D. (1989). Epidemiology of behavioral and emotional problems among Thai and American children: Teacher reports for ages 6–11. *Journal of Child Psychology and Psychiatry, 30*, 471–484.

Weisz, J.R., Suwanlert, S., Chaiyasit, W., Weiss, B., Achenbach, T.M., and Walter, B.A. (1987). Epidemiology of behavioral and emotional problems among Thai and American children: Parent reports for ages 6–11. *Journal of Child Psychology and Psychiatry, 26*, 890–898.

Werry, J.S. (1968). Developmental hyperactivity. *Pediatric Clinics of North America, 15*, 581–599.

Wittchen, H.-U. and Essau, C.A. (1990). Assessment of symptoms and psycosocial disabilities in primary care. In N. Sartorius, D. Goldberg, D., deGirolamo, G., Costa e Silva, J., Lebcrubier, Y., and H.-U. Wittchen (Eds.), *Psychological disorders in general medical settings* (pp. 111–136). Bern: Hogrefe and Huber Publishers.

Wittchen, H.-U., Robins, L.N., Cottler, L., Sartorius, N., Burke, J., Regier, D., and participants of the field trials (1991). Cross-cultural feasibility, reliability, and sources of variance of the Composite International Diagnostic Interview (CIDI) — Results of the multicenter WHO/ADAMHA Field Trials (Wave I). *British Journal of Psychiatry, 159*, 645–653.

Wittling, W., Schweiger, E., and Roschmann, R. (1995). Neuropsychologische Diagnostik. In R.S. Jäger and F. Petermann (Eds.), *Psychologische Diagnostik: Ein Lehrbuch* (pp. 575–602). Weinheim: Psychologie Verlags Union.

World Health Organization (1993). *The ICD-10 classification of mental and behavioral disorders*. Geneva: World Health Organization.

World Health Organization (1994). *SCAN: Schedules for Clinical Assessment in Neuropsychiatry*. Geneva: World Health Organization.

Yule, W. (1981). The epidemiology of child psychopathology. In B.B. Lahey and A.E. Kazdin (Eds.), *Advances in clinical psychology* (Vol. 4, pp. 1–51). New York: Plenum.

Zeichner, A. (1987). Neuropsychological, physiological, and biochemical assessment. In C.L. Frame and J.L. Matson (Eds.), *Handbook of assessment in childhood psychopathology: Applied issues in differential diagnosis and treatment evaluations* (pp. 107–129). New York: Plenum Press.

CHAPTER 3

RESEARCH METHODS AND DESIGNS

Cecilia Ahmoi Essau, Franz Petermann, and Michael Feehan

Various quantitative research methods have been used to obtain information on the prevalence, risk factors, and course and outcome of
psychiatric disorders in children and adolescents. Some of the more
commonly used methods are epidemiological studies and family-
genetic and twin studies. In this chapter, some examples of these studies
will be presented in detail.

RESEARCH METHODS

Epidemiological Studies

Epidemiologically based research is the cornerstone of developmental
psychopathology. Epidemiology can be defined as the study of the frequency of a disorder and its distribution in various populations (Lilienfeld
and Lilienfeld, 1980). However, the scope of epidemiology is wide and
includes: (i) establishing dimensions of morbidity and mortality as a function of person, place, and time; (ii) quantifying the risks of developing a
disease; (iii) identifying and defining syndromes; (iv) describing the
natural history of diseases in terms of onset, duration, recurrence, complications and disability; (v) identifying factors which influence or even
predict clinical course; (vi) searching for causes of disorder and related
disability; and (vii) evaluating specific methods of disease prevention and
control (Morris, 1975; von Korff and Eaton, 1989).

A major strength of epidemiological research using samples taken
from the general population is the ability to produce findings of greater
generalizability than studies of restricted clinical samples. Data from
clinical settings are generally not representative of children and adolescents with psychiatric disorders because of the bias in service attendance through restrictions in evaluating, access, and selection processes

in terms of help-seeking behaviour, symptoms, and chronicity (Wittchen and Essau, 1993).

Epidemiological studies can broadly be grouped under descriptive, analytic, and experimental (Boyle, 1995). Descriptive studies are generally used to give an estimate of the rates of disorders in a specific population. Knowing the baseline rate is important for understanding the burden of illness and the proportion of untreated cases in the population. Such information is useful for health planners to determine the kind of treatment services needed in the community. Analytic studies are used to examine the different rates of disorders in various groups so as to identify groups at a higher risk of developing an illness. Experimental studies are used to test the presumed association between a risk factor and a disorder. Once risk factors are identified, and their associations with a distal outcome quantified, preventive or therapeutic interventions can be designed to reduce the contribution of the risk factors in the development and outcomes of the illness.

A review of the literature regarding the epidemiology of mental health shows three approaches to classifying an individual with psychiatric disorders. These approaches include the assignment of a diagnosis to the respondents by a clinician (i.e., the clinical approach); the use of a checklist or a questionnaire to assess well-being or distress, and symptoms or syndromes of psychiatric disorders (i.e., the dimensional approach); and the administration of a standardized diagnostic interview (i.e., the categorical approach). Of course, various studies will often use combinations of the above.

The Clinical Approach

The clinical approach has been used frequently in European epidemiological studies. In such studies, the children and their parents are interviewed by a child psychiatrist and other clinicians with a standardized clinical interview. Some examples of studies using this approach are those done in Norway (Vikan, 1985), Germany (Esser *et al.*, 1990), and Australia (Connell *et al.*, 1982). The main disadvantage of this approach is the cost involved in having psychiatrists or clinicians do interviews on a large scale. An example of a study using the clinical approach will be described below.

In the Mannheim Study (Esser *et al.*, 1990), from the total 1444 8-year old German children who were born between March and September 1970, and who lived in Mannheim on March 1978, 361 were randomly selected to participate in the study (Esser *et al.*, 1990). Through refusal (36%), having low IQ (below 70), a chronic disease or severe handicap, or having had moved away, 216 (60%) children formed the final sample. Numerous instruments were used including the highly structured parent interview (modified from Graham and Rutter, 1968), neurological, neuropsychological and neurophysiological examinations, and tests of specific skills and abilities. The assessment of psychiatric disorders was arrived at by an expert rating following a two-hour highly structured parent interview.

During the second stage of the study when the children were 13 years old, cases were determined using an interview of the child. All interviews were done by child psychiatrists and experienced clinical psychologists. The disorders examined included: neurotic and emotional disorders (ICD 300 and 313); conduct disorder associated with emotional problems (ICD 312.3); antisocial and conduct disorder (ICD 312, excluding 312.3); hyperkinetic syndromes (ICD 314); and "other" specific symptoms and syndromes (ICD 307). Measures of potential risk factors included: (i) tests for neurological/neurophysiological, neuropsychological, and specific skills to assess minimal brain dysfunction; (ii) specific learning disabilities; (iii) Family Adversity Index (Rutter and Quinton, 1977); and (iv) adverse life events.

At age 8, the overall prevalence rate was 16.2%. The most frequent disorders were neurotic and emotional disorders (6%), followed by hyperkinetic syndromes (4.2%), and other specific symptoms and syndromes (4.2%). Antisocial and conduct disorders, and conduct disorders associated with emotional problems occurred least frequently — with rates of 0.9%. Boys had higher rates than girls for most individual symptoms. Risk factors for psychiatric disorders were high scores on Family Adversity and learning disabilities. The overall prevalence rates obtained during the follow-up investigation, conducted when the children were 13 years old, remained constant. Significant differences were noted for three disorders: The prevalence rate showed an increase for conduct disorder, but a decrease for hyperkinetic syndromes and specific symptoms and "other" syndromes.

The Dimensional Approach

The dimensional approach is associated with empirically derived approaches to assessment. Items from checklists and questionnaires are used to elicit symptomatology of broad classes of disorder, other items are also used to elicit a general sense of distress. Individuals with high problem counts or syndrome scores can be considered cases. A major problem with the dimensional approach is that it does not allow the formulation of a clinical diagnosis and cut-offs used to indicate caseness can be arbitrary.

One of the most widely used instruments for the assessment of disorder symptoms is the Child Behavior Checklist (Achenbach and Edelbrock, 1986). According to Achenbach and Brown's review (1991), over 1200 publications have used the CBCL in clinical research and services, from various centers around the world (Weisz and Eastman, 1995). Verhulst (1995) reviewed the prevalence of maladaptive functioning of children that used the CBCL published between 1965 and 1993. Forty-nine studies with a total of 243000 children were analysed. Verhulst (1995) estimated, about 12.3% of the children in the general population world wide have psychiatric dysfunction.

The Categorical Approach

The categorical approach involves identification of disorders within the DSM and ICD systems, and favours the use of standard diagnostic interviews which can be administered by lay interviewers. In recent years, a number of epidemiological studies have been conducted with children and adolescents using structured interview schedules and refined sampling techniques and provided DSM-III or DSM-III-R diagnoses. These studies include:

a)   The Isle of Wight Studies, UK

This seminal first large-scale epidemiological survey aimed to establish the prevalence of psychiatric disorders in children aged 10 and 11 years. It used a two-stage design (Graham and Rutter, 1973). Parents and teachers of all the 10–11-year old children who lived on the Isle of Wight completed a set of questionnaires about the child's emotional and behaviour problems. Children at high risk for psychiatric disorders were selected for more detailed assessment. Psychiatrists and other clinicians were used as interviewers for the detailed assessments, and made diagnosis based on the ICD. Based on a semi-structured interview between 6% and 7% of the children were identified as meeting criteria for a psychiatric disorder. Of these, about one-third had a neurotic or emotional disorder and two-thirds had "antisocial or mixed conduct-emotional disorder". During a follow-up interview done 4 to 5 years later, the overall prevalence of disorder was estimated at 21%; the most common was emotional disorder

(12.9%), followed by mixed conduct and emotional disorder (5.8%), and then conduct disorder (2.1%).

b) The New Jersey County Study, USA

This is a two-stage epidemiologic study designed to estimate the lifetime prevalence of selected psychiatric disorders (Whitaker *et al.*, 1990). The sample consisted of 5108 (2564 boys and 2544 girls) school children aged between 14 and 17 years who were recruited from 8 secondary schools (5 general public high schools, 1 public vocational-technical high school, 1 parochial school, 1 private day-boarding school) in the New Jersey County. Questionnaires used in the first stage included the Leyton Obsessional Inventory Child Version (Berg *et al.*, 1986), the Beck Depression Inventory (Beck *et al.*, 1961), Eating Symptoms Inventory, Eating Attitudes Test (Garner *et al.*, 1982), and items to elicit symptoms of panic disorder. Additionally, some items were developed to assess anxiety and some items were taken from the Framingham (Haynes *et al.*, 1978) and Tocorna Scales (Siegel *et al.*, 1981) to measure Type A and Type B behaviour patterns. Other questions included those used to elicit sociodemographic characteristics, school attendance and grades, and personal and family health. The questionnaires were administered by the teachers during the classroom hours.

Each participant had some probability of being chosen for the second stage. Those with positive results on more than one screening test had high chances of selection on the corresponding strate. Based on this specified screening criteria, 468 students were selected for the second stage interview. The interview for stage 2 was conducted by 13 clinicians (5 child psychiatrists, 2 child psychiatry fellows, 3 clinical psychologists, 2 social workers, 1 nurse) with experience in adolescent psychiatry. Most interviews were done in the school (90%), and the rest at home (10%). The interview, which averaged 75 minutes in duration, began with having each student complete the Youth Self-Report (Achenbach and Edelbrock, 1987). The interview comprised of separate sections to assess DSM-III criteria for eating disorders, depression, anxiety disorders, and obsessive-compulsive disorder. Following each interview, each student was scored by the clinician on the Children's Global Assessment Scale (Schaffer *et al.*, 1983).

The most common lifetime DSM-III disorders found were dysthymic disorder (4.9%), major depression (4.0%), and generalized anxiety disorder (3.7%). Bulimia, obsessive compulsive disorder, panic disorder, and anorexia nervosa occurred less frequently. Girls were significantly more likely than boys to meet criteria for major depression and generalized anxiety disorder. Based on clinician's ratings on the Children's Global Assessment Scale, 54% of students with a lifetime major diagnosis were currently impaired compared to 10.6% of those without a diagnosis. Students with dysthymic disorder, major depression, and generalized anxiety disorder were the most impaired. Overall, 35% of students with any kind of diagnosis had used some type of mental health service compared to 5.3% of those without diagnoses.

c) The Ontario Child Health Study, Canada

In 1989, a simple random sample was taken of 2317 6–16 year old children who attended public schools in an industralized, urban setting (Boyle *et al.*, 1987, 1993; Offord *et al.*, 1992). Out of the 2219 children who were eligible to participate in the study, 1751 parents completed problem checklists and gave informed consent to obtain teacher assessments; the reasons for not participating included refusal, language problems, and others. The questionnaires were mailed to the teachers to complete.

A stratified random sample of participants for stage 2 assessments, which took place 1–3 months after stage 1, were done on the basis of age (6–11, 12–16), sex, and high versus low symptom scores on the Ontario Child Health Study Scales (Boyle *et al.*, 1987). Altogether 251 of the 329 children who had been selected for stage 2 agreed to participate. During the stage 2 assessment, parents and children completed problem checklists and were administered the revised version of the Diagnostic Interview for Children and Adolescents (DICA-R; Reich and Welner, 1988) 2 times at 3 weeks apart. The families were randomly divided into two groups. In the first group, the first and the second DICA-R interviews were conducted by different trained lay interviewers. In the second group, the first and the second interviews were done either by two lay interviewers, a lay interviewer and a child psychiatrist, or two child psychiatrists. The lay interviewers consisted of 16 women with extensive interviewing experience. The clinicians consisted of five child psychiatrists. Both groups of interviewers had been trained in using the DICA-R interviewer manual and interview. The disorders covered in the DICA-R were conduct disorder, attention-deficit hyperactivity disorder, overanxious disorder, separation anxiety disorder, major depression, and dysthymia.

The overall rate, based on the child interview, in the 6–11 year olds were 25.8%, and in the 12–16 year old, 32%. The rates based on the parent interview were slightly lower, being 18.5% for the younger (6–11 year old) and 20.5% for the older children (12–16 year olds). The most frequent disorders, as reported by the children, were that of dysthymia, with rates of 21.3% in the older and 14.5% in the younger groups; and overanxious disorder with rates of 20.5% in the older and 11.1% in the younger groups.

d) The Puerto Rican Child Psychiatry Epidemiologic Study

This study investigated 4–16 (N = 777) year old children who had been randomly selected from households distributed across the island of Puerto Rico (Bird *et al.*, 1988). The study used a two-stage design. During the first stage, the Child Behavior Checklist — parent version (CBCL; Achenbach and Edelbrock, 1981) and the teacher version of the CBCL (Achenbach and Edelbrock, 1981) were used as screening instruments for case identification for children aged 6 to 16 years old. Children who scored above the cutpoint on either the parent or the teacher version of the CBCL were randomly selected from the total sample for a second-stage assessment. All interviewers had at least a bachelor's college degree, and had previous survey experience. The interview was done with the mother in her home. The type of information obtained during the interview included: family composition, the parent version of the CBCL, demographic data, and various variables for the studies of the risk factors of disorders. Clinical assessments in the second stage were based on parent and child interviews with the Spanish Diagnostic Interview Schedule for Children. The interview was done by four child psychiatrists who were knowledgeable about DSM-III nosology, and its application. For every psychiatric diagnosis in which the criteria were met, the psychiatrist also scored each child on the Children's Global Assessment Scale to measure adaptive functioning (Schaffer *et al.*, 1983).

The six-month prevalence based on the presence of DSM-III diagnoses plus meeting functional impairment criteria on the Children's Global Assessment Scale was estimated at 17.9%. The most common disorders were oppositional disorder (9.9%), attention deficit disorder (9.5%), and depression/dysthymia (5.9%). Being male and coming from low socioeconomic background were factors most strongly associated with psychopathology. The findings also showed high comorbidity between conduct/oppositional disorder and attention deficit disorder. More than half of the children with attention deficit disorder also had conduct/oppositional disorder, and almost half of those with conduct/oppositional disorder also had attention deficit disorder.

e) The Dunedin Multidisciplinary Health and Developmental Study, New Zealand

This study has followed a cohort from birth to age 21 with a comprehensive assessment frame including health, mental health and academic attainment (Silva, 1990; McGee *et al.*, 1994). Sample members belonged to a cohort born at the city's maternity hospital between April 1, 1972 and March 31, 1973. These children were first assessed at age 3 years (N = 1037), then reassessed every two years (5, 7, 9, 11, 13, 15) and three-yearly at ages 18 and 21 years. In childhood (ages 5, 7, and 9 years) the children were assessed with the Rutter Child Scales for completion by parents and teachers (Rutter *et al.*, 1970). The prevalence and characteristics of behaviour problems have been reported in detail (e. g., McGee *et al.*, 1983). Diagnostic interviews have been conducted with the children, using: the Diagnostic Interview Schedule for Children (DISC; Costello *et al.*, 1982) at age 11 (Anderson *et al.*, 1987); a modified DISC at 13 (Frost *et al.*, 1989) and 15 (McGee *et al.*, 1990); and a modified version of the adult Diagnostic Interview Schedule at age 18 (Feehan *et al.*, 1994). In addition, various measures have been included for assessing family, peer and school attachment, life stress and general background circumstances.

At age 11, 17.6% of children were classified as meeting DSM-III criteria based on the combined information for child, parent and teacher; the most common disorders were attention-deficit disorder and oppositional disorder (Anderson *et al.*, 1987). At age 15, the rate of disorder was estimated to be 22% (McGee *et al.*, 1990), and 36.3% when the adolescents were 18 years old (Feehan *et al.*, 1993). Continues in disorder between ages have been found to be strong (Feehan *et al.*, 1993, 1995; McGee *et al.*, 1992).

f) The Christchurch Health and Developmental Study, New Zealand

This is a longitudinal study of a birth cohort of 1265 New Zealand children born in the Christchurch urban region during mid-1977 who have been studied at birth, 4 months, 1 year, and annual intervals to the age of 15 years. Data were available from a combination of sources including maternal interview, child interview, and teacher report (Fergusson *et al.*, 1993). At ages 15 and 16 years, maternal reports and self-reports of different symptoms were obtained. Interviews were done separately with the child and the mother, with mothers being interviewed at home and children at school, as well as by different interviewers.

The abbreviated version of the DISC (Costello *et al.*, 1982; McGee *et al.*, 1990) was administered to the child to measure anxiety disorders (overanxious disorder, separation anxiety disorder, simple and social phobia), oppositional defiant disorder, and attention-deficit hyperactivity disorder, supplemented by additional items to meet DSM-III-R criteria. To assess conduct disorder, the Self-report Early Delinquency Scale (Moffitt and Silva, 1988) was used. Substance abuse behaviours (tobacco, alcohol, and illicit drug abuse) were measured using survey questions, supplemented by the Rutgers Alcohol Problems Index (White and Labouvie, 1989). Parallel to those used in children, maternal reports of the child's behaviour were obtained using the DISC interview for anxiety and mood disorders, and the Revised Behavior Problems Checklist (Quay and Petersen, 1987) to measure oppositional defiant disorder, and attention-deficit hyperactivity disorder. Conduct disorder was assessed using the parent version of the Self-report Early Delinquency Scale (Moffitt and Silva, 1988). Children's problems with tobacco, alcohol, and illicit drug were obtained from parent's report.

At age 15, a total of 25% had at least one DSM-III-R diagnosis. The most common disorders were the anxiety disorders with rates, ranging from 10.7 to 12.8%. Conduct and oppositional disorders also occurred frequently (ranges: 8.1 to 10.8%). The rates for substance use disorders ranged from 5.2 to 7.7%. High comorbidity rates were found between conduct disorder/oppositional defiant disorder and attention-deficit hyperactivity disorder, as well as between conduct disorder and substance use disorders. Additionally, there was a significant tendency for children with anxiety disorders to have increased rates of mood disorders. Those with mood or anxiety disorders also had high rates of conduct/oppositional disorders and substance use disorders. In terms of service utilization, the majority of children who met the criteria for at least one DSM-III-R disorder did not receive any form of assistance, counseling or therapy for these conditions. Only 21% of those meeting the diagnostic criteria on the basis of maternal or child report had received some assistance from school counselors, mental health professionals (psychiatrists, clinical psychologists, psychiatric social workers), or from other sources (social workers and lay support groups).

The extent to which children came to attention for problems varied with the child's symptomatology: 9% of the children with anxiety or mood disorders, 26% with conduct problems, attention deficit, or substance abuse, and 36% with both anxiety/mood disorders and disruptive behavior/substance use disorders had received some form of assistance.

g) The Northeastern Study, USA

This is a 14-year longitudinal study that began when a sample of 385 children entered kindergarten in Northeastern United States at age 5 years. The children were re-interviewed at ages 9, 15, and 18 years (Reinherz *et al.*, 1993a). The Diagnostic Interview Schedule, Version III-R (Robins *et al.*, 1989) was used to provide a lifetime diagnosis of major depression, anxiety disorders (simple phobia, social phobia, post-traumatic stress disorder), and substance use disorders (alcohol abuse/ dependence and drug abuse/dependence) according to DSM-III-R criteria. Parents completed questionnaires and/or interviews when the children were aged 5, 9, and 15 years old, and teachers comments and school records of grades were gathered for the period from ages 6 to 15 years. Multiple sources of information used included the structured clinical interview for assessing psychiatric disorders and ages of onset, self-report questionnaires for evaluating current functioning, and school records for academic performance and suspensions or explusions. The mother gave information about the children's health from the prenatal period to age 5 years. Teacher comments and school records of grade and grade retentions were obtained for the time when the children were between 6 to 15 years old. Ten trained interviewers with either research or clinical experience administered the DIS-III-R to the 18-year old adolescents.

Six indices of current behavioural, emotional, academic, and social functioning were assessed through self-report measures and school records: (i) The Youth Self-Report (Achenbach and Edelbrock, 1987) provided overall emotional and behavioural functioning; (ii) Self esteem was measured by the Rosenberg Self-Esteem Scale (Rosenberg, 1986); (iii) Interpersonal problems were assessed by the Interpersonal Problems Scale (Reinherz *et al.*, 1993b); (iv) Information about course grades were taken from school transcripts; (v) School suspensions or explusion in the preceding year were taken from school records and self-reports; and (vi) Arrests in past year or involvement in the juvenile justice systems were based on self-reports.

About 29% of adolescents had any six of the DSM-III-R disorders by as early as age 14 years. The most frequent disorders were alcohol abuse/dependence (32.4%), followed by social (13.7%) and simple phobia (11.1%). The disorder with the earliest onset was simple phobia beginning in early childhood, whereas major depression, post-traumatic stress disorder, and substance use disorders had an age of onset around mid-adolescence. During early childhood to late adolescence, females were more likely to have developed alcohol abuse/depression. Among depressed cases, females experienced an earlier (almost 1.5 years earlier) first depressive episode than males. The data on posttraumatic stress disorder was of interest since it indicated that more than 40% of the adolescents have experienced a qualifying trauma such as physical assault, rape or sudden injury by age 18. Adolescents with onset of any disorders had significantly higher risk for having comorbid disorder, as compared to those with later onset. Early onset of psychiatric disorder was associated with deficits in psychosocial functioning at age 18. A major problem of the study was that the adolescents were mostly white, and were recruited from a working class community. Thus, results should not be generalized to adolescents of other socioeconomic status or ethnic background. In addition, age of onset was based on retrospective reports which is subject to problem with recall.

h)   The New York Child Longitudinal Study, USA

Children in the age 1–10 year range were originally sampled in 1975 from the upstate New York counties (Cohen et al., 1993). A follow-up interview was done eight years later, when the children were aged 9–18 years old. The diagnoses determined using the DISC were attention deficit hyperactive disorder, conduct disorder, oppositional defiant disorder, overanxious disorder, alcohol abuse and major depression. The overall prevalence rate was 17.7%. There was a high level of diagnostic persistence over a period of 2.5 years, except for major depression.

For overanxious disorders, comparable rates were found for boys and girls in late childhood, after which there was a strong linear decline for boys from age 10 to 20; less decline was noted for girls. Both the rates and age trends of separation anxiety were similar for boys and girls; there was a 23% decline in the rate each year after the age 10. The prevalence of major depression in late childhood was low and comparable for both sexes. While the prevalence remained the same during the adolescent years in boys, there was a sharp increase in prevalence for girls during the post puberty years. The rates of attention deficit hyperactivity disorder and conduct disorder were about two times higher in boys and girls. Oppositional defiant disorder showed the same prevalence and age pattern for the two genders. Both alcohol and marijuana abuse showed an increased in rates with age, especially in boys. There was a strong overlap among different disorders. Among the cases with major depressive disorder 62% also had an additional disruptive disorder, and 43% had a comorbid anxiety disorder.

i) The Oregon Adolescent Depression Project, USA

A total of 1710 high school students (mean age = 16.6 years) in three cohorts (1987, 1988, 1989) were recruited for the study, of which 1508 participated in two sequential interviews (Lewinsohn *et al.*, 1993, 1994). The schools were located in two urban communities with a population of about 200 000, and three rural communities in West Central Oregon. The schools were chosen because of their locations, all being within 100 miles from the project center. The sampling frame used was designed based on parental consent and proportional stratification according to gender, grade and school size.

The diagnostic interview used at Time 1 was the Schedule for Affective Disorder and Schizophrenia for School-age Children (K-SADS; Puig-Antich and Chambers, 1983). At a follow-up investigation, done a year later, the Longitudinal Interval Follow-Up Evaluation (LIFE) interview (Shapiro and Keller, 1979) was used to determine the course of the psychiatric disorders present at Time 2 and the onset of new disorders since Time 1. The interviewers also made an Axis V Global Assessment of Functioning rating, to evaluate the participant's psychological, social, and occupational functioning and the need for treatment. The interview was done by 27 interviewers with advanced degrees in clinical or counseling psychology or social work, who had finished a 70-hour didactic and experiential course in diagnostic interviewing. To determine the clinical significance of episodes of affective disorders, all adolescents with a current diagnosis of affective disorders were rated by three child psychiatrists with respect to "current level of functioning", "highest level of functioning during the past year", the "severity of depression", and the "need for treatment".

The overall prevalence of any current diagnosis was about 10% and for any lifetime diagnosis was 37%. The most common disorder was major depressive disorder, followed by the anxiety disorders. High reoccurrence rates were found for all disorders. This was especially the case for major depressive and substance use disorders. Comorbidity between major psychiatric disorders was high. Females had significantly higher rates of major depressive disorders, anxiety disorders, eating disorders, and adjustment disorder, whereas, males had higher rates of disruptive behavior disorder.

j) The Cambridgeshire Study, UK

A total of 1060 11–16-year old girls were recruited from three secondary state schools within the county of Cambridgeshire (Cooper and Goodyer, 1993). One school was urban and two were rural. The Mood and Feelings Questionnaire (Costello and Angold, 1988), which was administered in the classroom, was used to identify mood disturbance. A stratified random procedure was used to select the subjects for a more detailed interview. For each year within each school, subjects were divided into three groups in terms of their score on the Mood and Feelings Questionnaire. All those in the top 10%, one in two of the next 10%, and one in ten of the remainder were selected for interview. All interviews were conducted by three trained interviewers who had experience in working with young people in health care, education, or both. Over the study period, a meeting was held every week between the interviewers and the principle investigators to discuss any problems encountered during the interview.

Based on a modified form of the DISC, the one-month prevalence of DSM-III-R major depressive disorder was 3.6%, the one-year prevalence was 6%. Symptoms with high rates were that of depressed mood, social withdrawal, and early insomnia — all with a prevalence of about 20%. Anxiety symptoms occurred less frequently when compared with depressed symptoms, except for phobias and anxiety associated with school attendance. Among cases of major depressive disorder, 40% also had anxiety, behavioural, and obsessional disorders. In these depressed cases, depressed mood, social withdrawal, agitation, early insomnia, and nihilistic ideas had similarly high rates across all ages. The rates for the items "hopeless" significantly decreased with increased age, whereas that of "weight loss" and "suicidal acts" increased with increasing age.

The above studies have highlighted a wide variation in the rates of disorders, with overall estimates ranging from 17.6 to 37%; these differences may be accounted for by differences in methodology and assessment techniques, ages of participants, case definition and varying diagnostic criteria. While direct comparability of findings across studies is not straight forward, the available data indicate at least one in five and as many as one in three children or adolescents can be reasonably considered to have a meaningful dysfunction of their mental health.

In addition to estimating the simple presence or absence of psychiatric disorders, epidemiological data which have been collected by means of structured diagnostic interviews have also been used to study the nature of those disorders, including patterns of comorbidity and the temporal sequencing of disorders, their age of onset, courses and outcomes. Detailed information on these issues will be reported for each specific disorder described in the chapters that follow.

Family-genetic Studies and Twin Studies

The role of genetic factors in the aetiology of psychiatric disorders have been examined using family, twin, adoption, and genetic linkage studies (Weissman *et al.*, 1986). Twin and family-genetic studies are nearly uniform in reporting: a strong degree of familial aggregation for most psychiatric disorders; a higher concordance rates among monozygotic than dizygotic twins; and a higher prevalence of disorders among biological offspring of affected individuals compared to biological offspring of unaffected individuals.

Family Study

The main aim of a family study is to collect detailed information regarding the disorder under investigation in biological relatives. Family studies generally comprise a group of probands, a group of individuals to act as a control, and relatives of each group. In almost all studies, probands with psychiatric disorder are recruited from a treatment setting. A control group is used to compare patterns of familial aggregation among the probands who may consist of those who are medically (but not psychiatrically) ill individuals without a psychiatric disorder, or those who have a psychiatric disorder other than the one under investigation (Weissman *et al.*, 1986). The proband's and control's relatives may consist of the spouse and first-degree relatives such as parents, siblings, and offspring.

Family case-control studies, top-down, bottom-up, and high-risk studies are examples of designs used in family studies. In the family case-control design, the prevalence of the disorder among the first degree relatives is compared with the prevalence among relatives in the control group. The *top-down design* begins with the adult probands who have been selected from treatment settings or case registers, and assess for the presence of disorders among their offspring (Puig-Antich, 1984). *Bottom-up studies* begin with children or adolescents (who have been selected from treatment settings) as the probands, and study psychopathology in their parents or adult relatives. *High-risk studies* are designed to determine the extent to which an illness runs in families. These studies involve studying children of ill probands to identify risk factors which are premorbid to the disorder (Weissman *et al.*, 1984). The development of the high risk paradigm for studying children of ill parents can be attributed largely to schizophrenia researchers in the 1970s. Findings generally show higher rates of schizophrenia and "manic-depressive" illness among family members of affected individuals than those in general population. Theoretically this design can potentially provide information on the early signs of illness and suggest factors which may protect vulnerable individuals from developing the disorder or by minimizing its impact.

In this section, we will discuss some examples of family studies.

a) Yale Family Study, USA

In the Yale Family Study, depressed probands who received treatment at the Yale University Depression Research Unit and normal controls who had been recruited from a community survey in New Haven and who had no history of psychiatric disorder were interviewed. The sample consisted of 220 participants between the ages of 6 and 23 at the first investigation. Of these, 153 had one or more depressed parents, and 67 children whose parents did not have depression (Weissman *et al.*, 1982). A follow-up interview was conducted two years later with a total of 174 offspring. About two-thirds of the sample (N = 121) were children of depressed parents, and one-third (N = 53) were children of non-depressed parents (Weissman *et al.*, 1992). Diagnostic assessment used with parents included the Schedule for Affective Disorders and Schizophrenia, and among their offspring the modified version of the Schedule for Affective Disorders and Schizophrenia for School-age Children — Epidemiologic Version (K-SADS-E). The K-SADS-E covered five DSM-III diagnostic groups including major depression, anxiety disorders (separation anxiety, panic disorder, phobia, obsessive-compulsive disorder, and overanxious disorder), conduct disorder, substance abuse (alcohol and drug abuse), and dysthymia.

Results from the first investigation indicated that, compared to children of control parents, children of depressed parent were more likely to have a lifetime diagnosis of major depression and substance abuse.

They were also likely to have been in treatment, and have experienced various types of health problems, injuries and accidents. Additionally, they experienced the first onset of major depression at an earlier age (Weissman, 1988). Children whose parents were both depressed were at a greater risk for a psychiatric disorder than those with only one depressed parent. The presence of major depression, dysthymia, or anxiety disorders among children of depressed parents at the first interview did not predict the presence of other disorders at the second interview (Weissman _et al._, 1992). By contrast, substance abuse at the first interview predicted substance abuse at the second interview. Family factors such as affectionless control, parental divorce, poor marital adjustment, and low family cohesion were associated with an increased incidence of substance abuse disorder and conduct disorder in the offspring, but not major depression or anxiety disorder (Weissman _et al._, 1992).

b) The Leckman _et al._'s study, USA

The Leckman _et al._'s study (1983) is an example of a case-control family study of psychiatric disorder. In this study, diagnostic estimates were made on 1331 first degree relatives (parents, siblings, and children) of 82 normal control probands (i.e., no current or past psychiatric disorders) and 133 probands with psychiatric disorders (52 had major depression without anxiety, 51 had depression with associated anxiety, 30 had depression with a separation anxiety episode). In about 40% of the sample, direct interviews were used. The modified Research Diagnostic Criteria (Mazure and Gershon, 1979) were used by multiple raters to make diagnostic estimates.

Relatives of individuals with major depression and anxiety disorder had the highest rate of both major depression and anxiety, whereas the lowest rates for these two disorders were found in relatives of normal control probands. Their data also indicated that the presence of anxiety symptoms during a major depressive episode was associated with higher rates of both depression and anxiety among first degree relatives, compared to those found in relatives of probands who had major depression with anxiety disorders.

c) The UCLA Family Stress Project, USA

The UCLA Family Stress Project is a study of high-risk children of unipolar depressed (N = 22), bipolar (N = 18), medically ill (insulin-dependent diabetes with juvenile onset and severe early onset rheumatoid arthritis (N = 18) mothers, and children of normal mothers (N = 38). Children were followed longitudinally, with families being contacted at 6-month intervals by telephone up to a period of three years. The functioning of mothers and children was assessed with several measures and through direct observations of interaction.

During the initial assessment, the mothers were administered the (i) Schedule for Affective Disorders and Schizophrenia-Lifetime version (Endicott and Spitzer, 1979), which was used to evaluate the lifetime psychiatric histories; (ii) Beck Depression Inventory (Beck *et al.*, 1961) which is a self-report questionnaire that measures severity of depressive symptoms; (iii) Social Adjustment Scale (Weissman and Bothwell, 1976) which assesses women's level of functioning in the areas of occupational, relationships with immediate family and children, extended family, and recreation. Children were administered the (i) K-SADS (Orvaschel *et al.*, 1982; Puig-Antich *et al.*, 1983) which was used to assess diagnoses of current and lifetime disorders; (ii) Mothers completed the Child Behavior Checklist (Achenbach and Edelbrock, 1983) for each child, in order to assess for behaviour problems and social competence; (iii) Children were also administered the Peabody Picture Vocabulary Test-Revised (Dunn and Dunn, 1981) to obtain their verbal IQ; (iv) To measure the children's cognitive abilities, the Piers-Harris Children's Self-Concept Scale (Piers and Harris, 1969) and the Children's Attribution Style Questionnaire (Seligman *et al.*, 1984) were used.

The overall rates of disorder were significantly higher in the offspring of unipolar depressed (72%) and bipolar (67%) mothers than in the children of medically ill mothers (44%) and those of normal mothers (24%). Major depressive episodes were reported in 41% of the children of mothers with unipolar depression. Children of mothers with unipolar depression also showed impairment of functioning in the areas of social and academic functioning, and in the mother-child relationship. Both unipolar women and their children tended to be exposed to a greater number of stressful life events compared to those in the other groups. Results of the Conflict Discussion Task showed unipolar women as being irritable and critical of their children, being less positive and have difficulty staying focused on constructive problem solving with the children. At follow-up, children of unipolar mothers, in contrast to children of bipolar mothers and comparison group children, displayed high rates of chronic and new disorders including dysthymic disorder, overanxious disorder, conduct disorder, and chronic substance abuse problems.

d)   The Western Psychiatric Institute and Clinic Family History Study, USA

The main aim of the study was to examine the presence of major psychiatric disorder in the biological relatives (adults) of prepubertal children with major depression (N = 48). The results were then compared to children with nonaffective psychiatric disorder (N = 20) and normal children (N = 27). The children were interviewed with the Schedule for Affective Disorders and Schizophrenia for School-age Children (Orvaschel *et al.*, 1982). Relatives were interviewed with the Schedule for Affective Disorders and Schizophrenia, Lifetime version (Endicott and Spitzer, 1978) and the Research Diagnostic Criteria (RDC; Spitzer *et al.*, 1978). Interviewers were also trained to use the Family History-RDC method (Andreasen *et al.*, 1977, 1986; Thompson *et al.*, 1982).

Prevalence rates for major depression and alcoholism were significantly higher (about twice) in relatives of prepubertal children with major depressive disorder than in relatives of normal children. This suggested that children who developed major depressive disorder came from families with rates for psychiatric disorders (especially major depressive disorder, alcoholism, and anxiety disorder) which are markedly higher than those in families of normal children. Highest familial rates of major depressive disorder were associated with never having suicidal behaviour or ideation, and not having a comorbid conduct disorder in children with major depressive disorder. These findings, however, should be interpreted with caution because of the partial blindness of the assessment of families. The use of depressed children from clinical settings could mean that some referral biases may have affected the results. For example, parents who have psychiatric disorders such as depression, anxiety disorders, or alcoholism, could have recognized depression in their children earlier and sought help more promptly than parents without any psychiatric disorders.

Twin Studies

In twin studies investigators seek to separate out genetic and environmental influences by comparing concordance rates in monozygotic (MZ) and dizygotic (DZ) twin pairs. It can be simply argued that if the disorder was due to environmental factors, individuals in both MZ and DZ pairs should be at equal risk. If, on the other hand, pathogenic genes are largely responsible for the manifestation of illness then a MZ co-twin would be at a higher risk than would a DZ co-twin. Difficulties in the design involve selecting participants to ensure that individuals within the MZ and DZ dyads are raised in similar familial environments. A more precise estimate of the importance of heredity and environment would be made in studies comparing MZ and DZ twins reared together and reared separately.

a) Torgersen's Twin Study, Norway

The main aim of Torgersen's study (1983) was to examine the frequency of anxiety disorder in monozygotic (MZ) and dizygotic (DZ) adult same-sex twins. The study was part of a nationwide study of same-sex twins who underwent treatment for neurotic and borderline psychotic disorders in all psychiatric settings in Norway before 1977. The pairs were interviewed with the Present State Examination (Wing *et al.*, 1974). Information regarding a developmental history (childhood, relationship to parents, closeness between the twins and similarity in childhood environment), and social development and psychologic strain in adult age were recorded. Out of the 318 probands, 32 MZ and 53 DZ individuals have a current or past anxiety disorder as their main psychiatric disorder.

MZ twins had two times higher rates of anxiety disorder than DZ co-twins. The frequency of anxiety disorders with panic attacks were about five times higher in MZ than in DZ co-twins. The concordance for anxiety disorders for those with anxiety disorders without generalized anxiety disorder, was three times higher in the MZ than in DZ twins. These findings were interpreted as indicating that the familial transmission of anxiety disorder is hereditary.

b) Thapar and McGuffin's Twin Study, UK

The main aim of Thapar and McGuffin's study (1994) was to assess parental and self-reports of depressive symptoms in an epidemiological sample of twins. Using the Cardiff Births Survey Register, 457 live twin pairs born between 1976 and 1984 were identified, of which 456 were traced. The general practitioners of all these twins were also contacted. Due to various reasons (emigration, contraindications specified by the general practitioners, death, adoption, and refusal of the general practioners to disclose the family's address), the final study sample consisted of 411 pairs. Parental ratings were obtained using a set of questionnaires (which was sent by post) including a standard twin similarity questionnaire used to determine zygosity (Nichols and Bilbro, 1966) and the Mood and Feelings Questionnaire (Costello and Angold, 1988). A total of 316 families completed and returned the questionnaires. The sample was made up of 124 same-sex MZ pairs and 94 same sex DZ pairs.

The overall estimates for the heritability of depressive symptoms was 79%. However, there were significant differences in genetic effects in different age groups. Genetic factors showed little importance in the 8–11 year old children; in this group, shared environmental effects account for much of the variation, with "common environmentality" estimated at 77%. Among the 11–16 year olds, depressive symptoms appear to be influenced by genetic factors rather than shared environment. Although depressive symptoms seemed largely heritable, the influence of genetic and environmental factors varied with age.

c) Kendler *et al.*'s Study, USA

The Kendler *et al.*'s study (1994a) examined self-reported symptoms of depression from two samples of twins and their families (i.e., spouses, parents, siblings, and offsprings). One sample of twins were solicited through an American Association of Retired Persons newsletter (N = 19, 203) and another from the Virginia Twin Registry (N = 11, 242). Twins provided names and addresses of spouses and their first-degree relatives. Questionnaires covering health and lifestyle issues were mailed to the twins and their families. Two questionnaires were used to determine the zygosity of twins, namely, those pertaining to their physical similarity and to how frequently people confused the twins when they were children. Symptoms of psychopathology were obtained using a subset of the SCL-90 (Derogatis *et al.*, 1973), and have included the subscales of depression, somatization, anxiety, and phobic anxiety.

Familial resemblance in depressive symptoms appeared moderate and due largely to genetic factors. The estimated heritability of depressive symptoms was 37% for the American Association of Retired Persons newsletter samples, and 30% for the Virginia sample. Sibling environment factors such as family social class, neighborhood, and school, did not play a significant role in influencing depressive symptoms in adulthood.

In another study, Kendler *et al.* (1994b), using data from the Virginia Twin Registry, examined the relationship between clinical features of 646 female twins with DSM-III-R criteria for major depression and the risk for major depression in their co-twins. For this analysis, 500 pairs of known zygosity where either one (N = 354) or both (N = 146) met the diagnosis of major depression. The major depression diagnosis was made using a modified version of the Structured Clinical Interview (SCID) for DSM-III-R (Spitzer *et al.*, 1987). Other diagnoses covered included panic disorder, generalized anxiety disorder, alcohol dependence, anorexia nervosa, and bulimia nervosa. The interviewers had been trained in using the SCID, and had a master degree in psychology or social work, or a bachelor degree and two year's clinical experience.

Based on stepwise proportional hazards regression, four clinical features in the proband twins were identified as predicting the risk of major depression in the co-twins. These include the number of episodes, degree of impairment during the episode, and comorbidity with panic disorder or bulimia; comorbidity with bulimia increased the risk for depression to 61% in co-twins and with panic disorder 53%. The number of episodes predicted an increased risk of 46% and the degree of impairment predicted a 33% increased risk of depression in the co-twins. Comorbidity with phobia predicted a decreased risk of depression in the co-twins. Age of onset, number and kind of depressive symptoms, treatment seeking, duration of the longest episode and comorbidity with generalized anxiety disorder and alcohol dependence failed to predict risk of major depression. These findings suggested that certain features of major depression such as its recurrence, impairment and comorbidity patterns can be related to the familial venerability to depression.

Adoption Studies

Adoption studies are concerned with investigating children who have been reared from infancy by non-related adoptive parents. Two comparisons can generally be made: First, comparing the frequency of disorder in adopted children whose biological parents had the illness and those whose biological parents did not have it. Higher rates will be obtained in the former if there is a genetic cause. Second, comparing the frequency of psychiatric disorders in adopted children among their biological and adoptive parents. The rate will be greater in the former if there is a genetic cause.

RESEARCH DESIGNS

Case-control Design

In case-control designs, individuals with disorder are identified at the time of the study, and are compared with those without the disorder, matched on important defining characteristics (Verhulst and Koot, 1992). Data can either be collected from the individuals' recollections or from secondary records (e. g., medical charts). This design is particularly vulnerable to biases in recall when extensive use is made of retrospective data. Also, by using referred cases, information on cases in the general population is missed (Verhulst and Koot, 1992).

Cross-sectional and Retrospective Designs

In cross-sectional research, participants are assessed at one-time point. Cross-sectional research can be used to test competing hypotheses regarding the correlates of disorder (Rutter, 1994) and may help to sort out causal hypotheses which warrant testing through longitudinal designs (Rutter, 1994). Cross-sectional studies often rely on retrospective information but they also can serve as a platform for prospective longitudinal studies. The problems of expense, attrition, repeated measurement, and researcher's long-term commitment to the project are minimized (Palinkas, 1985). A major disadvantage of cross-sectional research is related to the problem of tracing developmental change and determining causality (Rutter, 1994). Also, cross-sectional studies have low internal validity since it is not possible to measure and control for major factors which might influence the dependent variable; the effects of age and cohort are confounded in cross-sectional studies (Loeber and Farrington, 1995).

Prospective Longitudinal Design

Prospective longitudinal studies attempt to follow children over an extended period of time, with observations of several variables being recorded at certain intervals (Petermann, 1995; Rutter, 1989). Prospective studies can be classed as "concurrent" and "nonconcurrent" studies. In a concurrent study, the individuals with or without the characteristic of interest are followed for an extended period of time into the future. In a nonconcurrent study, a cohort was selected as it existed at some point in the past, and is followed over time, usually to the present.

The prospective longitudinal study is the ideal research strategy to examine the continuity of disorder of children and adolescents into adulthood (Christie *et al.*, 1988). It provides information about the natural histories of child psychopathology in terms of their frequencies, form and variety (comorbidity), severity, and ages of onset and offset. The developmental sequences and pathways by which early factors predict adult psychopathology can be charted. The efficacy of prevention and treatment can be determined and much can be learned about the intergenerational transmission of psychopathology (Loeber and Farrington, 1995; McGee *et al.*, 1995). To illustrate the importance of prospective longitudinal studies, Robins (1983) gave the example of fears of the dark being common in 6-year-old girls and depression being rare, while depression is more common in 15-year-olds. She then stated: "Without longitudinal studies, we will not know whether these are two unrelated disorders with different ages of risk, or whether childhood fears predict the onset of adolescent depression" (p. 201).

Other advantages of longitudinal studies have recently been summarized by Rutter (1994). Longitudinal studies make it possible to know who is missing from the sample. This is in contrast to cross-sectional studies in which subjects who have died are not eligible for inclusion, and thus may cause bias. They also provide multiple points of measurement over time which may help increase reliability and decrease biases due to reporting variations in situational data. Longitudinal data can be used to explore how chains of experiences led either to persistence of sequelae or to major later change.

Despite their advantages, longitudinal studies are not common given their cost, logistical difficulty, and potential problems with attrition (Rutter, 1994). The longer the duration of a longitudinal study, the more likely selective attrition will occur. As reported by Boyle *et al.* (1991), it is common to lose 20–30% of subjects in longitudinal studies of childhood psychopathology, and in studies of adolescent substance use, losses of 20% to 55% are common. In conducting longitudinal studies, attention must be paid to societal change over time which may lead to the manifestation of cohort effects. They may also be delay in reporting findings so that there is a danger that theories, methods, instrument used, and policy concerns may be out of date by the time main results are published (Rutter, 1994). There also can be problems in data storage and maintaining confidentiality.

Additionally, there are a number of issues which present some challenges for conducting longitudinal research, including (Loeber and Farrington, 1995) (a) *Source of data:* The choice of informant (i.e., source of data) which depends on the types of disorder investigated, can be confounded since not all informants have the same opportunity or ability to observe the children's behaviour. Thus, for example, most investigators use parents or teachers as informants for information regarding symptoms related to attention-deficit hyperactivity disorder or conduct disorders

(Loeber *et al.*, 1990); (b) *Types of sample:* Two common types of samples used are general population and high risk. The main advantage of the general population samples is the representativity of the data obtained. In high-risk samples, the yield of disordered cases is greater than those from general population samples; (c) *Study duration:* Length of longitudinal studies (i.e., study duration) depends on the duration and course (including onset and offset of the disorder) of the target disorders, as well as the comorbid disorders, and the available funding; (d) *Frequency of assessment:* The frequency of assessments should be determined by the expected developmental changes. Thus, the faster the speed of development, the more frequent measures need to be done so as to ascertain the process of change. By contrast, the slower the speed of development, the less frequent the assessment needs to be done. Participant's responses to the repeated assessments also need to be considered in determining the frequency of assessment; (e) *Distinguishing ageing, period, and cohort effects:* Another major challenge involves trying to disentangle ageing effects (i.e., changes that occur with age) from period (i.e., influence of specific event to a particular time) and cohort effects (i.e., group of individuals who experience the same event during the same period); (f) *Data analysis:* Choice of statistical methods is dependent on the type of data available. Problems can occur when the data gathered earlier may not be in a form suitable for some new analytic techniques, or measures changed over time; (g) *Causal effects of behavior:* A major difficulty is to determine which of the correlates or associated factors have causal effects on behaviour.

Accelerated Longitudinal Design

To partially solve the problem of the long periods needed to establish causal linkages across ages in longitudinal studies, accelerated longitudinal designs have been developed (Bell, 1953). In an accelerated longitudinal design, children or adolescents of different ages are assessed longitudinally beginning in the same year. That is, several age-cohorts of individuals are each followed up for the same number of years so that the age of onset cohort at the end of the assessments coincides with the age of the next cohort at the beginning. In recent years, a number of studies have used an accelerated longitudinal design including those by Loeber *et al.* (1993), McConaughy *et al.* (1992), and Verhulst *et al.* (1990). The accelerated longitudinal analyses allow testing of the stability of problems over time and by considering cohort and period effects, and age change (Stanger *et al.*, 1994).

Each research design has particular strengths and weaknesses. The decision as to which design to use depends on several factors, including the aim of the study; hypotheses to be tested; expected rates of disorder; available methods for data analysis; and availability of time, money, and personnel.

DATA ANALYSIS

Measures of Frequency

The most common measures of frequency used in an epidemiologic study are prevalence and incidence (Verhulst, 1995). Prevalence refers to the proportion of individuals ill in a given population. It is calculated by dividing the number of cases by the total population that include both cases and noncases. Prevalence can be grouped under lifetime, period, and point. *Lifetime prevalence* refers to the proportion of individuals in the population who have or have ever had the disorder up to the date of assessment. *Period prevalence* is the proportion of the population with the disorder at any time during a specified period, be it within the six months (called "six-month prevalence") or one month (called "one-month prevalence") before the assessment period. *Point prevalence* is the proportion of individuals with the disorder at a certain point in time. *Incidence* is the rate of new cases of a disorder in the population during a specified period of time (Verhulst, 1995). In psychiatric epidemiology, the most common time periods reported are lifetime, one year, and periods of three and six months. To calculate incidence, one needs at least two examinations of each person in the sample, namely, at the start and again at the end of the designated time period.

Measures of Risk

Common methods for measuring association in studies that used categorical data are relative risk and attributable risk. *Relative risk* is the likelihood of developing the disorder among a group of individuals who have a characteristic under study compared to another group of individual without the characteristic. *Attributable risk* refers to the proportion of the risk for developing a disorder when exposed to the factor which can be attributed to the exposure itself (Verhulst and Koot, 1992).

In case-control studies, measure of risk between the two disorders is quantified using the odds ratio. To compute the odds ratio for the co-occurrence of two disorders, the frequencies of the two concurrences are multiplied (i.e., both present and both absent) and then divided by the product of the frequencies of the two non-concurrences (i.e., one present and one absent).

Measures of Change

Life Table and Survival Analysis

Life table analyses are generally used to compute the rate of morbidity or mortality across a specified number of time intervals during the course of the follow-up period. As such, it can help to provide an estimation of the probability of developing or dying from a disease for a given period (Palinkas, 1985). A survival analysis can be used to characterize the survival time of an individual with an illness. In psychiatric epidemiology it can be used to define time to onset according to risk factors (i.e., survival to illness) as well as time to remission. Three functions commonly used to characterize the distribution of survival times in a cohort include the survivorship function, hazard function, and the probability density function (Palinkas, 1985). Burke and colleagues (1990, 1991) used life time survival analysis to compare the age of onset of some selected psychiatric disorders based on the ECA data (Epidemiologic Catchment Area Program) by birth cohorts. They used survival methods to examine the average yearly hazard rates for a specific 5-year age interval; a hazard rate refers to the estimated probability that a person who has not experienced an event at the beginning of an interval will experience that event during the interval (Boyle, 1995). Burke *et al.* (1990) showed adolescence and young adulthood as peak periods for the development of unipolar major depression, bipolar illness, phobias, and drug and alcohol abuse/dependence.

Multiple Logistic Regression

Multiple logistic regression is another widely used method to (i) describe the linear dependence of a disorder on a set of characteristics of a particular population; (ii) control for potential confounding factors as a means of evaluating the contribution of a specific variable; and (iii) to find structural relations among sets of variables and to provide causal explanations for these relationship (Palinkas, 1985). *Logistic regression analysis* is a common procedure to model the effects of certain variables in the etiology and continuity of the disorder. For example, Feehan *et al.* (1995) reported three logistic regression models to examine the influence of history of psychiatric problems, individual and family backgrounds, and the experience of major transition events on the continuity of disorder between ages 15 and 18. According to these analyses, none of the factors examined showed any significant influences on the strength of the association between disorder at ages 15 and 18 years.

Structural Equation Models

Structural equation models can be used to describe the measurement and structure of observed variables using simultaneous linear equations which represent the full causal structure of the observed data (Fergusson, 1995). As such, simultaneous linear equations can help protect against faulty causal inferences due to the lack of an explicit causal account of the structure of the predictor. However, in order to take the advantage of structural equation models, certain conditions need to be met, including: the availability of a well specified conceptual theory of the data that can be represented by a set of identified simultaneous linear equations, and the availability of data of sufficient quality and quantity that permits testing of theory (Fergusson, 1995). The used of structural equation models have recently gained increased popularity in epidemiological studies. As reviewed by Fergusson (1995), the models have been used in epidemiological studies of children and adolescents to estimate errors in reporting of substance use behaviours (Newcomb and Bentler, 1988), and to analyze cross-informant correlations in child behavioural data (Fergusson and Horwood, 1993).

CONCLUSION

As reviewed by Kazdin and Kagan (1994), there has been increased attention to studying the nature of psychiatric disorders in children and adolescents using various kind of research methods (e. g., epidemiological and family-genetic studies) and designs (cross-sectional and retrospective, and prospective longitudinal). This interest has been spurred by the finding of high prevalences of psychiatric disorders in these age groups, and by findings regarding the continuity of disorders or dysfunction over the course of development. As reported by recent epidemiological studies presented earlier, between 17 to 22% of those under 18 years of age have experienced some kind of psychiatric disorders. These studies have also indicated that the prevalence of psychiatric disorders in early life can not only predict future problems (e.g., dropping out of school, unemployment status), but can also increase the risk for having other disorders during adulthood. For this reason, more prospective longitudinal studies are needed to examine factors that may be involved in the development and maintenance of psychiatric disorders in children and adolescents.

REFERENCES

Achenbach, T.M., and Brown, J.S. (1991). *Bibliography of published studies using the Child Behavior Checklist and related materials.* Burlington: University of Vermont.

Achenbach, T.M., and Edelbrock, C. (1983). *Manual for the Child Behavior Checklist and Revised Child Behavior Profile.* Burlington: University of Vermont Department of Psychiatry.

Achenbach, T.M., and Edelbrock, C. (1981). Behavioral problems and competencies reported by parents of normal and disturbed children aged four through sixteen. *Monographs of the Society for Research in Child Development,* serial no. 188, 46.

Achenbach, T.M., and Edelbrock, C. (1986). *Manual for the Teacher's Report Form and teacher version of the Child Behavior Profile.* Burlington: University of Vermont Department of Psychiatry.

Achenbach, T.M., and Edelbrock, C. (1987). *Manual for the Youth Self-Report and Profile.* Burlington: University of Vermont Department of Psychiatry.

Anderson, J.C., Williams, S., McGee, R. and Silva, P.A. (1987). DSM-III disorders in preadolescent children. Prevalence in a large sample from the general population. *Archives of General Psychiatry,* **44**, 69–76.

Andreasen, N.C., Endicott, J., Spitzer, R.L., and Winokur, G. (1977). The family history method using diagnostic criteria. *Archives of General Psychiatry,* **34**, 1229–1235.

Andreasen, N.C., Rice, J., Endicott, J., Reich, T., and Coryell, W. (1986). The family history approach to diagnosis. *Archives of General Psychiatry,* **43**, 421–429.

Beck, A.T., Ward, C.H., Mendelson, M., Mock, J., and Erbaugh, J. (1961). An inventory for measuring depression. *Archives of General Psychiatry,* **4**, 53–63.

Bell, R.Q. (1953). Convergence: An accelerated longitudinal approach. *Child Development,* **24**, 145–152.

Berg, I., Rapoport, J.L., and Flament, M. (1986). The Leyton Obsessional Inventory — Child version. *Journal of the American Academy of Child Psychiatry,* **25**, 84–91.

Bird, H., Canino, G., Rubio-Stipec, M., Gould, M.S., Ribera, J., Sesman, M., Woodbury, M., Huertas-Goldman, S., Pagan, A., Sanchez-Lacay, A., and Moscoso, M. (1988). Estimates of the prevalence of childhood maladjustment in a community survey in Puerto Rico. *Archives of General Psychiatry,* **45**, 1120–1126.

Boyle, M.H. (1995). Sampling in epidemiological studies. In F.C. Verhulst and H.M. Koot (Eds.), *The epidemiology of child and adolescent psychopathology* (pp. 66–85). Oxford: Oxford University Press.

Boyle, M.H., Offord, D.R., Racine, Y., Fleming, J.E., Szatmari, P., and Sanford, M. (1993). Evaluation of the Revised Ontario Child Health Study Scales. *Journal of Child Psychology and Psychiatry,* **34**, 189–213.

Boyle, M.H., Offord, D.R., Racine, Y.A., and Catlin, G. (1991). Ontario Child Health Study follow-up: Evaluation of sample loss. *Journal of the American Academy of Child and Adolescent Psychiatry,* **30**, 449–456.

Boyle, M.H., Offord, D.R., Hofman, H.G., Catlin, G.P., Byles, J.A., Cadman, D.T., Crawford, J.W., Links, P.S., Rae-Grant, N.I., and Szatmari, P. (1987). Ontario Child Health Study: I. Methodology. *Archives of General Psychiatry,* **44**, 826–831.

Burke, K., Burke, J., Rae, D., and Regier, D. (1991). Comparing age at onset of major depression and other psychiatric disorders by birth cohorts in five U.S. community populations. *Archives of General Psychiatry,* **48**, 789–795.

Burke, K., Burke, J., Regier, D., and Rae, D. (1990). Age at onset of selected mental disorders in five community populations. *Archives of General Psychiatry*, **47**, 511–518.

Christie, K.A., Burke, J.D., Regier, D.A., Rae, D.S., Boyd, J.H., and Locke, B.Z. (1988). Epidemiologic evidence for early onset of mental disorders and higher risk of drug abuse in young adults. *American Journal of Psychiatry*, **44**, 971–975.

Cohen, P., Cohen, J., Kasen, S., Velez, C.N., Hartmark, C., Johnson, J., Rojas, M., Brook, J., and Streuning, E.L. (1993). An epidemiological study of disorders in late childhood and adolescence — I. Age- and gender-specific prevalence. *Journal Child Psychology and Psychiatry*, **34**, 851–866.

Connell, H.M., Irvine, L., and Rodney, J. (1982). Psychiatric disorder in Queensland primary school children. *Australian Pediatrics Journal*, **18**, 177–180.

Cooper, P.J., and Goodyer, I.M. (1993). A community study of depression in adolescent girls. I. Estimates of symptom and syndrome prevalence. *British Journal of Psychiatry*, **163**, 369–374.

Costello, E. J., and Angold, A. (1988). Scales to assess child and adolescent depression: Checklists, screens and nets. *Journal of the American Academy of Child and Adolescent Psychiatry*, **27**, 726–737.

Costello, A.J., Edelbrock, C., Kalas, R., Kessler, M., and Klaric, S. (1982). *The Diagnostic Interview Schedule for Children (DISC)*. Bethesda, MD: National Institute of Mental Health.

Derogatis, L.R., Lipman, R.S., and Covi, L. (1973). SCL-90: An outpatient Psychiatric rating scale-preliminary report. *Psychopharmacological Bulletin*, **9**, 13–28.

Dunn, L.M., and Dunn, L.M. (1981). *Peabody Picture Vocabulary Test-Revised*. American Guidance Service, Circle Pines, MN.

Endicott, J., and Spitzer, R. (1979). Use of Research Diagnostic Criteria and the Schedule for Affective Disorders and Schizophrenia to study affective disorders. *American Journal of Psychiatry*, **136**, 52–56.

Endicott, J., and Spitzer, R. (1978). A diagnostic interview: The Schedule for Affective Disorders and Schizophrenia. *Archives of General Psychiatry*, **35**, 837–844.

Esser, G., Schmidt, M.H., and Woerner, W. (1990). Epidemiology and course of psychiatric disorders in school-age children — results of a longitudinal study. *Journal of Child Psychology and Psychiatry*, **31**, 243–263.

Feehan, M., McGee, R., and Williams, S.M. (1993). Mental health disorders from age 15 to age 18 years. *Journal of the American Academy of Child and Adolescent Psychiatry*, **32**, 1118–1126.

Feehan, M., McGee, R., Nada-Raja, S., and Williams, S.M. (1994). DSM-III-R disorders in New Zealand 18-year-olds. *Australian and New Zealand Journal of Psychiatry*, **28**, 87–99.

Feehan, M., McGee, R., William, S.M., and Nada-Raja, S. (1995). Models of adolescent psychopathology: Childhood risk and the transition to adulthood. *Journal of the American Academy of Child and Adolescent Psychiatry*, **34**, 670–679.

Fergusson, D.M. (1995). A brief introduction to structural equation models. In F.C. Verhulst and H.M. Koot (Eds.), *The epidemiology of child and adolescent psychopathology* (pp. 122–145). Oxford: Oxford University Press.

Fergusson, D.M., and Horwood, L.J. (1993). The structure, stability and correlations of the trait components of conduct disorder, attention deficit and anxiety/withdrawal reports. *Journal of Child Psychology and Psychiatry*, **34**, 749–766.

Fergusson, D.M., Horwood, L.J., and Lynskey, M.T. (1993). Prevalence and comorbidity of DSM-III-R diagnoses in a birth cohort of 15 year olds. *Journal of the American Academy of Child and Adolescent Psychiatry*, **32**, 1127–1134.

Frost, L.A., Moffitt, T.E., McGee, R. (1989). Neuropsychological correlates of psychopathology in an unselected cohort of young adolescents. *Journal of Abnormal Psychology*, **98**, 307–313.

Garner, D.M., Olmstead, M.P., Bohr, Y., and Garfinkel, P.E. (1982). The Eating Attitudes Test: Psychometric features and clinical correlates. *Psychological Medicine*, **12**, 871–878.

Graham, P., and Rutter, M. (1968). The reliability and validity of psychiatric assessment of the child: II. Interview with the parent. *British Journal of Psychiatry,* **114**, 581–592.

Graham, P., and Rutter, M. (1973). Psychiatric disorders in the young adolescent: A follow-up study. *Proceedings of the Royal Society of Medicine,* **66**, 1226–1229.

Haynes, S.G., Levine, S., Scotch, N., and Feinlab, M. (1978). The relationship of psychosocial factors to coronary heart disease in the Framingham Study, I: Methods and risk factors. *American Journal of Epidemiology,* **107**, 362–383.

Kazdin, A.E. (1989). Identifying depression in children: A comparison of alternative selection criteria. *Journal of Abnormal Child Psychology,* **17**, 437–455.

Kazdin, A.E., and Kagan, J. (1994). Models of dysfunction in developmental psychopathology. *Clinical Psychological: Science and Practice, 1 (summer),* 35–52.

Kendler, K.S., Walters, E.E., Truett, K.R., Heath, A.C., Neale, M.C., Martin, N.G., and Eaves, L.J. (1994a). Sources of individual differences in depressive symptoms: Analysis of two samples of twins and their families. *American Journal of Psychiatry,* **151**, 1605–1614.

Kendler, K.S., Neale, M.C., Kessler, R.C., Heath, A.C., and Eaves, L.J. (1994b). The clinical characteristics of major depression as indices of the familial risk to illness. *British Journal of Psychiatry,* **165**, 66–72.

Leckman, J.F., Merikangas, K.R., Pauls, D.L., Prusoff, B.A., and Weissman, M.M. (1983). Anxiety disorders and depression: Contradictions between family study data and DSM-III conventions. *American Journal of Psychiatry,* **140**, 880–882.

Lewinsohn, P., Clarke, G., Seeley, J., and Rohde, P. (1994). Major depression in community adolescents: Age at onset, episode duration and time to recurrence. *Journal of the American Academy of Child and Adolescent Psychiatry,* **33**, 809–818.

Lewinsohn, P.M., Hops, H., Roberts, R.E., Seeley, J.R., and Andrews, J.A. (1993). Adolescent psychopathology: I. Prevalence and incidence of depression and other DSM-III-R disorders in high school students. *Journal of Abnormal Psychology,* **102**, 133–144.

Lilienfeld, A.M., and Lilienfeld, D.E. (1980). *Foundations of epidemiology.* New York: Oxford University Press.

Loeber, R., and Farrington, D.P. (1995). Longitudinal approaches in epidemiological research of conduct problems. In F.C. Verhulst and H.M. Koot (Eds.), *The epidemiology of child and adolescent psychopathology* (pp. 307–336). Oxford: Oxford University Press.

Loeber, R., Wung, P., Keenan, K., Giroux, B., Stouthamer-Loeber, M., Van Kammen, W.B., and Maughan, B. (1993). Developmental pathways in disruptive child behavior. *Development and Psychopathology,* **5**, 101–131.

Loeber, R., Green, S.M., and Lahey, B.B. (1990). Mental health professionals' perception of the utility of children, mothers and teachers as informants on childhood psychopathology. *Journal of Clinical Child Psychology,* **19**, 136–143.

Mazure, C., and Gershon, E.S. (1979). Blindness and reliability in lifetime psychiatric diagnosis. *Archives of General Psychiatry,* **36**, 521–525.

McConaughy, S.H., Stanger, C., and Achenbach, T.M. (1992). Three-year course of behavioral/emotional problems in a national sample of 4- to 16-year-olds: I. Agreement among informants. *Journal of the American Academy of Child and Adolescent Psychiatry,* **31**, 932–940.

McGee, R., Feehan, M., Williams, S., and Anderson, J. (1992). Mental health disorders from age 11 to age 15 years. *Journal of the American Academy of Child and Adolescent Psychiatry,* **31**, 50–59.

McGee, R., Silva, P.A., and Williams, S.M. (1983). Parents' and teachers' perceptions of behavior problems in seven year old children. *The Exceptional Child,* **30**, 151–161.

McGee, R., Williams, S., Anderson, J., McKenzie-Parnell, J.M., and Silva, P.A. (1990). Hyperactivity and serum and hair zinc levels in 11 year old children from the general population. *Biological Psychiatry,* **28**, 165–168.

McGee, R., Williams, S., and Feehan, M. (1994). Behavior problems in New Zealand children. In P.R. Joyce, R.T. Mulder, M.A. Oakley-Browne, J.D. Sellman and W.G.A. Watkins (Eds.), *Development, personality and psychopathology* (pp. 15–22). Christchurch: Christchurch School of Medicine.

McGee, R., Feehan, M., and Williams, S. (1995). Long-term follow-up of a birth cohort. In F.C. Verhulst and H.M. Koot (Eds.), *The epidemiology of child and adolescent psychopathology* (pp. 366–384). Oxford: Oxford University Press.

Moffitt, T.E., and Silva, P.A. (1988). Self-reported delinquency: Results from an instrument for New Zealand. *Australian and New Zealand Journal of Criminology, 21*, 227–240.

Morris, J.N. (1975). *Uses of epidemiology.* London: Churchill Livingstone.

Newcomb, M.D., and Bentler, P.M. (1988). *Consequences of adolescent drug use: Impact on the lives of young adults.* Beverly Hills: Sage.

Nichols, R.C., and Bilbro, W.C. (1966). The diagnosis of twin zygosity. *Acta Genetica, 16*, 265–275.

Offord, D.R., Boyle, M.H., Racine, Y.A., Fleming, J.E., Cadman, D.T., Blum, H.M., Byrne, C., Links, P.S., Lipman, E.L., MacMillan, H.L., Grant, N.I.R., Sanford, M.N., Szatmari, P., Thomas, H., and Woodward, C.A. (1992). Outcome, prognosis and risk in a longitudinal follow-up study. *Journal of the American Academy of Child and Adolescent Psychiatry, 31*, 916–923.

Orvaschel, H., Puig-Antich, J., Chambers, W., Tabrizi, M.A., and Johnson, R. (1982). Retrospective assessment of prepubertal major depression with the Kiddie-SADS-E. *Journal of the American Academy of Child Psychiatry, 21*, 392.

Orvaschel, H., Thompson, W.D., Belanger, A., Prusoff, B.A., and Kidd, K.K. (1982). Comparisons of the family history method to direct interview: Factors affecting the diagnosis of depression. *Journal of Affective Disorders, 4*, 49–59.

Palinkas, L.A. (1985). Techniques of psychosocial epidemiology. In P. Karoly (Ed.), *Measurement strategies in health psychology* (pp. 49–112). New York: Wiley.

Petermann, F. (1995). Methodische Grundlagen der Entwicklungspsychologie. In R. Oerter and I. Montada (Eds.), *Entwicklungspsychologie: Ein Lehrbuch* (pp. 1147–1176). Weinheim: Psychologie Verlags Union.

Piers, E., and Harris, D. (1969). *The Piers-Harris Children's Self-Concept Scale.* Nashville, TN: Counselor Recordings and Tests.

Puig-Antich, J. (1984). Affective disorders. In H.J. Kaplan and Sadock, B.J. (Eds.), *Comprehensive textbook of psychiatry* (pp. 1850–1861). Baltimore: Williams and Wilkins.

Puig-Antich, J., and Chambers, W. (1983). *The Schedule for Affective Disorders and Schizophrenia for School-aged Children* (6–18). New York: State Psychiatric Institute, New York.

Puig-Antich, J., Chambers, W., and Tabrizi, M.A. (1983). The clinical assessment of current depressive episodes in children and adolescents: Interviews with parents and children. In B.P. Cantwell and G.A. Carlson (Eds.), *Affective disorders in childhood and adolescence* (pp. 157–180). New York: SP Medical and Scientific Books.

Quay, H., and Peterson, D.R. (1987). *Manual for the revised behavior problem checklist.* Miami: Authors.

Reich, W., and Welner, Z. (1988). *Revised version of DICA for children ages 6–12.* St. Louis, MD: Washington University, Department of Psychiatry.

Reinherz, H.Z., Giaconia, R.M., Lefkowitz, E.S., Pakiz, B., and Frost, A.K. (1993a). Prevalence of psychiatric disorders in a community population of older adolescents. *Journal of the American Academy of Child and Adolescent Psychiatry, 32*, 369–377.

Reinherz, H.Z., Giaconia, R.M., Pakiz, B., Silverman, A.B., Frost, A.K., and Lefkowitz, E.S. (1993b). Psychosocial risks for major depression in late adolescence: A longitudinal community study. *Journal of the American Academy of Child and Adolescent Psychiatry, 32*, 1155–1163.

Robins, L.N. (1983). Continuities and discontinuities in the psychiatric disorders of children. In D. Mechanic (Ed.), *Handbook of health, health care and the health professions*. New York: Free Press.

Robins, L.N., Helzer, J.E., Cottler, L., and Goldring, E. (1989). *NIMH Diagnostic Interview Schedule version III revised*. St. Louis, MO: Washington University, Department of Psychiatry.

Rosenberg, M. (1986). *Conceiving the self*. Malabar, FL: Basic Books, Inc.

Rutter, M. (1989). Isle of Wright revisited: Twenty-five years of child psychiatric epidemiology. *Journal of the American Academy of Child and Adolescent Psychiatry*, **28**, 633–653.32,

Rutter, M. (1994). Beyond longitudinal data: Causes, consequences, changes and continuity. *Journal of Consulting and Clinical Psychology*, **62**, 928–940.

Rutter, M., Tizard, J., and Whitmore, K. (1970). *Education, health and behavior*. London: Longmans.

Rutter, M., and Quinton, D. (1977). Psychiatric disorder — ecological factors and concepts of causation. In M. McGurk (Ed.), *Ecological factors in human development* (pp. 173–187). Amsterdam: Nord-Hollandsche.

Seligman, M.E.P., Peterson, C., Kaslow, N.J., Tenenbaum, R.L., Alloy, L.B., and Abramson, L.Y. (1984). Attributional style and depressive symptoms among children. *Journal of Abnormal Psychology*, **93**, 235–241.

Shaffer, D., Gould, M.S., Brasic, J., Ambrosini, P., Fisher, P., Bird, H., and Aluwahlia, S. (1983). A children's global assessment scale (CGAS). *Archives of General Psychiatry*, **40**, 1228–1231.

Shapiro, R., and Keller, M. (1979). *Longitudinal Interval Follow-up Evaluation (LIFE)*. Unpublished manuscript.

Siegel, J.M., Matthews, K.A., and Leitch, C.J. (1981). Validation of the Type A interview assessment of adolescents: A multidimensional approach. *Psychosomatic Medicine*, **43**, 311–321.

Silva, P.A. (1990). The Dunedin Multidisciplinary Health and Developmental Study: A 15 year longitudinal study. *Paediatric and Perinatal Epidemiology*, **4**, 76–107.

Spitzer, R.L., Endicott, J., and Robins, E. (1978). Research diagnostic criteria: Rationale and reliability. *Archives of General Psychiatry*, **35**, 773–782.

Spitzer, R.L., Williams, J.B., and Gibbon, M. (1987). *Structured clinical interview for DSM-III-R*. New York: New York State Psychiatric Institute, Biometrics Research Department.

Stanger, C., Achenbach, T.M., and Verhulst, F.C. (1994). Accelerating longitudinal research in psychopathology. *Psychological Assessment*, **6**, 102–107.

Thapar, A., and McGuffin, P. (1994). A twin study of depressive symptoms in childhood. *British Journal of Psychiatry*, **165**, 259–265.

Thompson, W.D., Orvaschel, H., Prusoff, B., and Kidd, K.K. (1982). An evaluation of the family history method for ascertaining psychiatric disorders. *Archives of General Psychiatry*, **39**, 53–58.

Torgersen, S. (1983). Genetic factors in anxiety disorders. *Archives of General Psychiatry*, **40**, 1085–1089.

Verhulst, F.C. (1995). The epidemiology of child and adolescent psychopathology: Strengths and limitations. In F.C. Verhulst and H.M. Koot (Eds.), *The epidemiology of child and adolescent psychopathology* (pp. 1–21). Oxford: Oxford University Press.

Verhulst, F.C., and Koot, H.M. (1992). *Child psychiatric epidemiology: Concepts, methods and findings*. Beverly Hills: Sage Publications.

Verhulst, F.C., Koot, H.M., and Berden, G.F.M.G. (1990). Four-year follow-up of an epidemiological sample. *Journal of the American Academy of Child and Adolescent Psychiatry*, **29**, 440–448

Von Korff, M., and Eaton, W.W. (1989). Epidemiologic findings on panic. In R. Baker (Ed.), *Panic disorder: Theory, research and therapy* (pp. 35–50). New York: Wiley.

Vikan, A. (1985). Psychiatric epidemiology in a sample of 1510 ten-year-old children. I. Prevalence. *Journal of Child Psychology and Psychiatry,* **26,** 55–75.

Weissman, M.M. (1988). Psychopathology in the children of depressed parents: Direct interview studies. In D.L. Dunner, E.S. Gershon and J. Barret (Eds.), *Relatives at risk for mental disorder* (pp. 143–159). New York: Raven Press.

Weissman, M.M., and Bothwell, S. (1976). The assessment of social adjustment by patient self-report. *Archives of General Psychiatry,* **33,** 1111–1115.

Weissman, M.M., Fendrich, M., Warner, V., and Wickramaratne, P. (1992). Incidence of psychiatric disorder in offspring at high and low risk for depression. *Journal of the American Academy of Child and Adolescent Psychiatry,* **31,** 640–648.

Weissman, M.M., Kidd, K.K., and Prusoff, B.A. (1982). Variability in rates of affective disorders in relatives of depressed and normal probands. *Archives of General Psychiatry,* **39,** 1397–1403.

Weissman, M.W., Gershon, E.S., Kidd, K.K., Prusoff, J.F., Leckman, E., Dibble, E., Hamovit, J., Thompson, W.D., Pauls, D.L., and Guroff, J.J. (1984). Psychiatric disorders in the relatives of probands with affective disorders. *Archives of General Psychiatry,* **41,** 13–21.

Weissman, M.M., Merikangas, K.R., John, K., Wickramaratne, Prusoff, B.A., and Kidd, K.K. (1986). Family-genetic studies of psychiatric disorders. *Archives of General Psychiatry,* **43,** 1104–1116.

Weisz, J.R., and Eastman, K.L. (1995). Cross-cultural research on child and adolescent psychopathology. In F.C. Verhulst and H.M. Koot (Eds.), *The epidemiology of child and adolescent psychopathology* (pp. 42–65). Oxford: Oxford University Press.

Whitaker, A., Johnson, J., Shaffer, D., Rapoport, J.L., Kalikow, K., Walsh, B.T., Davies, M., Braiman, S., and Dolinsky, A. (1990). Uncommon troubles in young people: Prevalence estimates of selected psychiatric disorders in a nonreferred population. *Archives of General Psychiatry,* **47,** 487–496.

White, H.L., and Labouvie, E.W. (1989). Towards the assessment of adolescent problem drinking. *Journal of Stud. Alcohol,* **50,** 30–37

Wing, J.K., Cooper, J.E., and Sartorius, N. (1974). *The measurement and classification of psychiatric symptoms: An introduction manual for the Present State Examination and CATEGO programme.* London: Cambridge University Press.

Wittchen, H.-U., and Essau, C.A. (1993). Epidemiology of anxiety disorders. In P.J. Wilner (Ed.), *Psychiatry* (pp. 1–25). Philadelphia: J.B. Lippincott Company.

CHAPTER **4**

CONDUCT AND OPPOSITIONAL DEFIANT DISORDERS

Wendy M. Craig and Debra J. Pepler

The most common reason for referral to children's mental health or counselling services is for behaviours symptomatic of conduct disorder and oppositional defiant disorder (Offord *et al.*, 1987; Rutter, 1981). The term conduct disorder refers to the persistent display of serious antisocial actions (overt, covert, or both) that are extreme given the child's developmental level and that have a significant impact on the rights of others (American Psychiatric Association; APA, 1994). Oppositional defiant disorder (ODD) refers to negativistic, defiant, disobedient and hostile behavior toward authority figures (APA, 1994).

Children with conduct disorder and ODD are at risk for developing psychiatric disorders, chronic unemployment, divorce, motor vehicle accidents, dependence on welfare systems, and reduced levels of attainment and competence in adulthood (Caspi *et al.*, 1987; Kazdin, 1987a, 1993; Robins, 1966). Conduct disorder and ODD are not only chronic, but are often transmitted across generations (Huesmann *et al.*, 1984). Finally, these disorders often has severe effects on others such as siblings, peers, parents, teachers, and strangers who are victims of children's antisocial and aggressive acts. The monetary costs of conduct disorder are high: children with these disorders generate life-long costs because they are involved in multiple systems such as the mental health, juvenile justice, special education, and social services. Interrupting this pattern of behaviour is a critical issue. Consequently, over the last two decades there has been a surge of research on conduct disorder to understand its etiology and cause as a foundation for the development of prevention and intervention strategies. The goal of this chapter is to review the literature on the classification, epidemiology, etiology, course, and treatment research on conduct disorder and ODD. We contend that in order to advance research and prevention efforts in the area we need to examine the disorder from a developmental psychopathology perspective.

DEFINITION AND CLASSIFICATION

Conduct Disorder

The term conduct disorder encompasses a wide variety of behaviours such as aggression, disruptive behaviours, theft, vandalism, lying, truancy, delinquency, and running away. These behaviours can range in severity, chronicity, frequency, and in combinations among individuals. The DSM-IV (Diagnostic and Statistical Manual of Mental Disorders, Fourth Edition; APA, 1994) organizes these antisocial behaviours into four areas of functioning: aggression towards people or animals, destruction of property, deceitfulness or theft, and serious rule violation (Table 4.1). At least three criteria must have occurred during the previous year, with at least one of these present in the last 6 months. In addition, there must be significant impairment in social, academic, and/or occupational functioning. The symptoms are usually displayed across several contexts, such as home, school, and/or neighbourhood. A diagnosis of conduct disorder may occur for individuals older than eighteen, but only if the criteria for Antisocial Personality are not met. In the DSM-IV there is a distinction among individuals with mild, moderate, and severe forms of conduct disorder. Mild conduct disorder is characterized by few if any conduct problems which cause relatively minor harm to others. Symptoms of the mild type may include: lying, truancy, and staying out after dark without permission. Moderate conduct disorder is characterized by more problems and a greater effect on others than mild conduct disorder. Severe conduct disorder is characterized by conduct problems in excess of those required to make a diagnosis which cause considerable harm to others. Symptoms of the severe type may include: forced sex, physical cruelty, use of weapons, stealing while confronting a victim, and breaking and entering.

In the ICD-10, there is a general definition for the broad category of conduct disorder (designated as F91), followed by definitions of more specific subcategories, such as undersocialized conduct disorder-aggressive type, undersocialized conduct disorder — unaggressive type, and socialized conduct disorder (World Health Organization; WHO, 1993). The ICD-10 also defines these types as unspecified, mild, moderate, and severe. Both the DSM-IV and the ICD-10 share the general Kraepelinian model in that each disorder is assumed to be either present or absent and categorically distinct from every other disorder.

One of the problems in the literature on conduct disorder is that the behaviours which characterize conduct disorder change with development. The diagnosis of conduct disorder according to the DSM-IV requires

Table 4.1   DSM-IV diagnostic criteria for conduct disorder

A. A repetitive and persistent pattern of behavior in which the basic rights of others or major age-appropriate societal norms or rules are violated as manifested by the presence of three (or more) of the following criteria in the past 12 months, with at least one criterion present in the past 6 months:

Aggression toward people and animals
1. often bullies, or intimidates others
2. often initiates physical fights
3. has used a weapon that can cause serious harm to others
4. has been physically cruel to people
5. has been physically cruel to animals
6. has stolen while confronting a victim
7. has forced someone into sexual activity

Destruction of property
8. has deliberately engaged in fire setting
9. has deliberately destroyed others' property (other than by fire setting)

Deceitfulness or theft
10. has broken into someone else's house, building or car
11. often lies to obtain goods or favours or to avoid obligations (i.e., cons others)
12. has stolen items of nontrival value without confronting the victim

Serious rule violations
13. often stays out at night despite parental prohibition, beginning before the age of 13 years
14. has run away from home overnight at least twice while living in parental surrogate home (or once without returning for a lengthy period)
15. is often truant from school, beginning before the age of 13 years

B. The disturbance in behavior causes clinically significant impairment in social, academic, or occupational functioning

C. If the individual is age 18 years or older, criteria are not met for Antisocial Personality Disorder

Reprinted with permission from the Diagnostic and Statistical Manual of Mental Disorders, Fourth Edition. Copyright 1994 American Psychiatric Association.

the same number of criterion behaviour problems regardless of age and sex. This diagnostic approach does not take into account normative developmental changes and gender differences in behaviour. Consequently, the prevalence of conduct disorder may vary by sex and age as a function of the base rate of these particular behaviours at different stages in development (Achenbach, 1993). For example, a high proportion of adolescents engage in some deviant behaviour, but not all of these adolescents are at psychiatric risk (Elliot *et al.*, 1985). A developmental increase in the prevalence of conduct disorder may reflect an increase in the normative nature of the criterion behaviours rather than an increase in the actual number of individuals who have conduct disorder. Similarly, current criteria of conduct disorder comprise behaviours that may be more typical of boys than girls, such as cruelty to animals, physical attacks, and getting into fights. The lack of recognition of age and gender differences may obscure the developmental course of disorders for which specific manifestations change with age. These concerns highlight the importance of clarifying and defining more rigorously the taxonomy for conduct disorder.

Subtypes of Conduct Disorder

Conduct disorder is a heterogenous diagnostic category (Farrington, 1987; Kazdin, 1987a), consequently researchers have proposed subtypes of conduct disorder. For example, DSM-III-R (APA, 1987) allows for the distinction among three types of conduct disorder: group type, solitary aggressive type, and undifferentiated type. Individuals with conduct disorder who are capable of sustaining social relationships and commit antisocial acts with other deviant peers are classified as the socialized or group type. Individuals who do not maintain interpersonal relations and commit antisocial acts alone are referred to as undersocialized. Children with undifferentiated type of conduct disorder engage in both forms of antisocial behaviour. Although these subtypes have been specified, researchers rarely differentiate among subtypes of conduct disordered individuals. The undersocialized type tends to be more aggressive than the socialized type (Stattin and Magnusson, 1990). Lahey (1992) has speculated that the undersocialized classification of conduct disorder may characterize those individuals who have a childhood-onset of conduct disorder, while the socialized subtype characterizes those individuals with an adolescent-onset. The DSM-IV, however specifies childhood-versus adolescent-onset as the primary subtypes. These subtypes differ with respect to the nature of the presenting conduct problems, developmental course, prognosis, and gender ratio. Both subtypes can occur in mild, moderate, or severe severity.

Childhood-Onset. The childhood-onset type is defined by the presence of at least one criterion characteristic of conduct disorder before the age of 10 years. Individuals with a childhood-onset begin to demonstrate ODD in early childhood and they progress toward the early symptoms of conduct disorder (lying, fighting, stealing), and in some cases these individuals become involved in more serious antisocial behaviour such as property crimes and interpersonal violence (Farrington, 1993).

Adolescent-Onset. This subtype of conduct disorder is defined as the absence of any criteria characteristic of conduct disorder before the age of 10 years. Adolescent-onset of conduct disorder is the most common developmental pathway and it involves little antisocial or oppositional behaviour during childhood. The first delinquent offense occurs generally around age fourteen or fifteen for the adolescent-onset group, while for the childhood-onset it is usually between age ten and twelve. Individuals with an adolescent-onset of conduct disorder tend to be less severe in their offending and are more likely to desist from their offending after adolescence compared with individuals with a childhood-onset (Lahey, 1992).

Other taxonomies for classifying antisocial behaviour include differentiating between individuals with primary symptoms of aggression versus stealing (Patterson, 1982); reactive versus proactive aggression (Dodge, 1993a); and overt (e.g., fighting) versus covert (lying, stealing) antisocial acts (Loeber, 1990). The recognition of subtypes of conduct disorder is important because it suggests different developmental pathways leading to a conduct disorder diagnosis. As a result, there may be different points of maximal effectiveness in prevention and intervention efforts. Nonetheless, the first step in subtyping is validation and reliability of the classification system. This is an area requiring future research.

Features of Childhood- and Adolescent-Onset

The empirical evidence for distinguishing childhood- from adolescent-onset is mounting and it is becoming increasingly accepted that there are multiple pathways leading to a diagnosis of conduct disorder. The developmental progression, precipitating factors, and adult outcomes are different for those with a childhood-onset than for those with an adolescent-onset of conduct disorder.

Individuals with a childhood-onset of conduct disorder are likely to have more early negative socialization influences and training for antisocial behaviour, which are not part of the early experiences of adolescent-onset individuals. With less stressful formative differences, the adolescent-onset individual is less likely to experience academic failure or peer rejection compared to the childhood-onset. Recently researchers have argued that the childhood-onset and adolescent-onset forms of conduct disorder have different correlates and prognoses, as well as etiologies (e.g., Moffitt, 1993a). Moffitt (1993a) has suggested that childhood-onset of conduct disorder may be more related to neurological deficits, whereas adolescent-onset of conduct disorder may be more related to peer influences. Quay (1988) and Lahey *et al.* (1988) found that individual differences in sympathetic and neuroendrocrine functioning characterize the aggressive childhood-onset group but not the nonaggressive adolescent-onset. This research is in its infancy, and consequently the conclusion that there may be both neurological and physiological differences that contribute to the etiology, onset, and prognosis of conduct disorder which differentiate adolescent- and childhood-onset requires further research.

Individuals in the childhood-onset pathway tend to first develop ODD and then later add the aggressive and nonaggressive symptoms of conduct disorder. Individuals with the adolescent-onset do not exhibit ODD in childhood and tend not to develop symptoms of aggression (Lahey, 1992) suggesting that there are different factors in the etiology of nonaggressive conduct disorder behaviour with childhood-onset as compared to those with adolescent-onset. Children showing continuity and early disruptive behaviours are differentiated from those who later desist by the frequency of their early symptoms, the occurrence of their symptoms in multiple contexts, the variety of problems at an early age, and the co-occurrence of hyperactivity (Campbell, 1993; Moffitt, 1990).

Robins (1966) reported that individuals with an onset of conduct disorder before the age of 11 were twice as likely to receive an adult diagnosis of antisocial personality disorder than those with an onset after the age of 11. McGee *et al.* (1990) found that individuals with an adolescent-onset of conduct disorder were as likely to be arrested as individuals with an earlier onset, but they were less likely to be involved in highly aggressive offenses. They also found that the adolescent-onset cases of nonaggressive conduct disorder included more females than males. For females the average age of onset was 11 years of age compared to 15 for males. Thus, there are qualitative differences in the frequency, severity, and long-term outcomes between individuals with a childhood-onset and individuals with an adolescent-onset of conduct disorder and for males and females.

Although individuals with a childhood-onset of conduct disorder account for a small percentage of the population (about 3–5%), they account for a disproportionate number of delinquent acts (Hinshaw *et al.*, 1993). Elliot *et al.* (1985) found that these individuals account for almost half the crimes committed by children and adolescents.

Furthermore, these individuals tend to be more aggressive than those with an adolescent-onset hence, they are likely to be responsible for the majority of violent crimes. About half of the individuals with childhood-onset become delinquent adolescents, and approximately half to three quarters of adolescent delinquents become adult offenders (Farrington, 1987). Thus, children with a childhood-onset of conduct disorder are more likely to stay on the antisocial behaviour trajectory than those with a later onset.

Oppositional Defiant Disorder

ODD is characterized by a recurrent pattern of negativistic, defiant, disobedient, and hostile behaviour toward authority figures (Table 4.2). Negativistic and defiant behaviours are expressed by persistent stubbornness, resistance to follow directions, and unwillingness to

Table 4.2   DSM-IV diagnostic criteria for oppositional defiant disorder

---

A. A pattern of negativistic, hostile, and defiant behavior lasting at least 6 months, during which four (or more) of the following are present:

1. often loses temper
2. often argues with adults
3. often actively defies or refuses to comply with adults' requests or rules
4. often deliberately annoys people
5. often blames others for his or her mistakes or misbehavior
6. is often touchy or easily annoyed by others
7. is often angry and resentful
8. is often spiteful or vindictive

Note: Consider a criterion met only if the behavior occurs more frequently than is typically observed in individuals of comparable age and developmental level.

B. The disturbance in behavior causes clinically significant impairment in social, academic, or occupational functioning

C. The behaviors do not occur exclusively during the course of a psychotic or mood disorder

D. Criteria are not met for conduct disorder, and, if the individual is age 18 years or older, criteria are not met for Antisocial Personality Disorder

---

compromise (APA, 1994), and hostility is shown by annoying others purposely. The symptoms of ODD includes: losing temper, arguing with adults, actively defying or refusing to comply with adults' requests or rules, deliberately annoying people, blaming others for his or her mistakes or misbehavior, being touchy or easily annoyed by others, being angry and resentful, and being spiteful or vindictive. In order to meet the diagnosis, four or more of these symptoms must be frequently present when compared to that which is typically observed in individuals of comparable age and developmental level. These symptoms also cause major impairment in social, academic, or occupational functioning.

Unlike conduct disorder, very few studies have been devoted to ODD. Therefore, in the following sections we will concentrate on reporting results of studies on conduct disorder.

EPIDEMIOLOGY

Estimates of the prevalence of conduct disorder in the general population range from 2 to 9% for persons under age sixteen (Institute of Medicine, 1989). In the United States, this percentage translates into approximately 1.3 to 3.8 million cases. Population estimates using standardized diagnostic criteria indicate prevalence rates of 12% for moderate levels of conduct disorder and 4% for severe levels of conduct disorder (Cohen *et al.*, 1993). The prevalence of ODD is about 6%, with values ranging from 1.7% to 9.9% (Anderson *et al.*, 1987; Bird *et al.*, 1988; Lewinsohn *et al.*, 1993).

RISK FACTORS

There is controversy about whether certain behaviours are the causes or the result of antisocial behaviour. Several mechanisms associated with the regulation of emotion, cognition, and behaviour are thought to underlie the development and maintenance of conduct disorder behaviour (Greenberg *et al.*, 1993; Moffitt, 1993b; Quay, 1993). Below is a brief review of factors that may influence the development of conduct disorder. Because conduct disorder is multiply determined, it is important to remember that these factors, although presented separately in this chapter, interact to place a child at risk for conduct disorder. Moffitt (1993a) notes a contradiction in the developmental course of antisocial behaviour and neurological damage. Although antisocial behaviour gets worse over time, a frequent progression for neurological impairment is an improvement, if not recovery. She suggests that the effects of early neuropsychological vulnerabilities are amplified over time as children interact with their environment. In this way children with neurological impairments and conduct problems may be at particularly high risk.

Sociodemographic Factors

Gender

Conduct disorder is about twice as prevalent in preadolescent boys as in girls. This sex ratio, however, diminishes from studies in preadolescent children to adolescents (Zoccolillo, 1993). Cohen *et al.* (1993) found that for boys the prevalence of conduct disorder was highest in the youngest group studied (age 10) and declined over the ages 10 to 20. In contrast, there was a peak prevalence for girls around age 16, followed by a sharp decline. The prevalence rates for males under the age of eighteen range from 6 to 16%, while for females rates range from 2 to 9% (APA, 1994). For example, Esser *et al.* (1990) report a conduct disorder prevalence of 6% and 5% for 13-year-old males and females. Similarily, McGee *et al.* (1990) report a conduct disorder prevalence of 7.2% and 7.4% for conduct disorder for 15-year-old males and females. The Ontario Child Health Study (Offord *et al.*, 1987), a community survey indicated a decrease in the sex ratio in the prevalence of conduct disorder from childhood to adolescence: in childhood, the prevalence of conduct disorder was 6.5% and 1.8% for boys and girls, respectively (a ratio of 3.6: 1). In adolescence, the prevalence of conduct disorder were 10.4% and 4.1% for boys and girls, respectively (a ratio of 2.5:1). Although there was an increase in prevalence of conduct disorder for girls by adolescence, it was not equal to the males adolescent prevalence rate. The rate for ODD was also higher in boys than in girls, however, only in prepubertal age because the rate in adolescents is comparable in the two sexes (Anderson *et al.*, 1987; Bird *et al.*, 1988; Lewinsohn *et al.*, 1993).

Given the differences in prevalence rates of conduct disorder for males and females, some researchers argue that being a male increases the risk of a diagnosis of conduct disorder (Loeber *et al.*, 1991). There are, however, relatively few published studies of conduct disorder and related behaviours in girls (Zoccolillo, 1993). The paucity of research on females with conduct disorder is probably due to the fact that the majority of studies derive from a criminal justice perspective where there are more males than females. Males have higher arrest and imprisonment rates and also commit more serious crimes than females. The social costs of male aggression has focused research efforts on males with conduct disorder (Robins, 1991). By contrast, girls' transgressions are often dealt with outside the criminal justice system. In addition, the criteria for the conduct disorder according to the DSM-IV are largely derived from studies with males only.

Despite the gender bias in the research, conduct disorder is the second most common diagnosis in adolescent females, with prevalence rates varying from less than 1 to 16% (Zoccolillo, 1993). Furthermore, gender differences in the prevalence of conduct disorder diminishes from preadolescence to adolescence. One interpretation of this finding is that conduct disorder has a later onset than in males. The childhood-onset of conduct disorder is far more common in males than females, ranging from 3:1 to 4:1 (Anderson *et al.*, 1987). In contrast, the ratio for males to females in adolescent-onset is 1:1 (Esser *et al.*, 1990; McGee *et al.*, 1992).

A second interpretation is that we have not adequately assessed the developmental trajectories of females with conduct disorder which may differ from those of men. When males and females with conduct disorder are compared, there are sex differences in the manifestations of conduct disorder. Lewis and colleagues (1991) found that females are arrested less often and for less serious offenses than conduct disorder males. Robins (1986) found that females diagnosed with conduct disorder were more likely to experience internalizing problems in adulthood than men. Females are less likely to manifest criminal behaviour, and are more likely to report somatization disorder either alone or with antisocial symptoms or antisocial personality disorder than males (Lewis *et al.*, 1991).

These findings on sex differences in conduct disorder raise the question of using different criteria to diagnose males and females with conduct disorder. Zoccollilo (1993) argues for differential criteria because: (1) some behaviours are more common in one sex than in the other; and (2) on some criteria it makes no sense to have the same threshold. For example, males are more likely than females to be arrested; therefore, any criterion based on the frequency of arrests could be interpreted differently for males and females. Other researchers argue against using different criteria to identify conduct disorder in males and females (Zahn-Waxler, 1993).

At present, we lack a full understanding of gender differences in the manifestation of conduct disorder. As Zahn-Waxler (1993) suggested, the etiology of conduct disorder should be investigated further to provide data relevant to its diagnosis such as: the different forms of antisocial behaviour in males and females; gender differences in other domains that may contribute to differences in antisocial behaviour (e.g., temperament, emotionality, physical and language development); and differential socialization practices that are implicated in adaptive and maladaptive development. Traditionally, researchers have not examined sex differences in the mechanisms and processes implicated in the development of conduct disorder, consequently questions remain as to the significance of gender in the development of conduct disorder.

Biological Factors

Individual differences in the internal organization at the physiological, neurological, and neurophysiological levels are implicated in the development of conduct disorder. Some of these biological factors may be transmitted genetically, while others may be due to perinatal trauma, prenatal or childhood exposure to neurotoxin (e.g., drugs, alcohol), other physical traumas (e.g., head injury in childhood), or effects of environmental deprivation on neuroanatomical growth.

Neurological Functioning

Individual differences in neuropsychological functioning of children with conduct disorder may be a result of an interaction or a combination of the reviewed factors below. Moffitt (1993a) proposes that a disruption in the ontogenesis of the fetal brain (e.g., maternal drug abuse, pre-post natal nutrition, and/or exposure to toxic agents) or child abuse, neglect or heritability may result in a chain of interactions that accumulate to produce antisocial and acting out behaviour characteristic of conduct disorder.

Neuropsychological functioning has implications for motor and cognitive development as well as personality. For example, toddlers with neurological impairment may be delayed in reaching developmental milestones and consequently may be clumsy, awkward, and overactive. They may also experience a number of cognitive deficits such as inattention, poor verbal comprehension, and other language and cognitive difficulties. Moffitt (1993a) notes that it may be more difficult for parents of children with neurological difficulties to support their cognitive and social development. These children may be more likely to evoke a chain of negative parent-child interactions. Neurological functioning is related to risk for maltreatment and abuse, punitive and harsh disciplinary techniques, and coercive interactions. These negative early experiences may generalize to other settings and consolidate into conduct disorder symptoms. In summary, Moffitt (1993a) suggests that children with neuropsychological deficits may evoke dysfunctional reactions from parents, especially under conditions of family adversity. The child may become ensnared in interactions that accumulate in a diagnosis of conduct disorder. Compromised neurological functioning may put a child at risk for conduct disorder and this risk may be perpetuated or exacerbated by interactions with the social environment, with adults, peers, at home and at school. At present, however, the role of neurological deficits in stimulating or sustaining patterns of antisocial behaviour is mostly speculation.

Heredity

Twin studies are frequently conducted to demonstrate the role of genetic factors in placing an individual at risk for conduct diorder. Higher concordance rates (i.e., the likelihood that one twin has the disorder if the other twin does) among monozygotic versus dizygotic twins indicates that there is genetic loading for the disorder. Gottesman *et al.* (1983) have found that for conduct disorder the concordance rate is nearly twice as great among monozygotic twins compared to dizygotic twins. The concordance rates for delinquency among monozygotic and dizygotic twins are 87% and 72%, respectively (Plomin, 1991). Similarly, adoption studies have indicated that conduct disorder in an offspring is more likely when a relative has had conduct disorder (Cadoret, 1986). Taken together these results indicate that there is genetic contribution to the development of conduct disorder. The genetic factor may interact with environmental factors to contribute to the development of conduct disorder.

Cadoret and colleagues (1986) highlight the interaction between heredity and environment in the etiology of adolescent antisocial behaviour. Dodge (1990) recently criticized efforts to examine the main effects of nature or nurture in conduct disorder, and emphasized the importance of focusing on the mechanisms and how they interact during development to contribute to the diagnosis of conduct disorder. However, there is some evidence to suggest that heredity plays a role in conduct disorder. Antisocial behaviour was higher in monozygotic twins reared apart than dizygotic twins reared apart (Moffitt, 1993b). Moffitt (1993b) argues for a transactional model examining neuropsychological vulnerability in the executive and verbal functioning may interact with other known risk factors such as family adversity, school failure, and poverty.

Biochemical Factors

Research in biochemical psychophysiological, and experimental-based behaviour studies of undersocialized aggressive children with conduct disorder, suggests that there are possible efficiency deficits in the brain's noradrenenergic and serotonergic systems implicated in activation and inhibition of aggression. Krusesi *et al.* (1992) found that there were significantly lower levels of serotonin in children and adolescents hospitalized for disruptive behaviour (including conduct disorder) compared to matched controls. In addition, some studies report that electrodermal responses to external stimuli, an index of sympathetic functioning processes related to anxiety and inhibition, tend to be diminished in groups of aggressive children and adolescents (Raine *et al.*, 1990).

Daugherty and Quay (1991) found that children with conduct disorder have a specific learning deficit in which they are more likely to continue in the face of failure. Lewis (1991) has reported serotonergic dysfunction in sociopaths linking the inability of the psychopath to learn from experience to similar findings from animal learning research on low serotonin levels. Thus, these biochemical deficits may put an individual at risk for conduct disorder as well as contribute to their academic problems.

Psychological/Social Factors

Family Characteristics and Relationships

Family-based risk factors associated with conduct disorder are listed in the DSM-IV (APA, 1994) and include: parental rejection, inconsistent management with harsh discipline, early institutional living, frequent shifting of parental figures (e.g. from parents to step-parents, to grandparents, to friends), large family size, involvement in delinquent groups, and the presence of an alcoholic father. Parental and family risk factors for conduct disorder can be classified into four domains: family demographics, parental characteristics, parenting techniques and parent-child relationships (Loeber and Stouthamer-Loeber, 1986).

Family demographic characteristics such as race, neighbourhood, parental education, income, and occupation are related to the prevalence of conduct disorder (Elliot *et al.*, 1985). For example, low socioeconomic status is associated with increased prevalence of conduct disorder (Rutter *et al.*, 1970). Family stressors such as unemployment, family violence, marital discord, and divorce are also associated with higher rates of conduct disorder (Farrington, 1987; Lewis *et al.*, 1987). Other risk factors in this domain include an adverse early rearing environment or early traumas such as poor housing, poor parental job record (Farrington, 1993), single parenting (Webster-Stratton, 1985), domestic violence (Offord *et al.*, 1991), and child abuse (Widom, 1991; Dodge *et al.*, 1990).

Characteristics of the parents are also linked to conduct disorder. Longitudinal studies point to the consistency of aggressive behaviour patterns over three generations and punishment over two generations (Huesmann *et al.*, 1984). Individuals with conduct disorder tend to have depressed and irritable mothers (Forehand and Long, 1988), antisocial or drug abusing parents (Offord *et al.*, 1991). In an epidemiological study, Offord *et al.* (1991) found that parents of conduct disorder children are more likely to exhibit Antisocial Personality Disorder and abuse drugs than parents of children without conduct disorder. In addition, children with conduct disorder tend to have mothers who exhibit more depression or somatization disorder (Williams *et al.*, 1990). Frick and colleagues (1992) found that the father's psychopathology and not the behaviour problems of the child or the mother's psychological adjustment was predictive of future delinquency. Criminal behaviour and alcoholism of the father are two of the stronger and consistently demonstrated parental characteristics associated with conduct disorder in youth. Thus, parental psychopathology (particularly internalizing problems for the mother and externalizing problems for the father) is a risk factor for conduct disorder.

Inept parenting techniques such as poor monitoring, physical coercion, and little positive reinforcement with children (Patterson *et al.*, 1992) have also been identified as risk factors for conduct disorder. Researchers have documented an empirical relationship among family interaction styles and children's behavioral problems. Coercive and inconsistent disciplinary practices operate in the onset and maintenance of aggressive behaviour (e.g., Patterson, 1982). According to Patterson (1982), the effects of family demographic variables on the development of children's aggressive behaviour are mediated by parenting practices, which break down under stressful family circumstances. Stress within the family exacerbates parents' antisocial tendencies, which in turn lead to irritable discipline practices and children's aggressive behaviour problems. Patterson's model illustrates how parental and family influences may operate together to place the child at risk for developing conduct problems (Loeber, 1990).

In a meta-analysis of family factors, Loeber and Stouthamer-Loeber (1986) concluded that lack of parental supervision was one of the strongest predictors of the development of conduct disorder and delinquency. Patterson and his colleagues have described how the breakdown of parenting practices and family management may provide the background for aggressive behaviour problems (Patterson, 1982, 1986; Patterson *et al.*, 1989). Their research indicates that families of aggressive children support the use of aversive and aggressive behaviours in their children by inadvertently reinforcing aggressive behaviours and by failing to adequately reinforce prosocial behaviours (Patterson, 1982). Through these processes, parents of aggressive children fail in teaching compliance and appropriate social problem solving which leads to a process of coercive family interactions and the development of aggressive behaviour patterns in the children. A number of studies have also cited a lack of parent-child involvement and parental rejection of the child as predictors of later aggressive behaviour problems and delinquency (e.g., Farrington, 1993; Loeber and Stouthamer-Loeber, 1986).

Harsh physical punishment has been implicated in the development of aggressive behaviour patterns (e.g., Farrington, 1993). Dodge *et al.* (1990) found that early physical harm was associated with aggression toward peers, above and beyond any co-occurring family ecological factor or child health problem and temperament. Dodge and his colleagues found that children who received harsh physical punishment were likely to develop biased and deficient patterns of social information processing. These include a failure to attend to relevant cues, a bias to attribute hostile intentions to others, and a lack of competent behavioral strategies to solve interpersonal problems. Social information processing patterns were, in turn, found to predict the development of aggressive behaviour. These findings suggest a mechanism in the development of conduct disorder: abuse at the hands of parents leads children to think and solve problems in deviant ways that later lead to the development of aggressive behaviour patterns and a continuation of the cycle of violence (Dodge *et al.*, 1990).

Robins (1978) implicates the following parenting variables as risk factors in conduct disorder: a negative parent-child dyadic relationship, the role of poor attachment, the role of nonsynchrony (i.e., ability of parents to align or calibrate their behaviour to meet the needs of the child), the ability of the parents to behave in a concerned matter about others and provide their children with abstract reasons for doing things, and the willingness of the parents to impart social values through modelling, teaching, and sanctioning of values. Dysfunctional relations are reflected in families of troubled youth who tend to be less accepting of their children, less warm, affectionate, and emotional supportive, compared to parents of nonreferred youths (Kazdin, 1993). Individuals with conduct disorder tend to have families who are characterized by low support, defensive communication among family members, low participation in activities as a family, and dominance of a family member.

Greenberg and his colleagues (Greenberg *et al.*, 1993) suggest that individuals with conduct disorder have a history of inadequate caregiving and insecure attachment relationships. These inadequacies are likely reflected in children's representational models of attachment figures and of the self in relation to others. As a result, these children may perceive the world as hostile and thereby expect negative interactions and patterns of behaviour. Through these processes, insecure attachment is a risk factor for conduct disorder.

In summary, direct as well as indirect influences comprise the risk factors for conduct disorder. These include: child rearing practises (Pettit and Bates, 1989), family relationships, and psychopathology such as having a delinquent male sibling (Patterson, 1986), and fighting with siblings (Loeber *et al.*, 1983). These factors are not all present in individuals with conduct disorder, but rather some combination and interaction among them may put an individual at risk for conduct disorder.

Academic Performance

Academic deficiencies and lower levels of intellectual functioning are associated with conduct disorder. For example, West (1982) and Rutter and Giller (1983) found that intellectual and school performance as measures by verbal and nonverbal intelligence test, school grades, and achievement tests were positively correlated with measures of conduct disorder such as self-report, teacher-report, and official records. Poor academic success may be a risk factor as well as process factor. For example, children with conduct disorder may be less successful at school because they spend less time at school (because of truancy, expulsion) and they spend less time with the teacher. In addition, academic failure is also related to other variables such as socioeconomic status, and family size. However, even when these variables are controlled for, academic failure is a unique predictor of conduct disorder (West, 1982). Thus, while academic failure is a risk factor for conduct disorder, the relationship is not unidirectional. Conduct disorder predicts subsequent academic failure and a lower level of educational attainment (Ledingham and Schwartzman, 1984).

Verbal Deficits

Cognitive and linguistic problems precede the development of conduct disorder. White *et al.* (1990) found broad deficiencies in acculturational learning rather than narrow social cognitive differences. Meltzer *et al.* (1984) found significant differences in the kind and frequency of reading style and errors, spelling style and errors, the mechanics and organization of the formulation of writing and mathematical errors in delinquents and nondelinquents. As early as grade two, 45% of delinquents exhibited differences in reading and 35% had delays in handwriting.

Skoff and Libon (1987) found deficiencies in the executive functioning in approximately two-thirds of the juvenile delinquents in their sample. Brickman *et al.* (1984) found that expressive speech and memory scales differentiated delinquents from nondelinquents. In a review of the literature, Moffitt (1993a) concluded that two cognitive factors play an important role in the etiology of conduct disorder: lesions in the left frontal lobe and the lobe's involvement with the limbic system. These are related to specific verbal skill deficits (e.g., expression and comprehension) and executive dysfunction (e.g., poor inhibitory control).

Social Cognition

Aggressive children tend to have a variety of cognitive, perceptual, and attributional deficits (Dodge *et al.*, 1990). For example, they tend to inaccurately interpret peers' intentions (Dodge *et al.*, 1990), infer a hostile intent (Lochman, 1992), fail to attend to relevant social cues (Dodge *et al.*, 1990), misjudge aggression as a means to a positive outcome and have deficits in problem solving skills and verbal-assertive strategies (Dodge *et al.*, 1990). Slaby and Guerra (1988) found that antisocial adolescent offenders had a dysfunctional, predictable pattern of problem solving, which included a hostile definition of the problem, choosing hostile goals, low frequency of seeking facts, creating few alternatives, and poor anticipation of the consequences of their choices.

Self-control Deficits

Antisocial behaviour is associated with deficiencies in the brain's self-control functions. These executive functions include: sustaining attention and concentration, formulating goals, abstract reasoning and concept formation, anticipating and planning, programming and initiating purposeful sequences of behaviours, self-monitoring, self-awareness, inhibiting unsuccessful or impulsive behaviours (Moffitt, 1993a).

In summary, conduct disorder is multiply determined by interactions among these biological processes and other social and environmental processes (Moffitt, 1993a). There is likely to be considerable heterogeneity in the etiology, developmental course, and mechanisms operating within the population of children and adolescents with conduct disorder. Consequently, chronically antisocial behaviour is likely to be the end product of complex, multifactorial processes operating within and outside a given individual, but relevant causal processes are likely to differ across individuals (Cicchetti and Richters, 1993). Much more work is needed to understand the etiology, mechanisms, and developmental pathways of conduct disorder. Understanding these processes and their contribution to conduct disorder will increase the efficacy of prevention and treatment efforts.

COMORBIDITY

From the above discussion, it is apparent that children and adolescents with conduct disorder experience multiple problems in multiple domains. Epidemiological research indicates that among individuals who meet the criteria for conduct disorder, approximately half will meet the criteria for another type of diagnosis (Anderson *et al.*, 1987). Two important conditions which are often comorbid with conduct disorder are Attention Deficit/Hyperactivity Disorder (ADHD) (45–70% of the cases) (Hinshaw, 1987; Hinshaw *et al.*, 1993; Loney, 1987; Kazdin, 1993). Children displaying both ADHD and conduct disorder show more physical aggression, a greater range of antisocial behaviours, greater persistence of antisocial behaviours, more severe underachievement, and higher rates of peer rejection than those with either disorder alone (Farrington *et al.*, 1990; McGee *et al.*, 1992). Hence, children with both conduct disorder and ADHD are at heightened risk for more negative outcomes, compared to those with conduct disorder only.

It is important to understand the mechanisms associated with the heightened risks for antisocial behaviour with comorbid ADHD. In preschool years, the comorbidity of hyperactivity/impulsivity and defiant/ oppositional behaviours may present an inordinate challenge to parents who may ultimately resort to using coercive parenting strategies which in turn heighten the risk for accelerated development of their children's antisocial behaviour (Patterson, 1982). In the school years, ADHD may exacerbate the likelihood of school failure, which may in turn fuel children's frustration and increase their acting out, their school problems and alienation from school (Hinshaw, 1992). Thus, in the preschool and early school years, ADHD may incur familial, school-related, and interpersonal processes that instigate additional developmental processes in motion contributing to the further development and consolidation of higher levels of antisocial behaviour.

Approximately 90% of the clinically referred children diagnosed with conduct disorder also meet the criteria for oppositional defiant disorder (Faraone *et al.*, 1991; Loeber, 1988; Walker *et al.*, 1991). Some researchers postulate that there is a developmental and hierarchical relationship between ODD and conduct disorder (Lahey and Loeber, 1991). ODD is presumed to be a precursor of conduct disorder. That is to say that a subset of children with ODD advance to conduct disorder. Lahey and Loeber (1991) argue that ODD and conduct disorder should be distinguished in diagnostic terms, but are closely related in both taxonomic and developmental respects.

Youths with conduct disorder were more likely to exhibit anxiety and depression than youths without conduct disorder (Zoccolillo, 1992). Lahey and Loeber (1991) found that compared to boys with conduct disorder alone, prepubertal boys with conduct disorder and a comorbid anxiety disorder had significantly fewer symptoms of aggression, yet there were no significant group differences in the overt, nonaggressive symptoms of conduct disorder. Depression and conduct disorder co-occur at higher than chance levels in a clinically-referred sample (Kovacs *et al.*, 1988). Conduct disorder appears to be a precursor of depression in adolescence and early adulthood (Holmes and Robins, 1987). Some adolescents who experience a depressive episode engage in antisocial behaviours during or after that episode (Matsen, 1988). Depression may be an important precursor or concomitant in some cases of adolescent-limited conduct disorder. Conduct disorder and depression are associated with increased risk of suicidal behaviour, particularly when the two occur together.

Other behaviour problems that are comorbid with conduct disorder include: substance abuse, academic deficiencies, such as achievement level, grades, rates of being left behind in school, drop-out, and deficiencies in specific skill areas. Frick *et al.* (1992) found that although both ADHD and conduct disorder children have above chance comorbidity with academic underachievement, only ADHD had an independent association. For conduct disorder children academic problems appear to be a function of their attention deficits. By adolescence, however, clear linkages exist between antisocial behaviour and delinquency and severe underachievement. Moffitt (1993b) notes that academic failure may largely be characteristic of child-onset of conduct disorder.

Moffitt (1993b) in a review paper suggested that comorbid diagnoses predict increased severity of symptoms and may increase the probability of reoccurrence. In adulthood, approximately 31% of individuals diagnosed with conduct disorder qualify for the diagnosis of Antisocial Personality Disorder. Epidemiological research indicates that these individuals suffer numerous deficits including: employment problems (94%), violence (85%), multiple traffic offenses (72%), and severe marital difficulties (67%) (Robins, 1966). Over the lifespan the problems of children with conduct disorder compound and it becomes increasingly difficult for these individuals to accomplish the developmental tasks associated with adolescence and adulthood. This high rate of comorbidity has implications for understanding etiology, as well as implications for treatment and assessment.

Data are consistent with the developmental pathway of ODD to conduct disorder. Lahey *et al.* (1988) found in a study of clinic-referred boys aged 7–12, 96% of the sample who met the criteria for conduct disorder also met the criteria for ODD. Similarly, in clinical field trials for the DSM-III-R, 84% of clinic referred conduct disordered youth met the criteria for ODD. These researchers concluded that ODD consistently precedes childhood-onset of conduct disorder and furthermore children with childhood-onset of conduct disorder retain half of their symptoms of ODD. However, not all children with ODD progress to have childhood-onset of conduct disorder (Hinshaw and Lahey, 1993). They conclude by suggesting that ODD is a milder form of conduct disorder.

COURSE AND OUTCOME

Conduct disorder is a highly stable disorder across time and generations. There is a high probability that diagnostic criteria for conduct disorder will be met in one or more subsequent years (Hinshaw *et al.*, 1993). In general, the disorder progresses from less severe behaviour problems, followed by behaviours with increasing severity and frequency. To date there has been little systematic research examining the development of conduct disorder prospectively from infancy, but data are available for examining the development of conduct disorder from early childhood and onwards (Achenbach, 1993). Perhaps a more comprehensive understanding of the development, course, and stability of conduct disorder can come from a developmental psychopathological perspective. This perspective accentuates the evolving capacities and limitations of individuals across developmental stages (Cicchetti and Richters, 1993). From this perspective both proximal and distal causes of conduct disorder can be examined. Proximal causes might include antisocial peers whereas a distal cause may be marital discord. Research on the etiology, course, and sequelae of conduct disorder is extremely complex. Cicchetti and Richters (1993) suggest that there are multiple contributors to conduct disorder outcomes within any individual, and that the relevant causal processes may vary among individuals with conduct disorder. As a consequence there is heterogeneity in the underlying causes and the manifestations of conduct disorder, as well as numerous pathways to any particular manifestation of conduct disorder behaviour.

The pattern of early behaviour problems leading to later disorder is also referred to as the early starter model (Patterson *et al.*, 1989), life-course persistent (Moffitt, 1993b), or aggressive-versatile pathway (Loeber, 1988). There is high continuity in aggressive behaviours throughout childhood and into adolescence. In this developmental sequence, overt behaviours (e.g., defiance, fighting) appear before the covert behaviours (e.g., lying, stealing), which augment the repertoire of antisocial behaviours. Finally, over time, the antisocial behaviours become generalized over many contexts (e.g., from the home to school, to the broader community).

The developmental pathway for early starters begins with ineffective parenting, which leads to disruptive behaviour in childhood, which leads to academic failure and rejection by the peer group (Patterson *et al.*, 1989). This progression culminates in depressed mood and gravitation to defiant but accepting peers. Loeber (1990) suggests a similar pathway beginning with difficult temperament (post natal) and hyperactivity, which leads to overt conduct problems such as aggression, covert or concealing conduct problems such as truancy, stealing, substance abuse, association with deviant peers, delinquency, and recidivism. Individuals with childhood-onset of conduct disorder are characterized by both oppositional behaviour and hyperactivity in elementary school as well as academic problems, most notably reading (Patterson, 1986). The coercive behaviours learned in the family context are generalized to the school context in children's interactions with teachers and peers. Their aversive behaviour often results in peer rejection and denied access to positive socialization with peers.

Conduct disorder children who are rejected by the prosocial peer group may find a deviant peer group comprised of children who are similar to themselves in terms of antisocial behaviours (Cairns and Cairns, 1992). This peer group provides further socialization in antisocial behaviour as well as opportunities to engage in specific delinquent acts (Patterson *et al.*, 1989). These children are on an aggressive-versatile trajectory because there is increased diversity in their disruptive behaviours over time, with some behaviours becoming more covert as these children move into adolescence (Patterson *et al.*, 1989). Inherent in this developmental formulation is the notion that the oppositional and antisocial acts change during the course of development (Loeber, 1990): there is both similarity in antisocial behaviours over time (homotypic continuity) and diversification in antisocial behaviours over time (heterotypic continuity).

Development is shaped by an interaction of risk and protective factors, which reside both within individuals and their environments. Risk factors are those which lead directly to disorder, whereas protective factors operate to buffer the effects of the risk variable. There is a cumulative effect of risk both within and across time (Rutter, 1983). Over time, there is a progressive accumulation of the consequences of individual factors (cumulative continuity) and the responses they elicit during social interaction (interactional continuity) (Caspi *et al.*, 1987). Different developmental outcomes derive from a combination of risk and protective factors within the individual, family, and broader socialization contexts such as the peer group. Below is a discussion of factors which may influence the course of development of conduct disorder.

Early Behaviour Problems

Aggressive behaviours in preschool and early elementary school are risk factors for the development of conduct disorder (Patterson *et al.*, 1991; Serbin *et al.*, 1993; Eron *et al.*, 1991). Antisocial and oppositional behaviour characterize children with a childhood-onset of conduct disorder well before they enter preschool (Patterson, 1982). Children who are aggressive and noncompliant continue to present these similar problems at school. When these children begin school, the coercive behaviours and interaction styles that the child has learned in the home are transferred to the classroom and playground. The noncompliant and undercontrolled behaviour begins to interfere with learning and consequently, these children are at increased risk for poor academic achievement (Patterson *et al.*, 1989).

School Factors

The school context, in general, may create a milieu that is conducive to conduct disorder and conduct disorder-related behaviours such as aggression. The National Research Council Report on Violence (1993) cites four characteristics of the school milieu that may contribute to violence. These occur when: (a) a relatively high numbers of students occupy a limited amount of space, (b) the capacity to avoid confrontations is somewhat reduced, (c) the imposition of behavioural routines and conformity contribute to feelings of anger, resentment, and rejection, and (d) poor design features facilitate the commission of violent acts.

The incidence of aggression has been related to the heavy and inflexible use of school rules in the classroom (Pratt, 1973). There tend to be higher levels of aggression in classrooms where teachers are rigid and inflexible than in classrooms where teachers are flexible (Pratt, 1973). The interactions among teachers, teacher hostility and lack of rapport between staff members were found to affect the environment adversely for the students (Pratt, 1973). Frude and Gault (1984) found that a lack of consensus in approaches to classroom management can lead to major inconsistencies in the limits set for students' behaviours. Laslett (1977) found that increases in reported incidents of disruption in the classroom (refusal to cooperate, lying, stealing, and temper tantrums) were associated with an increase in the number of bullying incidents reported. The positive correlation between classroom behaviour problems and bullying suggests that some school contexts may support and perhaps exacerbate conduct disorder problems.

Externalizing and academic behaviour problems are highly correlated (Hinshaw, 1992). Misbehaviour in schools relates to poor school performance; a lack of interest in school is related to delinquent behaviour. Early disruptive behaviour often precedes academic difficulties (Patterson *et al.*, 1991; Tremblay *et al.*, 1992). Thus, children's behaviour problems may impede their success in school which in turn may engender a negative and hostile attitude towards school and school-related tasks. At the same time, problems in school-related tasks may exacerbate aggressive behaviour. At this point in time, the directionality of these effects is unclear. Nevertheless, the end result of the interaction between acting out and behaviour problems appears to be that conduct disorder and conduct disorder-related behaviours are consolidated within the school context. Elliot *et al.* (1985) concluded that weak conventional bonding in the home and school contributes to increased negative peer bonding. The peer context is an important inhibitor or reinforcer of conduct disorder behaviour problems.

Peer Influences

There are several mechanisms through which the peer group influences or contributes to the development of conduct disorder. A child who enters school with a rich repertoire of aggressive and antisocial behaviours will interact with others using these strategies. Aggressive children exhibit significantly more inappropriate play, insults, threats, hitting and exclusion of peers than average children (Dodge, 1993a). They are less likely to engage in social conversation or to continue in group activities than other children (Coie and Kupersmidt, 1983; Dodge, 1993a). Not only are conduct disorder children at risk for rejection, but their aggressive behaviour will provoke retaliation and provocations. In this way, the peer interactions of aggressive children tend to develop into mechanisms of positive and negative reinforcement that will escalate the development of antisocial behaviour (Patterson *et al.*, 1992).

The processes within the peer group start in the early stages of peer interaction. Among preschoolers, early peer rejection serves to isolate the aggressive child and may play an important role in the maintenance of aggression in conduct problem preschoolers (Olsen, 1992). Once aggressive children are rejected by their classmates their rejection and status are relatively stable and resistant to change (Bierman, 1990). Furthermore, when aggressive/rejected children interact with their peers in the playground, the interaction is likely to be significantly more aversive and reciprocal than that of nonaggressive children (Walker *et al.*, 1987; Pepler *et al.*, 1995). Repeated and reciprocal aggressive coercive interactions within the peer group at school escalates the development of aggressive behaviour through processes similar to those within the family. The limited opportunity for positive peer interaction places rejected children at risk for continuing to learn and employ aggressive behaviours (Parker and Asher, 1987).

Parker and Asher (1987) postulate that aggression leads to low acceptance by peers, which in turn leads to further development of deviant behaviours and association with deviant peers. For aggressive children, rejection by peers and association with deviant peers are presumed to be critical factors in setting the course towards maladjustment in adulthood. Rejected children are more at risk for exposure to deviant peer influences than nonrejected children (Elliot *et al.*, 1985). Patterson *et al.* (1989) refers to this process as the "shopping" hypothesis since they are marginalized with their peer groups, rejected children tend to select out other rejected children as peer associates. These children tend to share similar antisocial values, attitudes, and behaviours (Cairns *et al.*, 1989) and therefore, comprise a deviant peer group. Association with deviant peers is highly correlated with peer conflict, indicating that these friendships may reinforce coercive patterns of interaction and fail to teach these children the necessary prosocial skills in friendships (Dishion, 1990). The deviant peer group is presumed to provide a training ground for delinquent behaviours and drug and alcohol use in later childhood and adolescence (Patterson *et al.*, 1989, 1991). The link between involvement with antisocial peers and delinquency is well established and documented. In longitudinal analyses comparing violent and non-violent adults, Farrington (1993) reported that adolescent involvement in group violence and vandalism was associated with the maintenance of antisocial behaviours into adulthood.

Parental monitoring is an important factor in children's drift to a deviant peer group. Unsupervised time after school is correlated with children's exposure to deviant peers and susceptibility to peer pressure (Patterson, 1986). Thus, the conditions that precede the detrimental processes within the peer group are likely to be established early within the family context and subsequently reinforced within the school context. Dishion (1990) described a model in which poor parenting practices were found to be associated with peer rejection through two mediating variables: antisocial behaviour and academic failure. Boys who were rejected by their peers had been exposed to more coercive and hostile family experiences compared to average children. Poor parenting practices led to poorly developed interactional skills in children, which in turn inhibit the development of positive peer relations. Dishion (1990) suggests that during childhood parenting skills such as arranging contact with peers, selection of safe neighbourhoods, coaching on how to initiate and maintain friendships, and modelling of peer relations are related to prosocial friendships. Similarly, during adolescence, parent supervision and involvement have been shown to relate to prosocial friendships (Snider *et al.*, 1986).

This link between children's experiences within the family and at school points to the important relations among systems within the child's life. Patterns of social interaction are multiply determined and, therefore, assessments of causes and effects should encompass the full range of factors including: individual factors, interindividual interactions, social networks, inter-net-work relations, and cultural-ecological-economic conditions (Cairns and Cairns, 1992). Some mechanisms that propel children on an antisocial trajectory have been identified; however, more research is needed to elucidate the multiple processes and pathways involved in the development of aggression and violence.

In summary, the research to date indicates that there are a host of potential symptoms and risk factors associated with conduct disorder over the course of development. The child-parent-family-context includes multiple and reciprocal influences that affect each participant and the systems in which they operate. Early behaviour problems such as aggressive or disruptive behaviours, hyperactivity, or attention problems may become exacerbated in family, peer, and school interactions. These negative behaviours and interactions reciprocally influence each other and accumulate over time resulting in the development, consolidation, and maintenance of conduct disorder.

ASSESSMENT

Assessment of conduct disorder can rely on various types of measures such as self-report questionnaires, reports from significant others or peers, direct observation, institutional and societal records. Commonly used self-report measures include: Children's Action Tendency Scale (Deluty, 1979), Adolescent Antisocial Self-Report Behavior Checklist (Kulik *et al.*, 1968), Self-Report Delinquency Scale (Elliot *et al.*, 1987), Ontario Child Health Study Scales (Boyle *et al.*, 1993), Behavior Problem Checklist (Quay and Peterson, 1975), and the Child Behavior Checklist (Achenbach, 1978) (Table 4.3). Another method is through reports of significant others such as the Child Behavior Checklist (Achenbach, 1992), Eyberg Child Behavior Inventory (Eyberg and Robinson, 1983), and the Peer Nomination of Aggression (Lefkowitz *et al.*, 1977). Another common method used for the assessment of conduct disorder is diagnostic interview such as a section

Table 4.3   Items for assessing symptoms of conduct disorder from selected checklists and self-report questionnaires

Instruments	Examples of questions	Coding options
Child Behavior Checklist (Achenbach, 1978)	Argues a lot Stubborn, sullen, or irritable Temper tantrums or hot temper	"not true" to "very often true"
Behavior Problem Checklist (Quay and Peterson, 1975)	Fighting Temper tantrums Destructiveness in regard to own other's property	"does not constitute a problem" to "constitutes a severe problem"
Louisville Behavior Checklist (Miller, 1977)	Constantly fighting or beating up others Has temper tantrums; yells, screams, cries, kicks feet over the least thing Bullies or frightens others	True / False
Ontario Child Health Study Scales (Boyle et al., 1993)	I have a hot temper I set fires I get in many fights	"never or not true" to "often or very true"

on conduct disorder of the Diagnostic Interview Schedule for Children (DISC; Costello et al., 1984), the Diagnostic Interview for Children and Adolescents (DICA-R; Reich and Welner, 1988), and the Schedule for Affective Disorders and Schizophrenia for School-aged children (Puig-Antich and Chambers, 1978) (Table 4.4). Finally, some measures of direct observation include: Adolescent Antisocial Behavioral Checklist (Curtiss et al., 1983) and the Family Interaction Coding System (Reid, 1978).

TREATMENT

Effective interventions for conduct disorder correspond to the current understanding of its causes, risks, and developmental course. Although techniques in treatment vary greatly, promising interventions focus directly or symbolically on the actual social interaction fabric in which the child's conduct disorder problems emerged. Kazdin identified over 230 different treatment techniques currently in use for children and adolescents

Table 4.4 Items for assessing conduc disorder from selected diagnostic interviews

Instruments	Examples of questions	Coding options			
DISC (Costello et al., 1984)	In the past year, have you snatched someone's purse?	0	[2*]		9
	Have you held someone up or robbed someone?	0	[2*]		9
	Have you threatened someone in order to steal from them?	0	[2*]		9
	IF YES, ASK:				
	A. Have you [SNATCHED A PURSE/ROBBED SOMEONE/THREATENED SOMEONE] in the past 6 months?	0	2		9
	B. How old were you the first time you did this?				
	CODE EXACT AGE ············>				years
	In the past year, have you started any fires without permission?	0	2		9
	IF YES, ASK:				
	A. Did the fire cause any damage or hurt anyone?	0	2		9
	B. Did you mean for the fire to cause damage or hurt someone?	0	2		9
	IF YES, C. Have you started a fire like this in the last six months?	0	2		9
	D. How old were you the first time you started a fire like this?				
	CODE EXACT AGE ············>				years
DICA-R (Reich and Welner, 1988)	Do you often argue with your parents, your teachers, or other adults?	1	2	4	9
	IF YES, A. Who do you argue with the most? RECORD _____				
	B. How often does it happen?				
	1 to 7 days a week				
	1 to 3 times a month				
	less than once a month				

Table 4.4 *continued*

Instruments	Examples of questions	Coding options
DICA-R (Reich and Welner, 1988)	Do you usually feel angry or irritable when people ask you to do things for them? (Probe: Does it make you mad when your mom/dad ask you to run an errand, clean your room, come in earlier than usual on a Friday or Saturday, or do something for them?)	1 2 4 9
K-SADS (Puig-Antich and Chambers, 1978)	Do you ever hurt people? For what reason? What do you do to them? Do you enjoy watching people suffer? Have you ever tortured anyone? How? Have you ever set anyone up? How often have you ever done these things?	0 1 2 3 4
	Have you ever forced anyone to have sex with you against his/her will? How often? Did you threaten him/her? Did you use physical force?	

Note: (i) DISC: 0 = no, 1 = sometimes/somewhat, 2 = yes, 9 = don't know; (ii) DICA-R: 1 = yes, 2 = sometimes, 4 = no, 9 = don't know; (iii) K-SADS: 1 = no information, 1 = no, 2 = occasionally, 3 = often, 4 = most of time

(Kazdin, 1988). The current treatments of choice for children with conduct disorder comprise training parents in child management skills or behavioural family therapy (Kazdin, 1987b). Meta-analyses of outcome studies indicate that these approaches are generally efficacious (Kazdin, 1987b). Even when conduct disorder problems are not eliminated, these treatments produce at least temporary improvements in processes linked to conduct disorder such as cognitive processes, social and academic skills, and parenting skills (Kazdin, 1993). Interventions for children with conduct disorder are complex to develop. They must be tailored to the needs of individual children, given the variety of causal and risk factors. In addition, interventions must be systematic and address not only problem behaviours of conduct disorder children, but also the processes that continue to support their behaviour problems at home, at school, and in the community. At this point, little is known about which treatments are most effective with youths at different stages of development and when and how to incorporate parent, family, peer, and other influences. The following section briefly reviews several treatment strategies in preventing and treating conduct disorder.

Pharmacotherapy

Stimulant medication has been effective in reducing several symptoms of ADHD, a condition very often comorbid with conduct disorder (Hinshaw, 1991). As yet, medication is not established as a treatment for children and adolescents with conduct disorder primarily due to the fact that the mechanisms or processes through which the stimulant operates to influence antisocial behaviour are not clear.

Psychological Interventions

Almost a decade ago, Kazdin (1987b) concluded from an extensive review of the literature on treatments of conduct disorder that despite a number of promising treatment approaches to conduct disorder, no treatment approach had been demonstrated to be effective in the long run. Over time, this conclusion is still valid (Kazdin, 1993). Below is a brief review of some of the more current and successful treatments of conduct disorder.

Parent Training

Training parents in effective child management skills has demonstrated the most promising effects in the reduction of antisocial behaviour (Kazdin,

1993). Much of the work in this area has been conducted by Patterson and his colleagues (Forgatch, 1991; Patterson, 1982; Patterson *et al.*, 1991). This approach emphasizes the need to change the social context in which aggressive behaviour occurs by providing parents with effective child-rearing skills. The intervention is based on a social-interactional perspective with the basic premise that family members directly train the child to perform antisocial behaviours. Through their use of noncontingent reinforcements, inept parenting practices, and harsh and inconsistent discipline, parents unwittingly permit numerous interactions in which coercive behaviours are reinforced (Patterson *et al.*, 1989).

Parent Management Training (PMT)

The PMT comprises procedures in which parents are trained to alter their children's behaviour in the home. Parents are taught specific procedures to alter interactions with their children, to promote prosocial behaviours, and to decrease antisocial behaviours. Parents are trained to observe, identify, and define problem behaviours in new ways. Treatment sessions cover social learning principles and procedures and include skills such as: positive reinforcement, the use of social praise and tokens, mild punishment (e.g., loss of privileges), negotiation, and contingency contracting. The sessions provide opportunities for parents to see how well they are implementing their behaviour programs.

The effectiveness of PMT has been extensively researched with conduct problem children and to a lesser extent with adolescents. Outcome studies generally indicate behavioural improvements in the child at home and school. Furthermore, these positive treatment effects are visible up to ten years after completion of the program (Forehand and Long, 1988). Nonetheless, conclusions concerning treatment tend to vary by domain, setting, and informant (Kazdin *et al.*, 1992). In addition, a number of factors have been shown to moderate outcome, most notably parent characteristics and family social circumstances.

A central feature of PMT is active participation from the parents. This feature presents a challenge because the parents who need treatment most tend not to participate and have family characteristics which mitigate against engagement and participation in treatment (Reid, 1993). Some parents are simply not able to participate due to mental retardation, other psychopathology, substance abuse, or emotional stress due to marital discord or family dysfunction (Kazdin, 1987b). Therefore, parent compliance presents a significant dilemma in attempting to treat children with conduct disorder. Interventions for children with conduct disorder are further complicated by the referral process. In the majority of cases, treatment occurs as a result of problems at school, with the law, or involvement of social services (Kazdin, 1987b). Children and adolescents do not refer themselves for treatment nor do they identify themselves as experiencing stress or problems. Often their parents fail to seek help for these problems. Hence, the other adults in these children's lives, such as teachers, principals, and law enforcement staff provide the impetus for treatment. Thus, the motivation and participation of the child or adolescent with conduct disorder is often not by their choice. The lack of commitment of the children themselves to the treatment process may explain why in some cases the treatment effects do not generalize outside of the family to other social domains (Kazdin et al., 1992).

The effectiveness of treatment varies considerably according to individual, family and treatment factors. Parent and family characteristics have been related to treatment outcome. For example, families characterized by multiple risk factors (e.g., marital discord, socioeconomic disadvantage) are less likely to succeed with just PMT than those with single risks (Kazdin, 1993). Duration of treatment and therapist expertise have also been shown to influence treatment outcomes (Kazdin, 1987b). Researchers have rarely examined child, parent, family, and other characteristics in order to identify case characteristics by treatment interactions. As a result, currently we know little about the type of child and family for whom treatment is most effective. Future research needs to examine the components of treatment that contribute to and moderate effectiveness, parameters of treatment, the relative roles of various components of treatment and the client and therapist characteristics that facilitate change.

Cognitive (Problem Solving) Training

Cognitive training (perceptions, self-statements, attributions, and problem solving skills) is a popular intervention technique, which is based on the premise that aggression is partly a function of the way events are perceived and processed. Through a series of studies, Dodge and his colleagues (1990) have demonstrated that aggressive children have a predisposition to attribute hostile intent to ambiguous stimuli. Similarly, Spivak and Shure (1982) have identified several cognitive skill deficits that are central to aggressive behaviour. These include: interpersonal cognitive problem solving, means-end thinking, generating alternative solutions, and consequential thinking. Deficits and distortions in these processes have been related to disruptive behaviour problems typical of children with conduct disorder (Rubin *et al.*, 1991). Interventions based on the cognitive bases for impulsive and disruptive behaviour attempt to change and enhance cognition and affect thereby supporting improved behavioural adjustment. Interventions targeting cognitive problem solving have demonstrated modest symptom improvements (Lochman, 1992; Pepler *et al.*, 1991).

A cognitive-behaviour modification approach is a commonly used intervention for aggressive children in German speaking countries (Petermann and Petermann, 1994). The training typically consists of eight individual sessions and between 6 and 10 group sessions. During the training, the child is taught: relaxation techniques, to perceive the environment differently, to be assertive, prosocial skills (i.e., cooperation, helping behaviours, sympathy), and anger control. With the help of various materials (observation questionnaires, self-instruction, and videos) and role plays, these skills are systematically practised. Generalization of skills is encouraged through parent involvement.

A wide variety of intervention approaches have been developed including problem solving skills, anger control, coping skills, and social skills. Problem solving skills training consists of developing cognitive problem solving skills necessary for effective interactions. The emphasis is on helping children approach social problems; they are taught a step-by-step process to solve problems such as responding to teasing or joining in. The findings of many studies indicate that cognitively-based interventions provide a significant reduction in aggressive and antisocial behaviour (Kazdin *et al.*, 1989). In some cases, the positive effects may not be generalized or persistent (Kazdin, 1993). On a more encouraging note, a recent outcome study by Kazdin *et al.* (1989) showed that cognitive-behavioral interventions with preadolescent, school-aged children in a structured hospital setting produced clear and effective reductions in antisocial behaviour up to a year following treatment.

The basis for the therapeutic changes in cognitively-based treatments is unclear. The literature on the effectiveness of cognitive interventions is difficult to interpret due to the heterogeneity of children studied (e.g., type of disorder, age group, severity of disorder) and the range of intervention components and instructional methods. The strength of conclusions is further mitigated by the fact that although children may improve, their functioning is often not raised to within the normal range. Durlak *et al.* (1991) reviewed social-cognitive and cognitive-behavioural interventions and concluded that evidence for the effectiveness is mixed and the link between cognitive change and behavioural change has not been demonstrated.

Behaviour modification and cognitive behavioural techniques comprise approximately half of the treatment outcome literature (Kazdin *et al.*, 1989). These treatments are usually brief in duration (the mean duration of treatment is eight to ten weeks) (Casey and Berman, 1985). It is surprising that treatment length is short given the complexity and consistency of conduct problems, the severity of impairment, and the heterogeneous nature of conduct disorder. In addition, fifty-nine percent of the studies do not collect follow-up data past one year (Kazdin, 1993). There is a paucity of outcome research on eclectic or other nontraditional interventions for conduct disorder.

Kazdin (1993) summarized the knowledge to date on treatment of conduct disorders with the following three conclusions: (1) The majority of treatments indicate short-term symptom relief (up to follow-up periods of one year) but relatively few examine longitudinal outcomes; (2) Treatments with multiple interventions in a variety of domains (e.g., family, behaviours and cognitions of the child) have positive effects; (3) None of the treatments has demonstrated robust long-term effects.

Given the burden of suffering associated with conduct disorder, we need to continue our efforts to intervene with evaluations of success. Research on treatment effectiveness might be expanded to include: a wider range of outcome criteria (e.g., reduction of antisocial behaviour in the siblings; using broader social outcomes such as the use of mental health services) and examining clinical significance versus statistical significance in treatment outcomes.

The nature and effectiveness of treatment for conduct disorder depends on children's age, developmental level, risk status for poor long-term outcomes, and on the severity of child and parent dysfunction. More research is needed on the multiple processes related to conduct disorder (individual, family, peer, and school). Treatment can then be conceptualized and targeted to these developmental processes in specific domains. The relation between basic developmental theory and clinical intervention should be reciprocal, with theory guiding intervention design and intervention outcomes informing theory (Dodge, 1993b; Forgatch, 1991).

CONCLUDING REMARKS

Conduct disorder offers a challenge to both clinicians and researchers given its potential multiple domains of dysfunction, severity of dysfunction, continuity in dysfunction, and resistance to change. Conduct disorder presents a heavy burden of suffering in terms of its prevalence, morbidity, and potentially high personal and social costs. At this point, it is important to move beyond the assessment of the prevalence and incidence of conduct disorder to an articulation of how and why this behaviour pattern develops in some children and not others over the course of development. This direction of research is informed by a developmental perspective examining changes over time in child functioning and the interface of these changes with the interpersonal environment.

From a developmental perspective, it is possible to test formulations about individual factors that are characteristic of a particular developmental period and interactional processes influencing developmental capacities and attainments. In assessing the critical mechanisms in development, prior sequences of adaptation are evaluated in light of their potential contributions to outcomes in subsequent developmental periods. The processes involved in the development of conduct disorder discussed earlier in this chapter do not occur in isolation. There are substantial interrelations among biological factors (e.g., neuropsychological functioning, deficits in learning), cognitive factors (e.g., impulse control), social factors (e.g., child-parent attachment, social cognition), and emotional factors (e.g., emotional regulation). In some cases, those individuals who continue to exhibit conduct problems may be influenced by different mechanisms across developmental stages. For example, a child who enters school with conduct problems may be reinforced for these behaviours in late childhood by a deviant peer group. On the other hand, positive experiences may serve to divert similarly troubled children from the conduct disorder pathway. Thus, it is important to take a developmental perspective within longitudinal research designs to examine individuals who exhibit specific deficits and individuals who do not exhibit these symptoms to determine the critical processes that shape the development and cessation of conduct problems.

The specification of conduct disorder is complex. As indicated in this chapter, an individual with conduct disorder has many potential trajectories which are determined by many potential individual and interactional processes. Furthermore, there is more than one pathway in the development of conduct disorder and the manifestation of conduct disorder varies across individuals (Waters et al., 1993). Given the diversity in the potential processes and outcomes, it is not surprising that conduct disorder does not have a unitary etiology. Conduct disorder is best understood by examining children's current risk and protective factors with an understanding of their prior biological status and behavioural experiences that have interacted to lay the foundation for the development of conduct problems (Cicchetti and Richters, 1993). Research is now at a stage where the understanding of conduct disorder is moving beyond a description of individual differences to examine how these differences evolve. To achieve the next level of understanding, research must be multidimensional to examine simultaneously variables within and outside the individual across time. Thus, individual factors (e.g., sex) as well the contexts in which conduct disorder is embedded are necessary considerations.

The complexity of conduct disorder presents equally difficult challenges for clinicians. Given that conduct disorder is multivariately determined, treatment with a unitary focus on one aspect of the behaviour problem in a single context is not likely to be effective or generalizable. A developmental approach to the understanding of conduct disorder is critical to treatment efforts. Interventions must reflect the diversity in the development of conduct disorder which occurs along at least two distinct pathways that differ in the age of onset, etiology, course, comorbidities, and persistence. Clinical efforts will benefit substantially from research which examines the risk and protective factors associated with the development of conduct disorder over childhood and adolescence. This research will elucidate possible mechanisms implicated in conduct disorder and more importantly such information will identify points for intervention.

Perhaps the most effective means of increasing our understanding of conduct disorder is to conduct preventive intervention trials. The committee on the Prevention of Mental Disorders of the United States' Institute of Medicine has recently published recommendations for the design of preventive interventions (Mrazek and Haggerty, 1994). The committee differentiates between small scale studies which are either pilot, confirmatory, or replication trials and others which are large-scale field trials. They suggest starting with pilot studies to explore the feasibility of a given type of intervention. Following successful small-scale trials, large-scale trials may be implemented to assess the generalizability of the intervention efficacy and its costs. A second large scale trial is recommended to assess the effectiveness of intervention.

From a policy perspective money invested in early (e.g., at-birth) prevention efforts with at-risk families will give larger pay-offs than money invested later (e.g., adolescence). Nonetheless, because juveniles with conduct problems attract more attention and concern than high risk infants, this approach is not easily applied. It is clear, however, that in the long run, a prevention strategy should reduce the extent of resources needed for treatment services within the health, education, and justice systems. A large-scale prevention effort requires cooperation among academics, educators, health professionals, child-welfare workers, and government officials. Future efforts need to consider not only individual children at-risk, but also the broader family, social, school, cultural, and economic contexts in which those children develop. Such a developmental psychopathological perspective in prevention will increase our efforts in understanding, intervening, and preventing conduct disorder.

REFERENCES

Achenbach, T.M. (1978). The Child Behavior Profile: I. Boys aged 6–11. *Journal of Consulting and Clinical Psychology, 46*, 487–488.

Achenbach, T.M. (1992). *Manual for the Child Behavior Checklist/4–18 and 1991 Profiles*. Burlington: University of Vermont, Department of Psychiatry.

Achenbach, T.M. (1993). Taxonomy and comorbidity of conduct problems: Evidence from empirically based approaches. *Development and Psychopathology, 5*, 51–64.

American Psychiatric Association (1987). *Diagnostic and statistical manual of mental disorders* (3rd ed. rev.). Washington, DC: American Psychiatric Association.

American Psychiatric Association (1994). *Diagnostic and statistical manual of mental disorders* (4th ed.). Washington, DC: American Psychiatric Association.

Anderson, J.C., Williams, S., McGee, R., and Silva, P. (1987). The prevalence of DSM-III disorders in pre-adolescent children: Prevalence in a large sample from the general populations. *Archives of General Psychiatry, 44*, 69–76.

Bierman, K. (1990). Improving the peer relations of rejected children. In B.B. Lahey and A.E. Kazdin (Eds.), *Advances in clinical child psychology* (pp. 131–149). New York: Plenum Press.

Bird, H., canino, G., Rubio-Stipec, M., Gould, M.S., Ribera, J., Sesman, M., Woodbury, M., Huertas-Goldman, S., Pagan, A., Sanchez-Lacay, A., and Moscoso, M. (1988). Estimates of the prevalence of childhood maladjustment in a community survey in Puerto Rico. *Archives of General Psychiatry, 45*, 1120–1126.

Boyle, M.H., Offord, D.R., Racine, Y., Fleming, J.E., Szatmari, P., and Sanford, M. (1993). Evaluation of the revised Ontario Child Health Study Scales. *Journal of Child Psychology and Psychiatry, 34*, 189–213.

Brickman, A.S., McManus, M.A., Grapentine, W., and Alessi (1984). Neurological assessment of seriously delinquent adolescents. *Journal of the Academy of Child Psychiatry, 23*, 453–457.

Cadoret, R., Troughton, E., O'Gorman, T., and Heywood, E. (1986). An adoption of genetic and environmental factors in drug abuse. *Archives of General Psychiatry, 43*, 1131–1136.

Cairns, R.B. and Cairns, B.D. (1992). The sociogenesis of aggressive and antisocial behaviors. In J. McCord (Ed.), *Facts, frameworks, and forecasts: Advances in criminological theory* (Vol. 3, pp. 157–191). New Brunswick, NJ: Transaction Press.

Cairns, R.B., Cairns, B.D., and Neckerman, H.J. (1989). Early school dropout: Configurations and determinants. *Child Development, 60*, 1437–1452.

Campbell, A. (1993). *Men, women, and aggression*. New York: Basic Books.

Casey, R.J. and Berman, J.S. (1985). The outcome of psychotherapy research with children. *Psychological Bulletin,* **98,** 388–400.

Caspi, A., Elder, G.H., and Bem, D.J. (1987). Moving against the world: Life course patterns of explosive children. *Developmental Psychology,* **23,** 308–313

Cicchetti, D. and Richters, J.E. (1993). Developmental considerations in the investigation of conduct disorders. *Development and Psychopathology,* **5,** 331–344.

Cohen, P., Cohen, J., Kasen, S., Velez, C., Hartmark, C., Johnson, J., Rojas, M., Brook, J., and Streuning, J. (1993). An epidemiological study of disorders in late childhood and adolescence: I. Age-and-gender-specific prevalence. *Journal of Child Psychology and Psychiatry,* **34,** 851–867.

Coie, J.D. and Kupersmidt, J.B. (1983). A behavioral analysis of emerging social status in boys' groups. *Child Development,* **54,** 1400–1416.

Costello, A.J., Edelbrock, C., Dulcan, R.K., Kalas, R., and Klaric, S.H. (1984). *Development and testing of the NIMH Diagnostic Interview Schedule for Children in a clinic population.* Rockville, MD: National Institute of Mental Health.

Curtiss, G., Rosenthal, R.H., Marohn, R.C., Ostrov, E., Offer, D. and Trujillo, J. (1983). Measuring delinquent behavior in inpatient treatment settings: Revision and validation of the Adolescent Antisocial Behavior Checklist. *Journal of the American Academy of Child Psychiatry,* **22,** 459–466.

Daugherty, T.K. and Quay, H. (1991). Response preservation and delayed responding in childhood behaviour disorders. *Journal of Child Psychiatry and Psychology,* **32,** 453–461.

Deluty, R.H. (1979). Children's Action tendency scale: A self-report measure aggressiveness, assertiveness, and submissiveness in children. *Journal of Consulting and Clinical Psychology,* **46,** 1061–1071.

Dishion, T.J. (1990). The family ecology of boys' peer relations in middle childhood. *Child Development,* **61,** 874–892.

Dodge, K.A. (1990). Nature versus nuture in child conduct disorder: It is time to ask a different question. *Developmental Psychopathology,* **26,** 698–701.

Dodge, K.A. (1993a). Social-cognitive mechanisms in the development of conduct disorder and depression. *Annual Review of Psychology,* **44,** 559–584.

Dodge, K.A. (1993b). The future research on the treatment of conduct disorder. *Development and Psychopathology,* **5,** 311–319.

Dodge, K.A., Bates, J.E., and Pettit, G. (1990). Mechanisms in the cycle of violence, *Science,* **250,** 311–319.

Dodge, K.A., Coie, J.D., Pettit, G.S., and Price, J.M. (1990). Peer status and aggression in boys groups: Developmental and context analyses. *Child Development,* **61,** 1289–1309.

Durlak, J.A., Fuhrman, T., and Lampman, C. (1991). Effectiveness of cognitive-behavioral therapy for maladapting children: A meta-analysis. *Psychological Bulletin,* **110,** 204–214.

Elliot, D.S., Huizinga, D., and Ageton, S.S. (1985). *Explaining delinquency and drug use.* Newbury Park, CA: Sage.

Elliot, D.S., Dunford, F.W., 7 Huizinger, D. (1987). The identification and prediction of career offenders utilizing self-reported and official data. In J.D. Burchard and S.N. Burchard (Eds.), *Preventing Delinqent Behavior* (90–121). Newbury Park, CA: Sage.

Eron, L., Huesmann, L., and Zelli, A. (1991). The role of parental variables in the learning of aggression: Early precursors and later-life outcomes. In D.J. Pepler and K. Rubin (Eds.), *The development and treatment of childhood aggression* (pp. 5–29). New York: Guiford Press.

Esser, G., Schmidt, M.H., and Woerner, W. (1990). Epidemiology and course of psychiatric disorders in school-age children: Results of a longitudinal study. *Journal of Child Psychology and Psychiatry,* **31,** 243–263.

Eyberg, S.M. and Robinson, E.A. (1983). Conduct problem behavior: Standardization of a behavior rating scale with adolescents. *Journal of Clinical Child Psychology,* **12,** 347–354.

Faraone, S.V., Biederman, J., Keenan, K., and Tsuang, M.T. (1991). Separation of DSM-III attention deficit disorder and conduct disorder: Evidence from a family genetic study of American child psychiatric patients. *Psychological Medicine,* **21,** 109–121.

Farrington, D.P. (1993). Motivations for conduct disorders and delinquent. *Development and Psychopathology,* **5,** 225–241.

Farrington, D.P. (1987). Epidemiology. In H.C. Quay (Ed.), *Handbook of juvenile delinquency* (pp. 31–61). New York: Wiley.

Farrington, D.P., Loeber, R., and Van Kammen, W.B. (1990). Long-term criminal outcomes of hyperactivity-impulsivity-attention deficit and conduct problems in childhood. In L.N. Robins and M. Rutter (Eds.), *Straight and devious pathways to adulthood.* New York: Cambridge University Press.

Forehand, R. and Long, N. (1988). Outpatient treatment of the acting out child: Procedures, long-term follow-up data and clinical problems. *Advances in Behavioral Research and Therapy,* **10,** 129–177.

Forgatch, M. (1991). The clinical science vortex: A developing theory of antisocial behaviour. In D.J. Pepler and K. Rubin (Eds.), *The development and treatment of childhood aggression* (pp. 291–316). New York: Guiford Press.

Frick, P.J., Lahey, B.B., Loeber, R., Stouthamer-Loeber, M., Christ, M.A.G., and Hanson, K. (1992). Familial risk factors to oppositional defiant disorder and conduct disorder: Parental psychopathology and maternal parenting. *Journal of Consulting and Clinical Psychology,* **60,** 49–55.

Frude, N. and Gault, H. (1984). *Disruptive behaviour in schools.* Chichester: Wiley.

Greenberg, M.T., Speltz, M.L., and DeKlyen, M. (1993). The role of attachment in the early development of disruptive behaviour problems. *Development and Psychopathology,* **5,** 191–213.

Gottesman, I.I., Carey, G., and Hanson, D.R. 91983). Pearls and perils in epigenetic psychopathology. In S.B. Guze, E.J. Earls, and J.E. Barrett (Eds.), *Childhood Psychopathology and development* (pp. 287–300). New York: Raven.

Hinshaw, S.P. (1987). On the distinction between attentional deficits/hyperactivity and conduct problems/aggression in child psychopathology. *Psychological Bulletin,* **101,** 443–463.

Hinshaw, S.P. (1991). Stimulant medication and the treatment of aggression in children with attentional deficits. *Journal of Consulting and Clinical Psychology,* **20,** 301–312.

Hinshaw, S.P. (1992). Externalizing behaviour problems and academic underachievement in childhood and adolescence: Causal relationships and underlying mechanisms. *Psychological Bulletin,* **111,** 127–155.

Hinshaw, S.P., Lahey, B., and Hart, L. (1993). Issues of taxonomy and comorbidity in the development of conduct disorder. *Development and Psychopathology,* **5,** 31–49.

Holmes, S.J. and Robins, L.N. (1987). The influence of childhood disciplinary experience on the development of alcoholism and depression. *Journal of Child Psychology and Psychiatry,* **28,** 399–415.

Huesmann, L.R., Eron, L.D., Lefkowitz, M.M., and Walder, L.O. (1984). Stability of aggression over time and generations. *Developmental Psychology,* **20,** 1120–1134.

Institute of Medicine (1989). *Research on children and adolescents with behavioral, mental, and developmental disorders.* Washington, DC: National Academy Press.

Kazdin, A.E. (1993). Treatment of conduct disorder: Progress and direction in psychotherapy research. *Development and Psychopathology,* **5,** 277–310.

Kazdin, A.E. (1987a). *Conduct disorder in childhood and adolescence.* Homewood, IL: Dorsey Press.

Kazdin, A.E. (1987b). Treatment of antisocial behaviour in children: Current status and future directions. *Psychological Bulletin,* **102,** 187–203.

Kazdin, A.E. (1988). The diagnosis of childhood disorder: Assessment issues and strategies. *Behavioral Assessment,* **10**, 67–94.

Kazdin, A.E., Siegel, T., and Bass, D. (1992). Cognitive problem-solving skills and parent management training in the treatment of antisocial behaviour in children. *Journal of Consulting and Clinical Psychology,* **60**, 733–747.

Kazdin, A.E., Siegel, T., Bass, D., and Thomas, C. (1989). Cognitive-behavioral therapy and relationship therapy in the treatment of children referred for antisocial behaviour. *Journal of Consulting and Clinical Psychology,* **57**, 522–535.

Kovacs, M., Paulauskas, S., Gatsonos, C., and Richards, C. (1988). Depressive disorders in childhood: A longitudinal study of comorbidity with and risk factors for conduct disorders. *Journal of Affective Disorders,* **15**, 205–217.

Kruesi, M., Hibbs, E., Zahn, T., Keysor, C., Hamburger, S., Bartko, J., and Rapoport, J. (1992). A 2 year prospective follow-up study of children and adolescents with disruptive behaviour disorders. *Archives of General Psychiatry,* **49**, 429–435.

Kulik, J.A., Stein, K.B., and Sarbin, T.R. (1968). Dimensions and patterns of adolescent antisocial behavior. *Journal of Consulting and Clinical Psychology,* **32**, 375–382.

Lahey, B. (1992, February). *Tentative results from the DSM-IV field trial for disruptive behaviour disorders.* Invited address at the annual meeting of the Society for Research in Child and Adolescent Psychopathology, Sarasota, FL.

Lahey, B. and Loeber, R. (1991, June). A preliminary developmental-psychobiological model of conduct disorder. In J. Sergeant (Chair), *Relationships among the externalizing disorders.* Session at the annual meeting of the Society for Research in Child and Adolescent Psychopathology, Zandvoort, Holland.

Lahey, B., Piacentini, J., McBurnett, K., Stone, P., Hartdagen, S., and Hynd, G. (1988). Psychopathology in the parents of children with conduct disorder and hyperactivity. *Journal of the American Academy of Child and Adolescent Psychiatry,* **27**, 163–170.

Laslett, R. (1977). Disruptive and violent pupils: The facts and fallacies. *Educational Review,* **29**, 152–162.

Ledingham, J.E. and Schwartzman, A.E. (1984). A 3-year follow-up of aggressive and withdrawn behavior in children: preliminary findings. *Journal of Abnormal Child Psychology,* **12**, 157–168.

Lewinsohn, P.M., Hops, H., Roberts, R.E., Seeley, J.R., and Andrews, J.A. (1993). Adolescent psychopathology: I. Prevalence and incidence of depression and other DSM-III-R disorders in high school students. *Journal of Abnormal Psychology,* **102**, 133–144.

Lewis, C.E. (1991). Neurochemical mechanisms of chronic antisocial behaviour psychopathy: A literature review. *Journal of Nervous and Mental Disease,* **179**, 720–727.

Lewis, D.O., Yeager, C.A., Cobham-Portorreal, C.S., Klein, N., Showalter, C., and Anthony, A. (1991). A follow-up of female delinquents: Maternal contributions to the perpetuation of deviance. *Journal of the American Academy of Child and Adolescent Psychiatry,* **30**, 197–201.

Lewis, D.O., Pincus, J., Lovely, R., Spitzer, E., and Moy, E. (1987). Biopsychosocial characteristics of matched samples of delinquents and nondelinquents. *Journal of the American Academy of Child and Adolescent Psychiatry,* **26**, 744–752.

Lochman, J.E. (1992). Cognitive-behavioral interventions with aggressive boys: Three year follow-up and preventive effects. *Journal of Consulting and Clinical Psychology,* **52**, 915–916.

Loeber, R. (1990). Development and risk factors of juvenile antisocial behavior and delinquency. *Clinical Psychology Review,* **10**, 1–41.

Loeber, R. (1988). The natural histories of juvenile conduct problems, substance use and delinquency: Evidence for developmental progressions. In B.B. Lahey and A.E. Kazdin (Eds.), *Advances in clinical child psychology* (Vol. 11, pp. 73–124). New York: Plenum Press.

Loeber, R. and Stouthamer-Loeber, M. (1986). Family factors as correlates and predictors of juvenile conduct problems and delinquency. In N. Morris and M. Tonry (Eds.),

Crime and justice: An annual review of the research (Vol. 7). Chicago: University of Chicago Press.

Loeber, R., Lahey, B.B., and Thomas, C. (1991). Diagnostic conundrum of oppositional defiant disorder and conduct disorder. *Journal of Abnormal Psychology*, **100**, 379–390.

Loeber, R., Weissman, W., and Reid, J.B. (1983). Family interactions of assaultive adolescents, stealers and nondelinquents. *Journal of Child Psychology*, **11**, 1–14.

Loney, J. (1987). Hyperactivity and aggression in the diagnosis of attention deficit disorder. In B.B. Lahey and A.E. Kazdin (Eds.), *Advances in clinical child psychology* (Vol. 10, pp. 99–135). New York: Plenum Press.

Matsen, A.S. (1988). Toward a developmental psychopathology of early adolescence. In M.D. Levine and E.R. McArney (Eds.), *Early adolescent transitions* (pp. 261–278). Lexington, MA: Heath.

McGee, R., Feehan, M., Williams, S., and Anderson, J. (1992). DSM-III disorders from age 11–15 years. *Journal of the American Academy of Child and Adolescent Psychiatry*, **31**, 50–59.

McGee, R., Feehan, M., Williams, S., Partridge, F., Silva, P.A., and Kelly, J. (1990). DSM-III disorders in a large sample of adolescents. *Journal of the American Academy of Child and Adolescent Psychiatry*, **29**, 611–619.

Meltzer, L.J., Levine, M.D., Karniski, W., Palfreg, J., and Clarke, S. (1984). An analysis of learning style of adolescent delinquents. *Journal of Learning Disabilities*, **17**, 600–608.

Moffitt, T.E. (1990). Juvenile delinquency and attention-deficit disorder: Developmental trajectories from age 3 to 15. *Child Development*, **61**, 893–910.

Moffitt, T.E. (1993a). The neuropsychology of conduct disorder. *Development and Psychopathology*, **5**, 135–151.

Moffitt, T.E. (1993b). Life course persistent and adolescent limited antisocial behaviour: A developmental taxonomy. *Psychological Review*, **100**, 674–701.

Mrazek, P. and Haggerty, R. (1994). *Reducing risks for mental disorders: Frontiers for preventive intervention research*. Washington: National Academy Press.

National Research Council. (1993). *Understanding and preventing violence*. Washington, DC: National Academy Press.

Offord, D., Boyle, M.H., and Racine, Y.A. (1991). The epidemiology of antisocial behavior in childhood and adolescence. In D.J. Pepler and K. Rubin (Eds.), *The development and treatment of childhood aggression* (pp. 31–54). Hillsdale, NJ: Erlbaum.

Offord, D.R., Boyle, M.H., Szatmari, Rae-Grant, N.I., Links, P.S., Cadman, D.T., Byles, J.A., Crawford, J.W., Blum, H.M., Byrne, C., Thomas, H., and Woodward, C.A. (1987). Ontario Child Health Study: II. Six-month prevalence of disorder and rates of service utilization. *Archives of General Psychiatry*, **44**, 832-836.

Olsen, S.L. (1992). Development of conduct problems and peer rejection in preschool children: A social systems analysis. *Journal of Abnormal Child Psychology*, **20**, 327–350.

Parker, J.G. and Asher, S.R. (1987). Peer relations and later personal adjustment: Are low-accepted children at risk? *Psychological Bulletin*, **102**, 357–389.

Patterson, G.R. (1982). *A social learning approach: Vol. 3. Coercive Family Processes*. Eugene, Oregon: Castilia.

Patterson, G.R. (1986). Performance models for antisocial boys. *American Psychologist*, **41**, 432–444.

Patterson, G.R., Capaldi, D., and Bank, L. (1991). An early starter model for predicting delinquency. In D.J. Pepler and K.H. Rubin (Eds.), *The development and treatment of childhood aggression* (pp. 139–168). Hillsdale, NJ: Erlbaum.

Patterson, G.R., DeBaryshe, B.D., and Ramsey, E. (1989). A developmental perspective on antisocial behaviour. *American Psychologist*, **44**, 329–335.

Patterson, G.R., Reid, J.B., and Dishion, T.J. (1992). *Antisocial boys*. Eugene, Oregon: Castilia.

Pepler, D.J. , Craig, W.M., and Roberts, W. (1995). Social skills training and aggression in the peer group. In J. McCord (Ed.), *Coercion and punishment in long-term perspectives.* New York: Cambridge Press.

Pepler, D.J., King, G., and Byrd, W. (1991). A social-cognitively based social skills training program for aggressive children. In D.J. Pepler and K.H. Rubin (Eds.), *The development and treatment of childhood aggression* (pp. 361–379). Hillsdale, NJ: Erlbaum.

Petermann, F. and Petermann, U. (1994). *Training mit aggressiven Kindern: Einzeltraining, Kindergruppen, Elternberatung.* Weinheim: Psycholgie Verlags Union, 7th Edition.

Pettit, G.S. and Bates, J.E. (1989). Family interaction patterns and children's behaviour problems from infancy to 4 years. *Developmental Psychopathology, 2, 25,* 413–420.

Plomin, R. (1991). Genetic risk and psychosocial disorders: Links between the normal and abnormal. In M. Rutter and P. Casaer (Eds.), *Biological risks factors for psychological disorders* (pp.101–138). Cambridge, UK: Cambridge University Press.

Puig-Antich, J. and Chambers, W. (1978). *The Schedule for Affective Disorders and Schizophrenia for School-aged Children.* New York: State Psychiatric Institute.

Pratt, T.M. (1973). Positive approaches to disruptive behaviour. *Today's Education,* **62,** 18–19.

Quay, H.C. (1993). The psychobiology of undersocialized aggressive conduct disorder: A theoretical perspective. *Development and Psychopathology, 5,* 165–180.

Quay, H.C. (1988). The behavioral reward and inhibition system in childhood behaviour disorders. In M. Bloomingdale (Ed.), *Attention deficit disorder* (Vol. 3). New York: Pergamon Press.

Quay, H.C. and Peterson, D.R. (1975). *Manual for the Behavior Problem Checklist.* Privately printed.

Raine, A., Venables, P., and Williams, M. (1990). Autonomic orienting responses in 15-year-old male subjects and criminal behaviour at age 24. *American Journal of Psychiatry,* **147,** 933–937.

Reich, W. and Welner, Z. (1988). *Revised version of the Diagnostic Interview for Children and Adolescents (DICA-R).* St. Louis, MO: Department of Psychiatry, Washington University, School of Medicine.

Reid, J.B. (1993). Prevention of conduct disorder before and after school entry: Relating interventions to developmental findings. *Development and Psychopathology, 5,* 243–262.

Reid, J.B. (1978). *A social learning approach to family intervention. Volume 2: Observations in the home settings.* Eugene, OR: Castalia.

Robins, L.N. (1991). Conduct disorder. *Journal of Child Psychology and Psychiatry, 32,* 193–212.

Robins, L.N. (1986). The consequences of conduct disorder in girls. In D. Olweus, J. Block, and M. Radke-Yarrow (Eds.), *Development of antisocial and prosocial behavior: Research, theories and issues.* San Diego, CA: Academic Press.

Robins, L.N. (1978). Study childhood predictors of adult antisocial behavior: Replications from longitudinal studies. *Psychological Medicine, 8,* 611–622.

Robins, L.N. (1966). *Deviant children grow up.* Baltimore: Williams and Wilkens.

Rubin, K.H., Bream, L., and Rose-Krasnor, L. (1991). Social problem solving and aggression in childhood. In D.J. Pepler and K. Rubin (Eds.), *The development and treatment of childhood aggression* (pp. 303–309). Hillsdale, NJ: Erlbaum.

Rutter, M. (1981). Epidemiological/longitudinal strategies and causal roots in child psychiatry. *Journal of the American Academy of Child Psychiatry,* **20,** 513–544.

Rutter, M.and Giller, H. (1983) *Juvenile Delinquency: Trends and perspectives.* New York: Penquin.

Rutter, M., Tizard, J., and Whitemore, R. (1970). *Education, health, and behaviour.* London: Longmans.

Serbin, L.A., Marchessault, K. McAffer, V., Peters, P., and Schwartzman, A.E. (1993). Patterns of social behaviour on the playground in 9–11 year old girls and boys: Relation to teacher perceptions and to peer ratings of aggression, withdrawal, and likeability. In C. Hart (Ed.), *Children on the playground* (pp. 162–183). New York: SUNY Press.

Slaby, R.G. and Guerra, N.G. (1988). Cognitive mediators of aggression in adolescent offenders: I. Assessment. *Developmental Psychology*, **24**, 580–588.

Snider, J.J., Dishion, T.J., and Patterson, G.R. (1986). Determinants and consequences of associating with deviant peers during preadolescence and adolescence. *Journal of Early Adolescence*, **6**, 29–43.

Spivak, G. and Shure, M.B. (1982). The cognition of social adjustment: Interpersonal cognitive problem solving thinking. In B.B. Lahey and A.E. Kazdin (Eds.), *Advances in clinical child psychology* (Vol. 5, pp. 323–372). New York: Plenum Press.

Skoff, B. and Libon, J. (1987). Impaired executive functions in a sample of male juvenile delinquents. *Journal of Clinical and Experimental Neuropsychology*, **9**, 60–64.

Stattin, H. and Magnusson, D. (1990). *Pubertal maturation in female development.* Hillsdale, NJ: Erlbaum.

Tremblay, R.E., Masse, B., Perron, D., Leblanc, M., Schwartzman, A.E., and Ledingham, J.E. (1992). Early disruptive behavior, poor school achievement, delinquent behavior, and delinquent personality: Longitudinal analyses. *Journal of Consulting and Clinical*, **60**, 64–72.

Walker, J.L., Lahey, B.B., Russo, M.F., Christ, M.A., McBurnett, K., Loeber, R., Stouthamer-Loeber, M., and Green, S.M. (1991). Anxiety, inhibition, and conduct disorder in children: I. Relations to social impairment. *Journal of the American Academy of Child and Adolescent Psychiatry*, **30**, 187–191.

Walker, H.M., Shinn, M.R., O'Niell, R.E., and Ramsey, E. (1987). A longitudinal assessment of the development of antisocial behaviour in boys: Rationale, methodology, and first year results. *Remedial and Special Education*, **8**, 7–17.

Waters, E., Posada, G., Crowell, J., and Keng-Ling, L. (1993). Is attachment theory ready to contribute to our understanding of disruptive behaviour problems? *Development and Psychopathology*, **5**, 215–224.

Webster-Stratton, C. (1985). Predictors of treatment outcome in parent training for conduct-disordered children. *Behaviour Therapy*, **16**, 223–243.

West, D.J. (1982). *Delinquency: Its roots, careers, and prospects.* Cambridge, MA. Harvard University Press.

White, J., Moffitt, T., Earls, F., Robins, L., and Silva, P. (1990). How early can we tell? Predictors of conduct disorder and adolescent delinquency. *Criminology*, **28**, 507–533.

Widom, C.S. (1991). The intergenerational transmission of violence. In N.A. Weiner and M.E. Wolfgang (Eds.), *Pathways to criminal violence.* San Francisco: Sage Publications.

Williams, S., Anderson, J., McGee, R., and Silva, P. (1990). Risk factors for behavioral and emotional disorders in preadolescent children. *Journal of the American Academy of Child and Adolescent Psychiatry*, **29**, 413–419.

World Health organization (1993). *Mental disorders: Glossary and guide to their classification in accordance with the Ninth Revision of the International Classification of Diseases (9th and 10th eds.). Geneva: author.*

Zahn-Waxler, C. (1993). Warriors and worriers: Gender and psychopathology. *Development and Psychopathology*, **5**, 79–89.

Zoccolillo, M. (1992). Co-occurrence of conduct disorder and its adult outcomes with depressive and anxiety disorders: A review. *Journal of the American Academy of Child and Adolescent Psychiatry*, **31**, 547–556.

Zoccolillo, M. (1993). Gender and the development of conduct disorder. *Development and Psychopathology*, **5**, 65–78.

CHAPTER 5

ATTENTION-DEFICIT/ HYPERACTIVITY DISORDER

Cecilia Ahmoi Essau, Rob Mcgee, and Michael Feehan

Attention-Deficit/Hyperactivity Disorder (ADHD) represents one of the most common reasons for referral in school settings and mental health clinics (Ross and Ross, 1982; Rubenstein and Brown, 1984; Stewart *et al.*, 1981). The disorder is characterized by difficulty in sustaining attention, and displaying hyperactive and impulsive behaviours. Inattention is generally manifested in academic, occupational or social situations, with individuals having ADHD failing to give close attention to details or making careless mistakes at different tasks. Attentional problems at home are shown by failure to follow through on parental requests, and inability to stick to activities. At school, inattention is usually evidenced by a failure to complete academic assignments. Hyperactivity may be manifested by fidgetiness, twisting in one's seat, an inability to remain seated when expected to, by being often "on the go", or by talking excessively. Impulsivity may be manifested by impatience, so that individuals with the disorder show difficulty in delaying responses or in awaiting their turn. At home, it is expressed by difficulty remaining seated during meals, or completing homework. In the classroom, it is evidenced by blurting out answers.

DEFINITION AND CLASSIFICATION

Despite various changes in several of the diagnostic criteria for the disorder over recent years, the essential feature of ADHD remains a persistent pattern of inattention and/or hyperactivity-impulsivity that is more common and severe than is usually seen in individuals at a comparable developmental level (American Psychiatric Association; APA, 1994). Symptoms of ADHD vary with age (APA, 1994), so that among young children, symptoms of gross motor activity are prominent and are

141

typically difficult to manage. During late childhood and early adolescence, such activity becomes less common and may be confined to fidgetiness or an inner feeling of jitteriness or restlessness. Among school-age children, symptoms of inattention may affect classroom work and academic performance, while impulsive symptoms may lead to breaking of familial, interpersonal and educational rules.

In the fourth edition of the Diagnostic and Statistical Manual of Mental Disorders (DSM-IV; APA, 1994), symptoms of ADHD are categorized under *inattention* (e.g., often have difficulty in sustaining attention in tasks or play activity; is often being easily distracted by extraneous stimuli, or often forgetful in daily activities), *hyperactivity* (e.g., often fidgets with hands or feet or squirms in seat, often "on the go" or often acts as if "driven by a motor"), and *impulsivity* (e.g., often blurts out answers before questions have been completed, often has difficulty awaiting turn). To meet the diagnosis of ADHD, at least six symptoms of inattention or at least six symptoms of hyperactivity-impulsivity have to be present. These symptoms must have persisted for at least six months, must be maladaptive and not consistent with the person's developmental level (APA, 1994) (Table 5.1). Unfortunately, DSM-IV does not make any attempt to define the frequency of "often".

In addition to the above criteria, some hyperactive-impulsive or inattentive symptoms that cause impairment must have been present before age 7 years in order to make the diagnosis of ADHD. DSM-IV gives no indication as to why this age was chosen or the number of early onset symptoms necessary to meet this criteria, and no specific criteria are given for defining impairment. Further, impairment from the symptoms must be present in at least two settings, for example, at home and at school or work. Finally, there should be a clear evidence that these symptoms have impaired developmentally appropriate social, academic, or occupational functioning. Exclusionary criteria are applied in that symptoms do not occur exclusively during the course of a pervasive developmental disorder, schizophrenia, or other psychotic disorder and are not due to another mental disorder such as a mood disorder, anxiety disorder, dissociative disorder, or personality disorder. As with other DSM-IV disorder criteria, all symptoms are given equal weight in making a diagnosis.

Subtypes of ADHD

A number of authors have subgrouped children with the disorder by the concept of pervasive versus situational variants of the syndrome. The

Table 5.1 DSM-IV diagnostic criteria for Attention-Deficit/Hyperactivity Disorder

A) Either (1) or (2):
   1) six (or more) of the following symptoms of **inattention** have persisted for at least 6 months to a degree that is maladaptive and inconsistent with developmental level:

Inattention
   a) often fails to give close attention to details or makes careless mistakes in schoolwork, work, or other activities
   b) often has difficulty sustaining attention in tasks or play activities
   c) often does not seem to listen when spoken to directly
   d) often does not follow through on instructions and fails to finish schoolwork, chores, or duties in the workplace (not due to oppositional behavior or failure to understand instructions)
   e) often has difficulty organizing tasks and activities
   f) often avoids, dislikes, or reluctant to engage in tasks that require sustained mental effort (such as schoolwork or homework)
   g) often loses things necessary for tasks or activities (e.g., toys, school assignments, pencils, books, or tools)
   h) is often easily distracted by extraneous stimuli
   i) is often forgetful in daily activities

   2) six (or more) of the following symptoms of **hyperactivity-impulsivity** have persisted for at least 6 months to a degree that is maladaptive and inconsistent with developmental level:

Hyperactivity
   a) often fidgets with hands or feet or squirms in seat
   b) often leaves seat in classroom or in other situations in which remaining seated is expected
   c) often runs about or climbs excessively in situations in which it is inappropriate (in adolescents or adults, may be limited to subjective feelings of restlessness)
   d) often has difficulty playing or engaging in leisure activities quietly
   e) is often "on the go" or often acts as if "driven by a motor"
   f) often talks excessively

Impulsivity
   g) often blurts out answers before questions have been completed
   h) often has difficulty awaiting turn
   i) often interrupts or intrudes on others (e.g., butts into conversations or games)

Table 5.1 *continued*

B) Some hyperactive-impulsive or attentive symptoms that caused impairment were present before age 7 years

C) Some impairment from the symptoms is present in two or more settings (e.g., at school [or work] and at home)

D) There must be clear evidence of clinically significant impairment in social, academic, or occupational functioning

E) The symptoms do not occur exclusively during the course of a pervasive developmental disorder, schizophrenia, or other psychotic disorder and are not better accounted for by another mental disorder (e.g., mood disorder, anxiety disorder, dissociative disorder, or a personality disorder)

Reprinted with permission from the Diagnostic and Statistical Manual of Mental Disorders, Fourth Edition. Copyright 1994 American Psychiatric Association.

pervasive type is manifested by the presence of severe levels of impulsivity, inattention, and hyperactivity in various settings (Schachter, 1991). These children generally have intellectual, academic, and interpersonal deficits, and delayed language development (Ho *et al.*, 1996). Children with the situational type are identified by only one source, and in most cases are defined based on parental intolerance or transitory environmental events (Schachter, 1991). Because of this and the fact that situationally hyperactive children may be distinguishable from children without psychiatric disorders, it is an open question whether this subgroup consist of a valid disorder. The separation of pervasive and situational type has furthermore been critized due to methodologic issues and recent empirical findings (Schachter, 1991).

With the advent of DSM-III (APA, 1980), the following subtypes of ADHD were introduced: Attention deficit disorder with hyperactivity (ADDH) and attention deficit disorder without hyperactivity (ADD/WO). In ADD/WO there are significant problems in inattention and impulsivity, but not in hyperactivity, whereas in ADDH there are problems related to inattention, impulsivity, and overactivity. The main features that differentiate the ADD/WO from ADDH include parental psychopathology, symptoms, impairment, and treatment response (Schachter, 1991). In ADD/WO, parental psychopathology is characterized by the presence of internalizing disorders and in ADD/H of externalizing disorders. Symptoms commonly found in ADD/WO are those that show internalizing symptomatology, together with being sluggish, forgetful, drowsy, and apathetic; they also experience peer neglect and learning disabilities. In ADD/H, the most common symptoms are those related to oppositional and aggressive behaviors, a need to have close supervision, and failure to complete tasks; they also experience peer rejection, and are in frequent need of school supervision and special education placement. In terms of treatment, children with ADD/WO respond to low dosage of stimulant medication, and those with ADD/H to moderate dosages.

DSM-IV differentiated between three subtypes of ADHD, which are based on the predominant symptom pattern reported or observed over the previous six months: (i) *ADHD combined type* with the presence of at least six symptoms of inattention and at least six symptoms of hyperactivity-impulsivity which have persisted for a minimum of six months; (ii) *ADHD inattentive type* if at least six symptoms of inattention have persisted for at least six months; and (iii) *ADHD hyperactive-impulsive type* when at least six symptoms of hyperactive-impulsivity have persisted for a minimum of six months.

EPIDEMIOLOGY

According to DSM-IV the prevalence of ADHD in "school-age children" (presumably ages 5–18 years) is estimated to be between 3% and 5%. An increase from 3% noted in the earlier DSM-III-R. No distinction is made about prevalence at different ages.

Based on findings of recent epidemiologic studies, the prevalence of ADHD among school-aged children in Canada, the United States, Puerto Rico and New Zealand has been estimated to range from 3 to 10% (Anderson *et al.*, 1987; Bird *et al.*, 1988; Cohen *et al.*, 1987; Offord *et al.*, 1987). Additionally, it has been estimated that between 5 to 29% of the paediatric outpatients (Bhatia *et al.*, 1991) and about 50% of the children referred to child guidance clinics met the diagnosis of ADHD (Stewart *et al.*, 1981). Among adolescents in the general population, one estimate of the prevalence of the disorder suggests a range from 3 to 5% (Fergusson *et al.*, 1993). None of these studies reported on the prevalences of possible subtypes of ADHD as newly proposed in DSM-IV.

Variations in the prevalence of ADHD across studies may be explained by the use of different versions of the diagnostic criteria (i.e., DSM-III, DSM-III-R, DSM-IV), informant source of information (teacher vs parent), and the ages of the sample. For example, DSM-III requires eight symptoms out of 14 which included a mixture of inattentive and hyperactive-impulsive items. Also, the DSM-IV requirement that the behaviour be exhibited in two or more settings was not evident in DSM-III-R. Another possible cause of the differences in prevalence rates may be related to the different types of diagnostic systems (DSM versus the International Classification of Diseases: ICD, World Health Organization, 1993). For example, studies that used the ICD generally report lower rates of ADHD than studies based on DSM, probably because the ICD has a narrower concept of ADHD based upon cross-situational pervasiveness. Also, a lower prevalence of the disorder is to be expected if the diagnosis of conduct disorder is given priority over ADHD in the diagnosis of childhood behaviour disorders (Sandberg, 1985). It is a moot point whether other disorders such as conduct disorder should constitute exclusionary criteria for a diagnosis of ADHD although DSM-IV seems to envisage this where ADHD is clearly the outcome of another disorder.

RISK FACTORS

Sociodemographic Factors

Sex

ADHD is more common in boys than girls, with DSM-IV estimates ranging from a 4:1 to 9:1 ratio, depending on whether the estimates were from general population or clinic data. A review of the community literature indicates a slightly broader range of male to female ratios of 3:1 to 9:1 (Anderson et al., 1987; Cohen et al., 1993; Esser et al., 1990; Fergusson et al., 1993; Szatmari et al., 1989). However, evidence relating to sex differences in ADHD have been questioned by some authors (Berry et al., 1985; Henker and Whalen, 1989; McGee and Feehan, 1991). For example, the differences in prevalence estimates appear restricted to teacher reports of ADHD, and are not so apparent in parent or self-reports (McGee and Feehan, 1991; Schaughency et al., 1994). It may be that teachers underrecognize ADHD among girls, particularly when inattentive behaviour occurs in the absence of severe behavioural disruption and when they do not cause management problems in the classroom. It does seem to be possible to identify girls with marked symptoms of ADHD by reference to the distribution of ADHD behaviours among girls in general (McGee et al., 1987). So in this sense, girls may constitute a "silent minority", "neglected subgroup" or unidentified group at risk for long-term emotional, social and academic problems (Whalen, 1983). In addition, few studies which have tested for sex-specific correlates of ADHD have not found strong evidence for their existence; boys and girls do not differ in behavioural or cognitive correlates of the disorder, or risk factors for the disorder (McGee and Feehan, 1991; Szatmari *et al.*, 1989), and they have similar treatment responses (Barkley, 1989). Consequently, the issue of sex differences in the disorder is perhaps not as clear-cut as it has been made out to be. Certainly, more research should focus on ADHD among girls, particularly in identifying sex differences in the correlates of the disorder.

Social Factors

Family Factors

Findings have been consistent in indicating that compared with other children, those with ADHD come from families often characterized by marital dissatisfaction and separation of their parents, family relationships characterised by conflict, and experience of more stressful life events in the past year (Bafera and Barkley, 1985; Barkley *et al.*, 1991; Campbell *et al.*, 1991; Cohen and Minde, 1983; McGee *et al.*, 1984). In a recent study by Biederman *et al.* (1995a), the odds ratio for having ADHD increased with the increased number of adversity indicators (i.e., severe marital discord of parents, low social class, large family size, parental criminality, maternal mental disorder, and foster placement). Specifically, compared with children without adverse backgrounds, the odds of having a diagnosis of ADHD were 7.4 times greater in children with a single adversity indicator. However, none of these findings should be considered as specific to children with ADHD, as they are also frequently found in the families of children with other types of disorders. It may be, therefore that such family charateristics serve to sustain or intensify ADHD behaviours, but are probably not aetiological factors unique to ADHD.

Mothers of children with the disorder have been described as being more impatient, power assertive, and less consistent (Patterson *et al.*, 1989), and as experiencing more parental stress around child rearing than mothers of children without disorder (Mash and Johnston, 1983). Observational assessments of mother-child interaction indicate that children with ADHD tend to initiate less interaction with their mothers, were less compliant, and were more negative during free play as compared to children without disorder (Campbell *et al.*, 1994; Mash and Johnston,

1982). The mothers initiated fewer contacts, responded less and encouraged play less. When children with ADHD did try to initiate interaction, their mothers were less responsive than mothers of controls. Cunningham and Barkley (1979) reported that mothers of children with ADHD made fewer contacts and responded less than mothers of control children. They tended to be more controlling and gave more commands. The authors concluded that the intrusive and controlling styles of the mothers may contribute to the children's behaviour. A consistent problem in the literature with regard to parental influences on children's mental health or problem behaviour is the almost total emphasis on maternal behaviour and mental health (Phares, 1992; Phares and Compas, 1992). How paternal-child interactions or paternal mental health status may influence the development of disorders such as ADHD is unknown.

Social Interaction

Children with ADHD have been described as having an uncooperative and aggressive interpersonal style (Pelham and Bender, 1982). They have difficulties in establishing and maintaining relationships with other children, and are often viewed by their peers as deviant and having problems (Whalen and Henker, 1985). They receive more rejection and less positive attention from peers (Pelham and Bender, 1982; Whalen and Henker, 1985), are less responsive to communications from peers, and more likely to ignore them or to behave inappropriately (Whalen and Henker, 1985). Impulsivity and a lack of attention to social cues may interfere with the skills development in reciprocity, sharing, and turn taking, that are needed for successful social exchange.

In the classroom, those with ADHD tend to engage in more inappropriate behaviour including annoying peers and disrupting ongoing classroom activities, and becoming involved in aggressive interactions with others (Whalen and Henker, 1985). Flicek (1992) has argued that many of the problems experienced by children with ADHD may be related to accompanying learning disabilities, and associated deficits in social cognitive processing. A combination of ADHD and learning problems may also mediate the aggression shown by these children. Interactions with teachers tend to be characterized by more negative affect and poor compliance on the part of children. The presence of children with ADHD in a classroom seems to have an impact in the interaction pattern of the classroom as a whole, in that teachers tend to interact negatively with all other children, and not necessarily just those with ADHD (Campbell *et al.*, 1977).

Academic Achievement

An association between symptoms which might now be considered as characteristic of ADHD, and reading failure was commented upon by Blanchard as long ago as 1928 (Blanchard, 1928). Gates (1941) also noted the association between behaviours such as restlessness, squirmi-ness, aggression and worry, and reading problems. It is now widely recognized that children with ADHD generally do poorly on a variety of measures of academic achievement such as reading, spelling, and mathematical ability (Cantwell and Satterfield, 1978; Claude and Firestone, 1995; McGee *et al.*, 1984). Children with ADHD show more grade repetitions, poorer grades in academic subjects, more placement in special classes, and more tutoring (Edelbrock *et al.*, 1984). For example, in a recent study by Biederman *et al.* (1995b), children with ADHD whose parent(s) also had ADHD had significantly greater rates of school failure as evidenced by more need of tutoring, placement in special classes, and repeated grades, as compared to their non-ADHD siblings. Those with ADHD also perform more poorly than control chil-dren on standard measures of intelligence and achievement.

The general belief, although this is by no means universal, is that the learning difficulties associated with ADHD are secondary to the impairment of attention and mechanisms of behavioural control. The academic difficulties suffered by many ADHD children could be the consequences of their excessive motor activity which may interfere with the input of new learning (Keogh, 1971). Also, the core charater-istics of ADHD — inattention and impulsivity — could cause impover-ished cognitive schemas and problem-solving skills which could lead to a worsening of academic performance over time (Claude and Firestone, 1995; Douglas, 1983; Keogh, 1971). As noted above, for some children, symptoms of inattention and hyperactivity clearly appear to be a consequence of learning disabilities. Furthermore, the evidence that ADHD symptoms necessarily precede problems in reading, spelling and so on is not particularly strong (McGee and Share, 1988).

Poor language development and lower overall cognitive ability characterizes preschoolers with the disorder, suggesting that develop-mental impairments among those with ADHD may be recognizeable at an early age. McGee *et al.* (1991) reported that preschoolers with per-vasive symptoms of ADHD performed more poorly on measures of lan-guage vocabulary, comprehension, and expressive language than comparison children. However, they did not differ on preschool meas-ures of motor ability. Preschoolers with ADHD also performed more poorly, made more errors of omission and spent more time-off-task on the standard version of the continous performance task and a personal vigilance task (Harper and Ottinger, 1992). They performed poorly on complex rule-learning and concept-formation tasks which need careful processing of large amount of information (Douglas, 1983). In approaching problems, they may tend to be less organized, less thoughtful, and less thorough (Douglas and Peters, 1979). These preschool characteristics may be precursors to the academic failure experienced by children with ADHD at school entry and beyond.

Biological Factors

Biochemical Factors

Because of the comprehensiveness of several reviews (Hechtman, 1994) on the biochemistry of ADHD, we will cover this issue only in passing. Irregular metabolism of monoamines (dopamine, norepinphrine, serotonin) has been implicated in the causation of ADHD. This hypothesis is based on the finding that amphetamine stimulant drugs (e.g., methylphenidate) show improvement in the behaviour of children with ADHD and remediate deficient dopaminergic activity (Solanto, 1984). Also, it has been demonstrated that hyperactive behaviour may be induced in animals through the experimental depletion of brain dopamine (Shaywitz et al., 1978). Another view involves the underarousal of the reticular activating system (Satterfield et al., 1972), leading children to have decreased control of their motor and sensory functions.

It has also been hypothesized that an imbalance of adrenaline formation or alpha-2 adrenergic receptor number or affinity leads to the inability to maintain the appropriate threshold for discharge of locus coeruleus neurons (Mefford and Potter, 1989; Shaywitz and Shaywitz, 1987). This integrated defect leads to "hypervigilance", a state in which the threshold for orienting to sensory stimuli is lowered.

Genetic Factors

Twin Studies. Twin studies suggest that monozygotic twins have a higher concordance rate for hyperactivity than dizygotic twins (Goodman and Stevenson, 1989; Heffron et al., 1984). As reported by Gillis et al. (1992) and Gilger et al. (1992), the concordance rate was 81% for monozygotic twins and 29% for dizygotic twins. The concordance rates for reading disability and ADHD was 44% for monozygotic twins and

30% for dizygotic twins, suggesting that both disorders have strong but independent genetic components (Gilger *et al.*, 1992). On the symptom levels, monozygotic (59%) twins were more alike than their dizygotic twins (33%) on measures of attentiveness and hyperactivity.

Adoption Studies. Early studies have shown that adopted relatives of children with ADHD were less likely to have ADHD than the biological relatives of these children (Morrison and Stewart, 1973). In Cadoret and Stewart's study (1991), adult adoptees with childhood histories of ADHD were more likely to have had a biological parent with a history of criminality/delinquency, and to come from an adoptive home with lower socioeconomic status. These factors appear to increase the likelihood of the adoptee developing an antisocial personality disorder which suggests that there is an interplay between genetic and environmental factors.

Family Studies. About 20% of hyperactive children had a parent(s) who was diagnosed as having ADHD as compared to 2–5% of control children (Cantwell, 1972; Morrison and Stewart, 1971). In a study that examined the prevalence of ADHD and anxiety disorders among the first degree relatives of clinic children with ADHD, Biederman *et al.* (1991) found relatives of ADHD children to have an increased risk of ADHD, regardless of whether the ADHD proband had anxiety or not. In another study, Biederman *et al.* (1992) found that relatives of ADHD probands had a higher risk for not only ADHD, but also for antisocial disorder, major depression, substance dependence and anxiety disorders. It was suggested that ADHD and major depression may show common familial vulnerabilities, that ADHD and conduct disorder may be distinct subtypes and that ADHD and anxiety disorder are transmitted independently in families (Biederman *et al.*, 1991). More recently, Biederman *et al.* (1995a, b) reported that children of parents with ADHD were found to have a higher risk for ADHD; 57% of these children had ADHD, with 75% of them receiving treatment for the disorder. The authors concluded that ADHD with early onset in childhood, and persisting to adolescence and adulthood seems to have a strong familial component.

Nutrition

Feingold (1975) hypothesized that food containing artifical dyes and flavours, certain preservatives and naturally occurring salicylates may be related to hyperactivity. This hypothesis has received widespread publicity and it is apparent that many parents do attribute their children's behaviour to what they eat. An early study by Harley and

Matthews (1980) showed that about 25 to 50% of hyperactive children might respond favourably to diets that eliminated these substances. However, most later studies have failed to support these findings (Conners, 1980; Gross *et al.*, 1987; Harley and Matthews, 1980; Spring *et al.*, 1987).

While this early interest in additive and behaviour has waned to certain extend, an association between sugar and ADHD behaviours continues to receive considerable publicity. Early studies by Prinz *et al.* (1980) and Prinz and Riddle (1986) have suggested a significant correlation between the amount of sugar intake and destructive/aggressive and restless behaviour in ADHD children, and in "normal children" in terms of locomotor activity. However, several other studies have found no such effects associated with sugar intake (Kruesi *et al.*, 1987; Milich and Pelham, 1986; Rosen *et al.*, 1988; Wolraich *et al.*, 1994). While Rosen *et al.* (1988) found that high amounts of sugar were associated with small increases in children's activity, these increases were too small to be considered clinically significant. Despite the intuitive appeal of the sugar ADHD hypothesis, it seems unlikely that sugar in food accounts for a significant proportion of cases of ADHD, and it may well be time to lay this hypothesis to rest.

Allergies, Asthma, and Zinc

Colquhoun and Bunday (1981) hypothesized that hyperactive children suffered an excess of allergic disorders, zinc deficiency and problems of carbohydrate absorption, and that these were evidence of an overall deficiency in prostaglandin synthesis. Admittedly, this hypothesis was entirely speculative and relied on informal reports of parents with children who were hyperactive. However, there has been some research testing these authors' proposals. McGee *et al.* (1990) found no evidence for a zinc deficiency associated with ADHD symptoms. Parent and teacher ratings of ADHD behaviours were uncorrelated with both blood and hair zinc levels among 11 year olds in the Dunedin longitudinal study. Furthermore, children identified with attention deficit disorder did not differ from their peers in zinc levels.

There have been some reports in the literature of an association between ADHD and atopic disorder (Roth *et al.*, 1991) and asthma (Egger *et al.*, 1985), and this has been interpreted as evidence for an imbalance in neuronal transmitter systems associated with norepinephrine affecting both behaviour and immune response (Roth *et al.*, 1991).

However, Mitchell *et al.* (1987) found no evidence for increases in asthma, eczema or other allergies among 48 hyperactive children. Using general population data from the Dunedin study, McGee *et al.* (1993) found no evidence for any association between ADHD behaviour and physician diagnosed asthma, eczema, rhinitis and urticaria, and no evidence for an association with atopic responsiveness by skin test or serum IgE levels.

COMORBIDITY

Children with ADHD are likely to also experience other psychiatric disorders, particularly conduct disorder, oppositional-defiant disorder, and affective and anxiety disorders (Anderson *et al.*, 1987; Bird *et al.*, 1988; Fergusson *et al.*, 1993; Livingston *et al.*, 1990; Munir *et al.*, 1987; Rutter *et al.*, 1970; Schaughency *et al.*, 1994). In a comprehensive review of the comorbidity of ADHD, Biederman *et al.* (1991) reported the rates of comorbid ADHD with conduct/oppositional disorder to be in the range of 30–50%, with mood disorders between 15–75%, and with anxiety disorders about 25%. Methodological differences across studies, and the age groups under investigation may account for the wide variations in comorbidity rates.

There is some evidence for sex and age differences in the comorbidity patterns of children with ADHD. Girls exhibited less impulsivity and fewer conduct problems than boys (de Haas, 1986), but more severe cognitive deficits and learning problems (Berry *et al.*, 1985). As for age, ADHD is commonly comorbid with tic or elimination disorders in younger children (at 8 years) and in older children (at 11 years) with oppositional disorder. The age of onset of ADHD also has an impact on comorbidity. Based on the data from the Dunedin longitudinal study, Schaughency *et al.* (1994) found a higher percentage of adolescents in the early onset group had a comorbid disorder (72%) than those in the late onset group (46%).

It is unclear to what extent ADHD which is comorbid with another disorder differs from ADHD alone. For example, those with a comorbid anxiety or depressive disorder may differ from those with ADHD only in reporting higher life stress and parental psychiatric symptoms (Jensen *et al.*, 1993). According to Jensen *et al.* (1993), children with ADHD are vulnerable to environmental and familial stresses, and when so stressed become anxious and depressed. Others (Pliszka, 1992) consider children who have both ADHD and anxiety disorder as constituting a distinct subtype of children with ADHD who do not respond to stimulants as readily as children with ADHD only. It was presumed that ADHD symptoms are the result of their underlying anxious conditions, so that it may well be the case that when the underlying anxiety is treated, symptoms of ADHD would disappear.

COURSE AND OUTCOME

Age of Onset

The peak prevalence of ADHD is between ages 6 and 11 years (Bird *et al.*, 1988), and the rates of ADHD decrease with age thereafter (Esser *et al.*, 1990; Gomez-Beneyto *et al.*, 1994; McGee *et al.*, 1984; McGee *et al.*, 1985; Szatmari *et al.*, 1989), with an average decline of about 20% per year (Cohen *et al.*, 1993). DSM-III, DSM-III-R, and DSM-IV all specify onset of ADHD before age 7 as one of the criteria for diagnosis. However, in DSM-III it is stated that "onset is typically by age 3" while according to DSM-III-R, onset in about half of all cases occurs before age 4. ICD-10 considers onset by age 6 years. Other authors claim that the disorder arises in infancy or early childhood (Barkley, 1982) or during the preschool years (Ross and Ross, 1982).

According to several studies, the mean age of ADHD onset ranges from 3 to 7 years (Barkley *et al.*, 1990; Campbell, 1985; Green *et al.*, 1991; Keller *et al.*, 1992; Thorley, 1984). An earlier onset of ADHD is associated with more severe symptomatology (Sandberg *et al.*, 1978) and greater comorbidity with other disorders particularly conduct disorder (McGee *et al.*, 1992; Schaughency *et al.*, 1994). As reported by McGee *et al.* (1992), those with onset during the preschool years (age 3) or by age of school entry (age 5–6) had the poorest outcome in adolescence. Furthermore, the boys with onset at school entry showed a consistently poorer reading ability from 7 to 15 years compared with boys having preschool or later onset. By contrast, those boys with later onset by age 7 showed a pattern of disorder consistent with ADHD being an outcome of reading disability; they showed no early cognitive deficits and low comorbidity with other disorders. The unanswered question is whether ADHD presenting at different ages represents the same core disorder or qualitatively different forms of disorder. For example, other evidence from the Dunedin longitudinal study suggests that preschool hyperactivity places the child at risk of a variety of mental health problems and not necessarily ADHD (McGee *et al.*, 1991). Furthermore, sex differences were not strongly apparent among preschool hyperactives. More research is needed to examine possible differences between early and late onset ADHD in childhood to fully address this issue.

Schaughency *et al.* (1994) found a high level of self-reported symptoms of ADHD in the Dunedin cohort at age 15 years, although relatively few adolescents fulfilled the criteria for disorder at this age. For many of these adolescents, ADHD symptoms at this age reflected a residual effect of early childhood disorder. What is of some interest is that a significant number of adolescents reported high levels of ADHD symptoms in the absence of a behavioural history of the disorder in childhood, and continued to show similarly high levels of symptoms three years later. It may be that among older samples, a pattern of ADHD symptoms reflects a more general level of adjustment difficulties.

Outcome

It was originally thought that children "grew out of" ADHD at puberty, but according to several longitudinal studies up to three-quarters of ADHD cases may still have a disorder at follow-up (Barkley, 1990; Biederman *et al.*, 1996; Cohen *et al.*, 1993; Klein and Mannuzza, 1991; Thorley, 1984; Weiss and Hechtman, 1993). Keller and colleagues (1992) have estimated the mean duration of ADHD as 8 years, and while 50% of the children had remitted from ADHD, 71% of the remitted children experienced some form of psychopathology after remission. Also, about half of the children will still have the disorder 9 years after onset. In several other studies, 31 to 72% of the ADHD samples followed over up to 8-year period had ADHD (Barkley *et al.*, 1990).

Compared with other children, those with ADHD are much more likely to exhibit various types of disturbance in adolescence and early adulthood including antisocial and substance abuse disorders, poor peer relationships, low self-esteem, academic underachievement and continuing inattentiveness, impulsiveness and restlessness (Hechtman *et al.*, 1984; Satterfield *et al.*, 1982; Weiss *et al.*, 1985). With a clinic sample, Weiss and Hechtman (1993) showed that boys with ADHD had more impulsive personality traits and were involved in more accidents and geographic moves when interviewed 10 years later. About one-third of clinic-referred children with ADHD exhibit serious delinquency (Mendelson *et al.*, 1971), and are institutionalized for delinquent or criminal behaviour in adolescence (Satterfield *et al.*, 1982). Adolescents with

ADHD were more likely to have been arrested for theft or shoplifting than nonreferred adolescents (Barkley *et al.*, 1990). Based on official court records for the assessment of criminal behaviours, samples of children with ADHD are more likely to be arrested, convicted, or incarcerated for criminal offences as they get older (Mannuzza *et al.*, 1989). However, when self-reports of criminal activity were used, no significant differences could be found between ADHD samples and controls when they were assessed at ages 19 and 25 years (Weiss and Hechtman, 1993). It is likely that these poor outcomes in terms of antisocial activities are not the direct result of ADHD, but rather reflect the high degree of comorbidity between ADHD and conduct disorder in childhood. The finding that outcome is poorer for officially recorded offences than for self-reported ones, suggests that there may exist judical bias towards those with ADHD who come before the court. A similar finding has been reported for learning disability which appears to be correlated with adjudicated offending but not self-reported offending (Broder *et al.*, 1981; Williams and McGee, 1994).

The academic and learning problems of children with ADHD also follow them well into adolescence and are reflected in chronic under-achievement and school failure (Gittelman *et al.*, 1985; Wilson and Marcotte, 1996). Up to one-third of adolescents dropped out of school, and few went to college (Barkley, 1989). Adolescents with ADHD had more adjustment problems (Schaughency *et al.*, 1994), and higher frequencies of retention, suspension and expulsion in school (Gittelman *et al.*, 1985). Children with ADHD also lagged behind the control group in the number of completed grades by one year (Claude and Firestone, 1995).

The pattern of comorbid disorders associated with ADHD has also been studied longitudinally. There appears to be a high comorbidity of conduct disorder (Wilson and Marcotte, 1996), antisocial personality disorder, and the substance use disorders among ADHD children at follow-up (Schaughency *et al.*, 1994). The comorbidity of ADHD with internalizing disorders such as anxiety and depression are rarely seen at follow-up (Mannuzza *et al.*, 1991). In Schaughency *et al.*'s study (1994), adolescents who reported ADHD symptomatology with a history of behavioural disorder were more likely to experience academic difficulties at age 15, and boys in this group were also more likely to have had contact with the police.

The presence of comorbid disorder in children with ADHD is closely related to psychosocial impairment, poor outcome of the disorder, and to high rates of service utilization (Bird *et al.*, 1993; Wilson and Marcotte, 1996). As reported by Sanson *et al.* (1993), hyperactive-aggressive children are significantly more irritable, inflexible, reactively aggressive, and have more behavioural problems than children with only ADHD. In a recent study by Satterfield *et al.* (1994), this high aggression/defiance ADHD subgroup had a poorer outcome than a low aggression/defiance ADHD subgroup 10 years later. Of the high aggression/defiance ADHD group, 43% had been arrested for felony offences during adolescence compared to 26% of those in the low aggression/defiance ADHD group.

Predictors of Outcome

Perhaps the strongest predictor of outcome is the initial severity of ADHD itself, and associated problems. The severity of inattentiveness (Wallander, 1988), being socially disabled (Greene *et al.*, 1996), the presence of delay in language development (Stevenson *et al.*, 1985), and the extent to which the disorder is pervasive across different settings (Klein and Mannuzza, 1991) have all been associated with poor outcome. As noted previously, the presence of comorbid conduct problems in childhood is also a predictor of a more negative prognosis in adolescence and adulthood of ADHD (Biederman *et al.*, 1996; Farrington *et al.*, 1990; Hechtman *et al.*, 1984). In a prospective study by Fischer *et al.* (1993), duration of mental health therapy was negatively related to outcome. That is, the longer the treatment, the worse the outcome. While such a finding might suggest the intractability of the disorder to therapy, duration of mental health treatment in this study may be serving as a proxy measure for the severity of the child's disorder.

Poor outcome in hyperactive children is predicted by the presence of poor family relations, maternal depression, parental divorce, and paternal antisocial behaviour (Lambert, 1988; Wallander, 1988), lower social class, greater family stress, higher maternal ratings of child hyperactivity (Campbell *et al.*, 1986), and psychosocial adversity (Biederman *et al.*, 1996). Data from the Dunedin longitudinal study also suggests poorer outcome for those with an earlier onset of the disorder and a history of family disadvantage (McGee *et al.*, 1984). Similarly, Henker and Whalen (1989) reported that parental psychopathology appeared to be a negative predictor, while having a supportive significant other was a positive predictor of more favourable outcome. However, they felt these factors were predictive of long-term adjustment in general rather than to ADHD in particular.

Loney *et al.* (1981) found an interaction between various factors that predict each outcome domain of children with ADHD. The domain "hyperactivity" was predicted by family socioeconomic status, childhood aggression and perinatal complications, while the domain "inattention" was predicted by age at which parents first realized the child's problem. By contrast, Hechtman *et al.* (1984) found no single initial variable to be associated with any specific outcome. What they did find was an interaction between initial variables which acted in additive fashion to elevate the risks for any domain maladjustment. Certain childhood characteristics (IQ, emotional stability, low frustration tolerance), family factors (mental health of family members), and socioeconomic characteristics often interacted to predict certain areas of later adversity.

Health Service Utilization

Evidence from the Dunedin study suggests a continuing pattern of service utilization by parents of children with ADHD from the early school years to adolescence. McGee *et al.* (1984) reported that among children with significant behavioural problems in the first two years of schooling, parents had sought some form of help for about one in every five, compared with about one in every twenty for those without problems. However, rates of help seeking for those with ADHD-conduct problems were close to one in two (McGee *et al.*, 1984) suggesting that ADHD comorbid with conduct problems represents a particularly difficult combination for parents to manage. A high rate of help seeking (about one in every three) by parents of children with ADHD was also noted by Anderson *et al.* (1987) in preadolescence. By adolescence those with a high level of self-reported ADHD symptoms but no early history of the disorder were more likely to report self-medication for their difficulties than were adolescents without ADHD symptoms. Parents of girls in the late onset group also sought help for their daughters more frequently than parents of girls in the non-ADHD group. Again these differences between early and late onset patterns of ADHD symptoms may reflect different patterns of comorbidity between the two onset times. A recent study by Claude and Firestone (1995) showed that clinic-referred ADHD children with high levels of aggressiveness received the most individual and residential treatment for their behaviour problems.

ASSESSMENT

Barkley (1981) proposed that the following areas be considered when assessing children with ADHD: the social and academic deficits; the social context of the child's behavioural problem (e.g., the parent's responses to the child's hyperactive behaviour may exacerbate it); and gathering of information from multiple informants (e.g., parents, teachers, relatives) who have frequent contact with the child in different situation.

Rating Scales and Checklists

Numerous rating scales have been used for assessing ADHD with children (Table 5.2). The most commonly used scales are the parent-teacher Abbreviated Conners Ratings Scale and the full Conners Teacher and Parent Rating Scales (Conners, 1969; Goyette *et al.*, 1978), the IOWA Conners Teacher Rating Scale (Loney and Milich, 1982), the Child Behavior Checklist (CBCL) for parents and teachers (Achenbach, 1978; Achenbach and Edelbrock, 1979), the revised Behavior Problem Checklist (Quay and Peterson, 1983), and the ADD-H Comprehensive Teacher's Rating Scale (Ullman *et al.*, 1985). Most of these rating scales have been designed to evaluate a wide range of psychopathology, but they also contain items that assess attentional deficits and hyperactivity. Although rating scales are useful as a screening instrument for assessing the core symptoms of ADHD, they do not allow a diagnosis to be made.

Diagnostic Interviews

In recent years a number of diagnostic interviews have been developed to measure the presence of psychiatric disorders in children and adolescents, including ADHD. Diagnostic interviews, especially structured diagnostic interviews, are useful for ascertaining a diagnosis of ADHD and comorbid disorders. The most commonly used diagnostic interviews include the Diagnostic Interview Schedule for Children (Costello *et al.*, 1985), Schedule for Affective Disorders and Schizophrenia for School-aged Children (K-SADS; Puig-Antich and Chambers, 1978), and the Diagnostic Interview for Children and Adolescents (DICA; Herjanic *et al.*, 1975; Reich and Welner, 1988) (Table 5.3).

Other Assessment Methods

Several measures of cognitive, intellectual, and achievement-related functioning have often been indicated for children with ADHD because a large proportion of them do have difficulties with school performances (Table 5.4). These measures include the Wechsler Intelligence Scale for Children (WISC-III; Wechsler, 1991), and the Kaufman Assessment Battery for Children (Kaufman and Kaufman, 1983).

Table 5.2 Examples of questions to assess ADHD symptoms in some questionnaires and checklists

Instruments/Authors	Examples of questions	Responses
Ontario Child Health Study Scales (Boyle *et al.*, 1993)	– I can't concentrate and can't pay attention for long – I do dangerous things without thinking – I jump from one activity to another – I am easily distracted, have difficulty sticking to any activity	"ever or not true" to "often or very true"
Conners Parent Rating Scale (Conners, 1969)	– Excitable, impulsive – Restless in the "squirmy" sense – Restless, always up and on the go – Distractibility or attention span a problem	"not at all" to "very much"
Abbreviated Parent-Teacher Questionnaire (Conners, 1969)	– Restless or overactive – Excitable, impulsive – Constantly fidgeting – Inattentive, easily distracted	"not at all" to "very much"
Child Behavior Checklist (Achenbach and Edelbrock, 1979)	– Cannot stay still, restless, always moving – Behaves without thinking – Inattentive to studying	"not at all true" to "very frequent"
Child Attention/Activity Profile (Edelbrock, 1987)	– Fails to finish things he/she starts – Can't concentrate, can't pay attention for long – Can't sit still, restless, or hyperactive	"not true" to "very or often true"

Table 5.3 Examples of questions to assess ADHD in the selected diagnostic interviews

Interviews	Examples of questions	Rating options
DISC (Costello et al., 1984)	– In the past 6 months, have you moved your hands and feet a lot or squirmed around your seat [during class/at your job]?	0 1* 2* 8 9
	– Do you have more trouble sitting still than other [children/teenagers] your age?	0 1* 2* 9
	– If you are some place where you have to be still or stay put, like in church or riding in a car, do you get very restless and feel you have to move around?	0 1* 2* 9
DICA-R (Reich and Welner, 1988)	– Do you have trouble in school because it is hard for you to sit in your seat for a long time? (PROBE: IN THE CLASSROOM IS THE TEACHER ALWAYS TELLING YOU TO GO BACK TO YOUR SEAT?)	1 2 4 9
	– Are people always telling you to sit still or to stop moving or squirming about? (PROBE: FIDGETING IN YOUR SEAT, PLAYING WITH YOUR HANDS AND FINGERS, JUST NEVER ABLE TO SIT STILL)	1 2 4 9
	– Is it hard for you to play quietly, either by yourself or with other kids? (PROBE: ARE PEOPLE ALWAYS TELLING YOU THAT YOU'RE TOO NOISY, THAT YOU ARE ALWAYS RUNNING AROUND, OR THAT YOU NEVER PLAY QUIETLY?)	1 2 4 9
K-SADS (Puig-Antich and Chambers, 1978)	Do you lose things alot; things you need for school or for home? — At school, do you frequently find you forgot your pen or pencil, or that you left your books or homework in the wrong place? — Do people tell you, you'd even lose your head if it wasn't tied on?	0 1 2 3 4

DISC: 0 = no, 1 = sometimes/somewhat, 2 = yes, 8 = not applicable, 9 = don't know; DICA-R: 1 = yes, 2 = sometimes, 4 = no, 9 = don't know; K-SADS: 0 = no information, 1 = no, 2 = slight, 3 = mild/moderate, 4 = severe/extreme

Table 5.4   Some examples of tests used in children with ADHD

Test	Description
Bender Visual Motor Gestalt Test (Bender, 1938)	Measures perceptual accuracy and motor coordination Requires the child to plan and monitor his/her behaviour and to attend to details
Measures of attention • Serial Reaction Task (Sykes *et al.*, 1973) • Continous Performance Test (Rosvold *et al.*, 1956)	Measures the ability of ADHD children to sustain attention for prolonged periods of time
Intelligence Tests • Wechsler Intelligence Scale for Children — Revised (WISC-R; Wechsler, 1974)	Measures difficulties related to distracbility, inattention, short-term memory, judgement, and overall responsibility to structured tasks
Measures of cognitive styles • Matching Familiar Figures Test (Kagan, 1965) • The Children's Embedded Figures Test (Karp and Konstadt, 1963) • Colour Distraction Test (Santostefano and Paley, 1964)	Measures difficulties related to impulsivity, field dependence, and constricted control/ distractibility

Other instruments commonly used to help quantify the degree of difficulty in tasks related to school functioning, core symptoms of ADHD (i.e., problems with inattention, hyperactivity, and impulsivity), and to monitor treatment effects include: (a) Continous Performance Test (CPT) — a measure of vigilance or sustained attention; (b) The Matching Unfamiliar Figures Test — a measure of behaviourial inhibition and cognitive tempo while engaged in visual problem solving; (c) Paired Associate Learning Test — a measure of short-term memory; (d) Stimulus Equivalence Paradigm — a measure of higher-order learning and long-term recall. Although these tests have been used to monitor treatment or to adjust medication dosages, their actual utility is open to question: cognitive performance in a laboratory is not related in any simple manner to naturalistic behaviour.

Psychopharmacotherapy

Psychostimulant medication has been the most frequent treatment for ADHD (Vyse and Rapport, 1989), with methylphenidate, dextroamphetamine, and pemoline being the most commonly used (see Gittelmann and Kanner, 1986; Spencer *et al.*, 1996; Werry, 1993 for review). According to Wolraich *et al.*'s report (1990), 88% of children with ADHD had been treated with methylphenidates; it must be stressed that this data come from the United States and that it may not apply to other countries. Safer and Krager (1988) found the rate of methylphenidate use to have increased over the past 20 years. Many studies have indicated the short-term efficacy of stimulant treatment with up to 75% of ADHD children treated with psychostimulants showed increased attention, improvement of short-term memory and reduced impulsivity and activity levels, especially in structured, demanding situations (Dulcan, 1986; Rapport *et al.*, 1985; see Spencer *et al.*, 1996 for review). Stimulants also decreased children's disruptive, noncompliant, and oppositional behaviour (Dulcan, 1986; Hinshaw *et al.*, 1989; Whalen *et al.*, 1990; see Spencer *et al.*, 1996 for review). Peers rated children with ADHD more positively following medically related improvement (Whalen *et al.*, 1989). However, for many children, stimulant treatment is a short term solution because benefits rapidly dissipate upon withdrawal of the medication (Brown *et al.*, 1987). Another problem is that between 20 to 30% of children do not respond favourably to stimulant medication, or do not tolerate it well. Furthermore, there is little support for the long-term efficacy of stimulant medication (Jacobvitz *et al.*, 1990; Weiss and Hechtman, 1993). Even among children who do respond, stimulant treatment has not significantly showed improvement in the long-term outcome of their symptoms (Hechtman *et al.*, 1984; Whalen *et al.*, 1985). The use of medication during childhood does not alter the prognosis in adolescence or adulthood. As compared with those who did not receive stimulant medication during childhood, children who received stimulant medication did not differ significantly in the areas of school, work, and personal adjustment in adolescence (Hechtman *et al.*, 1984).

Many parents refuse stimulant therapy for their children, especially mothers with a comprehensive knowledge of ADHD (Rostain *et al.*, 1993); others discontinue treatment prematurely (Brown *et al.*, 1985; Firestone, 1982). Compliance with long- term stimulant therapy is poor, with estimates of noncompliance ranging from 25 to 50% (Brown *et al.*,

1987; Brown *et al.*, 1985; Firestone, 1982). A major concern with the use of psychostimulants is the possible adverse side effects. The most commonly reported side effects include insomnia, decreased appetite, weight loss, irritability, abdominal pain, headaches, and drowsiness (Dulcan, 1986). An adverse drug reaction associated with chronic use is growth suppression, although this phenomenon appears to be dose dependent and reversible upon cessation of treatment (Gittelman and Kanner, 1986).

Psychological Intervention

Behavioural Therapy

Behaviour therapies involve teaching parents and/or teachers to carry out contingency management programs with the child. Contingency management procedures are derived from the principles of operant conditioning so that the child's behaviours are shaped by the consequences that follow them. These procedures use different types of reinforcement (material and social) and punishment procedures. The latter include response-cost procedures which involve the child losing some preobtained reward due to inappropriate behaviour. Time-out procedures which involve removing the child from the environment that elicited and maintained the inappropriate responses have also been used. A number of studies have shown the efficacy of a response-cost program in managing and improving the children's behaviour in the classroom (Pelham *et al.*, 1988; Rapport *et al.*, 1982).

Parent Training

Parent training is a popular method for the management of ADHD. The main aims are to enhance parents' knowledge about the nature of ADHD in order to better understand and manage their child's behavioural problems (Weiss and Hechtman, 1993). Such training also gives parents an ongoing clinical supervision in the use of contingency management techniques to deal with their child's ADHD symptoms and helps facilitate parents' adjustment to having a child with ADHD. This is important since the disorder is often associated with disturbance in parent-child interaction. As reported by several authors, parents of children with ADHD not only report negative attitudes toward their child, but also report difficulties in child management (Mash and Johnston, 1983). These reports are confirmed by observational studies of negative mother-child interactions (Mash and Johnston, 1982, 1983).

Most parental training consists of 10 to 12 steps, and involves informing parents about the nature, course, prognosis and etiology of ADHD (Barkley, 1989; Ialongo *et al.*, 1993; Weiss and Hechtman, 1993). Parents are also trained to attend to their children, giving commands to optimize compliance in their children, and to set up a home token economy in order to reinforce the child's completion of home responsibilities, and to use response cost and time out procedures for noncompliant behaviour. To facilitate generalization of the child's problem solving and self-control skills, parents are provided with instructions to prompt and reinforce their child's use of the newly acquired self-control and problem-solving skills together with a rationale for their use, the various steps of the plan and the skills to be used (Ialongo *et al.*, 1993). The efficacy of the parent training for long-term management of ADHD is yet to be evaluated (Weiss and Hechtman, 1993).

Classroom Behavioural Management

This procedure has been used to help children with ADHD improve their classroom behaviours and academic functioning. For example, a widely used procedure is to train teachers in the use of a daily home report card system in which parents provide rewards or mild punishment based on the teacher's rating of the child's classroom behaviour for that day. Butross (1988) has listed several recommendations in dealing with ADHD children in the classroom including promoting understanding about the way ADHD interferes with classroom function; ignoring provocative behaviour and reinforcing appropriate ones; minimizing distracting stimuli by avoiding the "open classroom" and for example, having the child sit in front and to the centre of the classroom; increasing teacher availability by use of teacher aides or resource rooms; structuring classroom functions by having predictable daily routines, use of record books and writing instructions on the board; having children do one task at a time; and breaking assignments into segments and checking periodically with the child to ensure completion.

Cognitive Training Programs

The main aim of this treatment approach is to teach children with ADHD more effective problem-solving and self-control skills such as self-monitoring training and self-instruction training. *Self-monitoring training* involves teaching children with ADHD to observe and evaluate their performance from time to time to help promote greater attention to detail and awareness of the problem-solving process. *Self-control training* is used to teach ADHD children to "think before they act" by training them to "talk to themselves internally" to help focus and guide their behaviour on a task (Meichenbaum and Goodman, 1971). *Problem-solving training* has also been used to help children recognize and define an interpersonal problem when it arises, and to generate alternative solutions, to evaluate the consequences and implement the chosen solution. Kendall and Panichelli (1995), in their review of the effects of cognitive-behavioural treatments on ADHD suggest that they may be most effective in treating the impulsivity component of the disorder.

Combined Treatments

The most common treatment combinations are those of psychostimulant medication with social learning based approaches (Barkley, 1989), and/or cognitive behavioural interventions (Kendall and Braswell, 1985). Studies evaluating the effectiveness of combined interventions for the treatment of ADHD have given mixed results (Pelham and Murphy, 1986). In Cohen *et al.*'s study (1981), the effects of combined stimulant medication and cognitive-behavioural therapy were no greater than the control condition at a one-year follow-up. Ialongo *et al.* (1993) examined the effects of different dosages of stimulant medication alone and in combination with psychological interventions such as parent training, cognitive-behavioural therapy for the child, and classroom behavioural management. The combination of stimulant medication with the psychological intervention facilitated little maintenance over a 9-month follow-up. In fact, there was deterioration of treatment effects for all conditions.

By contrast, a number of studies (Carlson *et al.*, 1992; Pelham *et al.*, 1992) have shown psychostimulant therapy and psychological intervention to be superior to either intervention alone, and is also more cost-effective (Carlson *et al.*, 1992; Pelham *et al.*, 1992). As shown by Satterfield *et al.* (1987) combined treatment of psychostimulant and psychological interventions have positive long-term effects of up to 6 years. Also, compared to boys with ADHD who received psychostimulants only, those who received the combined treatment had lower rates of arrests for serious offences and institutionalization. Carlson *et al.* (1992) have shown that it is possible to achieve the same results with half the psychostimulant dose when medication is combined with behaviour therapy.

In addition to all these interventions, environmental management of sensory stimulation that involves reducing the amount of stimulation and distraction in the child's home and school setting may be necessary. For example, this might involve avoiding situations where there are lots of people (e.g., supermarket) and encouraging controlled physical activity or exercise. An individualized educational plan can be developed with the school to facilitate classroom arrangements, and perhaps with specialized interventions to take into account comorbid learning disorders.

CONCLUDING REMARKS

ADHD is a common disorder affecting significant numbers of school-aged children in the general population. Writing in mid-1980, Campbell and Werry (1986) ended their review of attention deficit disorder-hyperactivity by cautioning that issues of diagnostic specificity and the nature of the mechanisms underlying the disorder still need to be addressed. It could be argued that this disorder has been the most thoroughly investigated of all psychopathological disorders of childhood. Now ten years later, are we any further along the track to answering the questions these authors raised?

Recent research has focussed on the association between ADHD and conduct disorder on the one hand, and the relationship between ADHD and academic problems on the other. Part of the key to solving the issue of diagnostic specificity may be to fully explore the temporal relationships between these domains to identify the pattern(s) of sequencing of these disorders. Further longitudinal studies examining the age of onset of ADHD, conduct and literacy problems will be needed to enhance our understanding of the nature of the disorder. It is also important to examine the role of both biological and psychosocial factors in the onset and maintenance of ADHD, and how these might affect the course and outcome of the disorder.

REFERENCES

Achenbach, T.M. (1978). The Child Behavior Profile: I. Boys aged 6–11. *Journal of Counsulting and Clinical Psychology*, **46**, 478–488.
Achenbach, T.M. and Edelbrock, C. (1979). The Child Behavior Checklist Profile: II. Boys aged 12–16 and girls aged 6–11 and 12–15. *Journal of Consulting and Clinical Psychology*, **47**, 223–233.
American Psychiatric Association (1980). *Diagnostic and statistical manual of mental disorders (3rd ed.)*. Washington, DC: Author.

American Psychiatric Association (1987). *Diagnostic and statistical manual of mental disorders (3rd ed. rev.).* Washington, DC: Author.

American Psychiatric Association (1994). *Diagnostic and statistical manual of mental disorders (4th ed.).* Washington, DC: Author.

Anderson, J.C., Williams, S., McGee, R., and Silva, P.A. (1987). DSM-III disorders in preadolescent children. *Archives of General Psychiatry,* **44**, 69–76.

Bafera, M.S. and Barkley, R.A. (1985). Hyperactive and normal girls and boys: Mother-child interaction, parent psychiatric status and child psychopathology. *Journal of Child Psychology and Psychiatry,* **26**, 439–452.

Barkley, R.A. (1981). *Hyperactive children: A handbook for diagnosis and treatment.* New York: Guilford Press.

Barkley, R.A. (1982). Guidelines for defining hyperactivity in children. In B.B. Lahey and A.E. Kazdin (Eds.), *Advances in Clinical Child Psychology* (Vol. 5, pp. 137–180). New York: Plenum Press.

Barkley, R.A. (1989). Hyperactive girls and boys: Stimulant drug effects on mother-child interactions. *Journal of Child Psychology and Psychiatry,* **30**, 379–390.

Barkley, R.A. (1990). *Attention deficit hyperactivity disorder: A handbook for diagnosis and treatment.* Hove, East Sussex: Guilford.

Barkley, R.A., Fischer, M., Edelbrock, C.S., and Smallish, L. (1990). The adolescent outcome of hyperactive children diagnosed by research criteria: I. An 8-year prospective follow-up study. *Journal of the American Academy of Child and Adolescent Psychiatry,* **29**, 546–557.

Barkley, R.A., Fischer, M., Edelbrock, C.S., and Smallish, L. (1991). The adolescent outcome of hyperactive children diagnosed by research criteria: III. Mother-child interactions, family conflicts and maternal psychopathology. *Journal of Child Psychology and Psychiatry,* **32**, 233–255.

Bender, L. (1938). *A visual motor gestalt test and its clinical uses (Research monographs, no. 3).* New York: Academic Press.

Berry, C.A., Shaywitz, S.E., and Shaywitz, B.A. (1985). Girls with attention deficit disorder: A silent minority? *Pediatrics,* **26**, 439–452.

Bhatia, M.S., Nigam, V.R., Bohra, N., and Malik, S.C. (1991). Attention deficit disorder with hyperactivity among paediatric outpatients. *Journal of Child Psychology and Psychiatry,* **32**, 297–306.

Biederman, J., Faraone, S., Milberger, S., Curtis, S., Chen, L., Marrs, A., Ouellette, C., Moore, P., and Spencer, T. (1996). Predictors of persistence and remission of ADHD into adolescence: Results from a four-year prospective follow-up study. *Journal of the American Academy of Child and Adolescent Psychiatry,* **35**, 343–351.

Biederman, J., Faraone, S.V., Keenan, K., Steingard, R., and Tsuang, M.T. (1991). Familial association between attention deficit disorder and anxiety disorders. *American Journal of Psychiatry,* **148**, 251–256.

Biederman, J., Faraone, S., Keinan, K., Benjamin, J., Krifcher, B., Moore, C., Sprich, S., Ugaglia, K., Jellinek, M.S., Steingard, R., Spencer, T., Norman, D., Kolodny, R., Kraus, I., Perrin, J., Keller, M.B., and Tsuang, M.T. (1992). Further evidence for family-genetic risk factors in attention deficit hyperactivity disorders: Patterns of comorbidity in probands and relatives in psychiatrically and pediatrically referred samples. *Archives of General Psychiatry,* **79**, 728–738.

Biederman, J., Faraone, S.V., Mick, E., Spencer, T., Wilens, T., Kiely, K., Guite, J., Ablon, J.S., Reed, E., and Warburton, R. (1995a). High risk for attention deficit hyperactivity disorder among children of parents with childhood onset of the disorder: A pilot study. *American Journal of Psychiatry,* **152**, 431–435.

Biederman, J., Milberger, S., Faraone, S.V., Kiely, K., Guite, J., Mick, E., Ablon, S., Warburton, R., and Reed, E. (1995b). Family-environment risk factors for attention-deficit hyperactivity disorder: A test of Rutter's indicator of adversity. *Archives of General Psychiatry,* **52**, 464–470.

Bird, H., Canino, G., Rubio-Stipec, M., Gould, M.S., Ribera, J., Sesman, M., Woodbury, M., Huertas-Goldman, S., Pagan, A., Sanchez-Lacay, A., and Moscoso, M. (1988). Estimates of the prevalence of childhood maladjustment in a community survey in Puerto Rico. *Archives of General Psychiatry, 45,* 1120–1126.

Bird, H.R., Gould, M.S., and Staghezza, B.M. (1993). Patterns of diagnostic comorbidity in a community sample of children aged 9 through 16 years. *Journal of the American Academy of Child and Adolescent Psychiatry, 32,* 361–368.

Blanchard, P. (1928). Reading disabilities in relation to maladjustment. *Mental Hygiene, 12,* 772–788.

Boyle, H.M., Offord, R.D., Racine, Y., Fleming, J.E., Szatmari, P., and Sanford, M. (1993). Evaluations of the Revised Ontario Child Health Study Scales. *Journal of Child Psychology and Psychiatry, 34,* 189–213.

Broder, P.K., Dunivant, N., Smith, E.C., and Sutton, L.P. (1981). Further observations on the link between learning disabilities and juvenile delinquency. *Journal of Educational Psychology, 73,* 838–850.

Brown, R.T., Borden, K.A., and Clingerman, S.R. (1985). Adherence to methylphenidate therapy in a pediatric population: A preliminary investigation. *Psychopharmacology Bulletin, 21,* 192–211.

Brown, R.T., Borden, K.A., Wynne, M.E., Spunt, A.L., and Clingerman, S.R. (1987). Compliance with pharmacological and cognitive treatments for attention deficit disorder. *Journal of the American Academy of Child and Adolescent Psychiatry, 26,* 521–526.

Brown, R.T., Wynne, M.E., and Medenis, R. (1985). Methylphenidate and cognitive therapy: A comparison of treatment approaches with hyperactive boys. *Journal of Abnormal Child Psychology, 13,* 69–87.

Butross, S. (1988). Disorders of attention and vigilance. *Seminars in Neurology, 8,* 97–107.

Cadoret, R.J. and Stewart, M.A. (1991). An adoption study of attention decificit hyperactivity/aggression and their relationship to adult antisocial personality. *Comprehensive Psychiatry, 32,* 73–82.

Campbell, S.B. (1985). Hyperactivity in preschoolers: Correlates and prognostic implications. *Clinical Psychology Review, 5,* 405–428.

Campbell, S.B., Breaux, A.M., Ewing, L.J., and Szumowski, E.K. (1986). Correlates and predictors of hyperactivity and aggression: A longitudinal study of parent-referred problem preschoolers. *Journal of Abnormal Child Psychology, 14,* 217–234.

Campbell, S.B., Endman, M., and Bernfield, G. (1977). A three-year follow-up of hyperactive preschoolers into elementary school. *Journal of Child Psychology and Psychiatry, 18,* 239–249.

Campbell, S.B., Pierce, E., March, C., and Ewing, L.J. (1991). Noncompliant behavior, overactivity, and family stress as predictors of negative maternal control in preschool children. *Development and Psychopathology, 3,* 175–190.

Campbell, S.B., Pierce, E., March, C., Ewing, L.J., and Szumowski, E.K. (1994). Hard-to-manage preschool boys: Symptomatic behavior across contexts and time. *Child Development, 65,* 836–851.

Campbell, S.B. and Werry, J.S. (1986). Attention deficit disorder (hyperactivity). In H. Quay and J.S. Werry (Eds.), *Psychopathological disorders of childhood* (pp. 111–155). New York: Wiley.

Cantwell, D. (1972). Psychiatric illness in families of hyperactive children. *Archives of General Psychiatry, 27,* 414–423.

Cantwell, D.P. and Satterfield, J.H. (1978). The prevalence of underachievement in hyperactive children. *Journal of Pediatric Psychology, 3,* 168–171.

Carlson, C.L., Pelham, W.E., Milich, R., and Dixon, J. (1992). Single and combined effects of methylphenidate and behavior therapy on the classroom performance of children with attention-deficit hyperactivity disorder. *Journal of Abnormal Child Psychology, 20,* 213–232.

170   *Developmental Psychopathology*

Claude, D. and Firestone, P. (1995). The development of ADHD boys: A 12-year follow-up. *Canadian Journal of Behavioral Science*, **27**, 226–249.

Cohen, P., Cohen, J., and Brook, J. (1993). An epidemiological study of disorders in late childhood and adolescence — II. Persistence of disorders. *Journal of Child Psychology and Psychiatry*, **34**, 869–877.

Cohen, N.J. and Minde, K. (1983). The "hyperactive syndrome" in kindergarten children: Comparison of children with pervasive and situational symptoms. *Journal of Child Psychology and Psychiatry*, **24**, 443–456.

Cohen, N.J., Sullivan, J., Minde, K., Novack, C., and Helwig, C. (1981). Evaluation of the relative effectiveness of methylphenidate and cognitive behavior modification in the treatment of kindergarten-aged hyperactive children. *Journal of Abnormal Child Psychology*, **9**, 43–54.

Cohen, P., Velez, N., Kohn, M., Schwab-Stone, M., and Johnston, J. (1987). Child psychiatric diagnosis by computer algorithm: Theoretical issues and empirical tests. *Journal of the American Academy of Child and Adolescent Psychiatry*, **26**, 631–638.

Conners, C.K. (1980). *Food additives and hyperactive children.* New York: Plenum.

Conners, C.K. (1969). A teacher rating for use in drug studies with children. *American Journal of Psychiatry*, **126**, 152–156.

Colquhoun, I. and Bunday, S. (1981). A lack of essential fatty acids as a possible cause of hyperactivity in children. *Medical Hypotheses*, **7**, 673–679.

Costello, E.J., Edelbrock, C.S., and Costello, A.J. (1985). Validity of the NIMH Diagnostic Interview Schedule for Children: A comparison between psychiatric and pediatric referrals. *Journal of Abnormal Child Psychology*, **13**, 579–595.

Costello, A.J., Edelbrock, C., Dulcan, R.K., Kalas, R., and Klaric, S.H. (1984). *Development and testing of the NIMH Diagnostic Interview Schedule for Children in a clinic population.* Rockville, MD: National Institute of Mental Health.

Cunningham, C.E. and Barkley, R.A. (1979). The interactions of normal and hyperactive children with their mothers in free play and structured tasks. *Child Development*, **50**, 217–224.

de Haas, P. (1986). Attention styles and peer relationships of hyperactive and normal boys and girls. *Journal of Abnormal Child Psychology*, **14**, 457–467.

Douglas, V.I. (1983). Attentional and cognitive problems. In M. Rutter (Ed.), *Developmental neuropsychiatry*. New York: Guilford.

Douglas, V.I. and Peters, K. (1979). Toward a clearer definition of the attentional deficit of hyperactive children. In G. Hale and M. Lewis (Eds.), *Attention and the development of cognitive skills*. New York: Plenum.

Dulcan, M.K. (1986). Comprehensive treatment of children and adolescents with attention deficit disorders: The state of the art. *Clinical Psychology Review*, **6**, 539–569.

Edelbrock, C., Costello, A.J., and Kessler, M. (1984). Empirical corroboration of attention deficit disorder. *Journal of the American Academy of Child Psychiatry*, **23**, 285–290.

Egger, J., Carter, C.M., Graham, P.J., Gumley, D., and Soothill, J.F. (1985). Controlled trial of oligiantigenic treatment in the hyperkinetic syndrome. *Lancet i*, 540–545.

Esser, G., Schmidt, M.H., and Woerner, W. (1990). Epidemiology and course of psychiatric disorders in school-age children — Results of a longitudinal study. *Journal of Child Psychology and Psychiatry*, **31**, 243–263.

Farrington, D.P., Loeber, R., and Van Kammen, W.B. (1990). Long-term criminal outcomes of hyperactivity-impulsivity-attention-deficit and conduct problems in childhood. In L.N. Robins and M. Rutter (Eds.), *Straight and devious pathways to adulthood* (pp. 62–81). New York: Cambridge University Press.

Feingold, B. (1975). *Why your child is hyperactive.* New York: Random House.

Fergusson, D.M., Horwood, L.J., and Lynskey, M.T. (1993). Prevalence and comorbidity of DSM-III-R diagnoses in a birth cohort of 15 year olds. *Journal of the American Academy of Child Psychiatry*, **32**, 1127–1134.

Firestone, P. (1982). Factors associated with adherence to stimulant medication. *American Journal of Orthopsychiatry*, **52**, 447–456.

Fischer, M., Barkley, R.A., Fletcher, K.E., and Smallish, L. (1993). The adolescent outcome of hyperactive children: Predictors of psychiatric, academic, social, and emotional adjustment. *Journal of the American Academy of Child and Adolescent Psychiatry*, **32**, 324–332.

Flicek, M. (1992). Social status of boys with both academic problems and attention-deficit hyperactivity disorder. *Journal of Abnormal Child Psychology*, **20**, 353–366.

Gates, A.I. (1941). The role of personality maladjustment in reading disability. *Journal of Genetic Psychology*, **59**, 77–83.

Gilger, J.W., Pennington, B.F., and DeFries, J.C. (1992). A twin study of the etiology of comorbidity: Attention deficit hyperactivity disorder and dyslexia. *Journal of the American Academy of Child and Adolescent Psychiatry*, **31**, 343–348.

Gillis, J.J., Gilger, J.W., Pennington, B.F., and DeFries, J.C. (1992). Attention deficit disorder in reading-disabled twins: Evidence for a genetic etiology. *Journal of Abnormal Child Psychology*, **20**, 303–315.

Gittelman, R. and Kanner, A. (1986). Psychopharmacotherapy. In H. Quay and J.S. Werry (Eds.), *Psychopathological disorders of children*. New York: Wiley.

Gittelman, R., Mannuzza, S., Shenker, R., and Bonagura, N. (1985). Hyperactive boys almost grown up. I. Psychiatric status. *Archives of General Psychiatry*, **42**, 937–947.

Gomez-Beneyto, M., Bonet, A., Catala, M.A., Puche, E., and Vila, V. (1994). Prevalence of mental disorders among children in Valencia, Spain. *Acta Psychiatrica Scandinavica*, **89**, 352–357.

Goodman, R. and Stevenson, J. (1989). A twin study of hyperactivity-II. The aetiological role of genes, family relationships and perinatal adversity. *Journal of Child Psychology and Psychiatry*, **30**, 691–709.

Goyette, C.H., Conners, C.K., and Ulrich, R.F. (1978). Normative data on revised Conners parent and teacher rating scales. *Journal of Abnormal Child Psychology*, **6**, 221–236.

Green, R.W., Biederman, J., Faraone, S.V., Ouellette, C.A., Penn, C., and Griffin, S.M. (1996). Toward a new psychometric definition of social disability in children with attention-deficit hyperactivity disorder. *Journal of the American Academy of Child and Adolescent Psychiatry*, **35**, 571–578.

Green, S.M., Loeber, R., and Lahey, B.B. (1991). Stability of mothers' recall of the age of onset of their child's attention and hyperactivity problems. *Journal of the American Academy of Child and Adolescent Psychiatry*, **30**, 135–137.

Gross, M.D., Tofanelli, R.A., Butzirus, S.M., and Snodgrass, E.W. (1987). The effects of diets rich in and free from addictives on the behavior of children with hyperkinetic and learning disorders. *Journal of the American Academy of Child and Adolescent Psychiatry*, **26**, 53–55.

Harley, J.P. and Matthews, C.G. (1980). Food addictives and hyperactivity in children: Experimental investigations. In R.M. Knights and D.J. Bakker (Eds.), *Treatment of hyperactive and learning disordered children*. Baltimore: University Park Press.

Harper, G.W. and Ottinger, D.R. (1992). The performance of hyperactive and control preschoolers as a new computerized measure of visual vigilance: The preschool vigilance-task. *Journal of Child Psychology and Psychiatry*, **33**, 1365–1372.

Hechtman, L. (1994). Genetic and neurobiological aspects of attention deficit hyperactive disorder: A review. *Journal of Psychiatry Neuroscience*, **19**, 193–201.

Hechtman, L., Weiss, G., and Perlman, T. (1984). Young adult outcome of hyperactive children who received long-term stimulant treatment. *Journal of the American Academy of Child Psychiatry*, **23**, 261–269.

Heffron, W.A., Martin, C.A., and Welsh, R.J. (1984). Attention deficit disorders in three pairs of monozygotic twins: A case report. *Journal of the American Academy of Child Psychiatry*, **23**, 299–301.

Herjanic, B., Herjanic, M., Brown, F., and Wheatt, T. (1975). Are children reliable reporters? *Journal of Anormal Child Psychology*, **3**, 4–48.

Henker, B. and Whalen, C.K. (1989). Hyperactivity and attention deficits. *American Psychologist*, **44**, 216–223.

Hinshaw, S.P., Henker, B., Whalen, C.K., Erhardt, D., and Dunnington, R.E., Jr. (1989). Aggressive, prosocial, and non-social behavior in hyperactive boys: Dose effects of methylphenidate in naturalistic settings. *Journal of Counselling and Clinical Psychology*, **57**, 636–643.

Ho, T.P., Luk, E.S.L., Leung, P.W.L., Taylor, E., Lieh-Mak, F., and Bacon-Shone, J. (1996). Situational versus pervasive hyperactivity in a community sample. *Psychological Medicine*, **26**, 309–321.

Ialongo, N.S., Horn, W.F., Pascoe, J.M., Greenberg, G., Packard, T., Lopez, M., Wagner, A., and Puttler, L. (1993). The effects of a multimodal intervention with Attention-deficit Hyperactivity Disorder children: A 9-month follow-up. *Journal of the American Academy of Child and Adolescent Psychiatry*, **32**, 182–189.

Jacobvitz, D., Sroufe, L.A., Stewart, M., and Leffert, N. (1990). Treatment of attentional and hyperactivity problems in children with sympathomimetic drugs: Comprehensive review. *Journal of the American Academy of Child and Adolescent Psychiatry*, **29**, 677–688.

Jensen, P.S., Shervette, R.E., Xenakis, S.N., and Richters, J. (1993). Anxiety and depressive disorders in attention deficit disorder with hyperactivity: New findings. *American Journal of Psychiatry*, **150**, 1203–1209.

Kagan, J. (1965). Individual differences in the resolution of response uncertainty. *Journal of Personality and Social Psychology*, **47**, 365–395.

Karp, S.A. and Konstadt, N. (1963). *Manual for the Children's Embedded Figures Test.* New York: Cognitive Tests.

Kaufman, A.S. and Kaufman, N.L. (1983). *Kaufman Assessment Battery for Children — K-ABC.* Circles Pines, MN: American Guidance Service.

Keller, M.B., Lavori, P.W., Wunder, J., Beardslee, W.R., Schwartz, C.E., and Roth, J. (1992). Chronic course of anxiety disorders in children and adolescents. *Journal of the American Academy of Child and Adolescent Psychiatry*, **31**, 596–599.

Kendall, P.C. and Braswell, L. (1985). *Cognitive-behavioral therapy for impulsive children.* New York: Guilford Press.

Kendall, P.C. and Panichelli, S.M. (1995). Cognitive-behavioral treatments. *Journal of Abnormal Child Psychology*, **23**, 107–124.

Keogh, B.K. (1971). Hyperactivity and learning disorders: Review and speculation. *Exceptional Children*, **38**, 101–109.

Klein, R. and Mannuzza, S. (1991). Long-term outcome of hyperactive children: A review. *Journal of the American Academy of Child and Adolescent Psychiatry*, **30**, 383–387.

Kruesi, J.P., Rapoport, J.L., Cummings, M., Berg, C.J., Ismond, D.R., Flament, M., Yarrow, M., and Zahn-Waxler, C. (1987). Effects of sugar and aspartame on aggression and activity in children. *American Journal of Psychiatry*, **144**, 1487–1490.

Lambert, N.M. (1988). Adolescent outcomes for hyperactive children. Perspectives on general and specific patterns of childhood risk for adolescenct educational, social, and mental health problems. *American Psychologist*, **43**, 786–799.

Livingston, R.L., Dykman, R.A., and Ackerman, P.T. (1990). The frequency and significance of additional self reported psychiatric diagnoses in children with attention deficit disorder. *Journal of Child Psychology*, **18**, 465–478.

Loney, J., Kramer, J., and Milich, R.S. (1981). The hyperactive child grows up: Predictors of symptoms, delinquency and achievement at follow-up. In K.D. Gadow and J. Loney (Eds.), Psychosocial aspects of drug treatment of hyperactivity (pp. 318–415). Boulder, CO: Westview.

Loney, J. and Milich, R. (1982). Hyperactivity, inattention, and aggression in clinical practice. In M. Wolraich and D. Routh (Eds.), *Advances in developmental and behavioral pediatrics* (pp. 143–147). Greenwich, CT: JAI.

Mannuzza, S., Gittelman Klein, R., Honig, P., and Giampino, T.L. (1989). Hyperactive boys almost grown up. *Archives of General Psychiatry*, **46**, 1073–1079.

Mannuzza, S., Klein, R.G., and Addalli, K.A. (1991). Young adult mental status of hyperactive boys and their brothers: A prospective follow-up study. *Journal of the American Academy of Child and Adolescent Psychiatry*, **30**, 743–751.

Mash, E.J. and Johnston, C. (1982). Comparison of the mother-child interactions of younger and older hyperactive and normal children. *Child Development,* **53,** 1371–1381.

Mash, E.J. and Johnston, C. (1983). Parental perceptions of child behavior problems, parenting self-esteem, and mothers' reported stress in younger and older hyperactive and normal children. *Journal of Consulting and Clinical Psychology,* **51,** 86–99.

McGee, R. and Feehan, M. (1991). Are girls with problems of attention underrecognized? *Journal of Psychopathology and Behavioral Assessment,* **13,** 187–198.

McGee, R., Partridge, F., Williams, S., and Silva, P.A. (1991). A twelve year follow-up of preschool hyperactive children. *Journal of the American Academy of Child and Adolescent Psychiatry,* **30,** 224–232.

McGee, R. and Share, D.L. (1988). Attention deficit disorder-hyperactivity and academic failure: Which comes first and what should be treated? *Journal of the American Academy of Child and Adolescent Psychiatry,* **27,** 318–325.

McGee, R., Stanton, W.R., and Sears, M.R. (1993). Allergic disorders and attention deficit disorder in children. *Journal of Abnormal Child Psychology,* **21,** 79–88.

McGee, R., Williams, S., Anderson, J., McKenzie-Parnell, J.M., and Silva, P.A. (1990). Hyperactivity and serum and hair zinc levels in 11 year old children from the general population. *Biological Psychiatry,* **28,** 165–168.

McGee, R., Williams, S., and Feehan, M. (1992). Attention deficit disorder and age of onset of problem behaviors. *Journal of Abnormal Child Psychology,* **20,** 487–502.

McGee, R., Williams, S.M., and Silva, P.A. (1984). Behavioral and developmental characteristics of aggressive, hyperactive and aggressive-hyperactive boys. *Journal of the American Academy of Child and Adolescent Psychiatry,* **23,** 270–279.

McGee, R., Williams, S.M., and Silva, P.A. (1985). The factor structure and correlates of ratings of inattention, hyperactivity and antisocial behavior in a large sample of nine-year-old children from the general population. *Journal of Consulting and Clinical Psychology,* **53,** 480–490.

McGee, R., Williams, S.M., and Silva, P.A. (1987). A comparison of girls and boys with teacher-identified problems of attention. *Journal of the American Academy of Child and Adolescent Psychiatry,* **26,** 711–717.

Mefford, I.N. and Potter, W.Z. (1989). A neuroanatomical and biochemical basis for attention deficit disorder with hyperactivity in children: A defect in tonic adrenaline medicated inhibition of locus coeruleus stimulation. *Medical Hypotheses,* **29,** 33–42.

Meichenbaum, D. and Goodman, J. (1971). Training impulsive children to talk to themselves: A means of developing self-control. *Journal of Abnormal Psychology,* **77,** 115–129.

Mendelson, W., Johnson, N. M., and Stewart, M. (1971). Hyperactive children as teenagers: A follow-up study. *Journal of Nervous and Mental Disease,* **153,** 273–279.

Milich, R. and Pelham, W.E. (1986). Effects of sugar ingestion on the classroom and playground behavior of attention deficit disordered boys. *Journal of Consulting and Clinical Psychology,* **54,** 714–718.

Mitchell, E.A., Aman, M.G., Turbott, S.H., and Manku, M. (1987). Clinical characteristics and serum essential fatty acid levels in hyperactive children. *Clinical Pediatrics,* **26,** 406–411.

Morrison, J.R. and Stewart, M.A. (1971). A family study of hyperactive child syndrome. *Biological Psychiatry,* **3,** 189–195.

Morrison, J.L. and Stewart, M. (1973). The psychiatric status of legal families of adopted hyperactives. *Archives of General Psychiatry,* **28,** 888–891.

Munir, K., Biederman, J., and Knee, D. (1987). Psychiatric comorbidity in patients with attention deficit disorder: A controlled study. *Journal of the American Academy of Child and Adolescent Psychiatry,* **26,** 844–848.

Offord, D.R., Boyle, M.H., Szatmari, P., Rae-Grant, N.I., Links, P.S., Cadman, D.T., Byles, J.A., Crawford, J.W., Blum, H.M., Byrne, C., Thomas, H., and Woodward, C.A. (1987). Ontario Child Health Study: II. Six month prevalence of disorder and rates of service utilization. *Archives of General Psychiatry,* **44,** 832–836.

Patterson, G.R., DeBarsyshe, B.D., and Ramsey, E. (1989). A developmental perspective on antisocial behavior. *American Psychologist*, **44**, 329–335.

Pelham, W. and Bender, M.E. (1982). Peer relationships in hyperactive children: Description and treatment. In K.D. Gadow and I. Bialer (Eds.), *Advances in learning and behavioral disabilities*. Greenwich, CT: JAI.

Pelham, W.E., Gnagy, E.M., Greenslade, K.E., and Milich, R. (1992). Teacher ratings of DSM-III-R symptoms for the disruptive behavior disorders. *Journal of the American Academy of Child and Adolescent Psychiatry*, **31**, 210–218.

Pelham, W.E. and Murphy, H.A. (1986). Attention deficit and conduct disorders. In M. Hersen (Ed.), *Pharmacological and behavioral treatment: An integrative approach* (pp. 108–148). New York: Wiley.

Pelham, W.E., Schnedler, R.W., Bender, M.E., Nilsson, D.E., Miller, J., Budrow, M.S., and Ronner, M. (1988). The combination of behavior therapy and methylphenidate in the treatment of attention deficit disorder. A therapy outcome study. In L. Bloomingdale (Ed.), *Attention deficit disorder* (Vol. 3, pp. 29–48). Oxford: Pergamon.

Phares, V. (1992). Where's poppa? The relative lack of attention to the role of fathers in child and adolescent psychopathology. *American Psychologist*, **47**, 656–664.

Phares, V. and Compas, B.E. (1992). The role of fathers in child and adolescent psychopathology: Make room for daddy. *Psychological Bulletin*, **111**, 387–412.

Pliszka, St. R. (1992). Comorbidity of attention-deficit hyperactivity disorder and overanxious disorder. *Journal of the American Academy of Child and Adolescent Psychiatry*, **32**, 197–203.

Puig-Antich, J. and Chambers, W. (1978). *The Schedule for Affective Disorders and Schizophrenia for school-aged children*. New York: State Psychiatric Institute, New York.

Prinz, R.J. and Riddle, D.B. (1986). Associations between nutrition and behavior in five-year-old children. *Nutrition Reviews*, **44**, 151–157.

Prinz, R.J., Roberts, W.A., and Hartman, E. (1980). Dietary correlates of hyperactive behavior in children. *Journal of Consulting and Clinical Psychology*, **48**, 760–769.

Quay, H.C. and Peterson, D.R. (1983). *Interim manual for the Revised Behavior Problem Checklist*. Coral Gables, Florida: Unpublished Manuscript.

Rapport, M.D., DuPaul, G.J., Stoner, G., Birmingham, B.K., and Masse, G. (1985). Attention deficit disorder with hyperactivity: Differential effects of methylphenidate on impulsivity. *Pediatrics*, **76**, 938–943.

Rapport, M.D., Murphy, A., and Bailey, J.S. (1982). Ritalin versus response cost in the control of hyperactive children: A within-subject comparison. *Journal of Applied Behavioral Analysis*, **15**, 20–31.

Reich, W. and Welner, Z. (1988). *Revised version of the Diagnostic Interview for Children and Adolescents (DICA-R)*. St. Louis, MO: Department of Psychiatry, Washington University, School of Medicine.

Rosen, L.A., Booth, S.R., Bender, M.E., McGrath, M.L., Sorell, S., and Drabman, R.S. (1988). Effects of sugar (sucrose) on children's behavior. *Journal of Consulting and Clinical Psychology*, **56**, 583–589.

Ross, D.M. and Ross, S.A. (1982). *Hyperactivity: Current issues, research and theory*. New York: Wiley.

Rostain, A.L., Power, T.J., and Atkins, M.C. (1993). Assessing parents' willingness to pursue treatment for children with attention-deficit hyperactivity disorder. *Journal of the American Academy of Child and Adolescent Psychiatry*, **32**, 175–181.

Rosvold, H., Mirsky, A., Sarason, I., Bransome, E., and Beck, L. (1956). A continous performance test of brain damage. *Journal of Consulting and Clinical Psychology*, **20**, 343–350.

Roth, N., Beyreiss, J., Schlenzka, K., and Beyer, H. (1991). Coincidence of attention deficit disorder and atopic disorders in children: Empirical findings and hypothetical background. *Journal of Abnormal Child Psychology*, **19**, 1–13.

Rubenstein, R.A. and Brown, R.T. (1984). An evaluation of the validity of the diagnostic category of attention deficit disorder. *American Journal of Orthopsychiatry*, **54**, 398–414.

Rutter, M., Tizard, J., and Whitmore, K. (1970). *Education, health and behaviur.* London: Longmans.

Safer, D.J. and Krager, J.M. (1988). A survey of medication treatment for hyperactive/inattentive students. *Journal of the American Medical Association*, **260**, 2256–2258.

Sandberg, S. (1985). Hyperactive disorder of childhood: Some clinical implications of recent research. *Acta Paedriatrica Scandinavica*, **74**, 481–488.

Sandberg, S.T., Rutter, M., and Taylor, E. (1978). Hyperkinetic disorder in psychiatric clinic attenders. *Developmental Medicine and Child Neurology*, **20**, 279–299.

Sanson, A., Smart, D., Prior, M., and Oberklaid, F. (1993). Precursors of hyperactivity and aggression. *Journal of the American Academy of Child and Adolescent Psychiatry*, **32**, 1207–1216.

Santostefano, S. and Paley, E. (1964). Development of cognitive controls in children. *Child Development*, **35**, 939–949.

Satterfield, J.H., Cantwell, D.P., Lesser, L.I., and Podosin, R.L. (1972). Physiological studies of the hyperactive child: I. *American Journal of Psychiatry*, **128**, 1418–1424.

Satterfield, J.H., Hoppe, C.M., and Schell, A.M. (1982). A prospective study of delinquency in 110 adolescent boys with attention deficit disorder and 88 normal adolescent boys. *American Journal of Psychiatry*, **139**, 795–798.

Satterfield, J., Swanson, J., Schell, A., and Lee, F. (1994). Prediction of antisocial behavior in attention-deficit hyperactivity disorder boys from aggression/defiance scores. *Journal of the American Academy of Child and Adolescent Psychiatry*, **33**, 185–190.

Satterfield, J.H., Satterfield, B.T., and Schnell, A.M. (1987). Therapeutic interventions to prevent delinquency in hyperactive boys. *Journal of the American Academy of Child and Adolescent Psychiatry*, **26**, 56–64.

Schachter; R. (1991). Childhood hyperactivity. *Journal of Child Psychology and Psychiatry*, **42**, 155–191.

Schaughency, E., McGee, R., Raja, S.N., Feehan, M., and Silva, P.A. (1994). Self-reported inattention, impulsivity, and hyperactivity at ages 15 and 18 years in the general population. *Journal of the American Academy of Child and Adolescent Psychiatry*, **33**, 173–184.

Shaywitz, S.E., Cohen, D.J., and Shaywitz, B.A. (1978). The biochemical basis of minimal brain dysfunction. *Journal of Pediatrics*, **92**, 179–187.

Shaywitz, S.E. and Shaywitz, B.A. (1987). Attention deficit disorder: Current perspectives. *Pediatric Neurology*, **3**, 129–225.

Solanto, M.W. (1984). Neuropharmacological basis of stimulant drug action in attention deficit disorder with hyperactivity: A review and synthesis. *Psychological Bulletin*, **95**, 387–409.

Spencer, T., Biederman, J., Wilens, T., Harding, M., O'Donnell, D., and Griffin, S. (1996). Pharmacotherapy of attention-deficit/hyperactivity disorder across the life time. *Journal of the American Academy of Child and Adolescent Psychiatry*, **35**, 409–432.

Spring, B., Chiodo, J., and Bowen, D.J. (1987). Carbohydrates, tryptophan, and behavior: A methodological review. *Psychological Bulletin*, **102**, 234–256.

Stevenson, J., Richman, N., and Graham, P. (1985). Behavior problems and language abilities at three years and behavioral deviance at eight years. *Journal of Child Psychology and Psychiatry*, **26**, 215–230.

Stewart, M.A., Cummings, C., Singer, S., and DeBlois, C.S. (1981). The overlap between hyperactive and undersocialized aggressive children. *Journal of Child Psychology and Psychiatry*, **22**, 35–45.

Sykes, D.H., Douglas, V.I., Morganstern, G. (1973). Sustained attention in hyperactive children. *Journal of Child Psychology and Psychiatry*, **14**, 213–220.

Szatmari, P., Offord, D.R., and Boyle, M.H. (1989). Ontario Child Health Study: Prevalence of attention deficit disorder with hyperactivity. *Journal of Child Psychology and Psychiatry,* **30**, 219–230.

Ullman, R.K., Sleator, E.K., and Spraque, R.L. (1985). A change of mind: The Conners Abbreviated Rating Scales reconsidered. *Journal of Child Psychiatry,* **13**, 553–565.

Thorley, G. (1984). Review of follow-up and follow-back studies of childhood hyperactivity. *Psychological Bulletin,* **96**, 116–132.

Wallander, J.L. (1988). The relationship between attention problems in childhood and antisocial behavior eight years later. *Journal of Child Psychology and Psychiatry,* **29**, 53–61.

Wechsler, D. (1974). *Wechsler Intelligence Scale for Children — Revised.* New York: Psychological Corporation.

Wechsler, D. (1991). *Wechsler Intelligence Scale for Children.* Third edition. San Antonio, Tx: Psychological Corp.

Weiss, G. and Hechtman, L.T. (1993). *Hyperactive children grown up.* New York: Guilford Press.

Weiss, G., Hechtman, L., Milroy, T., and Perlman, T. (1985). Psychiatric status of hyperactives as adults: A controlled perspective 15-year follow-up of 63 hyperactive children. *Journal of the American Academy of Child Psychiatry,* **24**, 211–220.

Werry, J.S. (1993). Long-term drug use in psychiatric disorders in children. Facts, controversies and the future. *Acta Paedopsychiatrica,* **56**, 113–118.

Whalen, C.K. (1983). Hyperactivity, learning problems, and the attention deficit disorders. In T.H. Ollendick and M. Hersen (Eds.), *Handbook of childhood psychopathology* (pp. 151–200). New York: Plenum Press.

Whalen, C.K. and Henker, B. (1985). The social worlds of hyperactive (ADDH) children. *Clinical Psychology Review,* **5**, 447–478.

Whalen, C.K., Henker, B., Buhrmester, D., Hinshaw, S.P., Huber, A., and Laski, K. (1989). Does stimulant medication improve the peer status of hyperactive boys? *Journal of Consulting and Clinical Psychology,* **57**, 545–549.

Whalen, C.K., Henker, B., and Hinshaw, S.P. (1985). Cognitive-behavioral therapies for hyperactive children: Premises, problems, and prospects. *Journal of Abnormal Child Psychology,* **13**, 391–410.

Whalen, C.K., Henker, B., and Granger, D.A. (1990). Social judgement processes in hyperactive boys: Effects of methylphenidate and comparisons with normal peers. *Journal of Abnormal Child Psychology,* **18**, 297–316.

Williams, S. and McGee, R. (1994). Reading attainment and juvenile delinqency. *Journal of Child Psychology and Psychiatry,* **35**, 441–459.

Wilson, J.M. and Marcotte, A.C. (1996). Psychosocial adjustment and educational outcome in adolescents with a childhood diagnosis of attention deficit disorder. *Journal of the American Academy of Child and Adolescent Psychiatry,* **35**, 579–587.

Wolraich, M.L., Lindgren, S., Stromquist, A., Milich, R., Davis, C., and Watson, D. (1990). Stimulant medication use by primary care physicians in the treatment of attention deficit hyperactivity disorder. *Pediatrics,* **86**, 95–101.

Wolraich, M., Lindgren, S.D., Stumbo, P.J., Stegink, L.D., Appelbaum, L.I., and Kirtisy, M.C. (1994). Effects of diets high in sucrose or aspartame on the behavior and cognitive performance of children. *New England Journal of Medicine,* **330**, 301–307.

World Health Organization (1993). *The ICD-10 classification of mental and behavioural disorders.* Geneva: World Health Organization.

Vyse, S.A. and Rapport, M. (1989). The effects of methylphlenidate on learning in children with ADDH: The stimulus equivalence paradigm. *Journal of Consulting and Clinical Psychology,* **57**, 425–435.

CHAPTER 6
PERVASIVE DEVELOPMENTAL DISORDERS
Michael Kusch and Franz Petermann

The main features of pervasive developmental disorders (PDD) are the presence of severe and pervasive impairment in numerous areas of development, including reciprocal social interaction skills, communication skills, or the presence of stereotyped behavior, interests, and activities (APA, 1994). In DSM-IV, PDD include Autistic disorder, Asperger's disorder, Rett's disorder, Childhood disintegrative disorder, and Pervasive developmental disorder not otherwise specified (Table 6.1). Autistic disorder has an early onset of impairments in social interaction,

Table 6.1 Comparison of subcategories of Pervasive Developmental Disorder (PDD).

DSM-III-R	DSM-IV	ICD-10
Autistic disorder	Autistic Disorder	Childhood autism
		Atypical autism
	Asperger's disorder	Asperger syndrome
	Rett's disorder	Rett syndrome
	Childhood disintegrative disorder	Childhood disintegrative disorder
		Other childhood disintegrative disorder
		Overactive disorder associated with mental retardation and stereotyped movements
Pervasive developmental disorder not otherwise specified	Pervasive developmental disorder not otherwise specified	

communication deficits, restricted activities, and interest. In Asperger's disorder, there is a relative preservation of language skills and intellect. Rett's disorder shows some similarity with autistic disorder for a limited period during early childhood, and is often associated with mental retardation, generalized growth retardation, and multiple neurological symptoms. Childhood disintegrative disorder has similar symptoms to autistic disorder, with symptoms occurring about 2 years of normal development. After that, early development gains disappeared and a stable level of autistic-like functioning reached.

DEFINITION AND CLASSIFICATION

Autistic Disorder

Autistic disorder can be viewed as a "particular mode of existence" (Bosch, 1970, p. 3) because children with this condition seem to have a deviated course of development from birth on (Table 6.2). As suggested by Kanner (1943) autistic children were born "with an innate inability to form the usual, biologically provided affective contact with people" (p. 42). But Kanner also suggested that disturbances in parent-child interaction may lead to affective problems experienced by autistic children.

Table 6.2 Possible early symptoms of Autistic Disorder

The newborn	Does not seem to need mother
	Cries infrequently. Rarely fusses. "A very good baby"
	Intensely irritable. Overreactive to stimulation
	Indifferent to being held
	Muscle tone seems flaccid
The first six months	Undemanding. Fails to notice mother
	Delayed or absent smiling, cooing, babbling and anticipatory response
	Lack of interest in toys. Overreactive to sounds
The second six months	Unaffectionate. No interest in social games
	Indifferent, limp, or rigid when held
	Absent verbal and nonverbal communication
	Toys cast away, flicked at, or dropped
	Under- and overreactive to stimulation
	Aversion to solid foods
	Delayed or uneven motor milestones

Modified from Ornitz (1983)

Others have defined autistic disorder as the condition with behavioural or phenotypical symptoms such as social interaction and social communication (Fein *et al.*, 1986; APA, 1994). Both positions have received substantial empirical evidence since a biological basis in the sense of a genetic cause have been reported to account for more than 80% of the phenotypic variance (Szatmari and Jones, 1991), and a host of psychological abnormalities that could be explained by social or cognitive deficits (Baron-Cohen *et al.*, 1993; Fein *et al.*, 1986; Mundy and Hogan, 1994). Although no one would argue for a psychogenic basis of autistic disorder, the question of how the neurobiological origins of autistic disorder will lead to the autism-specific phenotype of social behaviour disturbances has yet to be answered. According to the available data, autistic disorder can be defined at three interdependent levels: (i) a neurobiological disorder with normal brain development (Rubinstein *et al.*, 1993); (ii) a psychological disorder of normal cognitive-emotional development (Baron-Cohen *et al.*, 1993; Frith *et al.*, 1991; Hobson, 1993); and (iii) a "failure of normal socialisation" (Cohen *et al.*, 1987). Consequently, autistic disorder may be defined as a disorder in a chain of causation leading to different developmental pathways which result in a unique disorder of social behaviour patterns (Wing, 1981).

In DSM-IV, the main characteristics of autistic disorder (APA, 1994) is an abnormal or impaired development in social interaction and communication, a restricted repertoire of activity and interests (Table 6.3). Problem in social interaction may be manifested in impairment in the use of nonverbal behavior, inability to develop peer relationship that is appropriate to the developmental level, lack of spontaneous seeking to share enjoyment, interest with other people, and a lack of social or emotional reciprocity.

Asperger's Disorder

Children with Asperger's disorder are of normal intelligent, clumsy, assiduous pursuer of idiosyncratic interests. Other clinical features of Asperger's disorder (Frith, 1991; Szatmari *et al.*, 1989) include: (i) poor nonverbal communication; (ii) pedantic and monotonic speech; (iii) paucity of empathy; (iv) inappropriate, one-sided social conversation; (v) reduced ability to form friendships with feelings of social isolation; (vi) preoccupation and intense absorption in narrow topics, and (vii) clumsy, ill-coordinated movements and odd posture. Three associated features of children with Asperger's disorder have been reported including later age of onset, correct formal language, and high cognitive ability (Szatmari,

Table 6.3 Diagnostic criteria for Autistic Disorder

A. A total of six (or more) items from (1), (2), and (3), with at least two from (1), and one each from (2) and (3):

1. Qualitative impairment in social interaction, as manifested by at least two of the following:
    a) marked impairment in the use of multiple nonverbal behaviors such as eye-to-eye gaze, facial expression, body postures, and gestures to regulate social interaction;
    b) failure to develop peer relationships appropriate to developmental level;
    c) a lack of spontaneous seeking to share enjoyment, interests, or achievements with other people (e.g., buy a lack of showing, bringing, or pointing out objects of interest).

2. Qualitative impairments in communication as manifested by at least one of the following:
    a) delay in, or total lack of, the development of spoken language (not accompanied by an attempt to compensate through alternative modes of communication such as gestures or mime);
    b) in individuals with adequate speech, marked impairment in the ability to initiate or sustain a conversation with others;
    c) stereotyped and repetitive use of language or idiosyncratic language;
    d) lack of varied, spontaneous make-believe play or social imitative play appropriate to developmental level.

3. Restricted repetitive and stereotyped patterns of behavior, interests, and activities, as manifested by at least one of the following:
    a) encompassing preoccupation with one or more stereotyped and restricted patterns of interest that is abnormal either in intensity or focus;
    b) apparently inflexible adherence to specific, nonfunctional routines or rituals;
    c) stereotyped and repetitive motor mannerisms (e.g., hand or finger flapping or twisting, or complex whole-body movements);
    d) persistent preoccupation with parts of objects.

B. Delays or abnormal functioning in at least one of the following areas, with onset prior to age 3 years: (i) social interaction, (ii) language as used in social communication, or (iii) symbolic or imaginative play.

C. The disturbance is not better accounted for by Rett's Disorder or Childhood Disintegrative Disorder.

Reprinted with permission from the Diagnostic and Statistical Manual of Mental Disorders, Fourth Edition. Copyright 1994 American Psychiatric Association.

1992; Frith, 1991), although cases with mild retardation have also been reported (Gillberg, 1985). Asperger's disorder is sometimes observed with general medical conditions or various neurological symptoms and signs. Motor development may be delayed, and clumsiness is often observed (APA, 1994).

Asperger's disorder is characterized by severe and sustained impairment and restricted repetitive and stereotyped patterns of behaviour, interests, and activities (APA, 1994); these behaviour patterns are similar to that of Asperger's. However, unlike autistic disorder, there are no clinically significant developmental delays in language, cognition and adaptive behaviour (Table 6.4). In the ICD-10, a set of symptoms constituting

Table 6.4 Diagnostic criteria for Asperger´s Disorder

A.   Qualitative impairment in social interaction, as manifested by at least two of the following:
1)   marked impairment in the use of multiple nonverbal behavior such as eye-to-eye gaze, facial expression, body postures, and gestures to regulate social interaction
2)   failure to develop peer relationships appropriate to developmental level
3)   a lack of spontaneous seeking to share enjoyment, interests, or achievements with other people (e.g., by a lack of showing, bringing, or pointing out objects of interest to other people)
4)   lack of social or emotional reciprocity

B.   Restricted repetitive and stereotyped patterns of behavior, interests, and activities, as manifested by at least one of the following:
1)   encompassing preoccupation with one or more stereotyped and restricted patterns of interest that is abnormal either in intensity or focus
2)   apparently inflexible adherence to specific, nonfunctional routines or rituals
3)   stereotyped and repetitive motor mannerisms (e.g., hand or finger flapping or twisting, or complex whole-body movements)
4)   persistent preoccupation with part of objects

C.   There is no clinically significant general delay in language (e.g., single words used by age 2 years, communicative phrases used by age 3 years)

E.   There is no clinically significant delay in cognitive development or in the development of age-appropriate self-help skills, adaptive behavior (other than in social interaction), and curiosity about the environment in childhood.

F.   Criteria are not met for any specific Pervasive Developmental Disorder or Schizophrenia

---

APA (1994, p. 77)

of Asperger syndrom are a lack of any clinically significant general delay in language acquisition, cognitive development and adaptive behaviour, impairments in social and emotional behaviour, and a restricted, repetitive and stereotyped pattern of interest. Not necessary, but associated symptoms involve isolated special skills and motor deficits (WHO, 1993).

Rett's Disorder

In its early stages, Rett's disorder is associated with loss of facial expression, decrease in social interest, stereotype movements and loss of purposeful hand use. Five features of Rett's disorder are: predominant rejection of caressing and tenderness, conspicuous physical hyperactivity in terms of continuous grabbing and concomitant locomobility, excessive attachment to certain objects, rotation of small objects, and stereotypic playing habits (Olsson and Rett, 1985, 1990). The most prominent associated feature of children with Rett's disorder is severe (IQ level 20–25 to 35–40) or profound (IQ level below 20–25) mental retardation, and a continuous disorder of sleep-wakefulness cycle characterised by more daytime sleep and less nighttime sleep than in normal children. Pizza and colleagues (1990) reported delayed sleep onset, night walking and early waking. Mental retardation is even more severe in children with Rett's disorder than in autism. During the school years, orthopaedic problems (Loder *et al.*, 1989) and scoliosis (Harrison and Webb, 1990) are common problems found in most children with Rett's disorder.

Rett's disorder is first introduced as a distinct and separate diagnostic subcategory of pervasive developmental disorders in DSM-IV (Table 6.5). Children with this disorder show head growth deceleration, loss of previously acquired purposeful hand skills, and the appearance of poorly coordinated gait or trunk movements and severe impairment in expressive and receptive language skills. In ICD-10, Rett's disorder is classified as a separate subcategory of PDDs (WHO, 1993).

Childhood Disintegrative Disorder

The childhood disintegrative disorder (CDD) is characterized through a initial period of normal functioning and loss of previously acquired skills in various areas of functioning including: expressive or receptive language, social skills, bowel or bladder control, play, and motor skills. Similar to individuals with autistic disorder, those with CDD show social, communicative deficits and behavioural features (Table 6.6). The disturbance is not accounted for by another pervasive developmental disorders or by schizophrenia.

Table 6.5   Diagnostic criteria for Rett´s Disorder

A. All of the following:
   (1) apparently normal prenatal and perinatal development
   (2) apparently normal psychomotor development through the first 5 months after birth
   (3) normal head circumference at birth

B. Onset of all of the following after the period of normal development:
   (1) declaration of head growth between ages 5 and 18 months
   (2) loss of previously acquired purposeful hand skills between ages 5 and 30 months with the subsequent development of stereotyped hand movements (e.g., hand-wringing or hand washing)
   (3) loss of social engagement early in the course (although often social interaction develops later)
   (4) appearance of poorly coordinated gait or trunk movements
   (5) severely impaired expressive and receptive language development with severe psychomotor retardation

APA (1994, p. 72–73)

Table 6.6   Diagnostic criteria for Childhood Disintegrative Disorder

A. Apparently normal development for at least the first 2 years after birth as manifested by the presence of age-appropriate verbal and nonverbal communication, social relationship, play, and adaptive behavior

B. Clinically significant loss of previously acquired skills (before age 19 years) in at least two of the following areas:
   (1) expressive or receptive language
   (2) social skills or adaptive behavior
   (3) bowel or bladder control
   (4) play
   (5) motor skills

C. Abnormalities of functioning in at least two of the following areas:
   (1) qualitative impairments in social interaction (e.g., impairment in non-verbal behaviors, failure to develop peer relationships, lack of social or emotional reciprocity)
   (2) qualitative impairments in communication (e.g., delay of lack of spoken language, inability to initiate or sustain a conversation, stereotyped and repetitive use of language, lack of varied make-believe play)
   (3) restricted, repetitive, and stereotyped patterns of behavior, interests, and activities, including motor stereotypic and mannerisms

D. The disturbance is not better accounted for by other specific Pervasive developmental Disorder or by Schizophrenia.

APA (1994, p. 74–75)

Pervasive Developmental Disorder Not Otherwise Specified

This is a heterogeneous group of conditions that share some features of an early onset developmental deviance in social reciprocity and attachment (Gillberg, 1992). This condition is called a "subthreshold" pervasive developmental disorder because affected children have some important but not many and not comparably severe impairments in common with other children with pervasive developmental disorder. In ICD-10 atypical conditions of autism are separately codified if there is a subthreshold condition of childhood autism, when cases fail to meet age of onset criteria or both (WHO, 1993). In DSM-IV atypical autism is subsumed under PDDNOS because of the same reasons (APA, 1994).

EPIDEMIOLOGY

The number of cases of autistic disorder in a general population have been estimated to range from 2 to 5 cases in 10,000 (Zahner and Pauls, 1987). Studies that used a broader definition of autistic disorder have estimated a prevalence rate of 10 to 11 cases per 10,000 (Bryson *et al.*, 1988; Cialdella and Mamelle, 1989). The male to female sex ratio is about 4–5 to 1; females with autistic disorder tend to be more impaired than males (Lord and Schopler, 1987). Although early epidemiological studies reported a high percentage of autistic disorder coming from the upper social class, later studies have failed to confirm this finding (Cialdella and Mamelle, 1989).

The prevalence of Asperger's disorder is 1 case in 10,000 (Frith, 1991), but higher rates may be expected (Szatmari, 1992). Although the condition is most often present in boys, girls may be affected too. The estimated prevalence of Rett's disorder is 1 in 10,000 to 15,000 (Hagberg and Witt-Engerström, 1986). It is considered as a female disorder (Hagberg *et al.*, 1985) although few cases of males with possible Rett's disorder have been reported (Coleman, 1990; Philippart, 1989). Rett's disorder is known to exist in all social classes, races and countries (Hagberg, 1993). The prevalence of CDD is estimated to be 0.11 in 10,000 for males (Burd *et al.*, 1987). Volkmar's (1992) review of reported cases suggests a male-to-female ratio (4:1) similar to that in autism. An overall estimate of PDDNOS is 16 to 21 in 10,000 (Gillberg, 1992; Wing and Gould, 1979).

Risk Factors

Autistic Disorder

Family and Genetic Factors

The rate of autistic disorder in siblings of individuals with this disorder is 50 to 100 times higher than the prevalence found in the general population (Folstein and Rutter, 1988; Ritvo *et al.*, 1989; Rutter *et al.*, 1990). The risk of having an autistic disorder is increased if the oldest child has an autistic disorder. Additionally, many siblings of autistic children show cognitive impairment even if they do not have any autistic disorder (August *et al.*, 1981).

An examination of 21 same-sex twins in which at least one twin has autistic disorder, Folstein and Rutter (1977, 1978) found concordance rates of 36% in the monozygotic twin (MZ) and 0% in the dizygotic twin (DZ). About 82% of the MZ twins are also concordant for language and cognitive impairments compared with only 10% in DZ twins (Folstein and Rutter, 1977). Ritvo *et al.* (1985) reported a concordance rate for autistic disorder being 95.7% in MZ twins and 23.5% in DZ twins. Rutter (1991) found 50% concordance for autistic disorder in MZ and 3% for DZ twins. Szatmari and Jones (1991) argue that the results from twin and family studies that the genetic causes for autistic disorder accounts for more than 80% of the phenotypic variance. Possible genetic subtypes in autistic disorder include non-familial chromosomal abnormalities, multifactorial inheritance, X-linked inheritance and autosomal recessive inheritance (Rutter, 1991; Folstein and Rutter, 1987). Although genetic factors may be the major cause for autistic disorder, there are other causal factors such as viral disease (Tsai, 1992).

Brain Mechanisms

Neurobiological studies of autistic disorder have focused on various aspects of the structure and function of the brain: the frontal lobes, the left hemisphere, the thalamus, the limbic system, the brain stem, and the cerebellum (Courchesne, 1989; Rubinstein *et al.*, 1993). According to structural neuroimaging studies (see Aitken, 1991 for a review; Filipek *et al.*, 1992) only about 15% of the findings of computer tomography (CT) or magnetic resonance imaging (MRI) could be interpreted as abnormal and focal lesions could be identified in less than 50%. Lesions have been found in the frontal lobes, the limbic system, the cerebellum, and some other brain regions. Ventricular enlargement is thought to be a developmental atrophy in adjacent limbic and frontal structures. Piven *et al.* (1990) conducted a MRI study in 13 high-functioning males and found cortical migrational anomalies in 7 subjects (54%); a much higher rate than reported in pediatric and retarded samples. Autopsy studies have found extensive Purkinje cell loss in the cerebellum (Ritvo *et al.*, 1986). Courchesne *et al.* (1987) conducted a MRI study and found cerebellar abnormalities, too. Hypoplasia was found in 84 to 92% of autistic patients and enlargement of the cerebellar verims (hyperplasia) in 8 to 19% (Courchesne *et al.*, 1994). It has been suggested that the neuron loss of cerebellar Purkinje cells is a prenatal event during the second trimester (Courchesne, 1991).

Brain hypermetabolism in autistic patients has been found in two functional neuroimaging studies (Horowitz *et al.*, 1988; Minshew *et al.*, 1993). Brain hypermetabolism would be consistent with a hypothesis of a disturbed integration of information processing in the neocerebellum (Courchesne, 1991) or the prefrontal cortex (Minshew *et al.*, 1993).

Controlled neurophysiological investigations similarly showed little difference between autistic and other children (Rubinstein *et al.*, 1993). EEG investigation for experience-correlated potential show a reduced P300 wave amplitude (Courchesne, 1989). Ornitz's study (1987) suggested a disturbance in the brain stem, especially an ascending reticular system (ARAS) which explains the hypo- and hyperactivity condition of the autistic children. Dawson's (1991) experiments showed that a disorder of autonomic regulation process is involved. Moreover, autistic children show an activity pattern of both brain hemispheres during the processing of verbal information.

It is generally accepted that autistic disorder is a neurodevelopmental disorder (Rubinstein *et al.*, 1993; Rutter and Schopler, 1987; Dawson, 1991). Autistic children are at risk of having associated mental retardation and medical conditions, they have diverse neuroanatomical abnormalities and neurophysiological dysfunctions. Despite these biological conditions, the findings account only for a minority of cases and many autistic children, even those with mental retardation, do not show detectable dysfunctions of the central nervous system (Schopler and Mesibov, 1987).

Neurological Models

Frontal Lobe and Executive Dysfunction

Damasio and Maurer (1978) proposed that the autistic disorder-specific deficits may be related to dysfunctions of the mesolimbic cortex, an area in the mesial frontal lobe and related limbic structures. Dysfunctions of this phylogenetically and neurochemically distinct structure may account for certain repetitive and stereotypic movements, verbal and nonverbal communication problems and a failure to attend to salient goal- and emotion-related stimuli found in autistic persons. Structural imaging studies (Aitken, 1991; Filipek *et al.*, 1992) support Damasio and Maurer's model (1978) in some instances, but the frontal lobe is considered as a cerebral structure that can produce various types of symptoms. Hence, frontal lobe dysfunctions will depend on the localization of the lesion and the affected connection between frontal lobe and mesolimbic structures. Rogers and Pennington (1991) proceed in the assumption of a frontal lobe disorder in which the primary lesion is localized in the non-motor regions like the dorso-lateral and orbito-frontal cortex. Associated with this disorder is an executive deficit defined as difficulties in appropriate goal-directed problem solving abilities. In a serial of neuropsychological studies, Pennington and colleges (McEvoy *et al.*, 1993; Ozonoff *et al.*, 1991) demonstrate that an executive deficit accounts for some problems of autistic children (i.e., perseverance and lack of planning ability).

Boucher (1989) and Bachevalier (1991) view autistic disorder as a developmental amnesia that results from early damage of limbic memory structures; the amygdala and hippocampus. Boucher (1989) who tested his assumptions using neuropsychological measures of memory found deficits in episodic memory. According to the available data it is impossible to conclude whether the primary neurological deficit of children with autistic disorder is located in frontal or limbic brain structures. Nevertheless, Damasio and Maurer's (1978) model could be supported because most neurological studies show that only those brain regions of the frontal lobe are affected that are intimately linked with the limbic system or vice versa.

Cerebellar Dysfunction

According to Courchesne (1989, 1991; Courchesne *et al.*, 1994) early prenatal loss of granule or Purkinje cells may lead to the cerebellar hypoplasia found in many persons with autistic disorder. Cell loss in the cerebellum may cause a failure of modulation of excitatory cerebellar output to other areas of the brain. Most of these brain regions seem to be involved in attentional processes. In conjunction with those functional impairments, unmodulated cerebellar excitatory output may lead to structural abnormalities in later developing brain regions. A primary subcortical dysfunction may have widespread negative consequences on other cortical regions such as the frontal cortex. Impairments in shifting or orienting attention early in postnatal development may lead to misattuned social interaction because of temporal and spatial gaps in social information processing of the infant (Dawson, 1991) and in deviant mental representations of event structures (Duchan, 1987). This in turn may result in problems of causal inferencing and joint attention skills and the subsequent autism-specific problems (Courchesne, 1989).

The attention/arousal modulation theory has been proposed to explain autistic disorder-specific symptoms using the so-called "bottom-up" model (Dawson, 1991; Dawson and Lewy, 1989). According to this model autistic children have difficulties in processing complex, context-dependent information contained in social interaction like imitation, joint attention or conceptual perspective taking. In Dawson's theoretical conception, autistic children have a primary deficit in arousal regulation and orientation to novelty that is evident in a various neurophysiological and psychological measures (Dawson and Lewy, 1989). Dawson (1991) proposed that the findings of cerebral hemispheric activation can be related to the underlying difficulties of arousal regulation. He argued that not only specific higher neural structures are necessary to produce the autistic disorder-specific phenotype but also reciprocal subcortical-cortical influences involving reticular, limbic, and cortical systems. According to Ornitz (1987) there is a complex anatomical relationship between brainstem-diencephalic centres and cortical structures. Subcortical neural networks are responsible for arousal and orientation and higher networks modulate and elaborate the excitatory outcome of the reticular formation.

It has been impossible to deduce the autistic phenotype from one neurological model; even a combination of models has been too weak to explain the complex picture of autistic behaviour. Nevertheless two or three working hypotheses can be derived: First, a "top-down" model suggest a primary cortico-limbic deficit in autistic disorder with involvement of only those cortical networks that are interwoven with limbic structures. Second, a "bottom-up" model argues for a primary deficit in subcortical neural networks and associated structures in the limbic and frontal cortex. Both models may give an appropriate explanation to a subgroup of autistic children, with differences in age of onset (Fein *et al.*, 1986; Kusch and Petermann, 1991). Third, it can be speculated that during brain development a cortical area or functional neural network may be affected and that the resulting dysfunction will become more and more independent from the primary deficit. Heterogeneous aetiological conditions in early prenatal or postnatal life may lead to disastrous effects within a short span of development or etiopathogenesis. In autistic disorder it may be the case that during neurodevelopment a cortical system responsible for a biologically preprogrammed interest of babies in the complex social context will be affected (Fein *et al.*, 1986). The phenotypical outcome may depend on the neurodevelopmental stage and the subsequent pathway of brain development than on the aetiological condition (Rubinstein *et al.*, 1993).

Neuropsychological Theories

Since the pioneering study by Baron-Cohen *et al.* (1985) it is widely accepted that children with autistic lack a "theory of mind", which is a cognitive ability to attribute independent mental state to self and others in order to predict and explain behaviour. A convincing demonstration of a "theory of mind" deficit involves the use of false belief tasks. In one such task, children with autistic disorder and younger children with language impairment were shown a well known box with sweets and were asked "What is in here?" All children gave the correct answer "sweets" or "candies". The children were then shown what was really in the box and were told that it was a pencil. In the next step, the pencil was put back into the candy-box and the children were asked to predict what other children would say was in the box and what really was in it. About 80% of the autistic children gave a wrong answer to the question and said "a pencil". Over 80% of the language-impaired children gave the correct answer and said "candies" (Perner *et al.*, 1989). Many investigations have attempted to replicate and expand these findings and to explain the other autistic disorder-specific symptoms according to what was assumed to be the underlying primary deficit (see Baron-Cohen, 1995; Baron-Cohen *et al.*, 1993 for review). It has been demonstrated that most normally developing 4-year-old children as well as more than 80% of children with other mental disorders (e.g., Down's Syndrome or language impairment) replied correctly to "theory of mind" tasks. Even those autistic children who passed false belief tasks could not pass advanced second order theory of mind tasks like "What does Mary think that John thinks?" (Baron-Cohen, 1989). These findings were taken as evidence for an autistic disorder-specific impairment in mentalising (i.e., "thinking about other thought"; Leslie, 1987).

The ability to mentalize is thought to develop without learning and manifest itself in overt behaviour during the first five years of life. During the first year of life infants become able to build an internal representation of the physical world; an ability called primary or first-order representations. During the second year of life children become increasingly able to, for example, pretend to drink water from one empty glass. Pretence behaviour is impossible to show without a process of decoupling one representation from another representation, that is to build meta- or second order representations. It is assumed that an autistic child has impairment to process his representations of the physical world in two instances: (i) to build a copy of the reality. This computational process is called EXPRAIS (expression raiser) and will lead, for example, to a primary representation "This cup is empty." (ii) to use the primary representation of pretence purposes. This computational process is called "manipulator" and will lead to a second order representation "This cup is full." Only if a child's computational process will lead to decoupled EXPRAISed representations is it able, for example, to distinguish between itself in the mirror and in reality. Children with autistic do have the capacity of mirror self-recognition (Sigman *et al.*, 1987) which makes a primary representation deficit incredible. Indeed, capacities that require primary representations of self and other, rote memory, object permanence or causal reasoning are not likely to be impaired in autistic children (Sigman *et al.*, 1987). What seems to be a computational problem for autistic children is the manipulation of primary representations in order to use it in another manner or context. The ability to anticipate or to direct another's behaviour, tool use or the use of objects (i.e., telephone) in a functional manner requires the computational capacity to manipulate the content of decoupled expressions. Even these capacities have been demonstrated as not autism-specific impaired in children with autistic disorder, as demonstrated in perceptual perspective taking, behaviour regulation or functional play (Sigman *et al.*, 1987). What seems to be a specific computational inability in autistic children is the manipulation of decoupled representation in order to use it in a personalized context (Leslie and Thaiss, 1992). Pretending that an empty cup is full of water only makes sense in a social situation in which one person conceals the reality (of an empty cup of water) so that the other falsely assumes the cup to be full of water. This construction of social reality is the outcome of internal propositional attitudes, that is, conceiving the other person to assume that the cup is full of water. As demonstrated in the above candy example, most autistic children are unable to recognize that other persons may have or not have constructions of a given situation like themselves; they have false beliefs about what is in another person's mind. The underlying mentalising or decoupling deficit is considered to be domain-specific, because it only affects the manipulator and leaves other computational processes relatively unaffected (Leslie and Thaiss, 1992). Many of the autism-specific symptoms can be explained according to this underlying deficit quite satisfactorily (see Baron-Cohen *et al.*, 1993).

Is the mentalising-deficit universal in autistic disorder? There are some investigators who propose alternative or additional theories of autistic disorder. One alternative to the mentalising-deficit explanation is given by Hobson (1993) who argued that many affective problems of autistic children (e.g., impaired expression, perception, and understanding of affect, deficit in affective sharing, emotion-perception or social referencing deficit) can be explained without reference to mentalising. According to Hobson (1993), the primary deficit in autistic disorder is a disturbance of affective contact or intersubjectivity. In normal infants the capacity for affective contact to the caregiver is innate and biological. Intersubjectivity has a continuous development from birth onward and leads to an emotional understanding of self and other people. In autistic disorder this developmental process is assumed to be deficient very early in life. Disruptions of the process can be found in joint attention (Hobson, 1993; Mundy *et al.*, 1986), especially in the coordination of attention and emotion involving in situations where the child, another person and an object are involved (Lord, 1984).

Huges and Russell (1993) suggested another alternative explanation of mentalising. They argued that autistic children maybe able to mentalize but fail false belief tasks because they cannot overcome the perceptual salience of the real object. Huges and Russell (1993) proposed an underlying executive function deficit to explain their findings. Ozonoff *et al.* (1991) conducted false belief, executive function and emotion perception tasks to demonstrate that looking for one primary impairment (i.e., a mentalising deficit) in order to explain all symptoms in autistic children may be misleading. In comparison to matched controls, autistic children showed deficits in all the three tasks, but over 80% of the autistic children failed the cognitive tasks; the "theory of mind" and executive function (Tower of Hanoi) task. Although it can be argued that a decoupling deficit is primary to executive function, Ozonoff *et al.* (1991) postulate a neurological dysfunction of the prefrontal cortex as the underlying impairment of both cognitive deficits. Fein *et al.* (1986) have suggested that human infants are biologically pre-programmed to develop social behaviours and that the prefrontal cortex may play a critical role in this developmental domain. In reference to this assumption, Rogers and Pennington (1991) proposed that autistic children are impaired in forming and coordinating specific social representations of self and other. This neuropsychological impairment can be seen in social capacities like imitation of other's body movements, emotion sharing, and "theory of mind". Secondary to this deficit, the development of pretend play, joint attention and pragmatic communication will also become impaired (Rogers and Pennington, 1991).

Mundy and colleagues (Mundy and Hogan, 1994; Mundy *et al.*, 1986; Mundy *et al.*, 1993) investigated the coherences between three aspects of deviant social behaviour in autistic disorder, namely: sharing intentions (i.e., the ability to communicate one's wishes, beliefs, desires or goals); joint attention (i.e., the ability to share one's visual perspective on objects or events); and affective sharing (i.e., the ability to share one's emotional response to objects or events). Normal infants as young as 7–12 months have developed the capacity to share these three aspects of mental states with others (intersubjectivity). Autistic children, independent of mental and chronological age are severely impaired in communicating false beliefs (Baron-Cohen *et al.*, 1985), referential looking (Mundy *et al.*, 1986), and socially directed smiling (Dawson, 1991). None of the existing theories of autistic disorder can sufficiently explain all these three aspects of intersubjectivity. Mundy and Hogan (1994) argued that each model does not reflect inadequacies of the model developers, but rather on our knowledge of early social development. The mentalising-deficit may sufficiently explain most symptoms of children with autistic disorder (Leslie and Thaiss, 1992). Nevertheless, investigators like Hobson and Pennington argued that some specific impairments of autistic children are not accounted for by a mentalising deficit.

The findings from neurological studies suggest that there are more than one neurological causes of the autistic behavioral phenotype. Wing and Attwood (1987) have similarly stated that there is never a straight pathway in the development of a mental disorder. According to this consideration many authors speculated on the possible causes and etiological factors in pervasive developmental disorders. Pennington and Ozonoff (1991, p. 118) stated that "it must be possible to trace a somewhat specific causal path across levels of analysis, from the etiology level up to the level of observable behaviors". They suggested many possible connections between the biotype (etiological level) and the phenotype (primary underlying observable deficit) working in the etiology and pathogenesis of autistic disorder and in other mental disorders: (a) *One-to-one correspondence.* Possible in the case of trisomie 21 or single major gene disorders leading to some cases of autistic disorder (Folstein and Rutter, 1988); (b) *One-to-many correspondence or pleiotropy* is possible because one cause can lead to various clinical manifestations (Rutter and Schopler, 1992); (c) *Many-to-one correspondence, aetiologic heterogenity or multifactoriality*: autistic disorder may be seen as the final common pathway of many aetiological conditions (Steffenburg, 1991); (d) *Many-to-many correspondence or interaction* account for about 37% of autistic disorder and other pervasive developmental disorders (Gillberg, 1992); (e) *Reciprocal causation.* A biotype initially causes a behavioural phenotype that affects future development of the biotype (developmental correspondence). This may be also the case in autistic disorder, if one considers the possibility that many neurobiological factors may have a shaping effect in the pre-, peri-, and even in the postnatal period of brain development (Tsai, 1987), and that several different neuropathological mechanisms are involved in the pathogenesis leading to an autistic spectrum disorder (Coleman, 1987; Rubinstein *et al.*, 1993).

COMORBIDITY

Many autistic children exhibit associated mild to profound mental retardation (Volkmar *et al.*, 1990). Infact, approximately 75% of children with autistic disorder function at a retarded level (APA, 1994). The profile of cognitive skills is uneven, regardless of the general level of intelligence. Some children show hyperlexia, others may have a better IQ in performance skills than in verbal intelligence, and some of the more intelligent children may have better language comprehension skills than speech (Yirmiya and Sigman, 1991). Abnormalities in behavioural symptoms include hyperactivity, short attention span, impulsivity, aggression, self-injurious behaviour, and, particularly in young children, temper tantrums.

Abnormalities in response to sensory stimuli can be found in odd or overselective reactions to pain, touch, sound, light, and other stimuli (Dawson, 1991). Autistic children with mental retardation have a higher rate of medical problems as compared to those with autistic disorder only (Rutter *et al.*, 1994).

Between 28 to 33% of autistic children have central nervous conditions (Bryson *et al.*, 1988; Cialdella and Mamelle, 1989). The prevalence of seizures among individuals in autistic disorder increases from preadolescence to adulthood, with rates ranging from 5 to 14% in preadolescent children and about 26% in young adults (Cialdella and Mamelle, 1989; Gillberg and Steffenburg, 1987). As reviewed by Wing (1993), the prevalence of neurological conditions in autism ranges from 27 to 80% across studies. Approximately 70 to 85% of autistic children exhibit associated mental retardation (Volkmar *et al.*, 1990). About 66% had IQ levels below 70, 37% between 10 and 50, and only 12% had IQ scores of 90 and above (Ritvo *et al.*, 1989). Other studies reported 5 to 30% of autistic children to function within the normal intelligence level (Yirmiya and Sigman, 1991). IQ scores of autistic children seem to be quite stable after the age of five and are a good predictor of later performance outcome (Paul, 1987).

In the course of development and in dependence on cognitive capacities, autistic children may show some comorbid disorders, like learning difficulties, hyperactivity, anxiety and depression (Rutter, 1970). During the preschool period autistic children exhibit symptoms of hyperactivity that are persistent during early school years and generally become less persistent in adolescence. Hyperreagibility in preschool and symptoms of anxiety in school age are often observed in autistic children. Autistic adolescents with some capacity to realize their social isolation from peers may show depressive symptomatology.

COURSE AND OUTCOME

Course

Autistic Disorder

Features of autistic disorder vary in the age at which they are detected (Rutter and Schopler, 1987). Short and Schopler (1988) argue that the severity of autism could be related to age of onset; 94% of cases can be recognized by the age of 3 years and 74% within the second year of life.

Some aspects of the early social and communicative developmental of autistic children are presented in Table 6.2.

The First and Second Year.   There is some uncertainty about the age of onset of autistic disorder. However, according to retrospective parental reports some autistic children have delays in the development during their first and second years of life (Gillberg *et al.*, 1990; Ornitz, 1983). Some autistic children may even have unusual characteristics during the first year of life (Ornitz, 1983). The features discriminating one- to two-year old autistic children from other children are their isolated behaviour, lack of play, strange reactions to sound, failure to attract attention to their own activity, lack of smile at times when it is expected, and the empty gaze (Gillberg *et al.*, 1990) and a lack of interest in other children, enjoying to play peek-a-boo or hide-and-seek games, and engagement in pretend play, restricted use of an index finger to point at something of interest or to show objects to parents (Baron-Cohen *et al.*, 1993).

The Preschool and Early Childhood Years.   The prototypic picture of autistic disorder include aloofness, muteness or echolalia, and preservation of sameness associated with stereotypic motor behaviours. In early childhood the social behaviour of mentally retarded and intelligent autistic children is fairly similar. Three interactional styles can be differentiated in the preschool and early childhood years: social aloofness (e.g., aloof and indifferent in most situations, little apparent interest in social aspects of contact, poor eye contact, moderate to severe cognitive deficiency), passive interaction (e.g., limited spontaneous social approaches, little pleasure derived from social contact with active rejection being infrequent, varying degrees of cognitive deficiency), and active-but-odd interaction (e.g., spontaneous social approaches, poor role taking skills) (Borden and Ollendick, 1992; Prizant and Schuler, 1987; Wing and Attwood, 1987).

The interactional styles of autistic children may be a phenomenon of social-cognitive functioning and development because of two factors. First, the subgroups defined by Wing and Gould (1979) seem to vary depending on the severity of autistic disorder and intelligence (Castelloe and Dawson, 1993; Volkmar *et al.*, 1989). Symptoms of autistic disorder were more severe for the aloof group than the active-but-odd children, with passive children in the middle. Aloof children had lower IQ scores than both passive and active-but-odd children. Individuals with higher levels of cognitive functioning show a progression from aloofness to passive acceptance to active-but-odd social interaction. Among those with IQs in the retarded range, progression from aloofness to passivity is common, but not for the active-but-odd social interactions (Wing and Attwood, 1987). Second, there seems to be a characteristic developmental course within the domain of social behaviour (Borden and Ollendick, 1992). Lord (1984) proposed a developmental sequence in social interaction from "aloof" to "passive" in response to social interactions, and from "aloof" or "passive" to "active-but-odd" in initiating social interaction. Wetherby (1986) suggested a similar developmental sequence in the domain of intentional communication. In the first step autistic children show communicative attempts to regulate other people's behaviour to achieve environmental ends such as requesting objects or action and protesting. In the second step the autistic child is able to attract other people's attention. The child is able to request social interaction, to greet other's in a ritualistic manner, to use calling to obtain objects or actions, to request permission, and to show-off. In the third step, communication for social ends occurs in the communicative functions being focussed on interaction and sharing a topic. The child is able to direct other people's attention to an object or event by requesting information about it, commenting on it, and interactive labelling (Wetherby, 1986; Stone and Caro-Martinez, 1990). Children at the first step of intentional communication and social interaction may impose "aloof", children at the third step impose "active-but-odd".

There is ample evidence that a simple deviant view of autistic children should be abandoned and replaced by focusing on developmental issues. The deviance model does not take into account that the behaviour of autistic children does change and that they reach uneven developmental levels in different domains (Volkmar *et al.*, 1990). Thus, according to Burack (1992), behaviour development among autistic children can best be understood within the framework of typical development. This framework seems to be a precondition to differentiate the deviated and delayed characteristics of autistic children development (Volkmar *et al.*, 1990).

Pauls (1987) summarizes the findings of long-term outcome studies of autistic disorder as: (i) two-thirds are unable to lead an independent life; (ii) 15 to 20% of autistic individuals gain full employment; (iii) about 14% of autistic children improve in social behaviour, although they continue to show lack empathy and social "know how"; and (iv) only 1 to 2% will have a very good outcome. Autistic children with full-scale IQ scores of 50 or less have the worst long-term prognosis, exhibit seizures, are likely to be mute, have severe behaviour problems (e.g., stereotype, auto-aggression), and are most likely to stay in residential care (Rutter and Garmezy, 1983).

Asperger's Disorder

Children with Asperger's disorder have a somewhat later onset of the disorder then children with autism (Tantam, 1988). In early stages of development children with Asperger's disorder show an unusual fascination with letters and numbers, and some children can talked before they could walk. Some of the children may be able to decode words, although with little or no understanding. Other may develop toe walking and finger flicking. These symptoms diminish in adolescence or appear only in especially anxiety-provoking situations. The preschool and early school age child often shows marked physical symptoms like visible awkwardness, odd posture, rigid gait patterns, a delay in the acquisition of motor skills, poor manipulative skills, and significant deficits in visual-motor coordination. A delay in acquisition of motor milestones and the presence of motor clumsiness are typical symptoms of the early childhood period of children with Asperger's disorder. Odd attachment patterns to family members and inappropriate approaches to peers and other persons are more characteristic of children with Asperger's disorder than social aloofness. Some children continually attempt to initiate contact with their parents or peers. They hug or scream at them or ask them repeatedly the same questions about an unusual topic. Older children express some interest in other people and in making friendship, but their approaches may be inappropriate and peculiar. The often one-sided conversation seems like they were unaware of the presence of their communication partner and insensitive to his feelings, intentions and communicative attempts.

In adolescence idiosyncratic interests in factual information may become very salient as they shift to unusual and narrow topics (e.g., names of animals). The facts are learned in rote fashion and reflect poor understanding. The factual information about circumscribed topics (e.g., of the underground traffic-network) appears to be an all-absorbing preoccupation of many children and adolescents with Asperger's disorder. In contrast, children with autistic disorder display savant talents or isolated skills in manipulative, visuo-spatial and musical areas. Life history of children with Asperger's disorder always show no clinically significant general delay in language acquisition, cognitive development, and adaptive behaviour. The condition is highly stable and may have a better long-term outcome than is typically observed in autism (Frith, 1991).

Rett's Disorder

Rett's disorder has its onset prior to age four years, usually in the first or second year of life (DSM-IV; APA, 1994). A four-stage model of the developmental course of Rett's disorder indicates (Hagberg and Witt-Engerström, 1986): (i) early-onset stagnation stage that is present between six to 18 months of age; (ii) rapid developmental regression stage beginning at one to two years of age; (iii) pseudostationary stage that usually occurs at three to four years of age; and (iv) late motor deterioration stage occurring during school age or early adolescence (Table 6.7). The long-term outcome is very poor, leading to severe invalidation and a loss of mobility in about 80% of the cases (Hagberg, 1993).

Childhood Disintegrative Disorder

An essential feature of CDD is a period of prolonged normal functioning during the first two or three years of life (Volkmar, 1992; Volkmar and Cohen, 1989). Because of these prolonged period most children

Table 6.7 The developmental course of Rett-syndrome

Stage	Clinical symptoms
Stage 1	Declaration of headgrowth Hypotonia Loss of interest in play
Stage 2	Autistic-like symptoms (prominent) Self-abusive behavior Development of seizures EEG-abnormalities
Stage 3	Autistic-like features (less prominent) Abnormal wake-sleep cycles Respiratory dysfunctions Bruxism (habitual, purposeless clenching and grinding of the teeth) Truncal ataxia (blunted coordination of the muscles) Decline of neuromotor functioning
Stage 4	Improvement in social interest and interactions Tetraparetic weakness Muscle wasting Limb distortion Severe scoliosis More or less complete immobilisation

Modified from Hagberg and Witt-Engerström (1986).

should speak in sentences and reach the capacity for symbolic play. A premonitory phase can be observed in some cases. The children may become nonspecifically agitated, anxious, or dysphoric during this phase. CDD typically have an onset after age two years (median age = 3.36 years). A few cases were reported to have a onset after school entry at nine years. This very late onset conditions maybe associated with some diagnosable medical condition (Corbett *et al.*, 1977).

Two distinctive patterns of onset of CDD can be distinguished. In some children CDD develops gradually over a period of weeks or months. In other cases there is a relatively abrupt onset within days or weeks. Once the full clinical picture is established, the feature is similar to autism, but somewhat less severe. In school-age, the most prominent autistic-like features include social disturbances, stereotype behavior and resistance to change, overactivity and affective symptoms (agitation, apparent anxiety). Speech deterioration and deterioration in self-help skills are common in CDD, and even total loss of the capacity to speak or marked deterioration in communication skills. Children who regain some communicative speech have similar difficulties as those found in children with autistic disorder. Different patterns of syndrome progression have been recognized (Volkmar, 1992): in about 75% of cases, the child deteriorates to some markedly lower level of functioning but development then stabilises. As many as 40% of patients may regain the ability to speak in single words, with 20% regaining the capacity to speak in sentences. In some cases of CDD the regression is progressive with a continuously deteriorating course. In about three-fourths of cases, the course is static with only minimal improvement in rare cases (Corbett *et al.*, 1977). A marked degree of recovery may be absent.

Psychosocial Impairment

Before the age of 30 months, the development of children who received the diagnosis of autistic disorder appears impaired or distorted (Rutter and Schopler, 1987). Social abnormalities that reflect a basic deficit in the ability of autistic children to form relationships became evident in early childhood. Disturbances in social relationships can be found in autistic children's inadequate appreciation of socioemotional cues, in their lack of response to other people's emotions and a lack of modulation of behaviour according to social context, in their poor use of social signals and weak integration of social, emotional, and communicative behaviours, and especially in their lack of socioemotional reciprocity. These deficits are shown in features such as: (i) a failure to use eye-to-eye contact, facial expression, body posture, and gestures to regulate social interaction; (ii) rarely seeking others for comfort or affection; (iii) rarely imitating interactive play with others; (iv) rarely offering comfort to others or responding to other people's distress or happiness; (v) rarely greeting others, and (vi) no peer friendship in terms of a mutual sharing of interests, activities, and emotions despite ample opportunities.

The capacity of autistic children to use language for social communication appears to be a deviance rather than a delay in development. This is evident in their lack of social usage of language, in poor synchrony and lack of reciprocity in conversational interchange, in a poor flexibility in language expression, an inadequate response to other people's verbal and nonverbal overtures, and an impaired use of variations in cadence or emphasis to reflect communicative modulation. These features may be shown by: (i) a delay in or a lack of the development of spoken language that is not compensated for by use of gesturing as alternative modes of communication (often preceded by a lack of communicative babbling); (ii) a failure to respond to other people (e.g., not responding when called by name); (iii) a failure to initiate or sustain conversational interchange; (iv) stereotyped and repetitive use of language; (v) use of you when I is meant; (vi) idiosyncratic use of words, and (vii) abnormalities in pitch, stress, rate, rhythm, and intonation of speech.

The lack of creativity and spontaneity in autistic children's use of social language is paralleled to their deficits in preverbal skills. Thus, a lack of varied spontaneous "make-believe" play is especially characteristic. Another set of impairment concerns restricted, repetitive, and stereotyped patterns of behaviour. This tendency to impose rigidity on various day-to-day functioning appears to be a general tendency since it applies to both routine and novel activities. The stereotyped patterns may include: (i) an encompassing preoccupation with stereotyped and restricted patterns of interest; (ii) attachment to unusual objects; (iii) compulsive rituals; (iv) stereotyped and repetitive motor mannerisms; (v) preoccupation with part-objects or non-functional elements of play materials; and (vi) distress over changes in small details of the environment.

ASSESSMENT

Numerous questionnaires, checklists, and diagnostic interviews have been developed to detect and diagnose autistic disorder. The most commonly used among infants are the Schedule for Autistic Behavior in

Children 0–2 years of age (Dahlgren and Gillberg, 1989) and Checklist for Autism in Toddlers (Baron-Cohen *et al.*, 1992). Among preschool and school-age children, these include the Autism Behavior Checklist (Krug *et al.*, 1980), Autism Diagnostic Interview (Le Couteur *et al.*, 1989), Autism Diagnostic Observation Schedule (Lord *et al.*, 1989), and the Childhood Autism Rating Scale (Schopler *et al.*, 1988). Among school-age children, the most frequently used instruments are the Asperger Syndrome (and related problems) Screening Questionnaire (Ehlers and Gillberg, 1993) and the Asperger Syndrome Diagnostic Interview (Gillberg and Gillberg, 1989).

TREATMENT

Pharmacotherapy

Advances in the pharmacotherapy of autistic disorder are reviewed by Gualtieri *et al.* (1987) and recently by McDougel *et al.* (1994). According to Gillberg and Steffenburg (1987) about 25% of all autistic children and 75% of all autistic adolescents are treated with medication. The pharmacotherapy is generally used among children with autistic disorder to threat: (i) primary and autism-specific symptoms to promote the normal development of social, cognitive, and language skills; and (ii) secondary symptoms such as epilepsy, stereotype behaviour, and aggression (Campbell *et al.* (1987).

Megavitamins

A high dose of Vitamin B_6 with magnesium is a common therapy for autistic patients (Rimland, 1987). Among 200 patients who were treated in this way, 20 showed improvement in their behaviour; 8 of the 16 patients who took part in a double-blind study showed deterioration of their behaviour (Rimland *et al.*, 1978). In a study by LeLord *et al.* (1982), 10 of the 44 patients showed some improvement in autistic behaviour, and three children showed an increase of autistic symptoms when treated with a high dosage of Vitamin B_6. However, later studies have failed to replicate these findings (Coleman and Gillberg, 1987). Since Rimland's study (1987) dealt with withdrawal attempt, Gualtieri *et al.* (1987) raised the question of whether the deterioration of behaviour is based on withdrawal symptoms after a long-term consumption of a high dose of vitamin. Although Vitamin B_6 and magnesium are often used, there are no definite results to prove their success whilst it is often said that vitamin treatment has no or little side effects it is important to realize that vitamins are not always harmless (Gualtieri *et al.*, 1987).

Fenfluramine Therapy

Fenfluramine (Ponderase) is a medicine for weight reduction which reduces serotonin levels. Since elevated levels of serotonin have been found in 30 to 40% of the autistic persons, a number of clinicians have given fenfluramine to autistic children. In a study by Geller *et al.* (1982), three autistic children showed significant improvement in their behaviour and increased serotonin levels when treated with fenfluramine; upon withdrawal of the medication they showed a deterioration in the symptoms.

Rutter (1986) indicated that 27% of the 81 autistic children treated with fenfluramine showed a significant improvement in symptoms. However, in a systematic behavioural observation for measuring changes in severely retarded autistic children, no positive effect of fenfluramine was observed (Campbell *et al.*, 1987; Yarbrough *et al.*, 1987). Gualtieri *et al.* (1987) have indicated the side effects of fenfluramine and considered the current treatment to be not justified. The negative effects such as weight reduction and disturbance of the metabolism of serotonin in the brain argue against the use of fenfluramine (Gualtieri *et al.*, 1987).

Therapy with Opiatantagonist

The discovery that the body can produce opiate has led to the introduction of numerous theories and studies which try to explain psychiatric disorder as being caused by endogenous opiate metabolism. Panksepp and Sahley (1987) consider the social problems of autistic children to be caused by overactivity of the endogenous opiate system; furthermore, opiatantagonists (e.g., Nahaxon and Naltrexon) could lead to an improvement of autistic behaviour. Endogenous opiate should lead to a sensitivity to pain and to self-aggressive behaviour in these children (Coleman and Gillberg, 1987). Campbell *et al.* (1987) treated one 5-year old severely impaired autistic child with Naltrexon. After receiving a low dose of Naltrexon, the aggressive, hyperactive child became more calm; the withdrawal behaviour was reduced with a high dose (2–3 mg/kg/day). A major limitation of the study is that the child's behaviour before the treatment was variable and that the improvement at the end of Naltrexon treatment was not maintained.

The idea that some autistic children have an elevated body-produced opiate was supported by Gillberg *et al.* (1985) who showed an increased body-produced opiate in liquor of 10 of the 20 autistic children in their study. Among these 10 children, nine were clearly sensitive to pain, and seven showed self-aggressive behaviour either during the liquor intake or in their life time. Several trials have shown successful outcomes of auto-aggressive behaviour in mentally retarded autistic children who have been treated with opiatantagonist. Others showed a dose-dependent reduction in the self-aggressive behaviour (Herman *et al.*, 1985). Since the self-aggressive behaviour often occurs in mentally-retarded autistic children, the use of opiatantagonist in this group of children needs special attention.

Neuroleptic Therapy

Neuroleptic is the most commonly used treatment for autistic patients (Campbell *et al.*, 1987; Gualtieri *et al.*, 1987), which works specifically on various "psychotic" symptoms. In one controlled study with neuroleptic haloperidol, Campbell *et al.* (1978) found that: (i) haloperidol affects two main symptoms — withdrawal and stereotype behaviour — of autistic children more than placebo; and (ii) the combination of haloperidol and a behavioural therapy for speech training is more effective than with only medication or behavioural therapy.

Campbell and Anderson (Campbell *et al.*, 1982; Anderson *et al.*, 1984) studied the effects of haloperidol on the behaviour and learning skills of autistic children in a naturalistic environment and in a highly structured experimental setting. The children were divided into one of two 4-week treatment sequences: haloperidol-placebo-haloperidol-sequence, and placebo-haloperidol-placebo-sequence. The haloperidol treatment caused improvement in different areas. The positive effect of haloperidol in a structured learning situation is based on the improved attentional and/or cognitive processes.

When considering that autistic children have problems in the dopaminergic system (Coleman and Gillberg, 1987), and haloperidol affects the sensory axis of the dopaminergic nervous system, one can conclude that the hypothesis of the impaired sensory modulation by Ornitz (1987) is supported. The affected dopaminergic nervous system which controls the selected attention and the cognitive function, and also controls the motoric behaviour, seems to be impaired at the sensory axis. Furthermore, psychological experiments have shown perception problems in autistic disorder (Frith and Baron-Cohen, 1987). Campbell *et al.* (1982) also found positive changes among treated autistic children not only in a natural situation, but also in structured learning situation with discrimination tasks. Compared to children in the placebo-therapy, children treated with haloperidol showed higher developmental levels (Anderson *et al.*, 1984).

Although haloperidol showed no side effects in the short-term treatment, the side effects in long-term use are similar to those of the other neuroleptic therapies (e.g., dyskinesia). Problems also appear during the acclimatise phase and during overdose (Gualtieri *et al.*, 1987). Experimental studies showed that autistic children with symptoms of hyperactivity, aggressivity, low frustration tolerance level, agitation or short attentional span have a good response to haloperidol. Social isolation, stereotypic behaviour, negativism and lability can be reduced. Neuroleptic does not seem appropriate for use in hypoactivity. The dose of neuroleptic should be given in such a way that it can reduce the symptoms with little side effects (Campbell *et al.*, 1987; Gualtieri *et al.*, 1987). For the treatment of echolalia, a combination of neuroleptic therapy and developmentally oriented behavioural therapy is effective in communication problems and in reducing speech activity of autistic children (Anderson *et al.*, 1984).

Neuroleptic has been used to reduce autistic symptoms such as stereotype behaviour, hyperactivity, and restlessness. This makes it easier for the children to learn both in therapy and in the classroom. With careful supervision and examination for improvement and side effects, pharmacotherapy can be useful for individual cases even in younger children. However, using a high dose of haloperidol, the children can react quickly with massive sedation so that an early and individual adjustment is necessary (Gualtieri *et al.*, 1987). In a prospective study, about one-fifth of the children showed medically-dependent dyskinesia (Campbell *et al.*, 1987). Acute extrapyramidal symptoms and other symptoms during treatment with neuroleptic can appear in autistic patients.

Psychological Intervention

Behaviour Therapy

The use of behavioural therapy to help autistic children lead an independent life has increased enormously in the last years. A major problem with behavioural therapy is related to the ability to generalise the short-term therapeutic effects (Koegel and Koegel, 1987). These include the problem of generalising the learned behaviour: (i) on other relevant conditions than the one under which the behavioural patterns are acquired the first time; (ii) over a long-term period; and (iii) to another, similar behaviour.

The difficulties of autistic children to show the learned behaviour under different stimulus is related to its problem of decontextualisation (Kusch and Petermann, 1991; Wetherby, 1986). According to several studies, the behaviour of autistic children can be dependent on the social context such as the therapist, the therapeutic situation or the therapy room, and the specific reinforcer or a specific motoric movement of the therapist. Other studies have shown that the acquired behavioural competence can be lost immediately after the intervention. These studies have given some insight as to why autistic children do not automatically generalise a learned behaviour to other areas (Koegel and Koegel, 1987).

The treatment of autistic disorder has been rather ineffective (Kazdin, 1994), probably because these children are often treated after their fifth year (Lovaas and Smith, 1989). Children who are treated before the fifth year generally show greater improvement in their social behaviour and school achievements (Simeonson *et al.*, 1987). Despite these findings, only a few models of early intervention are available for children with an early form or an increased risk of autistic disorder (Greenspan, 1992; Prizant and Wetherby, 1988). This is not surprising because the therapy-oriented diagnostic procedure and intervention methods for treating such children are unknown (Greenspan, 1992; Kusch, 1993; Wetherby and Prizant, 1993).

It is only in recent years that new behavioural therapy techniques with autistic children have been developed (Duchan, 1986; Koegel *et al.*, 1987). These new techniques are based on an increased consideration of the developmental psychological knowledge, in which what is learned generally makes sense to the children when they know the structure of the event (event-script), what is learned can be applied (decontextualisation), when the behavioural reprimands which are relevant for those events (conceptualisation) are learned, and when they are the reasons for the children's action (intrinsic motivation, intention). The problem of generalising the learned knowledge will not occur when the children are aware of all three aspects (Kusch and Petermann, 1991; Prizant and Schuler, 1987).

Developmentally Related Behavioural Therapy

The therapy uses developmentally related procedures for prevention, early management, and treatment (Kusch and Petermann, 1995). The aims are to: (a) treat autistic children at an early stage and not when they are at a pre-school age (Greenspan, 1992), and to train the caretaker in adjusting to the child's problem; (b) prevent the development of autistic disorder during certain developmental period (Prizant and Wetherby, 1988); (c) act as a treatment model which is related to symptoms of autistic disorder such as imitation, attentional problem, and intentional communication (Prizant and Schuler, 1987); and to (d) deal with the impairments under various conditions (Kusch, 1993).

Since toddlers with a high risk of pervasive developmental disorder experience difficulties in carrying out social interaction and communication (Borden and Ollendick, 1992; Wetherby and Prizant, 1993), the basic requirement for each intervention involves the establishment of the so called fine-tuning for social competence (Duchan, 1986). Social interaction with autistic children includes: (i) the establishment psychophysiological regulation (i.e., the child should not be either hypo- or hyperactive); (ii) focus on the sensory motor attention by observing the child's focus of attention when the child is in a well-balanced state; (iii) pay attention to the child's sensory and motoric reaction; (iv) repeat the communication offer; (v) initiate daily interaction using signals such as physical and eye contact, clapping hands, and then varying the signals the child uses to communicate by changing its intensity, frequency or its duration; and (vi) each social interaction sequence has to be ended formally.

These aspects of social behaviour make use of the "scaffolding" concept for the therapy with families of an autistic child. The parents built a temporary social context favorable for the child's development, which have to be learned first before the next step of adult-child interaction. The corresponding aspects of the therapy-oriented diagnosis and the therapy for social competence are demonstrated by means of the parent-child interaction training *in-vivo* (Kusch and Petermann, 1991).

Parent-child Interaction Training *In-vivo* with Autistic Preschool children: *In-vivo* trainings are based on the idea that assessment and intervention can only be made successfully when aspects of mood congruence and state dependent learning are considered. That means that: (i) assessment has to be undertaken only in situations in which the child and his parent(s) actually present problematic behaviour. This helps ensure that the trainer observe the behavioural, intellectual and emotional reactions of both interaction partners; (ii) the behaviour problems have to be treated in situations where both interaction partners are in a (assessment-situation) congruent mood of interaction. Learning and behavioural change can only take place in this mood-congruent state (Kusch, 1993).

The parent-child interaction training *in-vivo* for diagnostic and therapeutic procedures are elucidated through: (a) *Construction of interaction sequence.* The first step of the parent-child interaction training involves an analysis of a social context in which the problem occurs (Wetherby and Prizant, 1993). During the second step, an interaction sequence is constructed by the trainer that reflects the natural situation in which the problem occurs. The third step involves deciding which person, under which condition (interaction situation), and with what style (interaction style) will interact with the child; (b) *Audio-visual recording and video-analysis* allows practice control of the data collected, as well as for selecting and modifying the therapeutic strategy (Kusch, 1993; Kusch and Petermann, 1991); (c) *Therapy planning* includes identification of the problem for which treatment is needed, and characteristics of the sequence of interaction. The therapy planning is completed when the behavioural problems are specified, and when the characteristics of the interaction are defined; (d) *Training construction and performance.* After knowing which behaviour of the child and/or parents, which situational characteristics and/or which behavioural competence of the child are to be changed, the diagnostic interaction sequence of the child and mother/father will be used for intervention purposes by giving feedback over an ear phone and through behavioural correction by the trainer. After one interaction sequence, the therapist and the parents discuss the therapeutic situation. On the basis of the cognitive-emotional restructuring from a concrete example, the parents can have a perspective on an interaction partner (emotional experience) and observer (cognitive information processing). The results of the video-analysis of the therapeutic interaction sequence and the cognitive restructuring on a concrete example will be considered in the planning of the next therapy session; (e) *Control of the therapeutic process.* The audio-visual recording, the protocol of the video-analysis and the analysis of the parent conversation over the whole therapy session allows a continual control of the course of the therapy; (f) *Therapy effect control.* A comparison between the first diagnostic and the last therapeutic interaction sequence shows the treatment success. The comparison of the different recordings show the effect of the parent-child interaction training. The concluding parental discussion allows the evaluation of the whole therapy course. A follow-up investigation is possible at any time.

Educational Programms

Sophisticated treatment and education programmes for autistic children have been developed (Schopler and Mesibov, 1994). One such program is *facilitated communication,* which strives to expand vocabulary, refining syntax, and to train autistic children to use their language effectively in social interactions (Prizant and Schuler, 1987). Prizant and Schuler (1987) introduced developmentally based prelanguage and language approaches to facilitate communication, including theoretical considerations, intervention oriented assessment techniques, and intervention strategies. Although empirical evidence showing its effectiveness is lacking, this treatment method is worth examining because of its use of developmental principles.

In a treatment program developed by Greenspan (1992), infants, toddlers, and preschool children are trained to reestablish the developmental sequences. Treatment involves teaching children and their parents in an interactive process essential for the first three aspects of emotional development. In the first step, the capacity for self-regulation of the child and shared attention between child and the parent is fostered. In the second step, the parents are educated in the "special" emotional engagement of their child and to build a reliable social signaling system with the child. The third step involves the establishment of reciprocal social communication between child and caretaker.

The treatment and education of autistic and other children with communication handicaps (TEACCH)

This training was initiated in 1968 by parents of autistic children (Schopler, 1994). TEACCH was the first statewide program in the United States that provides training to teachers and give supports to families of autistic children. All members of the TEACCH are also engaged as social advocators of the children, in development, empirical research, and all day practice of diagnostic and intervention strategies and programs (Schopler *et al.,* 1990).

Psychoeducational programms

These programms with individualized teaching activities are one of the most impressive support activities for children with autistic disorders (Schopler, 1994). The treatment usually is carried out in a highly structured classroom or in a room at home (Schopler *et al.,* 1984). Structure is most important in the setting because the child's environment has to be as predictable and comprehensive as possible, to facilitate communication and minimize "aberrant" behaviour, to ease stimulus and response generalization and to promote a child's independence.

Individualized teaching activities are developed in four steps. The first step involves assessment of social, cognitive and/or communicative skills based on naturalistic observation. The aim is to gain a picture of the child's strengths and weaknesses in various domains of behaviour and social context. In a second step, an interview assesses the child's parents point of view concerning the behaviour of their child and priorities for change. This information is used in step three to translate the priorities into concrete treatment objectives. In step four, these objectives form the basis for designing individual teaching activities (Schopler and Mesibov, 1984, 1985, 1987, 1992, 1994).

CONCLUDING REMARKS

Children with autistic disorders can be sufficiently differentiated from children with other developmental disorders (APA, 1994). A major problem is related to early identification since there is lack of criteria available to identify the cases with autistic disorder. It should be possible in the near future to identify autistic children during the first year of life. This seems realistic considering three aspects of early identification: (i) investigation of large sample size in high-risk children; (ii) analyses of video-recording of autistic children during the first year of life; and (iii) identification of developmental areas in which autism-specific deficits (e.g., mentalising-deficit and "theory of mind") are present. Prospective studies are needed in each of these domains of investigation.

Developmental psychopathology deals mainly with the third point in which the normal and deviated development of children are compared (Dawson, 1991). This domain of investigation may contribute to the attempt to identify autistic children at an early stage, and thus allowing successful early-intervention. Reports of parents with autistic children have confirmed that autistic children often show some signs of the disorder during the first two years of life (Ornitz, 1983; Gillberg *et al.*, 1990).

Although behavioural problems that occur in the early developmental phase are most often non-specific, they may lead to the occurrence of more severe disorders (Cicchetti, 1990). However, the problems of non-specificity of "early symptoms" remains and hamper early identification and intervention of autistic children. A possible solution to this problem has been developed by Wetherby and Prizant (Prizant and Wetherby, 1987, 1988; Wetherby and Prizant, 1993), who investigate behavioural problems in social context by analyzing distortions of the social interchange between the child and his parent. Kusch and Petermann (1991, 1995) have developed a diagnostic procedure in which various aspects of social interaction can be varied systematically. The aspects can be traced back to the results and assessment procedures used in research of autistic disorder (Lord, 1993; McEnvoy *et al.*, 1993) and developmental psychopathology (Cicchetti, 1990) so that the interaction situation can be constructed and autistic symptoms of toddlers investigated.

The importance of new attempts of early identification and early intervention with autistic children cannot be underestimated if one takes into consideration the concept of sensitive periods and corresponding concepts of human brain development (Cicchetti and Tucker, 1994). Intrinsic factors affecting brain development and infant communication in the first years of life may give rise to autistic disorder (Trevarthen and Aitken, 1994). An underlying disorder of an infant may lead to different symptomatology depending on brain development and the sensitive period the infant is in. Therefore early identification of, and early intervention with autistic children has to be sensitive to the sensitive period. Different long term intervention effects may occur if an intervention takes place during a sensitive period or afterwards. Consequently, we should not wait until we can diagnose a distinct psychopathology but intervene if social and communicative competences are impaired (Greenspan, 1992; Mundy and Hogan, 1994; Prizant and Wetherby, 1988).

REFERENCES

Aitken, K.J. (1991). Examining the evidence for a common structural basis to autism. *Developmental Medicine and Child Neurology*, **33**, 930–938.

American Psychiatric Association (1980). *Diagnostic and statistical manual of mental disorders* (3rd ed.). Washington, DC: American Psychiatric Association.

American Psychiatric Association (1987). *Diagnostic and statistical manual of mental disorders* (3rd ed. rev.). Washington, DC: American Psychiatric Association.

American Psychiatric Association (1994). *Diagnostic and statistical manual of mental disorders* (4th ed.). Washington, DC: American Psychiatric Association.

Anderson, L.T., Campbell, M., Grega, D.M., Perry, R., Small, A.M., and Green, W.H. (1984). Haloperidol in infantile autism: Effects on learning and behavioral symptoms. *American Journal of Psychiatry*, **141**, 1195–1202.

August, G.J., Stewart, M.A., and Tsai, L. (1981). The incidence of cognitive disabilities in the siblings of autistic children. *British Journal of Psychiatry*, **138**, 416–422.

Bachevalier, J. (1991). An animal model for childhood autism: Memory loss and socio-emotional disturbances following neonatal damage to the limbic system in monkeys. In C.A. Tamminga and S.C. Schulz (Eds.), *Advances in neuropsychiatry and psychopharmacology,* Vol. 1 (pp. 129–140). New York: Raven Press.

Baron-Cohen, S. (1989). The autistic child's theory of mind: A case of specific developmental delay. *Journal of Child Psychology and Psychiatry,* **30**, 285–297.

Baron-Cohen, S. (1995). *Mindblindness.* Cambridge, MA: MIT Press.

Baron-Cohen, S., Allen, J., and Gillberg, C. (1992). Can autism be detected at 18 months? The needle, the haystack and the CHAT. *British Journal of Psychiatry,* **161**, 839–843.

Baron-Cohen, S., Leslie, A.M., and Frith, U. (1985). Does the autistic child have a theory of mind. *Cognition,* **21**, 37–46.

Baron-Cohen, S., Tager-Flusberg, H., and Cohen, D.J. (Eds.) (1993). *Understanding other minds. Perspectives from autism.* Oxford: Oxford University Press.

Borden, M.C. and Ollendick, T.H. (1992). The development and differentiation of social subtypes in autism. *Advances in Clinical Psychology,* **14**, 61–106.

Bosch, G. (1970). *Infantile autism.* New York: Springer.

Boucher, J. (1989). The theory of mind hypothesis of autism: Explanation, evidence and assessment. *British Journal of Disorders of Communication,* **24**, 181–198.

Bryson, S.E., Clark, B.S., and Smith, I.M. (1988). First report of a Canadian epidemiological study of autistic syndromes. *Journal of Child Psychology and Psychiatry,* **29**, 433–445.

Burack, J.A. (1992). Debate and argument: Clarifying developmental issues in the study of autism. *Journal of Child Psychology and Psychiatry,* **33**, 617–621.

Burd, L., Fischer, W., and Kerbeshian, J. (1987). A prevalence study of pervasive developmental disorders in North Dakota. *Journal of the American Academy of Child Psychiatry,* **26**, 700–703.

Campbell, M., Anderson, L.T., Green, W.H., and Deutsch, S.I. (1987). Psychopharmacology. In D.J. Cohen and A.M. Donnellan (Eds.), *Handbook of autism and pervasive developmental disorders* (pp. 545–565). New York: Wiley.

Campbell, M., Anderson, L.T., Small, A.M., Perry, R., Green, W.H., and Caplan, R. (1982). The effects of halperidol on learning and behavior in autistic children. *Journal of Autism and Developmental Disorders,* **12**, 167–175.

Campbell, M., Hardesty, A.S., Breuer, H., and Dolevòy, N. (1978). Childhood psychosis in perspective: A follow-up of 10 children. *Journal of the American Academy of Child Psychiatry,* **17**, 14–28.

Cantor, S., Evans, J., and Pezzot-Pearce, T. (1982). Childhood schizophrenia: Present but not accounted for. *American Journal of Psychiatry,* **139**, 758–762.

Cantwell, D., Backer, L., and Rutter, M. (1987). A comparative study of infantile autism and specific developmental receptive language disorder. IV. Analysis of syntax and language function. *Journal of Child Psychology and Psychiatry,* **19**, 351–362.

Castelloe, P. and Dawson, G. (1993). Subclassification of children with autism and pervasive developmental disorder: A questionnaire based in Wing's subgrouping system. *Journal of Autism and Developmental Disorders,* **23**, 229–241.

Cialdella, P. and Mamelle, N. (1989). An epidemiological study of infantile autism in French department (Rhone): A research note. *Journal of Child Psychology and Psychiatry,* **30**, 165–175.

Cicchetti, D. (1990). The organization and coherence of socio-emotional, cognitive and representational development: Illustrations through a developmental psychopathology perspective on Down's Syndrome and child maltreatment. In R.A. Thompson (Ed.), *Nebraska symposium on motivation: Socio-emotional development* (pp. 275–382). Lincoln: University of Nebraska Press.

Cicchetti, D. and Tucker, D. (1994). Development and self-regulatory structures of the mind. *Development and Psychopathology,* **6**, 533–549.

Cohen, D.J., Paul, R., and Volkmar, F.R. (1986). Issues in the classification of pervasive and other developmental disorders: Toward DSM-IV. *Journal of the American Academy of Child Psychiatry,* **25**, 213–220.

Cohen, D.J., Paul, R., and Volkmar, F.R. (1987). Issues in the classification of perva-sive developmental disorders and associated conditions. In D.J. Cohen and A.M. Donnellan (Eds.), *Handbook of autism and pervasive developmental disorders* (pp. 20–40). New York: Wiley.

Cohen, D.J., Paul, R., and Volkmar, F.R. (1988). The diagnosis and classification of autism: Empirical studies relevant to nosology. In J. Mezzich and M. von Carnach (Eds.), *International Classification in Psychiatry*. Cambridge: At the University Press.

Coleman, M. and Gillberg, C. (1987). *The biology of the autistic syndromes*. New York: Praeger.

Coleman, M. (1987). The search for neurological subgroups in autism. In E. Schopler and G. Mesibov (Eds.), *Neurobiological issues in autism* (pp. 163–189). New York: Plenum Press.

Coleman, M. (1990). Is classical Rett syndrome ever present in males? *Brain Develop-ment*, **12**, 31–32.

Corbett, J., Harris, R., Taylor, E. *et al.* (1977). Progressive disintegrative psychosis of child-hood. *Journal of Psychology and Psychiatry*, **18**, 211–219.

Courchesne, E. (1989). Neuroanatomical systems involved in infantile autism: The impli-cations of cerebellar abnormalities. In G. Dawson (Ed.), *Autism: Nature, diagnosis, and treatment* (pp. 119–143). New York: Guilford Press.

Courchesne, E. (1991). Neuroanatomic imaging in autism. *Pediatrics*, **87**, 781–790.

Courchesne, E., Hesselink, J.R., Jernigan, T.L., and Yeung-Courchesne, R. (1987). Abnormal neuroanatomy in a nonretarded person with autism: Unusual findings with magnetic resonance imaging. *Archives of Neurology*, **44**, 335–341.

Courchesne, E., Townsend, J., Akshoomoff, N.A., Yeung-Courchesne, R., Press, G., Murakami, J., Lincoln, A., James, H., Saitoh, O., Haas, R., and Schreibman, L. (1994). A new finding: Impairment in shifting attention in autistic and cerebellar patients. In S.H. Broman and J. Grafman (Eds.), *Atypical cognitive deficits in developmental dis-orders: Implications for brain function* (pp. 160–393). Hillsdale, NJ: Erlbaum.

Dahlgren, S.O. and Gillberg, C. (1989). Symptoms in the first two years of life. A pre-liminary population study of infantile autism. *European Archives of Psychiatry and Neurological Sciences*, **238**, 169–174.

Damasio, A.R. and Maurer, R.G. (1978). A neurological model for childhood autism. *Archives of Neurology*, **35**, 777–786.

Dawson, G. (1991). A psychobiological perspective on the early socio-emotional development of children with autism. In D. Cicchetti and S.L. Toth (Eds.), *Rochester symposium on developmental psychopathology: Models and integrations*, Vol. 3 (pp. 207–234). Hillsdale, NJ: Erlbaum.

Dawson, G. and Lewy, A. (1989). Arousal, attention, and the socioemotional impairments of individuals with autism. In G. Dawson (Ed.), *Autism: Nature, diagnosis, and treat-ment* (pp. 49–74). New York: Guilford Press.

Denckla, M.B. (1986). New diagnostic criteria for autism and related behavioral disor-ders: Guidelines for research protocols. *Journal of the American Academy of Child and Adolescent Psychiatry*, **25**, 221–230.

Duchan, J.F. (1986). Language intervention through sensemaking and finetuning. In R. Schiefelbusch (Ed.), *Communicative competence: Assessment and language inter-vention* (pp. 187–212). Baltimore: University Park Press.

Duchan, J.F. (1987). Functionalism: A perspective on autistic communication. In D.J. Cohen and A.M. Donnellan (Eds.), *Handbook of autism and pervasive devel-opmental disorders* (pp. 703–709). New York: Wiley.

Ehlers, S. and Gillberg, C. (1993). The epidemiology of Asperger syndrome. A total population study. *Journal of Child Psychology and Psychiatry*, **34**, 1327–1350.

Fein, D., Pennington, B., Markowitz, P., Braverman, M., and Waterhouse, L. (1986). Towards a neuropsychological model of infantile autism: Are the social deficits primary? *Journal of the American Academy of Child Psychiatry*, **25**, 198–212.

Filipek, P.A., Kennedy, D.N., and Caviness, V.S. (1992). Neuroimaging in child neuropsychology. In I. Rapin and S.J. Segalowitz (Eds.), *Handbook of neurology: Child neuropsychology,* Vol. 6. New York: Elsevier.

Folstein, S.E. and Rutter, M. (1988). Autism: Familial aggregation and genetic implications. *Journal of Autism and Developmental Disorders,* **18,** 3–30.

Frith, U. and Baron-Cohen, S. (1987). Perception in autistic children. In D.J. Cohen and A.M. Donnellan (Eds.), *Handbook of autism and pervasive developmental disorders* (pp. 85–102). New York: Wiley.

Frith, U. (Ed.) (1991). *Autism and Asperger syndrome.* Cambridge: Cambridge University Press.

Frith, U., Morton, J., and Leslie, A.M. (1991). The cognitive basis of a biological disorder: Autism. *Trends in Neurosciences,* **14,** 433–438.

Geller, E., Ritvo, E.R., Freeman, B.J., and Yuwiler, A. (1982). Preliminary observations on the effects on fenfluramine on blood serotonin and symptoms in three autistic boys. *New England Journal of Medicine,* **370,** 165–169.

Gillberg, C. (1985). Asperger's syndrome and recurrent psychosis: A case study. *Journal of Autism and Developmental Disorders,* **15,** 389–398.

Gillberg, C. (1992). Autism and autistic-like conditions: Subclasses among disorders of empathy. *Journal of Child Psychology and Psychiatry,* **33,** 813–842.

Gillberg, C., Ehlers, S., Schauman, H., Jakobsson, G., Dahlgren, S., Lindblom, R., Bagenholm, A., Tjuus, T., and Blidner, E. (1990). Autism under age 3 years: A clinical study of 28 cases referred for autistic symptoms in infancy. *Journal of Child Psychology and Psychiatry,* **31,** 921–934.

Gillberg, I.C. and Gillberg, C. (1989). Asperger syndrome — some epidemiological considerations: A research note. *Journal of Child Psychology and Psychiatry,* **30,** 631–638.

Gillberg, C. and Steffenburg, S. (1987). Outcome and prognostic factors in infantile autism and similar conditions. A population based study of 46 cases followed through puberty. *Journal of Autism and Developmental Disorders,* **17,** 273–287.

Gillberg, C., Terenius, L., and Lonnerholm, G. (1985). Endorphin activity in childhood psychosis. *Archives in Genetic Psychiatry,* **42,** 780–783.

Greenspan, S. (1992). Reconsidering the diagnosis and treatment of very young children with autistic spectrum or pervasive developmental disorder. *Zero to Three,* **13,** 1–9.

Gualtieri, T., Evans, R.W., and Patterson, D.R. (1987). The medical treatment of autistic people. In E. Schopler and G.B. Mesibov (Eds.), *Neurobiological issues in autism* (pp. 373–387). New York: Plenum.

Hagberg, B.A. (1993). *Rett syndrome: Clinical and biological aspects.* Cambridge: Cambridge University Press.

Hagberg, B.A., Goutieres, F., Hanefeld, F. *et al.* (1985). Rett syndrome: Criteria for inclusion and exclusion. *Brain Development,* **7,** 372–373.

Hagberg, B.A. and Witt-Engerström, I. (1986). Rett syndrome: A suggested staging system for describing impairment profile with increasing age toward adolescence. *American Journal of Medicine Genetics,* **24,** 47–59.

Harrison, D.J. and Webb, P.J. (1990). Scoliosis in the Rett syndrome: Natural history and treatment. *Brain Development,* **12,** 154–156.

Herman, B.M., Hammock, M.K., Egan, N., Feinstein, L., Chatoor, R., Boeckx, N., Zelnick, M., Jack, R., and Rosenquist, J. (1985). Naltrexone induces dose-dependent decreases in self-injurious behavior. *Neuroscience Abstracts,* **11,** 468.

Hermelin, B. and O'Connor, N. (1985). Logico-affective states and non-verbal language. In E. Schopler and G.B. Mesibov (Eds.), *Communication problems in autism* (pp. 283–301). New York: Plenum.

Hobson, R.P. (1993). *Autism and the development of mind.* Hillsdale, NJ: Erlbaum.

Horowitz, B., Rumsey, J.M., Gradey, C.L., and Rapoport, S.I. (1988). The cerebral metabolic landscape in autism: Intercorrelations of regional glucose utilation. *Archives of Neurology,* **45,** 749–755.

Huges, C.H. and Russell, J. (1993). Autistic children's difficulty with mental disengagement from an object: Its implications for theories of autism. *Developmental Psychology,* **29**, 498–510.

Jarrold, C., Boucher, J., and Smith, P. (1993). Symbolic play in autism: A review. *Journal of Autism and Pervasive Developmental Disorder,* **23**, 281–306.

Kanner, L. (1943). Autistic disturbance of affective contact. *Nervous Child,* **2**, 217–250.

Kazdin, A.E. (1994). Psychotherapy for children and adolescents. In A.E. Bergin and S.L. Garfield (Eds.), *Handbook of psychotherapy and behavior change* (pp. 543–594). New York: Wiley.

Koegel, R.L. and Koegel, L.K. (1987). Generalization issues in the treatment of autism. *Seminars in Speech and Language,* **8**, 241–256.

Koegel, R.L., O'Dell, M., and Koegel, L. (1987). A natural language teaching paradigm for nonverbal autistic children. *Journal of Autism and Developmental Disorders,* **17**, 187–200.

Krug, D.A., Arick, J., and Almond, P. (1980). Behavior checklist for identifying severely handicapped individuals with high levels of autistic behavior. *Journal of Child Psychology and Psychiatry,* **21**, 221–229.

Kusch, M. (1993). *Entwicklungspsychopathologie und Therapieplanung in der Kinderverhaltenstherapie.* Frankfurt: Peter Lang.

Kusch, M. and Petermann, F. (1991). *Entwicklung autistischer Störungen.* Bern: Huber.

Kusch, M. and Petermann, F. (1995). Tiefgreifende Entwicklungsstörungen. In F. Petermann (Ed.), *Lehrbuch der Klinischen Kinderpsychologie* (pp. 325–350). Göttingen: Hogrefe.

Le Couteur, A. *et al.* (1989). Autism diagnostic interview: A standardized investigator-based instrument. *Journal of Autism and Developmental Disorders,* **19**, 33–387.[1]

LeLord, G., Callaway, E., and Muh, J.P. (1982). Clinical and biological effects of high doses of vitamin B6 and magnesium on autistic children. *Acta Vitaminologica et Enzymologica,* **4**, 27–44.

Leslie, A.M. (1987). Pretense and representation: The origin of "theory of mind". *Psychological Review,* **94**, 412–426.

Leslie, A.M. and Thaiss, L. (1992). Domain specificity in conceptual development: Neuropsychological evidence from autism. *Cognition,* **43**, 225–251.

Loder, R.T., Lee, C.L., and Richards, B.S. (1989). Orthopedic aspects of Rett syndrome: A multicenter review. *Journal of Pediatric Orthopaedics,* **9**, 557–562.

Lord, C. (1984). Peer relation in autism. In F.J. Morrison, C. Lord, and D.P. Keating (Eds.), *Applied developmental psychology,* Vol. 1 (pp. 165–229). New York: Academic Press.

Lord, C. (1993). The complexity of social behavior in autism. In S. Baron-Cohen, U. Tager-Flusberg, and D.J. Cohen (Eds.), *Understanding other minds. Perspectives from autism* (pp. 292–316). Oxford: Oxford University Press.

Lord *et al.* (1989). Autism diagnostic observation schedule: A standardized observation of communicative and social behavior. *Journal of Autism and Developmental Disorders,* **19**, 185–212.

Lord, C. and Schopler, E. (1987). Neurobiological implications of sex differences in autism. In E. Schopler and G.B. Mesibov (Eds.), *Neurobiological issues in autism* (pp. 191–211). New York: Plenum Press.

Lovaas, O.I. and Smith, T. (1989). A comprehensive behavioral theory of autistic children: Paradigm for research and treatment. *Journal of Behavior Therapy and Experimental Psychiatry,* **20**, 17–29.

McDougel, C.J., Price, L.H., and Volkmar, F.R. (1994). Recent advances in the pharmacotherapy of autism and related conditions. *Child and Adolescent Psychiatric Clinics of North America,* **3**, 71–89.

McEnvoy, R.E., Rogers, S.J., and Pennington, B.F. (1993). Executive function and social communication deficits in young autistic children. *Journal of Child Psychology and Psychiatry,* **34**, 563–578.

Minshew, N.J., Dombrowsky, S.M., Panchalingam, K., and Pettegrew, J.W. (1993). A preliminary 31P MRS study of autism: Evidence for undersynthesis and increased degregation of brain membranes. *Society of Biological Psychiatry*, **33**, 762–773.

Mundy, P. and Hogan, A. (1994). Intersubjectivity, joint attention, and autistic developmental psychopathology. In D. Cicchetti and S.L. Toth (Eds.), *Disorders and dysfunctions of the self. Rochester symposium on developmental psychopathology* (pp. 1–30). New York: University of Rochester Press.

Mundy, P., Sigman, M., and Kasari, C. (1993). The theory of mind and joint-attention deficits in autism. In S. Baron-Cohen, U. Tager-Flusberg, and D.J. Cohen (Eds.), *Understanding other minds. Perspectives from autism* (pp. 181–203). Oxford: Oxford University Press.

Mundy, P.C., Sigman, M., Ungerer, J.A., and Sherman, T. (1986). Defining the social deficits of autism: The contribution of nonverbal-communication measures. *Journal of Child Psychology and Psychiatry*, **27**, 657–669.

Olsson, B. and Rett, A (1990). A review of the Rett syndrome with a theory of autism. *Brain Development*, **12**, 11–15.

Olsson, B. and Rett, A. (1985). Behavioral observations concerning differential diagnosis between the Rett syndrome and autism. *Brain development*, **7**, 281–289,

Ornitz, E.M. (1983). The functional neuroanatomy of infantile autism. *International Journal of Neuroscience*, **19**, 85–124.

Ornitz, E.M. (1987). Neurophysiological studies in infantile autism. In D.J. Cohen and A.M. Donnellan (Eds.), *Handbook of autism and pervasive developmental disorders* (pp. 148–165). New York: Wiley.

Ozonoff, S., Pennington, B.F., and Rogers, S.J. (1991). Executive function deficits in high-functioning autistic individuals: Relationship to theory of mind. *Journal of Child Psychology and Psychiatry*, **32**, 1081–1105.

Panksepp, J. and Sahley, T. (1987). Possible brain opioid involvement in disturbed social intent and language development of autism. In E. Schopler and G.B. Mesibov (Eds.), *Neurobiological Issues in Autism* (pp. 357–371). New York: Plenum.

Paul, R. (1987). Natural history. In D.J. Cohen and A.M. Donnellan (Eds.), *Handbook of autism and pervasive developmental disorders* (pp. 121–132). New York: Wiley.

Pauls, D. (1987). The familiarity of autism and related disorders: A review of the evidence. In D.J. Cohen and A.M. Donnellan (Eds.), *Handbook of autism and pervasive developmental disorders* (pp. 192–198). New York: Wiley.

Pennington, B.F. and Ozonoff, S. (1991). A neuroscientific perspective on continuity and discontinuity in developmental psychopathology. In D. Cicchetti and S.L. Toth (Eds.), *Rochester symposium on developmental psychopathology*, Vol. 3: models and integrations (pp. 117–160). Hillsdale, NJ: Erlbaum.

Perner, J., Frith, U., Leslie, A.M., and Leekmann, S.R. (1989). Exploration of the autistic child's theory of mind: Knowledge, belief and communication. *Child Development*, **60**, 689–700.

Philippart, M. (1990). The Rett syndrome in males. *Brain development*, **12**, 33–36.

Piven, J., Berthier, M.L., Starkstein, S.E., Nehme, E., Pearlson, G., and Folstein, S. (1990). Magnetic reasoning imaging evidence for a deficit of cerebral cortical development in autism. In S. Chase and M.E. Hertzig (Eds.), *Annual progress in child psychiatry and child development* (pp. 455–465). New York: Brunner/Mazel.

Pizza, C.C., Fisher, W., Kiesewetter, K. *et al.* (1990). Aberrant sleep patterns in children with the Rett syndrome. *Brain development*, **12**, 488–493.

Prizant, B. and Schuler, A. (1987). Facilitating communication: Theoretical foundations. In D.J. Cohen and A.M. Donnellan (Eds.), *Handbook of autism and pervasive developmental disorders* (pp. 289–300). New York: Wiley.

Prizant, B.M. and Wetherby, A.M. (1987). Communicative intent: A framework for understanding social-communicative behavior in autism. *Journal of the American Academy of Child Psychiatry*, **26**, 472–479.

Prizant, B. and Wetherby, A.M. (1988). Providing service to children with autism (0–2 years) and their families. *Topics in Language Disorders*, **9**, 1–13.

Rimland, B. (1987). Megavitamin B6 and magnesium in treatment of autistic children and adults. In E. Schopler and G.B. Mesibov (Eds.), *Neurobiological Issues in Autism* (pp. 357–375). New York: Plenum.

Rimland, B., Callaway, E., and Dreyfus, P. (1978). The effect of high doses of vitamin B6 on autistic children: A double-blind crossover study. *American Journal of Psychiatry*, **135**, 472–475.

Ritvo, E.R., Freeman, B.J., Mason-Brother, A., Mo, A., and Ritvo, A.M. (1985). Concordance for the syndrome of autism in 40 pairs of afflicted twins. *American Journal of Psychiatry*, **142**, 74–77.

Ritvo, E.R., Freeman, B.J., Scheibel, A.B., Doung, P.T., Robinson, H., and Guthrie, D. (1986). Decreased Purkinje cell density in four autistic patients: Initial findings of the UCLAN-NSAC Autopsy Research Project. *American Journal of Psychiatry*, **43**, 862–866.

Ritvo, E.R., Jorde, L.B., Mason-Brothers, A., Freeman, B.J. *et al.* (1989). The UCLA-University of Utah epidemiology survey of autism: Recurrence estimates and genetic counseling. *American Journal of Psychiatry*, **146**, 1032–1036.

Rogers, S.J. and Pennington, B.P. (1991). A theoretical approach to the deficits in infantile autism. *Development and Psychopathology*, **3**, 137–162.

Rubinstein, J.L., Lotspeich, L., and Ciaranello, R.D. (1993). The neurobiology of developmental disorders. In B.B. Lahey and A.E. Kazdin (Eds.), *Advances in clinical child psychology* (pp. 1–52), New York: Plenum.

Rutter, M. (1970). Autistic children: Infancy to adulthood. *Seminars in Psychiatry*, **2**, 435–450.

Rutter, M. (1986). Child psychiatry: Looking 30 years ahead. *Journal of Child Psychology and Psychiatry*, **27**, 803–840.

Rutter, M. and Garmezy, N. (1983). Developmental Psychopathology. In E.M. Hetherington (Ed.), *Handbook of child psychology*, Vol. 4 (pp. 775–911). New York: Wiley.

Rutter, M. and Mawhood, L. (1991). The long-term psychosocial sequelae of specific developmental disorders of speech and language. In M. Rutter and P. Casaer (Eds.), *Biological risk factors for psychosocial disorders* (pp. 233–259). Cambridge: Cambridge University Press.

Rutter, M. and Schopler, E. (1987). Autism and pervasive developmental disorders: Concepts and diagnostic issues. *Journal of Autism and Developmental Disorders*, **17**, 159–186.

Rutter, M. and Schopler, E. (1992). Classification of pervasive developmental disorders: Some concepts and practical considerations. *Journal of Autism and Developmental Disorders*, **22**, 459–182.

Rutter, M., Bailey, A., Bolton, P., and LaCouteur, A. (1994). Autism and known medical conditions. Myth and substance. *Journal of Child Psychology and Psychiatry*, **35**, 311–322.

Schopler, E. (1983). New developments in the definitions and diagnosis of autism. In: B.B. Lahey and A.E. Kazdin (Eds.), *Advances in Clinical Psychology*. New York: Plenum.

Schopler, E. (1987). Specific and non-specific factors in the effectiveness of a treatment system. *American Psychologist*, **42**, 376.

Schopler, E. (1994). A statewide program for the treatment and education of autistic and related communication handicapped children (Teacch). *Child and Adolescent Psychiatric Clinics of North America*, **3**, 91–103.

Schopler, E. and Mesibov, G.B. (Eds.) (1984). *The effects of autism on the family.* New York: Plenum.

Schopler, E. and Mesibov, G.B. (Eds.) (1985). *Communication problems in autism.* New York: Plenum.

Schopler, E. and Mesibov, G.B. (Eds.) (1987). *Neurobiological issues in autism.* New York: Plenum Press.

Schopler, E. and Mesibov, G.B. (Eds.) (1992). *High-functioning individuals with autism*: New York: Plenum Press.

Schopler, E. and Mesibov, G.B. (Eds.) (1994). *Behavioral issues in autism*. New York: Plenum Press.

Schopler, E., Mesibov, G.B., Shigley, H., and Bashford, A. (1984). Helping autistic children through their parents: The TEACCH model. In E. Schopler and G.B. Mesibov (Eds.), *The effects of autism on the family* (pp. 65–81). New York: Plenum Press.

Schopler, E., Reichler, R., Bashford, A. *et al.* (1990). Individualized assessment and treatment for autistic and developmentally disabled children. Vol. 1: *Psychoeducational profile revised*. Austin, TX: Pro-Ed.

Schopler, E., Reichler, R.J., and Renner, B.R. (1988). *The childhood autism rating scale (CARS; revised)*. Los Angeles: Western Psychological Services.

Sigman, M., Ungerer, J.A., Mundy, P., and Sherman, T. (1987). Cognition in autistic children. In D.J. Cohen and A.M. Donnellan (Eds.), *Handbook of autism and pervasive developmental disorders* (pp. 103–120). New York: Wiley.

Simeonson, R.J., Olley, J.G., and Rosenthal. S.L. (1987). Early intervention for children with autism. In M. Guralnick and F. Bennett (Eds.), *The effectiveness of early intervention for at-risk and handicapped children*. New York: Academic Press.

Steffenburg, S. (1991). Neuropsychiatry assessment of children with autism: A population-based study. *Developmental Medicine and Child Neurology*, **33**, 493–551.

Stone, W.L. and Caro-Martinez, L.M. (1990). Naturalistic observations of spontaneous communication in autistic children. *Journal of Autism and Developmental Disorders*, **20**, 437–453.

Szatmari, P. (1992). The validity of autistic spectrum disorders: A literature review. *Journal of Autism and Developmental Disorders*, **22**, 583–600.

Szatmari, P., and Jones, M.B. (1991). IQ and the genetics of autism. *Journal of Child Psychology and Psychiatry*, **32**, 897–908.

Szatmari, P., Bartoluci, G., and Bremner, R. (1989). Asperger's syndrome and autism: Comparisons on early history and outcome. *Journal of Developmental Medicine and Child Neurology*, **31**, 709–720.

Tantam, D. (1988). Asperger's syndrome. *Journal of Child Psychology and Psychiatry*, **29**, 245–255.

Trevarthen, S. and Aitken, K.J. (1994). Brain development, infant communication, and empathy disorders: Intrinsic factors in child mental health. *Development and Psychopathology*, **6**, 597–634.

Tsai, L. (1987). Pre-, peri-, and neonatal factors in autism. In E. Schopler and G. Mesibov (Eds.), *Neurobiological issues in autism* (pp. 180–191). New York: Plenum Press.

Tsai, L. (1992). Is Rett syndrome a subtype of pervasive developmental disorder? *Journal of Autism and Developmental Disorders*, **22**, 551–561.

Volkmar, F.R. (1992). Childhood disintegrative disorder: Issues for DSM-IV. *Journal of Autism and Developmental Disorders*, **22**, 625–642.

Volkmar, F.R. and Cohen, D.J. (1989). Comorbid association of autism and schizophrenia. *American Journal of Psychiatry*, **148**, 1705–1710.

Volkmar, F.R., Burack, J.A., and Cohen, D.J. (1990). Deviance and developmental approach in the study of autism. In R.M. Hodapp, J.A. Burack, and E. Zigler (Eds.), *Issues in the developmental approach to mental retardation* (pp. 246–270). Cambridge: Cambridge University Press.

Volkmar, F.R., Cicchetti, D.V., Cohen, D.J., and Bergman, J. (1992). Developmental aspects of DSM-III-R criteria for autism. *Journal of Autism and Developmental Disorders*, **22**, 657–662.

Volkmar, F.R., Cohen, D.J., Bergman, J.D., Hooks, M.Y., and Stevenson, J.M. (1989). An examination of social typologies in autism. *Journal of the American Academy of Child Psychiatry*, **28**, 82–86.

Waterhouse, L., Wing, L., Spitzer, R., and Siegal, B. (1992). Pervasive developmental disorders: From DSM-III to DSM-III-R. *Journal of Autism and Developmental Disorders*, **22**, 525–549.

Wetherby, A.M. (1986). Ontogeny of communicative functions in autism. *Journal of Autism and Developmental Disorders*, **16**, 295–316.

Wetherby, A. and Prizant, B. (1993). *Communication and Symbolic Behavior Scales — Normed Edition*. Chicago, IL: Riverside Publishing.

Wing, L. (1981). Language, social and cognitive impairments in autism and severe mental retardation. *Journal of Autism and Developmental Disorders*, **11**, 31–44.

Wing, L. (1993). The definition and prevalence of autism: A review. *European Journal of Adolescent Psychiatry*, **2**, 61–74.

Wing, L. and Attwood, A. (1987). Syndromes of autism and atypical development. In D.J. Cohen and A.M. Donnellan (Eds.), *Handbook of autism and pervasive developmental disorders* (pp. 3–19). New York: Wiley.

Wing, L. and Gould, J. (1979). Severe impairments of social interaction and associated abnormalities in children: Epidemiology and classification. *Journal of Autism and Developmental Disorders*, **9**, 11–30.

Witt-Engerström, I. and Gillberg, C. (1987). Rett syndrome in Sweden. *Journal of Autism and Developmental Disorders*, **17**, 149–150.

World Health Organization (1993). *International Classification of Diseases — tenth edition*. Geneva: WHO.

Yarbrough, E., Santa, U., Pret, I., Webster, C., and Lombardi. (1987). Effects of fenfluramine on autistic individuals residing in state developmental center. *Journal of Autism and Developmental Disorders*, **17**, 303–314.

Yirmiya, N. and Sigman, M. (1991). High functioning individuals with autism: Diagnosis, empirical findings, and theoretical issues. *Clinical Psychology Review*, **11**, 669–683.

Zahner, G.E.P. and Pauls, D.L. (1987). Epidemiological surveys of infantile autism. In D.J. Cohen and A.M. Donnellan (Eds.), *Handbook of autism and pervasive developmental disorders* (pp. 199–207). New York: Wiley.

CHAPTER 7
ANXIETY DISORDERS

Paul M.G. Emmelkamp
and Agnes Scholing

Childhood anxiety disorders have only recently received the attention they deserve. Until the 1980s most scholars viewed anxiety in childhood as normal and high levels of anxiety in adolescence were viewed as a result of the psychological challenges involved in the developmental process. The epidemiological findings available at that time were in line with the view of anxiety in adolescence being a transient phenomenon. Agras and colleagues (1972) reported that all individuals who had phobias in adolescence were found to be improved 5 years later. Since the introduction of the third edition of the Diagnostic and Statistical Manual of Mental Disorders (DSM-III, American Psychiatric Association; APA, 1980), which provided diagnostic guidelines for anxiety disorders in childhood and adolescence, a number of methodologically sound epidemiological studies have been conducted, demonstrating that anxiety disorders are much more prevalent than previously thought. As a result of these diagnostic guidelines, research is gradually appearing investigating characteristics of the various anxiety disorders. Research into the etiology of childhood anxiety disorders and into the effects of pharmacological and psychological treatment is still in an embryonic stage.

DEFINITION AND CLASSIFICATION

In the child and adolescent section of DSM-III-R (APA, 1987) the following disorders were distinguished: separation anxiety disorder, avoidant disorder, and overanxious disorder. Any diagnosis of the anxiety disorders of the adult section of the manual could also be applied to children or adolescents: panic disorder, social phobia, generalized anxiety disorder, simple phobia, obsessive-compulsive disorder and posttraumatic stress disorder.

In DSM-IV only separation anxiety disorder is contained in the child and adolescent section. In the adult section, social phobia now subsumes avoidant disorder of childhood, and the criteria have been changed to facilitate the classification in children. Generalized anxiety disorder now subsumes overanxious disorder of childhood. For compatibility with the tenth edition of the International Statistical Classification of Diseases, Inquiries and Causes of Death (ICD-10; World Health Organization; WHO, 1993) the term simple phobia was changed to specific phobia. Further, the threshold for panic disorder has been revised. In DSM-IV recurrent unexpected panic attacks accompanied by a month or more of persistent concern about having additional panic attacks are required for the diagnosis of panic disorder. The differences between DSM-III-R (APA, 1987) and DSM-IV (APA, 1994) are shown in Table 7.1.

Table 7.1 Classification of anxiety disorders in DSM-III-R and DSM-IV

DSM-III-R		*DSM-IV*	
Anxiety disorders in childhood		*Anxiety disorders in childhood*	
309.21	Separation anxiety disorder	309.21	Separation anxiety disorder
313.21	Avoidant disorder		
313.00	Overanxious disorder		
Anxiety disorders		*Anxiety disorders*	
300.01	Panic disorder without agoraphobia	300.01	Panic disorder without agoraphobia
300.21	Panic disorder with agoraphobia	300.21	Panic disorder with agoraphobia
300.22	Agoraphobia without history of panic disorder	300.22	Agoraphobia without history of panic disorder
300.29	Simple phobia	300.29	Specific phobia
300.23	Social phobia	300.23	Social phobia
300.30	Obsessive-compulsive disorder	300.3	Obsessive-compulsive disorder
309.81	Posttraumatic stress disorder	309.81	Posttraumatic stress disorder
		308.3	Acute stress disorder
300.02	Generalized anxiety disorder	300.02	Generalized anxiety disorder
		293.89	Anxiety disorder due to medical condition or substances
300.00	Anxiety disorder NOS	300.00	Anxiety disorder NOS

Since DSM-IV has been introduced only recently (APA, 1994), no research has yet been reported that has followed these diagnostic guidelines. Therefore, research reviewed in this chapter is based on DSM-III or DSM-III-R.

Avoidant Disorder

Avoidant disorder is characterized by excessive fearfulness and avoidance of social interactions with unfamiliar individuals. In contrast, avoidant disordered children appreciate the company of familiar people such as family members. Avoidant disorder tends to have an early onset and had a relatively equal gender distribution in one study (Last *et al.*, 1992), but was more common among girls in another (Francis *et al.*, 1992). In the latter study a remarkable degree of similarity between avoidant disorder and social phobia was found, thus offering support for the inclusion of avoidant disorder in social phobia in DSM-IV. Overanxious disorder was often a comorbid condition both in social phobia and in avoidant disorder (Francis *et al.*, 1992).

Separation Anxiety Disorder

A child with separation anxiety disorder demonstrates extreme worry and distress concerning separation from home or a major attachment figure (Table 7.2), usually (one of) the parent(s). The distress must last for more than four weeks and cause significant impairment in social, academic or other important areas of functioning before the diagnosis can be made. Homesickness is extremely common. A child with separation anxiety disorder is often reluctant to go to school. Such children may fear that their parents will die, often have difficulty in falling asleep, and a number of them have recurrent nightmares involving the theme of separation. Separation anxiety disorder is characterized by an early age of onset (7.5 years) and has an equal sex distribution (Last *et al.*, 1987; Last *et al.*, 1992; Keller *et al.*, 1992). As reported by Last *et al.* (1992), these children tend to come from a single parent home. In clinical samples separation anxiety disorder is more prevalent before puberty than in adolescence, but results of community studies are inconclusive. There are some differences in the symptomatology of younger and older children with separation anxiety disorder. In preadolescence, nightmares and fears about harm befalling attachment figures are quite prevalent, whereas in adolescents with separation anxiety disorder school refusal and somatic complaints dominate the picture (Clark *et al.*, 1994).

Table 7.2   Diagnostic criteria for separation anxiety disorder

A. Developmentally inappropriate and excessive anxiety concerning separation from home or from those to whom the individual is attached, as evidenced by three (or more) of the following:

1) Recurrent excessive distress when separation from home or major attachment figures occur or is anticipated

2) Persistent and excessive worry about losing, or about possible harm befalling, major attachment figures

3) Persistent and excessive worry that an untoward event will lead to separation from a major attachment figure (e.g., getting lost or being kidnapped)

4) Persistent reluctance or refusal to go to school or elsewhere because of fear of separation

5) Persistently and excessively fearful or reluctant to be alone or without major attachment figures at home or without significant adults in other settings

6) Persistent reluctance or refusal to go to sleep without being near a major attachment figure or to sleep away from home

7) Repeated nightmares involving the theme of separation

8) Repeated complaints of physical symptoms (such as headaches, stomachaches, nausea, or vomiting) when separation from major attachment figures occurs or is anticipated

B. The duration of the disturbance is at least 4 weeks.

C. The onset is before age 18 years.

D. The disturbance causes clinically significant distress or impairment in social, academic (occupational), or other important areas of functioning.

E. The disturbance does not occur exclusively during the course of a pervasive developmental disorder, schizophrenia, or other psychotic disorder and, in adolescents and adults, is not better accounted for by panic disorder with agoraphobia.

Specify if:

Early onset: if onset occurs before age 6 years.

Reprinted with permission from the Diagnostic and Statistical Manual of Mental Disorders, Fourth Edition. Copyright 1994 American Psychiatric Association.

Overanxious Disorder

Overanxious disordered children feel tense and are often unable to relax due to excessive worrying, for a period of at least 6 months, that is not triggered solely by an identifiable situation or psychosocial stressor. In contrast to separation anxiety and specific phobia the worry is generalized and not restricted to separation or a specific situation or object. The worry concerns primarily future event and about their competence in a number of areas (e.g., school, peer relationships, athletics). Some may worry about their behaviour in the past. Most of the children are extremely self-conscious and need continuing reassurance from parents and teachers. Children or adolescents who are overanxious often have multiple somatic complaints, such as stomachaches, dizziness, palpitations, and headaches. In DSM-IV this disorder is included in the generalized anxiety disorder. Now the excessive anxiety and worry must be present most of the time (occurring more days than not) and concern more than one situation. Further, the child needs to have hardly any control over the worry before the diagnosis can be applied; in children only one of six somatic symptoms is required (as compared with at least three in adults).

Overanxious disorder may start early in childhood (Last *et al.*, 1992: onset age 8.8 years). However, in other studies the onset of this disorder was somewhat later, being 10.5 years (Last *et al.*, 1987; Keller *et al.*, 1992) and 13.4 years (Last *et al.*, 1987). Comorbidity with other anxiety disorders is extremely high. There is some evidence that the content of the worries differs from childhood to adolescence; in older children the worries concern more past behaviour than in younger children (Kashani and Orvaschel, 1990; Strauss *et al.*, 1988). In the Last *et al.* (1992) study nearly all of the overanxious children had a lifetime history of at least one additional anxiety disorder, social phobia being the most common. This high comorbidity of social phobia in overanxious children corroborates previous findings (Last *et al.*, 1989; Last *et al.*, 1987). Overanxious children are often characterized by social isolation, shyness, and inadequate social skills (Strauss *et al.*, 1988). As noted before, in DSM-IV (APA, 1994) generalized anxiety subsumes overanxious disorder. However, given the specific clinical picture of overanxious disorder often involving social anxiety, we wonder whether this was a wise decision.

Obsessive-compulsive Disorder

Either recurrent obsessions or compulsions have to occur for a diagnosis of obsessive-compulsive disorder. Essential for the diagnosis is that the complaints cause marked distress, are time consuming (take more than one hour) and interfere with social relationships, school or work performance. Obsessions are repetitive, recurring thoughts, ideas, images or impulses that are experienced as intrusive. The child recognizes that the obsessions are the product of his or her own mind. Obsessions are experienced as senseless or repugnant. Compulsions are repetitive, excessive behaviours that are performed according to certain rules, or in a stereotyped fashion. Compulsions have the function of neutralizing or preventing discomfort and/or anxiety. The picture of obsessive-compulsive disorder in children is comparable to that in adults: Pure obsessions are rare, most children have multiple rituals, and washing is the most common compulsion. Other compulsions include grooming, checking, and doubting (Swedo *et al.*, 1989).

Obsessive-compulsive disorder in children starts usually between 10 and 14 years (Last and Strauss, 1989a; Swedo *et al.*, 1989). Results with respect to sex distribution are mixed: while some (Last and Strauss, 1989b; Swedo *et al.*, 1989) found obsessive-compulsive disorder to be more common among boys, this was not confirmed in a recent study (Last *et al.*, 1992). Simple phobia is the most common comorbid anxiety disorder (Last *et al.*, 1992; Swedo *et al.*, 1989), followed by overanxious disorder. In contrast with adults, where depression is a common comorbid diagnosis (Emmelkamp and Van Oppen, 1994) depression is less often diagnosed in obsessive-compulsive children. (Last and Strauss, 1989b; Last *et al.*, 1992)

Specific Phobia

The term specific phobia (in DSM-III-R simple phobia) refers to a broad scale of phobias associated with specific situations. According to the diagnostic criteria of DSM-IV, specific phobia should be diagnosed in the case of a persistent excessive or irrational fear of a circumscribed object or situation, which is avoided or endured with intense anxiety. The fear or the avoidance behaviour has to interfere significantly with the child's normal life. The fear-related stimulus of the specific phobia has to be different from stimuli associated with panic disorder/ agoraphobia or social phobia and unrelated to the content of the obsessions of obsessive-compulsive disorder or the trauma of acute or post-traumatic stress disorder. Common phobias in childhood are fear of darkness, school, dogs or other animals and insects, heights, and closed places (e.g., elevator or toilet).

According to a study conducted in a clinical setting, children with simple phobia had a mean age of onset of approximately 8 years (Last *et al.*, 1992; Strauss and Last, 1993). The mean onset age in specific phobias is related to the type of situation or object feared. The mean onset age for animal phobia is 7 years, for blood phobia 9 years, and for dental phobia 12 years (Öst, 1987).

Social Phobia

In DSM-IV, social phobia is described as a persistent fear of one òr more social or performance situations in which the child is exposed to possible scrutiny by others, and fears to behave in a way that will be humiliating and embarrassing. In children, there must be the capacity for age-appropriate social relationships with familiar people. Further, the anxiety must occur in social situations with other children, not just in interaction with adults. Children and adolescents with social phobia are usually very tense and anxious when confronted with the feared social situation and those situations will generally be avoided or endured only with intense anxiety, if avoidance is impossible. Typical situations feared by social phobic children are school, public speaking, blushing, crowds, eating, drinking or dressing in front of others (Strauss and Last, 1993).

The mean onset age of social phobia in adult samples is around 18 years (Emmelkamp *et al.*, 1992), indicating that social phobia usually starts in late adolescence. In child clinic samples, the mean onset of social phobia has been reported to be 11.3 years (Last *et al.*, 1992) and 12.3 years (Strauss and Last, 1993). In adolescence, fears of blushing and fears of being looked at peaked in girls on the average about two years earlier than in boys (Abe and Masui, 1981).

Panic Disorder

Panic disorder is characterized by recurrent unexpected panic attacks, during which the child experiences a number of somatic symptoms such as shortness of breath (dyspnea), dizziness or unsteady feelings, palpitations (tachycardia), trembling or shaking, sweating, choking, nausea or abdominal distress, depersonalization or derealization, paresthesias, (hot) flushes or chills, chest pain or discomfort, fear of dying, and fear of losing control. Many adult patients with panic disorder avoid situations or activities that trigger panic attacks (agoraphobia), but agoraphobia has been less well documented in children. In a paediatric primary care sample the prevalence of agoraphobia was found to be 1.2% among children of age 7–11 years (Costello *et al.*, 1989). Although agoraphobia may develop in adolescence, it usually starts later, the mean onset age being around 27 years (Emmelkamp *et al.*, 1992).

Although panic disorder does occur in childhood and adolescence, its prevalence is much lower than in adults. Only 9.6% of patients referred to a clinic specializing in the treatment of anxiety disorders received a primary diagnosis of panic disorder (Last and Strauss, 1989a; Last *et al.*, 1992). In adults who are referred for treatment of anxiety disorders, panic disorder is in most cases the primary diagnosis (Emmelkamp *et al.*, 1992). The mean age of onset in adolescents ranged from 14.1 years (Last *et al.*, 1992) to 15.6 years (Last and Strauss, 1989a), indicating that this disorder hardly occurs in early childhood. Panic symptoms occurring before adolescence are usually associated with another anxiety disorder rather than a panic disorder.

Generalized Anxiety Disorder

Generalized anxiety disorder is defined by excessive, unrealistic, and persistent anxiety and worry about two or more life circumstances and has to last for at least 6 months. In addition one somatic symptom is required, reflecting vigilance, scanning, motor tension or autonomic hyperactivity. In DSM-IV, the childhood equivalent of generalized anxiety, *overanxious disorder*, is included in generalized anxiety disorder. In a clinic-referred sample of anxious children, aged 5 to 18, no case of generalized anxiety was found.

Posttraumatic Stress Disorder

In posttraumatic stress disorder the child experienced or was confronted with a serious threatening event which resulted in intense fear, helplessness or horror, which in children may be expressed by disorganized or agitated behaviour. The DSM-IV criteria include re-experience of the traumatic event, which in children may be expressed in repetitive play in which (parts of) the trauma is expressed, in re-enactment behaviour, or in frightening dreams without recognizable content. Further, the child may show avoidance of stimuli related to the trauma, numbing of general responsivity (e.g., diminished interest in activities and feelings of detachment) and increased arousal. If these symptoms disappear within four weeks the diagnosis is acute stress disorder rather than posttraumatic stress disorder. In DSM-IV, symptoms of acute stress disorder are experienced during or immediately after the trauma, last for at least two days and are either resolved within four weeks after the traumatic event or the diagnosis is changed, usually to posttraumatic stress disorder.

Hardly any research has been conducted into posttraumatic stress disorder in children. The few studies that are available suggest that the symptoms of children are different from those of adults, as has been acknowledged by the DSM-IV criteria. Most notable in children are the lack of amnesia, flashbacks and numbing (Lyons, 1987; Terr, 1983). Sexual abuse may lead to posttraumatic stress disorder in a substantial number of victims (McLeer *et al.*, 1988), being abused by the biological father leading to the highest risk. Of children abused by their biological father 75% met DSM-III-R criteria for posttraumatic stress disorder.

Other Phobia and Anxiety

School Phobia. Although school phobia is not a separate category in DSM-IV, it deserves some discussion, given the diagnostic complexity of school avoidance. School refusal has to be distinguished from truancy. In the latter case the child attempts to conceal not going to school from the parents. The prevalence of school phobia has been estimated at about 1% in children from the normal community (de Aldaz *et al.*, 1987). In DSM-IV school phobia is mentioned as a possible manifestation of separation anxiety disorder. In a study (Berg *et al.*, 1993) among children of age 14 and 15 who attended school less than 40% of the time, 8% was found to have a separation anxiety disorder. In three studies (Berg *et al.*, 1993; Bernstein, 1991; Bools *et al.*, 1990) about half of the school refusers had an anxiety disorder, separation anxiety disorder being the most common. In a study by Last (1991) of clinic-referred anxious children, school refusal was more common among youngsters with somatic anxiety symptoms than among youngsters with non-somatic anxiety.

Test Anxiety. Although test anxiety may be related to social phobia, given the fact that fear of evaluation is central in both conditions, a number of clinicians and researchers consider it a separate category. Test anxiety is a common disorder in children. In a study of Beidel and Turner (1988) 60% of test-anxious children received a diagnosis of an anxiety disorder. Beidel *et al.* (1991) found that about half of the children with test anxiety fulfilled the criteria for an anxiety disorder. Taken the results of these studies together most children met the criteria for social phobia, followed by overanxious disorder and simple phobia. Children with test anxiety reported significantly more somatic complaints than normal controls, children with test anxiety plus social phobia having most symptoms. The results of the studies of Beidel and colleagues (1991) suggest that test anxiety is not a simple fear but a manifestation of a more pervasive anxiety state. Children with test anxiety not only worry about their performance on academic tasks, but the worrying is much more pervasive, including their appearance and performance in social situations and their own health and the health of family members. In comparison with non-test anxious children, test-anxious children engaged more in solitary activities and scored higher on trait anxiety (Beidel and Turner, 1988). In a study of Turner *et al.* (1991) test-anxious children did not show physiological habituation to repeated presentations of both fearful (picture of snake) and novel neutral stimuli (tone), whereas normal children adapted to these stimuli.

EPIDEMIOLOGY

Anxieties and fears are very common in children, but a number of these fears wax and wane and are associated with different developmental phases. Many young children go through phases of fearing hard noises, strangers, the dark and animals, but most of these fears dissipate without any intervention (Emmelkamp, 1982). In this section the epidemiological studies with respect to the prevalence of anxiety disorders will be reviewed for clinical and community samples.

Clinical Samples

In a clinic sample of 188 anxiety disordered children and adolescents in Pittsburgh (Last *et al.*, 1992) separation anxiety disorder was the most common reason for referral (27%), followed by simple phobia (20%), social phobia (15%) and overanxious disorder (13%). Panic disorder (10%) and obsessive-compulsive disorder (7%) were less common and posttraumatic stress disorder (3%) and avoidant disorder (3%) were relatively rare. Generalized anxiety disorder was never given as a primary diagnosis. Many children received one or more additional anxiety disorder diagnoses, separation anxiety disorder, simple phobia, social phobia and overanxious disorder being the most common. In previous studies, obsessive-compulsive disorder and panic disorder were also less common among anxious children referred for treatment (Last and Strauss, 1989a; 1989b).

Although a number of studies using clinical samples have produced figures about the relative prevalence of anxiety disorders, it is not possible to generalize from these clinical studies to the normal population, since referral may be influenced by other factors than having a disorder *per se*, for example, the impairment associated with the disorder and comorbidity with other (anxiety) disorders.

Community Studies

Studies using diagnostic interviews with parents, children, or both found DSM-III anxiety disorders ranging from 8% to as high as 26% (Bell-Dolan *et al.*, 1990; Brandenburg *et al.*, 1990). This broad range is due to the different measures used and the source (parent versus child). Furthermore, not all studies investigated the prevalence of all anxiety disorders.

Earlier studies that investigated the prevalence of anxiety in childhood were reviewed by Weissman (1988). Anxiety symptoms tended to decline with age. In these studies the prevalence of fears and worries ranged from 4 to 43%. Since then a number of studies have reported the prevalence of DSM-III anxiety disorders in childhood. In most studies simple phobia was the most common disorder (Anderson *et al.*, 1987; Benjamin *et al.*, 1990; Costello *et al.*, 1989). Based on these studies the mean prevalence for simple phobia is 6.1%, for separation anxiety disorder 3.9%, for overanxious disorder 3.2% and for social phobia 1.0%. Figures on the prevalence of avoidant disorder were not presented or were rather low (e.g., 1.6%; Costello *et al.*, 1989).

A number of community studies have been reported investigating the prevalence of anxiety disorders in adolescence. These studies include community studies from the USA (Kashani and Orvaschel, 1988, 1990; Whitaker *et al.*, 1990), Canada (Bergeron *et al.*, 1992) and New Zealand (Ferguson *et al.*, 1993; McGee *et al.*, 1990). One major problem is that in these various studies not all anxiety disorders have been assessed and that the disorders which were assessed varied from study to study. Based on these studies overanxious disorder/generalized anxiety disorder (mean prevalence 7.6%) is the most common disorder in the normal adolescent population, followed by simple phobia (mean prevalence 5.3%), separation anxiety disorder (mean prevalence 3.6%) and social phobia (mean prevalence 1.4%). Few studies investigated the prevalence of panic disorder and obsessive-compulsive disorder and when assessed these disorders were found to be rare (Whitaker *et al.*, 1990).

Anxiety disorders were found to be more prevalent in females than in males (e.g., Benjamin *et al.*, 1990; Kashani *et al.*, 1989; Weissman, 1988).

RISK FACTORS

Few studies have investigated risk factors associated with anxiety disorders in childhood (Benjamin *et al.*, 1990; Werry *et al.*, 1987). Summarizing the results of studies so far, it appears that anxious children come from normal homes, have a normal intellectual and motor development, but have more mental illness in the family than normal children. In a community study among nearly 800 children, lower socioeconomic status was found to be associated with separation anxiety disorder (Velez *et al.*, 1989). A number of other risk factors that are of potential interest will be discussed in some detail, including behavioural inhibition, parental anxiety and mood disorders, parental rearing practices and attachment and genetic factors.

Biological Factors

Behavioural Inhibition

"Behavioural inhibition to the unfamiliar" (Kagan, 1989) is a temperamental construct that refers to the tendency of toddlers and preschool children to be shy and withdrawn in unfamiliar situations. A number of children remain inhibited over the years. Children who remained inhibited up to 7.5 years showed more physiological arousal than uninhibited children (Kagan, 1989). Since behavioural inhibition bears some similarity to the social discomfort associated with avoidant disorder and social phobia, behavioural inhibition may be related to the development of anxiety in childhood. Children that had been characterized as behaviourally inhibited at about age 2 had higher rates of phobic disorders than uninhibited children (Biederman *et al.*, 1990; Biederman *et al.*, 1992). However, in a study of Hirshfeld *et al.* (1992) it was revealed that nearly all cases of anxiety disorders were found in children who remained inhibited up to 7.5 years. Such "stable" behavioural inhibition was also associated with continuing anxiety disorders in parents, that is both childhood anxiety disorder and adult anxiety disorder (see below). Whether behavioural inhibition is controlled by genetic factors or by environmental factors is yet unclear.

Family Studies: Parental Anxiety and Mood Disorders

Clearly there are familial influences on fears during childhood. Positive correlations have been found routinely between the fears of children and their mothers (Barrios and Hartman, 1987). The influence of mothers' and siblings' fears on the fear of children is probably greater among younger than among older children (McGlynn and McNeil, 1990). Further, there is considerable evidence that parents of children with anxiety disorders manifest anxiety disorders themselves. We will restrict the discussion here to studies that directly assessed the children of anxious parents.

Crowe and colleagues (1983) found a morbidity risk for panic disorder among the first degree relatives of patients with an anxiety disorder of 17.3% compared to 1.8% for controls. Turner *et al.* (1987) found an increased risk of anxiety disorders in children from anxious parents: twice as high as children of dysthymics and seven times as high as children of normal parents. Last *et al.* (1991) found an increased risk of anxiety disorders in the first degree relatives of children with anxiety disorders. In a study of Mufson *et al.* (1992), an increased risk was found of anxiety disorder and depression in children of parents with panic disorder and major depression. There was some evidence for specificity of transmission in that the risk for both major depression and anxiety disorder associated with having a parent with major depression and panic disorder was higher than the risk associated with having a parent with major depression only. A shortcoming of this study is that parents with panic disorder without depression and their children were not investigated.

In a study on clinic-referred anxious children with panic disorder, Last and Strauss (1989a) found a rate of 33% for panic disorder in the mother. Last *et al.* (1987) examined the prevalence of childhood anxiety disorders in the mothers of children with overanxious and separation anxiety disorders. Results of this study suggested that there was no specific relationship in separation anxiety, but there was a specific relationship in overanxious disorder. Mothers of children with separation anxiety disorder reported no separation anxiety in their own childhood. In contrast, 42% of mothers of children with overanxious disorder had suffered from overanxious disorder themselves at childhood.

A number of studies investigated whether the parents of obsessive-compulsive children had an obsessive-compulsive disorder themselves. As reviewed by Last and Strauss (1989b) the prevalence of obsessive-compulsive disorder in the parents is not particularly striking. Studies in a non-clinical sample of behaviourally inhibited children is also of interest. Rosenbaum *et al.* (1991) and Hirschfeld *et al.* (1992) found that parents of children who were inhibited at 21 months had increased risk for both childhood anxiety disorders and adult anxiety disorders compared with parents of uninhibited children.

The results of these studies suggest that some familial factors may be involved in the transmission of anxiety. How the anxiety is transmitted and whether this familial factor is environmental, biological, or a combination of these factors is still not clear.

Twin Studies: Genetic Factors

As discussed above, there is some evidence that anxiety disorders are familial, although there is less evidence for a specific transmission of a particular anxiety disorder from parent to child. While it is tempting to assume that a genetic basis is involved, the results from the studies discussed above are far from conclusive. There is, however, some evidence for a genetic factor in anxiety disorders provided by studies on monozygotic and dizygotic twins. Research among twins provide some insight into the possible role of a genetic factor, as both monozygotic and dizygotic twins growing up in the same family are exposed to more or less the same environmental influences, while the genetic material of only monozygotic twins is identical. In a study by Torgersen (1979) the concordances of blood-injury phobias and animal phobias were higher among monozygotic than among dizygotic twins. Skre *et al.* (1993), however, found similar prevalence of specific phobia in monozygotic and dizygotic twins. As for agoraphobia and panic disorder, a significantly higher concordance rate has been found in monozygotic than in dizygotic twins (Skre *et al.*, 1993; Torgersen, 1983). Torgersen (1988) garnered some support in twin studies for a genetic contribution to social fears in normals. Skre *et al.* (1993) found no evidence for a genetic contribution in social phobia. In obsessive-compulsive disorder the concordance for obsessions and compulsions was higher in monozygotic than in dizygotic twins (Torgersen, 1988), but results are still inconclusive (Skre *et al.*, 1993). Especially patients with both major depression and panic seem to display a strong evidence of a genetic etiology (Torgersen, 1990). Earlier studies found no evidence of a genetic component in generalized anxiety disorder (Torgersen, 1983, 1986), but in more recent studies there was a slightly higher prevalence of generalized anxiety disorder in co-twins of monozygotic than dizygotic twins

(Andrews *et al.*, 1990; Kendler *et al.*, 1992; Skre *et al.*, 1993). Research among twins has not been reported with respect to the specific anxiety disorders in childhood: separation anxiety, overanxious and avoidant disorders. In the Torgersen studies reviewed above, the overall concordance rate was twice as high for monozygotic (34%) than for dizygotic twins (17%) which is in support of an interaction between environmental and genetic contributions. However, the variance explained by this genetic factor is generally small.

Recently, a study (Boomsma and Verhulst, 1995) was published among normal twins of three years old, using the Child Behavior Checklist (CBCL, Achenbach and Edelbrock, 1983), rated by the parents. The correlation between monozygotic twins on the anxiety scale was .69, whereas the correlation between dizygotic twins was only .36. Subsequent analyses revealed that 72% of the variance was explained by genetic factors, whereas only 28% was explained by environmental factors. Although this study is clearly in support of a genetic contribution to anxiety in early childhood, there are some problems in the interpretation of these data. First, the behaviour of the twins was rated by their parents, who of course were not blind with respect to the specific twin status, which may have confounded the results. If parents believe that monozygotic twins are more similar than dizygotic twins, as most parents probably do, this may have influenced their rating. Second, a large genetic contribution at an early age does not rule out the possibility that environmental factors may become more influential later on in the developmental process. Further, while this study shows a clear genetic contribution on anxiety as rated on the CBCL, this does not necessarily imply a relationship between genetic factors and the development of subsequent anxiety disorders in childhood or adolescence.

On the basis of the knowledge available now, it is best to conclude that genetic factors may provide a risk factor which makes individuals vulnerable to the development of an anxiety disorder.

Familial and Psychological Factors

Parental Rearing Practices

Parental rearing factors have often been held responsible for the development of anxiety disorders. A number of studies have found an association between specific parental rearing characteristics and anxiety disorders. In a recent meta-analysis of studies that investigated this issue, Gerlsma *et al.* (1991) concluded that anxiety disorders were associated with parental overprotection and control as compared to healthy controls. Most of this research has been conducted on adult anxious patients who retrospectively recalled parental rearing characteristics. Nevertheless, the results of these studies suggest that parental rearing practices may be related to the development of anxiety disorders. These findings may be related to the attachment theory of Bowlby (1973). According to Bowlby, anxiety disorders are the result of prolonged and frequent separations during childhood or the threat of an impending separation. Bowlby's theory has led to considerable research. Ainsworth (1984), for instance, pointed out that safely attached children react differently from anxiously attached children when their mothers leave them behind in a strange room. Safely attached children demonstrate explorative behaviour when their mother is present; as soon as their mother leaves they become tense and when she returns they seek contact and approach. Anxiously attached children, on the other hand, demonstrate some explorative behaviour before, during and after separation from their mother, but often appear to avoid contact when she comes back. It can be assumed that a child uses the adult to whom it is attached as a safe base from which it can explore the world. If this safety figure is no longer present, separation anxiety arises; consequently, attachment behaviour is evoked and explorative behaviour is reduced. Bowlby holds that there is a striking similarity between school phobia in children and agoraphobia in adults. In his view the fear of leaving home is involved in both cases and both can be regarded as examples of separation anxiety. Research that has investigated the relationship between school phobia in childhood and later agoraphobia is inconclusive (Casat, 1988). As yet, no study has been reported that investigated attachment problems in early childhood and the development of anxiety disorders in childhood or adolescence.

Learning Theories

In the last decades several studies have been conducted on the acquisition of fear, most of them on adult patients with anxiety disorders. A major problem in studies on these subjects is that they are based on retrospective data; when patients are asked to remember how and in what situation their fears began, their answers are likely to be biased by memory distortions. In that respect, it is surprising that so little research is conducted on the development of fear in children. Future studies will have to demonstrate whether the results of the studies discussed below do generalize to children.

The two-stage theory (Mowrer, 1947, 1960) of fear acquisition has been highly influential and despite some serious criticisms (e.g., Mineka, 1979), it still plays a prominent role in current thinking on the development of phobias. Mowrer distinguished between classical conditioning, responsible for the acquisition of fear and operant conditioning or instrumental learning, responsible for the acquisition of the avoidance response. Since that time several criticisms, amplifications and modifications have been proposed. Given the aim of this chapter only a brief review will be given; for more details the reader is referred to Emmelkamp and Scholing (1994) and Menzies and Clarke (1995).

The classical conditioning paradigm states that neutral stimuli, once associated with fear or pain, elicit fear reactions and that the strength of the fear is determined by (i) the number of repetitions of the association between the stimuli and the emotional reactions and (ii) the intensity of the emotion experienced. Central to the model are one or more traumatic experiences in which the association between stimulus and fear reaction is learned.

Some experiments showed that a phobia can be acquired by means of classical conditioning. One of the most famous was conducted by Watson and Rayner (1920), who succeeded in changing a healthy one year old baby (Albert) into a phobic child through classical conditioning. Albert, who was afraid of nothing except of loud noises (which is normal at that age), was allowed to play with a laboratory rat. Initially, he showed no fear at all. A dramatic change took place when a loud noise was produced at the moment Albert approached the rat. After this had happened seven times, Albert became anxious by only seeing the rat without hearing the noise, which they interpreted as a classically conditioned fear reaction (although Delprato and McGlynn in 1984 correctly pointed at the fact that an instrumental contingency existed between Albert's behaviour and the presentation of the noise).

It must be noted, however, that several researchers have tried to replicate this study in other children, but mostly failed (e.g., Bregman, 1934; English, 1929). Moreover, studies on the impact of traumatic experiences showed that such events *per se* are not sufficient for the development of a phobia and many phobic patients do not recall traumatic experiences. In view of these problems with the two-stage-theory Rachman (1991) introduced the "three pathways to fear". In this notion it is posed that fear can be acquired in three ways: (i) by own experiences in the feared situations, (ii) through imitation of others (referred to as "vicarious learning") and (iii) by transmission of information.

Indirect evidence in favour of a vicarious learning interpretation for the acquisition of phobias came from studies demonstrating that children often share the fears of their parents. Particularly mothers (or presumably the children's most significant caretaker) may be an important etiological factor in children's fear (Emmelkamp, 1982). On the other hand, it should be noted that a relationship between fears of mother and child can also be the result of processes other than vicarious learning; for example, informational processes, genetic influences, or similar traumatic experiences. Other indirect evidence in favour of the vicarious transmission of fear came from retrospective patient reports (e.g., Kipper, 1977).

That fears can be acquired through modeling was demonstrated by Mineka and colleagues. For example, laboratory reared monkeys who initially were not fearful of snakes, developed a snake phobia as a result of observing wild monkeys displaying fear in the presence of a snake (Cook and Mineka, 1991). Other studies yielded unequivocal results (e.g., Rimm *et al.*, 1977; Murray and Foote, 1979; Öst and Hugdahl, 1981, 1985). Results of a study by Merkelbach *et al.* (1989) suggested that in most phobic patients both conditioning factors and vicarious learning are involved.

The assumption of the two-stage theory that avoidance is mediated by fear is neither supported by everyday experiences nor by experimental results. There is ample evidence that avoidance behaviour can be acquired and maintained in the absence of fear as a mediating factor (Gray, 1975). If the first stage of the theory is correct, it would be expected that rapid extinction of fear, and hence of avoidance behaviour, should occur when the UCS is no longer present. However, there is abundant evidence that avoidance behaviour, when established, is highly resistant to extinction.

Some behaviourists (e.g., Hekmat, 1987) hold that phobias are not acquired exclusively through a first-order conditioning process. In their view phobic reactions are not only acquired through aversive classical conditioning but may also be acquired by higher-order semantic conditioning processes. Thus, language conditioning is assigned an important role in the development of human fear reactions. In this view, a snake phobia does not necessarily develop through classical conditioning or vicarious learning but "The word 'snake' by virtue of being semantically accrued to negatively valued words such as 'ugly, poison, disgusting, slimy, etc.' may have indirectly acquired negative reactions through higher-order semantic conditioning" (Hekmat, 1987, p. 201).

Other authors have attempted to amplify the conditioning hypotheses with recent insights into cognitive theories (Martin and Levey, 1983; Baeyens *et al.*, 1992; Davey, 1992; Menzies and Clarke, 1995). Levey and Martin (1983) distinguished between two ways of learning, the first being a relatively immediate registration of stimuli associated with (positive or negative) events, the second being a more cognitive process, in which experiences of the past are summarized and repeated. Baeyens *et al.* (1992) described signal learning versus evaluative learning, the second being conceived as a kind of referential learning in which the CS activates a (cognitive) UCS-representation. Davey (1992) proposed a model of human conditioning, in which outcome expectancy, expectancy evaluation, cognitive representations of the UCS and revaluation processes play a major role.

The last construct to be mentioned here is preparedness. Some experiments showed that the nature of a conditioned stimulus is of paramount importance for conditioning of fear to occur: fear is much more easily conditioned to animals and furry objects than to wooden objects, shapes, and clothes (e.g., Bregman, 1934; English, 1929). This finding suggests that there might be an innate base for some fear development. According to Seligman (1971) the majority of clinical phobias concern objects of natural importance to the survival of the species. In his view evolution has preprogrammed the human species to easily acquire phobias of potentially dangerous situations. Such "prepared" learning is selective, highly resistant to extinction, probably non-cognitive, and can be acquired in one trail. This theory was partially supported in experiments by Öhman (1988) and Mineka (1987), although the results of studies by Merkelbach (1989) did not corroborate these findings.

Summarizing the results, development of fear seems to be determined by a combination of conditioning processes and other factors, for example neuroticism (Eysenck and Rachman, 1965; Lautch, 1971) or expectations (DiNardo *et al.*, 1988), interpretations (Rachman, 1991) and, more generally spoken, cognitive representations of the feared stimulus (Davey, 1992).

We finish this section with discussing studies that were concentrated on fear acquisition in childhood. For specific phobias, in various studies corresponding ages of onset are found, at least for animal phobias. According to some authors this suggests that children of ages eight to ten are more sensitive to such fears than older children. A minor traumatic experience at this stage could be sufficient for developing an animal phobia. In toddlers there are hardly any sex differences relating to animal phobias, whereas the animal phobias that develop later in life occur predominantly in women. Persons at an older age suffering from an animal phobia are more often able to recall traumatic experiences. Both findings advocate the hypothesis that a late-onset phobia differs from a childhood-onset phobia. On the other hand, however, it may well be that traumatic experiences are better remembered at an older age.

McNally and Steketee (1985) reported data on the etiology of severe animal phobias. All patients (22 adults) stated that the phobia had begun in early childhood and had remained stable or worsened with age. The majority of the patients (77%) could not remember the onset of the phobia, the others attributed it to conditioning events (frightening encounters, but no pain). In a study by DiNardo *et al.* (1988) on fear of dogs, conditioning events during childhood were reported by 56% of the fearful subjects and 66% of non-fearful subjects. Interestingly, all fearful subjects believed that fear and physical harm were likely consequences of confrontation with a dog, while few non-fearful subjects had such expectations. Summarising the results of these and other studies (e.g., Hekmat, 1987) no evidence was found for etiological significance of painful or frightening experiences because they were equally common among non-fearful subjects. Exaggerated expectation of harm, a cognitive factor, may play a role in the maintenance of the fear.

Lautch (1971) found that patients with a dental phobia (n = 34) reported having had a traumatic dental experience on at least one occasion in childhood. However, all patients were diagnosed as generally neurotic, whereas 10 control subjects with comparable traumatic experiences showed little sign of dental fear. Milgrom *et al.* (1995) found that dental fear in children was influenced both by direct conditioning experiences and modelling from the parents (especially the mother). Among 50 children with a fear of water only one mother could remember her child having had a traumatic experience involving water (Menzies and Clarke, 1993). Ollendick and King (1991) obtained data from 556 female and 536 male Australian and American children and adolescents. The majority attributed onset of their fears to vicarious and instructional factors, although these indirect sources of fear were often combined with direct conditioning experiences. The findings suggested that the three pathways to fear are interactive rather than independent. In sum, although the results suggest that conditioning processes play a significant role in the onset of some simple phobias, it is more and more recognized that other factors seem to be important as well.

Although the age of onset of social phobia generally begin at an early adolescence (Marks and Gelder, 1966; Öst, 1987), it has been suggested that factors predisposing such fears originate from early socialization processes. In Windheuser's study (1977), the similarity between phobias of children and those of their mothers applied especially for social phobics. Bruch *et al.* (1989) also reported that parents of social phobics themselves avoided several social situations, which could be explained in terms of vicarious learning.

Life Events

In most studies, children with anxiety disorders reported more life events compared to those without anxiety disorders. The most common life events were: an increased number of arguments with parents, trouble with a brother or a sister or classmates, receiving failing grades, losing a friend and breaking up with a boyfriend or girlfriend (Bernstein *et al.*, 1989; see Essau and Petermann, 1995 for review). Among those with panic disorder, the first panic attacks were often preceded by life events in form of interpersonal conflict, loss-related events such as parent separation or divorce, problems with grades, and family or peer conflict (Bradley and Hood, 1993; Macaulay and Kleinknecht, 1988; Warren and Zgourides, 1988).

COMORBIDITY

Anxiety Disorders

In a study (Benjamin *et al.*, 1990) among children aged 7–11 years from a normal population, 2.6% fulfilled criteria for two or more anxiety disorders. However, in clinical samples the comorbidity among anxiety disorders is much higher. In the Pittsburgh clinic sample of 188 anxiety disordered children and adolescents (Last *et al.*, 1992) many children received one or more additional anxiety disorder diagnoses, with separation anxiety disorder, simple phobia, social phobia and overanxious disorder being the most common. There is a high co-occurrence of avoidant disorder, social phobia and overanxious disorder (Francis *et al.*, 1992; Last *et al.*, 1987, 1992; Strauss and Last, 1993). The substantial comorbidity between avoidant disorder and social phobia suggests that these are no separate disorders and justifies the changes in DSM-IV, where social phobia now subsumes avoidant disorder of childhood.

Behavioural Disorder

A controversial issue is the relationship between anxiety disorders and conduct disorders. In a number of studies high rates of co-occurrence of anxiety disorders and conduct disorders have been found (e.g., Benjamin *et al.*, 1990; Bird *et al.*, 1993; Brandenburg *et al.*, 1990; Woolston *et al.*, 1989; Zoccolillo, 1992). There is some evidence that anxiety disorders occur more commonly than expected in children and adolescents with conduct disorder. In the Benjamin *et al.*'s study (1990), behavioural disorders (conduct disorder, oppositional disorder, and attention deficit disorder) were twice as common among children with an anxiety disorder as in youngsters without an anxiety disorder. Since this conclusion is based on general population studies, it is unaffected by referral biases.

Depression

Depression is often a comorbid condition in children and adolescents with a primary diagnosis of an anxiety disorder. Studies that investigated this issue have found the comorbidity of depression and anxiety disorders in childhood and adolescence to range from 50 to 72% (reviewed by Woolston *et al.*, 1989). In a community study (Benjamin *et al.*, 1990) the risk of depression was over six times as high in children with anxiety disorders as in children without. In the study by Last *et al.* (1992) nearly half of the social phobic children and adolescents had a lifetime history of major depression.

Depression is also often diagnosed in children with overanxious disorder. In a study by Last *et al.* (1987) one third of the children with overanxious disorder received an additional diagnosis of major depression. Brent *et al.* (1986) found increased suicidal ideation among overanxious children. In panic disorder children and in children with obsessive-compulsive disorder few children received an additional diagnosis of depression (Last and Strauss, 1989a, 1989b; Swedo *et al.*, 1989), which is in contrast with the much higher prevalence of depression in adults with panic disorder and obsessive-compulsive disorder (Emmelkamp and Van Oppen, 1994). Major depression is also rare in children with simple phobia and social phobia (Strauss and Last, 1993). In school phobic children who were diagnosed as suffering from an anxiety disorder, nearly half of the children had a comorbid depressive disorder (Bernstein, 1991).

Kovacs *et al.* (1989) studied the comorbidity with and risk for anxiety disorders in depressed children. They found that the anxiety disorder preceded the depression in most cases. In a substantial number of cases when the depression remitted, the anxiety disorder persisted. In the study by Last *et al.* (1992) in three-quarters of the social phobic children and adolescents the onset of the social phobia preceded the onset of the major depression.

COURSE AND OUTCOME

Course

Few studies are available that provide insight in the course of anxiety disorders in childhood. In Germany, Laucht and Schmidt (1987) found that three-quarters of the children with emotional and neurotic problems at age 8 still had problems 5 years later. However, 91% of children with conduct disorder at age 8 had still problems 5 year later. Other studies suggest that subclinical phobic fears remit with the passage of time (Emmelkamp, 1982; Morris and Kratochwill, 1983). There is no evidence, however, that the same is true for the more serious clinical childhood anxiety disorders. In a study by Keller *et al.* (1992) a protracted course of childhood anxiety disorders was found among children of parents with an affective disorder: in nearly half of the children the anxiety disorder lasted at least 8 years, indicating that anxious disorders in childhood may be more chronic than once believed.

It has been suggested that separation anxiety disorder in childhood or adolescence may result in panic disorder with agoraphobia in later life, but results of studies that investigated this issue are inconclusive (Casat, 1988; Thyrer, 1993). In adolescents with panic disorder there was only a small relationship with separation anxiety disorder in childhood: only 12% of the adolescents with panic disorder had had separation anxiety disorder in childhood (Last *et al.*, 1992).

Psychosocial Impairment

In an epidemiological study by Benjamin *et al.* (1990), the psychosocial impairment of children with anxiety disorders was compared with the impairment of children with behavioural disorders only and normal children. Parents of anxious children did not judge their children as more impaired than parents of normal children in social functioning, level of social activities and performance at school. In contrast, teachers found the anxious children to be markedly more impaired than normal children and equally as impaired as the children with behavioural disorders.

Clinicians, on the other hand, rated the anxious children as more impaired than the normal children, but as less impaired than the children with behavioural problems. In contrast, McGee *et al.* (1990) found no relationship between anxiety disorders and social functioning. An important difference between the Benjamin *et al.* (1990) study and the McGee *et al.* (1990) study is the age of the youngsters: Benjamin *et al.* worked with the 7–11 years age group whilst McGee *et al.*'s group were 15 years. The social impairment associated with anxiety disorders may be greater in younger children than in adolescents.

Two studies evaluated the peer social status of children with clinical anxiety disorders. Puig-Antich *et al.* (1985) found that anxiety disordered children and depressive children showed impaired peer relationships relative to normal children. Strauss *et al.* (1988) found that the social relationships of children with an anxiety disorder were as disrupted as those of children with a conduct disorder. Children with anxiety disorders tended to be lonely, were infrequently liked and often socially neglected by their classmates. Finally, generalized anxiety disorder in adolescence is often associated with substantial impairment, comparable to the impairment in adolescents with depressive disorders or externalizing disorders (Bowen *et al.*, 1990).

Health Services Utilization

Suffering from an anxiety disorder is often no reason to use a mental health facility, as can be concluded from the high prevalence of anxiety disorders in the community. There is some evidence that comorbidity is associated with mental health service utilization (Bird *et al.*, 1993). Whitaker and colleagues (1990) found that among adolescents diagnosed as generalized anxiety disorder 60% made use of health services. Other authors (Bowen *et al.*, 1990; Fergusson *et al.*, 1993) have reported that between 9–16% of the children with anxiety had used mental health or social services. Another 10.3% (Bowen *et al.*, 1990) perceived themselves as having had emotional or behavioural problems for which professional help is or was needed.

ASSESSMENT

A review of the literature shows that assessment of anxiety symptoms in children is a neglected topic. Only a few instruments have been developed, including structured and semi-structured diagnostic interviews (both for the anxious children themselves and for their parents), self-report questionnaires and behavioural checklists. Most of them measure anxiety symptoms in a global way. This situation is gradually changing, but although in some recently developed instruments attempts are made to measure specific anxiety symptoms, such as obsessions and compulsions, data on the validity and reliability of these devices are almost completely lacking. It has become common place to consider anxiety as a constellation of three response channels (verbal-cognitive, behaviour-motoric, and psychophysiological, Lang, 1971). Some authors have described these aspects in children (e.g., Kendall and Chansky, 1991; Francis, 1988; Beidel, 1989; Ollendick and Francis, 1988) but, again, for children no instruments are available that measure these aspects separately.

Self-report Questionnaires and Behavioural Checklists

Self-report questionnaires have been used to identify the children's specific fear stimuli, and are generally used to provide an overall index of fearfulness. These instruments generally contain lists of specific fear stimuli, and ask the children to rate their fear to each stimulus. Examples of such instruments include the Fear Survey Schedule for Children (Scherer and Nakamura, 1968) and the Revision of the Fear Survey Schedule for Children (Ollendick, 1983). Another type of self-report questionnaire has been developed to determine the child's anxiety level associated with fearful situations. The most commonly used anxiety measure is the Revised Children's Manifest Anxiety Scale (Reynolds and Richmond, 1978).

Numerous behavioural checklists and rating scales have also been developed to measure symptoms of psychopathology, including that of anxiety. Such checklists can either be administered by the children themselves, or by significant others, like parents and teachers. Some examples of checklists are the Child Behavior Checklist (Achenbach, 1978), the Revised Behavior Problem Checklist (Quay and Peterson, 1983), and the Louisville Fear Survey for Children (Miller *et al.*, 1971).

Diagnostic Interviews

A number of structured and semi-structured diagnostic interview schedules have been designed to assess anxiety disorders in children and adolescents. These include:

(a) *Anxiety Disorders Interview Schedules for Children and for Parents* (ADIS-C and ADIS-P, Silverman and Nelles, 1988). This instrument was adapted according to criteria of DSM-IV (Silverman, Albano, and Barlow, 1994) and permits differential diagnoses among the anxiety disorders, affective disorders, and externalizing disorders of childhood. The interview also provides screening questions for psychotic symptomatology. Both child and adult anxiety disorders are included. The parent and child versions show significant overlap, but the parent schedule is more detailed in questions about the history of the problem and the consequences that occur to the child after he or she engages in the problem behaviour. In addition to a diagnosis, the interviews provide data about anxiety symptomatology, cause, course, and a functional analysis of the problems. Administration of each interview takes about 90 minutes. Data about interrater agreement and 10–14 days test-retest reliability of the DSM-III-R version were satisfactory (Silverman and Eisen, 1992; Silverman and Nelles, 1988). Data on the reliability and validity of the DSM-IV version are currently being collected;

(b) The *Children's Anxiety Evaluation Form* (CAEF; Hoehn-Saric *et al.*, 1987) contains three areas of information: the history of the present illness, symptoms, and signs. Part I is scored on the basis of the admission note, which is reviewed on the presence or absence of symptoms suggestive of anxiety in the present illness. Ratings on parts II and III are obtained in a semi-structured interview, lasting about 30 minutes. Each part is rated on a 5-point scale, and the total CAEF score is the summation of the global scores from the three parts (0–12). Part II starts with an assessment of target anxiety symptoms, followed by an inventory of 11 other anxiety symptoms (e.g., tension, sleep difficulty, somatic signs), and of the focus of the anxiety symptoms (generalized, social, performance, separation, phobias, and panic attacks). Part III contains 18 signs that must be observed and rated during the interview, such as tenseness, closeness to tears, tics, and nail biting. Directions are given for administration of the interview. Although the CAEF has not been used in other studies, it seems promising because it takes relatively little time.

(c) The *Yale Brown Obsessive-Compulsive Scale-Child version* (CY-BOCS; Riddle *et al.*, 1992) aimed for assessment of obsessive-compulsive symptomatology, is modeled after the Y-BOCS for adults (Goodman *et al.*, 1989a). In both instruments the clinician is asked to rate obsessions and compulsions separately on time occupied, distress, impairment, resistance, and control. Each item is rated on a 5-point scale, from 0 (no symptoms) to 4 (serious symptomatology). Although the instrument has been used in some recent studies, psychometric data on the child version are lacking. The adult version has shown satisfactory reliability and validity (Goodman *et al.*, 1989b).

More general diagnostic interviews that were designed to measure various types of mental disorders, including anxiety disorders, are the Diagnostic Interview for Children and Adolescents (DICA-R; Reich and Welner, 1988), the Diagnostic Interview Schedule for Children (DISC; Costello *et al.*, 1984), and the Schedule for Affective Disorders and Schizophrenia for School-aged Children (K-SADS; Puig-Antich and Chambers, 1978) (Table 7.3).

Other Assessment Methods

Other assessment methods include behavioural observation, in which fearful behaviour is observed in the situation in which it occurs. For this purpose, behavioural observation systems have been developed, such as the Preschool Observation Scale of Anxiety (Glennon and Weisz, 1978). Other methods include self-monitoring procedures and physiological assessment, but, both methods have rarely been used in children and adolescents.

TREATMENT

Psychological Interventions

Pharmacotherapy

Psychopharmacologic treatment most commonly used in children and adolescents with anxiety disorders include tricyclic antidepressants (e.g., imipramine), benzodiazepines (e.g., alprazolam, clonazepam), and buspirone or fluoxetine. Although there is a considerable number of publications on the effects of psychopharmaca for anxiety disorders, most of them were case reports or open studies, some conducted retrospectively (e.g., Apter *et al.*, 1994; Birmaher *et al.*, 1994, Geller *et al.*, 1995). Some recent controlled studies on the use of psychopharmaca for DSM-III or later anxiety disorders in children and adolescents with anxiety disorders are included in Table 7.4.

Earlier studies (e.g., Gittelman-Klein and Klein, 1971, 1973; Berney *et al.*, 1981) are not discussed here. Summarizing the results it can be said that most studies were conducted on obsessive-compulsive disorder, and

Table 7.3   Examples of anxiety questions from some selected general diagnostic interviews

Instruments	Examples of items	Coding options				
DICA-R (Reich and Welner, 1988)	Did you ever go away from home for a few days, like visiting relatives and be so upset and worried that you came back home right away?	1	2	4		9
	Do you feel so shy that you can't make friends even though you want to?	1	2	4		9
	Are you a worrier — do you worry more than most children?	1	2	4		9
DISC (Costello et al., 1984)	In the past 6 months, have you been very afraid of going to places					
	A. where there will be a lot of people, like a party?	0	1	2		9
	B. or very afraid of meeting new people?	0	1	2		9
	In the past 6 months, have you had to count things over and over?					
	IF YES, A. Do you feel nervous or uneasy if you don't count this way?	0	1	2		9
	B. Do you think something bad might happen if you don't count like that?	0	1	2		9
	C. Do you like counting things this way?	0	1	2		9
	D. Is counting something you would like to stop but can't?	0	1	2		9
K-SADS (Puig-Antich and Chambers, 1978)	Do you have silly habits you have to do over and over again? Do you have habits you can't resist repeating like touching or counting things, washing your hands many times, checking locks, or collecting things?	0	1	2	3	4

Note: (i) DICA-R: 1 = yes, 2 = sometimes, 4 = no, 9 = don't know; (ii) DISC: 0 = no, 1 = sometimes/somewhat, 2 = yes, 9 = don't know; (iii) K-SADS: 0 = no information, 1 = no, 2 = slight, 3 = moderate, 4 = severe/extreme

Table 7.4 Controlled studies on pharmacological treatment in children

Study	Primary Diagnosis	Age	Treatment	Duration	Design	Results
DeVeaugh-Geiss et al. (1992)	OCD (54)	10–17	1. clomipramine 2. placebo	8 weeks	double blind, parallel groups	1. 37% improved, 2. 8% improved
Flament et al. (1985)	OCD (19)	10–18	1. clomipramine 2. placebo	10 weeks	double blind cross-over	1 > 2
Graae et al. (1994)	SAD (11) OAD (1)	7–13	1. CZP + ST 2. placebo + ST	8 weeks	cross-over	1 = 2, 3 dropouts (in CZP) 3 patients not improved 5 moderately improved
Klein et al. (1992)	SAD (20)	6–15	1. imipramine 2. placebo	6 weeks	double blind placebo controlled	1 = 2
Leonard et al. (1989)	OCD (49)	6–18	1. pla-CMI-DMI 2. pla-DMI-CMI	12 weeks (2–5–5)	cross-over	2 > 1; CMI > DMI relapse on DMI, not on CMI
Riddle et al. (1992)	OCD (14)	8–15	1. fluoxetine 2. placebo	20 weeks	double blind cross-over	1 > 2. Reduction in mean obsessive compulsive symptoms in 1: 30–45%, in 2: 12–27%
Simeon et al. (1992)	OAD (21) AD (9)	8–16	1. alprazolam 2. placebo	4 weeks	double blind placebo controlled	1 = 2; clinical judgement: 3 patients (very) much improved 7 patients not/minimally improved

Note: AD = avoidant disorder, FU = follow-up, OAD = overanxious disorder, OCD = obsessive-compulsive disorder, pla = placebo, SAD = separation disorder, WL = waitlist, CZP = clonazepam, CMI = clomipramine, DMI = desipramine all of them used antidepressants. Mean improvement during the treatments varied from 30–45%, but this result has to be qualified in view of the considerable improvements that were also found in the placebo conditions (from 8 to 27%). A number of side effects were reported, especially tremors, dry mouth, dizziness, and constipation. For the overanxious and separation anxiety disorders no evidence was found for a beneficial effect of benzodiazepines or antidepressants in comparison with placebo. For a more detailed review on pharmacotherapy for anxiety disorders in children and adolescents the reader is referred to Popper (1993).

Relapse. In earlier studies on psychological treatment of anxiety in children (mainly on specific fears such as fear of the dark) the sparse long-term follow-up data that were collected showed that the results were stable. As was described on the previous pages, only a few controlled studies have been conducted that evaluated the effects of psychological treatment in the other anxiety disorders. Studies on long-term follow-up results of these treatments are totally lacking. As far as data are available on long-term results of psychopharmacological treatment, they showed that many patients relapsed after discontinuation of the medication (64% in the study of Flament *et al.*, 1985; Leonard *et al.*, 1989).

Since the report of Jones (1924) about the successful treatment of Peter's fear of rabbits, many reports have been published about psychotherapy in children, but only a few of them (predominantly in the last decade) have been conducted on more homogenous groups of anxious or fearful children. In order to provide a framework for interpretation of these results, we shortly present the findings of older studies, summarized in two meta-analyses. We limit our scope to meta-analyses that presented separate data for children with anxiety problems.

Casey and Berman (1985) reviewed all studies published between 1952 and 1983 in which some form of psychotherapy for children was compared with a control group or another treatment. Studies were excluded if (a) the mean age of the subjects at the start of treatment was 13 or older, (b) no proper control groups were used, and (c) treatment was not aimed at a clinical problem, but at improving some aspect of normal functioning. On the whole, behavioural therapies appeared to be more effective than nonbehavioural therapies (Table 7.5).

Casey and Berman (1985) distinguished four categories of target problems: social adjustment (25 studies), impulsivity/hyperactivity (10 studies), phobia (9 studies) and somatic problems (3 studies); in the other 14 studies the problems were too heterogenous to be classified. Mean effect sizes of the active treatments are given in Table 7.5. Most treatments for the latter

Table 7.5 Effectiveness of psychotherapy in children: Results of meta-analyses

Study	Total number of studies	Age of subjects	Treatments (Number of studies)	Effect size	Target Problems	Effect size
Casey and Berman (1985)	64	mean < 13 (range 3–15)	Behavioural (37)* cognitive-behavioural (14) other behavioural (26) Nonbehavioural (29) client centred (20) dynamic (5)	0.91 0.81 0.96 0.40 0.49 0.21	Social adjustment Impulsivity/ hyperactivity Phobia Somatic problems	0.55 1.10 1.16 1.66
Weisz et al. (1987)	108	< 19	Behavioural (126) Nonbehavioural (27)	0.88 0.44	Overcontrolled – phobias/anxiety – social withdrawal Undercontrolled – delinquency – noncompliance – self-control – aggressive	0.88 0.74 1.07 0.79 0.66 1.33 0.75 0.74
Weisz et al. (1995)	150	mean 10.5	Behavioural (197) Nonbehavioural (27)	0.76 0.35	Overcontrolled – phobias/anxiety – social withdrawal Undercontrolled – delinquency – noncompliance – self-control – aggression	0.69 0.57 0.71 0.62 0.42 0.42 0.87 0.34

* Some studies examined more than one form of treatment

Note: AD = avoidant disorder, CBT = cognitive behaviour therapy, FU = follow-up, OAD = overanxious disorder, OCD = obsessive compulsive disorder, SAD = separation disorder, WL = wait list three categories of problems were behaviourally oriented; only for problems in social adjustment were behavioural and nonbehavioural methods used equally often. On the basis of these data it can be concluded that (cognitive) behaviour methods are effective in reducing fear and anxiety in general; no conclusions can be drawn about the possible effectiveness of nonbehavioural methods for these complaints. Given the character of the treated fears (specific phobias, like fear of the dark, fear of snakes, night time fear, or unspecified phobic disorders) the relevance of the results for the DSM-IV anxiety disorders other than specific phobia is unclear.

Weisz and colleagues (1987) also conducted a meta-analysis on the effectiveness of psychotherapy for children. They reviewed 108 studies (only 32 of which were also included in Casey and Berman's analysis) and were guided by four questions. First, they wondered whether the effects of psychotherapy for adolescents (12 years and older) are comparable to those for children. They came to this question through the consideration that

> "... various cognitive and social developments, including the advent of formal operations, make adolescents more cognitively complex than children, less likely to rely on adult authority, and seemingly less likely to adjust their behaviour to fit societal expectations. Thus, it is possible that adolescents may be more resistant than children to therapeutic intervention. On the other hand, adolescents are more likely than children to comprehend the purpose of therapy and to understand complex, interactive psychological determinants of behavior, which would make them better candidates for therapy than children..." (p. 542).

Interestingly, they found that, in general, children appeared to have profited significantly more from treatment than adolescents (mean effect sizes 0.92 versus 0.58). Second, they reexamined the question whether therapy methods differ in effectiveness, disagreeing with Casey and Berman's notion that the results for behavioural methods were flattered because the outcome measures in studies on these methods only measured what was exercised during the treatment. The "raw" mean effect sizes they found were in line with the findings of Casey and Berman. Omission of only the "unnecessary therapy-like outcomes" made no significant difference (mean effect sizes for behavioural and non-behavioural were 0.93 and 0.45 respectively), again indicating that, in general, behavioural interventions are clearly more effective than nonbehavioural interventions. This finding was stable across differences in age of the subjects, target problem and therapist experience. Third, unlike Casey and Berman (1985) and in line with factor analytic research, they distinguished two large categories of target problems: overcontrolled and undercontrolled behaviour. Of the 163 treatment groups, 67 contained subjects with overcontrolled problems, divided into phobias and anxiety (39 groups) versus social withdrawal/isolation (28 groups). The effectiveness of psychotherapy for these problems is given in Table 7.5. Finally, they addressed the question whether therapist experience mediates treatment success. On the whole, paraprofessionals, graduate students and professionals were equally effective. However, two interaction effects were found. First, paraprofessionals and graduate student therapists were more effective with younger than with older children, whereas trained professionals were equally effective for both groups. Second, all therapists were equally effective in the treatment of undercontrolled behaviour, whereas experienced therapists were more effective than the other two groups in the treatment of overcontrolled behaviour.

Weisz *et al.* (1995) reviewed recent studies, excluding studies reviewed in Casey and Berman (1985) and Weisz *et al.* (1987). The results confirmed earlier findings: treatment was more effective than waitlist, and behavioural interventions were about twice as effective as nonbehavioural interventions. In contrast with earlier results, they found no differences between the effects on overcontrolled versus undercontrolled problems. Further, in contrast with Weisz *et al.* (1987) they found better outcomes for adolescents than for children. Finally, trained paraprofessionals (mostly parents) appeared to be more effective than students and fully trained clinicians.

In summarizing these results it becomes obvious that psychotherapy is effective in decreasing children's fears, that behavioural methods are clearly more effective than nonbehavioural methods, and that the magnitude of the behavioural effects closely parallel those obtained from outcome research with adults (Kazdin, 1994). Given the fact that in most studies no formal classification system for target problems was used, the implications of the findings for the different anxiety disorders are unclear. Recently, a few studies have been conducted on psychotherapy for properly diagnosed anxiety disorders (Table 7.6).

Thyer and Sowars-Hoag (1988) reviewed the literature on behaviour therapy for separation anxiety disorder. They found 11 publications between 1960 and 1984, most of them being case reports. We discuss

Table 7.6 Studies (no case-reports) on psychological treatment of anxiety disorders in children (DSM-III or later)

Study	Primary Diagnosis	Age	Treatment	Modality	Sessions (months)	Follow-up	Design	Results
Blagg and Yule (1984)	SAD (66)	8–14	1. BT 2. Hosp 3. Ps + Sch	indiv.	2 weeks 45 weeks 72 weeks	12	no random assignment	1 > 3 >> 2
Kane and Kendall* (1989)	OAD (4)	9–13	1. CBT	indiv.	16–20 twice weekly	3–6	multiple baseline	all patients improved at follow-up two patients with slight relapse
Kendall (1994)	OAD (30) SAD (8) AD (9)	9–13	1. CBT (27) 2. WL (20)	indiv.	16–20	12 weekly patients in 2. treated in 1. after WL	random assignment to conditions	1 > 2; improvement on all measures; maintained at FU 13 dropouts (initial group n = 60)
March et al.* (1994)	OCD (15)	8–18	1. CBT (15) (7 with medication)	indiv.	3–21	1–21 study	uncontrolled	overall improvement no control groups maintained at FU; 4 markedly improved

* uncontrolled studies

Note: AD = avoidant disorder, BT = behaviour therapy, CBT = cognitive-behaviour therapy, FU = follow-up, Hos = hospitalization, OAD = overanxious disorder, OCD = obsessive-compulsive disorder, Ps + Sch = Psychotherapy + Schooling, SAD = separation anxiety disorder, indiv. = individually administered, WL = waiting list only the study by Blagg and Yule (1984), who compared behaviour therapy, hospitalization, and psychotherapy + home schooling. Subjects were 66 patients with separation anxiety. The behaviour therapy was clearly the most effective on all outcome measures, and very cost-efficient as well (given the length of treatment).

Kane and Kendall (1989) treated four children with an overanxious disorder in a multiple baseline study. The treatment focused on four major components: (a) recognizing anxious feelings and somatic reactions to anxiety; (b) clarifying cognitions in anxiety-provoking situations; (c) developing a plan to help cope with the situation; and (d) evaluating the success of the coping strategies and self-reinforcement as appropriate. Several behavioural strategies were included, such as modelling, exposure *in vivo*, and relaxation training. All children were significantly improved at the end of the treatment. At 3 to 6 months follow-up, two children had maintained their improvements as was confirmed by their parents. The other two children reported continued gains, but their parents reported return of some previous difficulties.

March *et al.* (1994) treated 15 children with obsessive-compulsive disorder with a cognitive behaviour therapy. Treatment was given according to an elaborate treatment protocol. The factual cognitive behavioural treatment was preceded by three steps (each covering one session): establishing obsessive-compulsive disorder as an illness, mapping obsessive-compulsive disorder, and teaching the "transition zone" (the area in which the child already has some success in resisting obsessive-compulsive disorder). The cognitive behaviour therapy consisted of a combination of anxiety management and exposure *in vivo* with response prevention, exercised in weekly homework assignments. Treatments were individually administered, although the parents were frequently involved in the treatment. The majority of the patients made substantial improvement, which was maintained or further improved at 18-months follow-up. Although both studies suggest that cognitive behavioural treatments are useful in decreasing anxiety disorders in children, it must be kept in mind that both studies were uncontrolled.

Kendall (1994) published the first study in which behaviour therapy (16 weeks) was compared with a wait-list condition (8 weeks). Patients were 47 children (9–13 years) with childhood anxiety disorders according to DSM-III-R. Treatment was comparable to that in the study of Kane and Kendall (1989). On all measures the active treatment appeared to be superior to the wait-list. As far as the clinical significance of the results is concerned, 64% of the patients in the active treatment no longer met diagnostic criteria for an anxiety disorder at posttreatment, in contrast to 5% of the wait-list condition. Results were stable or further improved at a 2–5 years follow-up investigation (Kendall and Southam-Gerow, 1996).

March (1995) reviewed the literature on cognitive-behavioural psychotherapy for obsessive-compulsive disorder in children and adults. He found 32 articles (from 1967–1994) describing a nonpharmacological treatment of obsessive-compulsive disorder (although in some studies psychopharmaca were added) in one or more child and adolescent subjects; 25 were case reports (little or no quantitative data), the remaining were single case studies, some of them on several patients. Not one controlled comparison of different treatment conditions was conducted. Divergent treatment strategies were used, most of them behaviourally oriented. Almost all studies used exposure and/or response prevention, sometimes amplified with other strategies, such as anxiety management or operant techniques. All authors stated that their treatment had been more or less effective, but these results are difficult to evaluate given the uncontrolled nature of the studies.

CONCLUDING REMARKS

An attempt has been made to describe the phenomenology of anxiety disorders in childhood and adolescence and the characteristics associated with them. Consensus on the diagnostic guidelines starting with DSM-III has led to considerable amount of work in this area. Both community and clinical studies have enhanced our knowledge of the epidemiology and characteristics of the various anxiety disorders in childhood and adolescence. What we still do not know is which factors are associated with referral to treatment agencies. Anxiety disorders in childhood are often chronic and much more prevalent than once thought, but very few of the children or adolescents who meet the criteria for an anxiety disorder are referred to a treatment agency. Although it is tempting to assume that comorbidity and impairment may be related to treatment seeking, more mundane reasons might also be involved such as the availability and accessability of treatment in the community.

Given the results of behaviour therapy in adults with anxiety disorders (e.g., Emmelkamp *et al.*, 1992), it is astonishing that so few controlled studies have been conducted on behaviour therapy in children. Most attention has been spent on pharmacological interventions, and direct comparisons between both types of treatments have not been conducted yet. Given this state of research, definite conclusions about the respective effectiveness of behavioural and pharmacological treatments in children can not be drawn yet. However, indirect evidence suggests that the results of psychological treatments are better and more stable than those of pharmacological treatments, at least for obsessive-compulsive disorder (March, 1995).

REFERENCES

Abe, K. and Masui, T. (1981). Age-sex trends of phobic and anxiety symptoms in adolescents. *British Journal of Psychiatry*, **138**, 297–302.

Achenbach, T.M. (1978). The child behavior profile: I. Boys aged 6–11. *Journal of Consulting and Clinical Psychology*, **46**, 478–488.

Achenbach, T.M. and Edelbrock, C.S (1983). *Manual for the Child Behaviour Checklist and Profile*. Burlington: University of Vermont.

Agras, W.S., Chapin, H.N., and Oliveau, D.C. (1972). The natural history of phobia: Course and prognosis. *Archives of General Psychiatry*, **26**, 315–317.

Ainsworth, M.D.S. (1984). Attachment. In N.S. Endler and J.Mc. Hunt (Eds.), *Personality and the behavioral disorders*, Vol. 1. New York: Wiley.

American Psychiatric Association (1980). *Diagnostic and statistical manual of mental disorders (3rd ed.)*. Washington, DC: American Psychiatric Association.

American Psychiatric Association (1987). *Diagnostic and statistical manual of mental disorders (3rd rev. ed.)*. Washington, DC: American Psychiatric Association.

American Psychiatric Association (1994). *Diagnostic and statistical manual of mental disorders (4th ed.)*. Washington: American Psychiatric Association.

Anderson, J.C., Williams, S., McGee, R., and Silva, P.A. (1987). DSM-III disorders in preadolescent children. *Archives of General Psychiatry*, **44**, 69–80.

Andrews, G., Stewart, S., Allen, R., and Henderson, A.S. (1990). The genetics of six neurotic disorders: A twin study. *Journal of Affective Disorders*, **19**, 23–29.

Apter, A., Ratzoni, G., King, R.A., Weizman, A., Iancu, I., Binder, M., Riddle, M.A. (1994). Fluvoxamine open-label treatment of adolescent inpatients with obsessive-compulsive disorder or depression. *Journal of the American Academy of Child and Adolescent Psychiatry*, **33**, 343–353.

Baeyens, F., Eelen, P., Crombez, G., and Van den Bergh, O. (1992). Human evaluative conditioning: Acquisition trials, presentation schedule, evaluative style and contingency awareness. *Behaviour Research and Therapy*, **30**, 133–142.

Barrios, B.A. and Hartman, D.P. (1987). Fears and anxieties. In E.J. Mash and L.G. Terdal (Eds.), *Behavioral assessment of anxiety disorders* (pp. 196–262). New York: Guilford Press.

Beidel, D.C. (1989). Determining the reliability of psychophysiological assessment in childhood anxiety. Special Issue: Assessment of childhood anxiety disorders. *Journal of Anxiety Disorders*, **5**, 139–150.

Beidel, D.C., Christ, M.A.G., and Long, P.J. (1991). Somatic complaints in anxious children. *Journal of Abnormal Child Psychology*, **19**, 659–670.

Beidel, D.B. and Turner, S.M. (1988). Comorbidity of test anxiety and other anxiety disorders in children. *Journal of Abnormal Child Psychology*, **16**, 275–287.

Bell-Dolan, D.J., Last, C.G., and Strauss, C.C. (1990). Symptoms of anxiety disorders in normal children. *Journal of the American Academy of Child and Adolescent Psychiatry*, **29**, 759–765.

Benjamin, R.S., Costello, E.J., and Warren, M. (1990). Anxiety disorders in a pediatric sample. *Journal of Anxiety Disorders*, **4**, 293–316.

Berg, I., Butler, A., Franklin, J., Hayes, H., Lucas, C., and Sims, R. (1993). DSM-III-R disorders, social factors and management of school attendance problems in the normal population. *Journal of Child Psychology and Psychiatry*, **34**, 1187–1203.

Bergeron, L., Valla, J.P., and Bretton, J.J. (1992). Pilot study for the Quebec Child Mental Health Survey. Part I. Measurement of prevalence estimates among six to 14 years olds. *Canadian Journal of Psychiatry*, **37**, 373–380.

Bernstein, G.A. (1991). Comorbidity and severity of anxiety and depressive disorders in a clinic sample. *Journal of the American Academy of Child and Adolescent Psychiatry*, **30**, 43–50.

Berney, T., Kolvin, S.R., Bhate, R.F., Garside, J., Jeans, B., Scarth, K., and Scarth, L. (1981). School phobia: A therapeutic trial with clomipramine and short-term outcome. *British Journal of Psychiatry*, **138**, 110–118.

Bernstein, G.A., Garfinkel, B.D., Hoberman, H.M. (1989). Self-reported anxiety in adolescents. *Journal of Psychiatry*, **146**, 384–386.

Biederman, J., Rosenbaum, J.F., Bolduc-Murphy, E.A., Faraone, S.V., Chaloff, J., Hirshfeld, D.R., and Kagan, J. (1992). A 3-year follow-up of children with and without behavioral inhibition. *Journal of the American Academy of Child and Adolescent Psychiatry*, **32**, 814–821.

Biederman, J., Rosenbaum, J.F., and Hirshfeld, D.R. (1990). Psychiatric correlates of behavioral inhibition in young children of parents with and without psychiatric disorders. *Archives of General Psychiatry*, **47**, 21–26.

Bird, H.R., Gould, M.S., and Staghezza, B.M. (1993). Patterns of diagnostic comorbidity in a community sample of children aged 9 through 16 years. *Journal of the American Academy of Child and Adolescent Psychiatry*, **32**, 361–368.

Birmaher, B., Waterman, S., Ryan, N., Cully, M., Balach, L., Ingram, J., and Brodsky, M. (1994). Fluoxetine for childhood anxiety disorders. *Journal of the American Academy of Child and Adolescent Psychiatry*, **33**, 993–999.

Blagg, N.R. and Yule, Y. (1984). The behavioural treatment of school refusal: A comparative study. *Behaviour Research and Therapy*, **22**, 119–127.

Bools, C., Forster, J., Brown, I., and Berg, I. (1990). The identification of psychiatric disorders in children who fail to attend school: A cluster analysis of a non-clinical population. *Psychological Medicine*, **20**, 171–181.

Boomsma, D.I. and Verhulst, F.C. (1995). Genetisch onderzoek naar psychopathologie bij jonge tweelingen. In C.A.L. Hoogduin, P. Schnabel, W., Vandereycken, K. van der Velden, and F.C. Verhulst (Eds.), *Jaarboek psychiatrie en psychotherapie* (Vol. V, pp. 90–102). Houten: Bohn Stafleu Van Loghum.

Bowen, R.C., Offord, D.R., and Boyle, M.H. (1990). The prevalence of overanxious disorder and separation anxiety disorder: Results from the Ontario Child Health Study. *Journal of the American Academy of Child and Adolescent Psychiatry*, **29**, 753–758.

Bowlby, J. (1973). *Attachment of loss: Vol. II: Separation, anxiety and anger*. New York: Basic Books.

Bradley, S. and Hood, J. (1993). Psychiatrically referred adolescents with panic attacks: Presenting symptoms, stressors and comorbidity. *Journal of the American Academy of Child and Adolescent Psychiatry*, **32**, 826–829.

Brandenburg, N.A., Friedman, R.M., and Silver, S.E. (1990). The epidemiology of childhood psychiatric disorders: Prevalence findings from recent studies. *Journal of the American Academy of Child and Adolescent Psychiatry*, **29**, 76–83.

Bregman, E. (1934). An attempt to modify the emotional attitude of infants by the conditioned response technique. *Journal of Genetic Psychology*, **45**, 169–198.

Brent, D.A., Kalas, R., Edelbrock, C., Costello, A.J., Dulcan, M.K., and Conover, N. (1986). Psychopathology and its relationship to suicidal ideation in childhood and adolescence. *Journal of the American Academy of Child and Adolescent Psychiatry*, **25**, 666–673.

Bruch, M.A., Heimberg, R.G., Berger, P., and Collins, T.M. (1989). Social phobia and perception of early parental and personal characteristics. *Anxiety Research*, **2**, 57–65.

Casat (1988). Childhood anxiety disorders: A review of the possible relationship to adult panic disorder and agoraphobia. Special issue: Perspectives in panic related disorders. *Journal of Anxiety Disorders*, **2**, 51–60.

Casey, R.J. and Berman, J.S. (1985). The outcome of psychotherapy with children. *Psychological Bulletin*, **98**, 388–400.

Clark, D.B., Smith, M.G., Neighbors, B.D., Skerlec, L.M., and Randall, J. (1994). Anxiety disorders in adolescence: Characteristics, prevalence, and comorbidities. *Clinical Psychology Review*, **14**, 113–137.

Cook, M. and Mineka, S. (1991). Selective associations in the origins of phobic fears and their implications for behavior therapy. In P.R. Martin (Ed.), *Handbook of behavior therapy and psychological science: An integrative approach* (pp. 413–434). New York: Pergamon.

Costello, A.J., Edelbrock, C., Dulcan, R.K., Kalas, R., and Klaric, S.H. (1984). *Development and testing of the NIMH Diagnostic Interview Schedule for Children in a clinic population.* Rockville, MD: National Institute of Mental Health.

Costello, E.J., Costello, A.J., Edelbrock, C., Burns, B.J., Dulcan, M.K., Brent, D., and Janiszewski, S. (1989). Psychiatric disorders in pediatric primary care. *Archives of General Psychiatry*, **45**, 1107–1116.

Crowe, R.R., Noyes, R., Pauls, D.L., and Slyman, D. (1983). Family study of panic disorder. *Archives of General Psychiatry*, **40**, 1065–1069.

Davey, G.C.L. (1992). Classical conditioning and the acquisition of human fears and phobias: A review and synthesis of the literature. *Advances in Behavior Research and Therapy*, **14**, 29–66.

De Aldaz, E.G., Feldman, L., Vivas, E., and Gelfland, D. (1987). Characteristics of Venezualan school refusers. *Journal of Nervous and Mental Diseases*, **175**, 402–407.

Delprato, D.J. and McGlynn, F.D. (1984). Behavioral theories of anxiety disorders. In S.M. Turner (Ed.), *Behavioral theories and treatment of anxiety* (pp. 1–49). New York: Plenum.

DeVeaugh, G.J., Moroz, G., Biederman, J., Cantwell, D.P. *et al.* (1992). Clomipramine hydrochloride in childhood and adolescent obsessive-compulsive disorder: A multicenter trial. *Journal of the American Academy of Child and Adolescent Psychiatry*, **31**, 45–49.

DiNardo, P.A., Guzy, T., Jenkins, J.A., Bak, R.M., Tomasi, S.F., and Copland, M. (1988). Etiology and maintenance of dog fears. *Behaviour Research and Therapy*, **26**, 241–244.

Emmelkamp, P.M.G. (1982). *Phobic and obsessive-compulsive disorder.* New York: Plenum.

Emmelkamp, P.M.G., Bouman, T.K., and Scholing, A. (1992). *Anxiety disorders.* Chichester: Wiley.

Emmelkamp, P.M.G. and Van Oppen, P. (1994). Anxiety disorders. In V.B. Van Hasselt and M. Hersen (Eds.), *Advanced abnormal psychology* (pp. 273–293). New York: Plenum.

Emmelkamp, P.M.G. and Scholing, A. (1994). Behavioral interpretations. In B.B. Wolman and G. Stricker (Eds.), *Anxiety and related disorders: A handbook* (pp 30–56). New York: Wiley.

English, H.B. (1929). Three cases of the "conditioned fear response". *Journal of Abnormal and Social Psychology*, **34**, 221–225.

Essau, C.A. and Petermann, U. (1995). Depression. In F. Petermann (Ed.), *Lehrbuch der klinischen Kinderpsychologie* (pp. 241–264). Hogrefe: Göttingen.

Eysenck, H.J. and Rachman, S. (1965). *The causes and cures of neurosis.* London: Routledge and Kegan Paul.

Fergusson, D.M., Horwood, J., and Lynskey, M.T. (1993). Prevalence and comorbidity of DSM-III-R diagnoses in a birth cohort of 15 year olds. *Journal of the American Academy of Child and Adolescent Psychiatry*, **32**, 1127–1134.

Flament, M.F., Rapoport, J.L., Berg, C.J., Sceery, W., Kilts, C., Mellstrom, B., and Linnoila, M. (1985). Clomipramine treatment of childhood obsessive-compulsive disorder. *Archives of General Psychiatry*, **42**, 977–963.

Francis, G. (1988). Assessing cognitions in anxious children. Special Issue: Behavioral assessment and treatment of childhood anxiety disorders. *Behavior Modification*, **12**, 267–280.

Francis, G., Last, C.G., and Strauss, C.C. (1992). Avoidant disorder and social phobia in children and adolescents. *Journal of the American Academy of Child and Adolescent Psychiatry*, **31**, 1086–1089.

Geller, D.A., Biederman, J., Reed, E.D., Spencer, T., and Wilens, T.E. (1995). Similarities in repsonse to fluoxetine in the treatment of children and adolescents with obsessive-compulsive disorder. *Journal of the American Academy of Child and Adolescent Psychiatry*, **34**, 36–44.

Gerlsma, C., Emmelkamp, P.M.G., and Arrindell, W.A. (1991). Anxiety, depression, and perception of early parenting: A meta-analysis. *Clinical Psychology Review*, **10**, 251–277.

Gittelman-Klein, R. and Klein, D.F. (1971). Controlled imipramine treatment of school phobia. *Archives of General Psychiatry*, **25**, 204–207.

Gittelman-Klein, R. and Klein, D.F. (1973). School phobia: Considerations in the light of imipramine effects. *Journal of Nervous and Mental Diseases*, **156**, 199–215.

Glennon, B. and Weisz, J.R. (1978). An observational approach to the assessment of anxiety in young children. *Journal of Consulting and Clinical Psychology*, **46**, 1246–1257.

Goodman, W.K., Price, L.H., Rasmussen, S.A., Mazure, C., Delgado, P., Heninger, G.R., and Charney, D.D. (1989a). The Yale-Brown Obsessive-Compulsive Scale: II validity. *Archives of General Psychiatry*, **46**, 1012–1016.

Goodman, W.K., Price, L.H., Rasmussen, S.A., Mazure, C., Fleischmann, R., Hill, C.L., Heninger, G.R., and Charney, D.D. (1989b). The Yale-Brown Obsessive-Compulsive Scale: I. Development, use and reliability. *Archives of General Psychiatry*, **46**, 1006–1011.

Graae, F., Milner, J., Rizzotto, L., and Klein, R.G. (1994). Clonazepam in childhood anxiety disorder. *Journal of the American Academy of Child and Adolescent Psychiatry*, **33**, 372–376.

Grad, L.R., Pelcovitz, D., Olson, M., Mathews, M., and Grad, G.J. (1987). Obsessive-compulsive symptomatology in children with Tourette's syndrome. *Journal of the American Academy of Child and Adolescent Psychiatry*, **26**, 69–73.

Gray, J.A. (1975). *Elements of a two-process theory of learning.* New York: Academic Press.

Hekmat, H. (1987). Origins and development of human fear reactions. *Journal of Anxiety Disorders*, **1**, 197–218.

Hirshfeld, D.R., Rosenbaum, J.F., Biederman, J., Bolduc, E.A., Faraone, S.V., Snidman, N., Reznick, J.S., and Kagan, J. (1992). Stable behavioral inhibition and its association with anxiety disorders. *Journal of the American Academy of Child and Adolescent Psychiatry*, **31**, 103–111.

Hoehn-Saric, E., Maisami, M., and Wiegand, D. (1987). Measurement of anxiety in children and adolescents using semistructured interviews. *Journal of the American Academy of Child and Adolescent Psychiatry*, **26**, 541–545.

Jones, M.C. (1924). A laboratory study of fear: The case of Peter. *Journal of Genetic Psychology*, **31**, 308–315.

Kagan, J. (1989). Temperamental contributions to social behavior. *American Psychologist*, **44**, 668–674.

Kane, M.T. and Kendall, P.C. (1989). Anxiety disorders in children: A multiple-baseline evaluation of a cognitive-behavioral treatment. *Behavior Therapy*, **20**, 499–508.

Kashani, J.H. and Orvaschel, H. (1990). A community study of anxiety in children and adolescents. *American Journal of Psychiatry*, **147**, 313–318.

Kashani, J.H., Orvaschel, H., Rosenberg, T.K., and Reid, J.C. (1989). Psychopathology in a community sample of children and adolescents: A developmental perspective. *Journal of the American Academy of Child and Adolescent Psychiatry*, **28**, 701–706.

Kazdin, A. (1994). Psychotherapy with children and adolsecents. In A.E. Bergin and S.L. Garfield (Eds.), *Handbook of psychotherapy and behaviour change* (pp. 19–71). New York: Wiley.

Keller, M.B., Lavori, P.W., Wunder, J., Beardslee, W.R., Schwartz, C.E., and Roth, J. (1992). Chronic course of anxiety disorders in children and adolescents. *Journal of the American Academy of Child and Adolescent Psychiatry*, **31**, 595–599.

Kendall, P.C. (1994). Treating anxiety disorders in children: Results of a randomized clinical trial. *Journal of Consulting and Clinical Psychology*, **62**, 100–110.

Kendall, P.C. and Chansky, T.E. (1991). Considering cognition in anxiety-disordered children. Special Issue: Assessment of childhood anxiety disorders. *Journal of Anxiety Disorders*, **5**, 167–185.

Kendall, P.C., and Southam-Gerow, M.A. (1996). Long-term follow-up of a cognitive-behavioural therapy for anxiety-disordered youth. *Journal of Consulting and Clinical Psychology*, **64**, 724–730.

Kendler, K.S., Neale, M.C., Kessler, R.C., Heath, A.C., and Eaves, L.J. (1992). Generalized anxiety disorder in women. A population based twin study. *Archives of General Psychiatry*, **49**, 267–272.

Kipper, D.A. (1977). Behavior therapy for fears brought on by war experiences. *Journal of Consulting and Clinical Psychology*, **45**, 216–221.

Klein, D.F., Mannuzza, S., Chapman, T., and Fyer, A. (1992). Child panic revisited. *Journal of the American Academy of Child and Adolescent Psychiatry*, **31**, 112–113.

Kovacs, M., Gatsonis, C., Paulauskas, S., and Richards, C. (1989). Depressive disorders in childhood. IV. A longitudinal study of comorbidity with and risk for anxiety disorders. *Archives of General Psychiatry*, **46**, 776–782.

Lang, P.J. (1971). The application of psychophysiological methods to the study of psychotherapy and behavior modification. In A.E. Bergin and S.L. Garfield (Eds.), *Handbook of psychotherapy and behaviour change* (pp. 75–125). New York: Wiley.

Last, C.G. (1991). Somatic complaints in anxiety disordered children. *Journal of Anxiety Disorders*, **5**, 125–138.

Last, C.G., Francis, G., Hersen, M., Kazdin, A.E., and Strauss, C.C. (1987). Separation anxiety and school phobia: A comparison using DSM-III criteria. *American Journal of Psychiatry*, **144**, 653–657.

Last, C.G., Francis, G., and Strauss, C.C. (1989). Assessing fears in anxiety disordered children with the revised Fear Survey Schedule for Children (FSSC-R). *Journal of Clinical Child Psychology*, **18**, 137–141.

Last, C.G., Hersen, M., Kazdin, A.E., Finkelstein, R., and Strauss, C.C. (1987). Comparison of DSM-III separation anxiety and overanxious disorders: demographic characteristics and patterns of comorbidity. *Journal of the American Academy of Child and Adolescent Psychiatry*, **26**, 527–531.

Last, C.G., Hersen, M., Kazdin, A.E., Orvaschel, H., and Perrin, S. (1991). Anxiety disorders in children and their families. *Archives of General Psychiatry*, **48**, 928–934.

Last, C.G., Perrin, S., Hersen, M., and Kazdin, A.E. (1992). DSM-III-R anxiety disorders in children: Sociodemographic and clinical charateristics. *Journal of the American Academy of Child and Adolescent Psychiatry*, **31**, 1070–1076.

Last, C.G., Phillips, J.E., and Statfeld, A. (1987). Childhood anxiety disorders in mothers and their children. *Child Psychiatry and Human Development*, **18**, 103–109.

Last, C.G. and Strauss, C.C. (1989a). Panic disorder in children and adolescents. *Journal of Anxiety Disorders*, **3**, 87–95.

Last, C.G. and Strauss, C.C. (1989b). Obsessive-compulsive disorder in childhood. *Journal of Anxiety Disorders*, **3**, 295–302.

Last, C.G., Strauss, C.C., and Francis, G. (1987). Comorbidity among childhood anxiety disorders. *Journal of Nervous and Mental Diseases*, **175**, 726–730.

Laucht, M.E. and Schmidt, M.H. (1987). Psychiatric disorders at the age of 3: Results and problems of a long-term study. In Cooper (Ed.), *Psychiatric epidemiology*. London: Croom Helm.

Lautch, H. (1971). Dental phobia. *British Journal of Psychiatry*, **119**, 151–158.

Leonard, H.L., Swedo, S.E., Rapoport, J.L., Koby, E.V., Lenane, D.L., and Hamburger, S.D. (1989). Treatment of Obsessive-Compulsive disorder with clomipramine and desipramine in children and adolescents. *Archives of General Psychiatry*, **46**, 1088–1092.

Levey, A.B. and Martin, I. (1983). Cognitions, evaluations and conditioning: Rules of sequence and rules of consequence. *Advances in Behaviour Research and Therapy*, **4**, 181–195.

Lyons, J.A. (1987). Posttraumatic stress disorder in children and in adolescents: A review of the literature. *Developmental and Behavioral Pediatrics*, **8**, 349–356.

Macaulay, J.L. and Kleinknecht, R.A. (1989). Panic and panic attacks in adolescents. *Journal of Anxiety Disorders*, **3**, 221–241.

March, J.S., Mulle, K., and Herbel, B. (1994). Behavioral psychotherapy for children and adolescents with obsessive-compulsive disorder: An open trial of a new protocol-driven treatment package. *Journal of the American Academy of Child and Adolescent Psychiatry*, **33**, 333–341.

March, J.S. (1995). Cognitive-behavioural psychotherapy for children and adolescents with OCD: A review and recommendations for treatment. *Journal of the American Academy of Child and Adolescent Psychiatry*, **34**, 7–18.

Marks, I.M. and Gelder, M.G. (1966). Different ages of onset in varieties of phobias. *American Journal of Psychiatry*, **123**, 218–221.

Martin, I. and Levey, A.B. (1983). Cognitions, evaluations and conditioning. Rules of sequence and rules of consequence. *Advances in Behaviour Research and Therapy*, **4**, 181–195.

McGee, R., Freehan, M., Williams, S., Partridge, F., Silva, P.A., and Kelly, J. (1990). DSM-III disorders in a large sample of adolescents. *Journal of the American Academy of Child and Adolescent Psychiatry*, **29**, 611–619.

McGlynn, F.D. and McNeil, D.W. (1990). Simple phobia in adulthood. In M. Hersen and C.G. Last (Eds.), *Handbook of child and adult psychopathology* (pp. 197–208). New York: Pergamon.

McLeer, S.V., Deblinger, E., Atkins, M.S., Foa, E.B., and Ralphe, D.L. (1988). Post-Traumatic Stress Disorder in sexually abused children. *Journal of the American Academy of Child and Adolescent Psychiatry*, **27**, 650–654.

McNally, R.J. and Steketee, G.S. (1985). The etiology and maintenance of severe animal phobias. *Behaviour Research and Therapy*, **23**, 431–435.

Menzies, R.G. and Clarke, J.C. (1993). The etiology of childhood water phobia. *Behaviour Research and Therapy*, **31**, 499–501.

Menzies, R.G. and Clarke, J.C. (1995). The etiology of phobias: A nonassociative account. *Clinical Psychology Review*, **15**, 23–48.

Merkelbach, H. (1989). *Preparedness and classical conditioning of fear: A critical inquiry*. Dissertation, University of Limburg, The Netherlands.

Merkelbach, H., de Ruiter, C., Van den Hout, M.A., and Hoekstra, R. (1989). Conditioning experiences and phobias. *Behaviour Research and Therapy*, **27**, 657–662.

Milgrom, P., Mancl, L., King, B., and Weinstein, P. (1995). Origins of childhood dental fear. *Behaviour Research and Therapy*, **33**, 313–319.

Miller, L.C., Barrett, C.L., Hampe, E., and Noble, H. (1971). Revised anxiety scales for the Louisville Behavior Checklist. *Psychological Reports*, **29**, 503–511.

Mineka, S. (1979). The role of fear in theories of avoidance learning, flooding, and extinction. *Psychological Bulletin*, **86**, 985–1010.

Mineka, S. (1987). A primate model of phobic fears. In H.J. Eysenck and I. Martin (Eds.), *Theoretical foundations of behavior therapy* (pp. 81–111). New York, Plenum Press.

Morris R.J. and Kratochwill, T.R. (1983). *Treating children's fears and phobias.* New York: Pergamon.

Mowrer, O.H. (1947). On the dual nature of learning — a reinterpretation of "conditioning" and "problem solving". *Harvard Educational Review,* **17**, 102–148.

Mowrer, O.H. (1960). Learning theory and behavior. New York: Wiley.

Mufson, L., Weissman, M.M., and Warner, V. (1992). Depression and anxiety in parents and children: A direct interview study. *Journal of Anxiety disorders,* **6**, 1–13.

Murray, E.J. and Foote, F. (1979). The origins of fear of snakes. *Behaviour Research and Therapy,* **17**, 489–493.

Öhman, A. (1988). The psychophysiology of emotion: An evolutionary-cognitive perspective. In P.K. Ackles, J.R. Jennings, and M.G.H. Coles (Eds.), *Advances in Psychophysiology* (Vol. 2, pp. 79–127). Greenwich: JAI Press.

Ollendick, T.H. (1983). Reliability and validity of the revised Fear Survey Schedule for Children (FSSC-R). *Behaviour Research and Therapy,* **21**, 685–692.

Ollendick, T.H. and Francis, G. (1988). Behavioral assessment and treatment of childhood phobias. Special Issue: Behavioral assessment and treatment of childhood anxiety disorders. *Behavior Modification,* **12**, 165–204.

Ollendick, T.H. and King, N.J. (1991). Origins of childhood fears: An evaluation of Rachman's theory of fear acquisition. *Behaviour Research and Therapy,* **29**, 117–123.

Öst, L-G. (1987). Age of onset in different phobias. *Journal of Abnormal Psychology,* **96**, 223–229.

Öst, L-G. and Hugdahl, K. (1981). Acquisition of phobias and anxiety response patterns in clinical patients. *Behaviour Research and Therapy,* **19**, 439–447.

Öst, L-G. and Hugdahl, K. (1985). Acquisition of blood and dental phobia and anxiety response patterns in clinical patients. *Behaviour Research and Therapy,* **23**, 27–34.

Popper, C.W. (1993). Psychopharmacologic treatment of anxiety disorders in adolescents and children. *Journal of Clinical Psychiatry,* **54**, 52–63.

Puig-Antich, J. and Chambers, W. (1978). *The Schedule for Affective Disorders and Schizophrenia for School-aged Children.* New York: State Psychiatric Institute.

Puig-Antich, J., Lukens, E., Davies, M., Goetz, D., Brennan-Quattrock, J., and Todak, G. (1985). Psychosocial functioning in prepubertal major depressive disorders: Interpersonal relationships during the depressive episode. *Archives of General Psychiatry,* **42**, 500–507.

Quay, H.C. and Peterson, D.R. (1983). *Manual for the Revised Behavior Problem Checklist.* Unpublished Manuscript.

Rachman, S. (1991). Neo-conditioning and the classical theory of fear acquisition. *Clinical Psychology Review,* **11**, 155–173.

Rasmussen, S.A. and Tsuang, M.T. (1986). Clinical characteristics and family history in DSM-III obsessive-compulsive disorder. *American Journal of Psychiatry,* **143**, 317–322.

Reich, W. and Welner, Z. (1988). *Revised version of the Diagnostic Interview for Children and Adolescents (DICA-R).* St. Louis, MO: Department of Psychiatry, Washington University, School of Medicine.

Reynolds, C.R. and Richmond, B.O. (1978). What I think and feel: A revised measure of children's manifest anxiety. *Journal of Abnormal Child Psychology,* **6**, 271–280.

Riddle, M.A., Scahill, L., King, R.A., Hardin, M.T., Anderson, G.M., Ort, S.I., Smith, J.C., Leckman, J.F., and Cohen, D.J. (1992). Double blind crossover trial of fluoxetine and placebo in children and adolescents with obsessive-compulsive disorder. *Journal of the American Academy of Child and Adolescent Psychiatry,* **31**, 1062–1069.

Rimm, D.C., Janda, L.H., Lancaster, D.W., Nahl, M., and Ditmar, K. (1977). An exploratory investigation of the origin and maintenance of phobias. *Behaviour Research and Therapy,* **15**, 231–238.

Rosenbaum, J.F., Biederman, J., Hirschfeld, D.R., Bolduc, E.A., Faraone, S.V., Kagan, J., Snidman, N., and Reznick, J.S. (1991). Further evidence of an association between behavioral inhibition and anxiety disorders: Results from a family study of children from a non-clinical sample. *Journal of Psychiatric Research*, **25**, 49–65.

Scherer, M.W. and Nakamura, C.Y. (1968). A Fear Survey Schedule for Children (FSSC-FC): A factor-analytic comparison with manifest anxiety (CMAS). *Behavior Research and Therapy*, **6**, 173–182.

Seligman, M.E.P. (1971). Phobias and preparedness. *Behavior Therapy*, **2**, 307–320.

Silverman, W.K., Albano, A.M., and Barlow, D. (1994). *The Anxiety Disorders Interview Schedule for Children: Parent, and child versions.* Albany, Center for Stress and Anxiety Disorders.

Silverman, W.K. and Eisen, A.R. (1992). Age differences in the reliability of parent and child reports of child anxious symptomatology using a structured interview. *Journal of the American Academy of Child and Adolescent Psychiatry*, **31**, 117–124.

Silverman, W.K. and Nelles, W.B. (1988). The Anxiety Disorders Interview Schedule for Children. *Journal of the American Academy of Child and Adolescent Psychiatry*, **27**, 772–778.

Simeon, J.G., Ferguson, H.B., Knott, V., Roberts, N. *et al.* (1992). Clinical, cognitive and neurophysiological effects of alprazolam in children and adolescents with overanxious and avoidant disorder. *Journal of the American Academy of Child and Adolescent Psychiatry*, **31**, 29–33.

Skre, I., Onstad, S., Torgersen, S., Lygren, S., and Kringlen, E. (1993). A twin study of DSM-III-R anxiety disorders. *Acta Psychiatrica Scandinavia*, **88**, 85–92.

Strauss, C.C., Lahey, B.B., Frick, P., Frame, C.L., and Hynd, G.W. (1988). Peer social status of children with anxiety disorders. *Journal of Consulting and Clinical Psychology*, **56**, 137–141.

Strauss, C.C. and Last, C.G. (1993). Social and simple phobias in children. *Journal of Anxiety Disorders*, **7**, 141–152.

Strauss, C.C., Lease, C.A., Last, C.G., and Francis, G. (1988). Overanxious disorder: An examination of developmental differences. *Journal of Abnormal Psychology*, **16**, 433–443.

Swedo, S.E., Rapoport, J.L., Leonard, H., Leane, M., and Cheslow, D. (1989). Obsessive-compulsive disorder in children and adolescents: Clinical phenomenology of 70 consecutive cases. *Archives of General Psychiatry*, **46**, 335–341.

Terr, L.C. (1983). Chowchilla revisited: The effects of psychic trauma four years after a schoolbus kidnapping. *American Journal of Psychiatry*, **140**, 1543–1550.

Thyer, B.A. and Sowars-Hoag, K.M. (1988). Behavior Therapy for separation anxiety disorder. *Behavior Modification*, **12**, 205–233.

Thyrer, B.A. (1993). Childhood separation anxiety disorder and adult onset agoraphobia: Review of evidence. In C.G. Last (Ed.), *Anxiety across the lifespan: A developmental perspective* (pp. 128–147). New York: Springer.

Torgersen, S. (1979). The nature and origin of common phobic fears. *British Journal of Psychiatry*, **134**, 343–351.

Torgersen, S. (1983). Genetic factors in anxiety disorders. *Archives of General Psychiatry*, **40**, 1085–1089.

Torgersen, S. (1986). Childhood and family characteristics in panic and generalized anxiety disorders. *American Journal of Psychiatry*, **143**, 630–632.

Torgersen, S. (1988). Genetics. In C.G. Last and M. Hersen (Eds.), *Handbook of anxiety disorders* (pp. 159–170). New York: Pergamon Press.

Torgersen, S. (1990). Comorbidity of major depression and anxiety disorders in twin pairs. *American Journal of Psychiatry*.

Turner, S., Beidel, D.C., and Costello, A. (1987). Psychopathology in the offspring of anxiety disorder patients. *Journal of Consulting and Clinical Psychology*, **55**, 229–235.

Turner, S., Beidel, D.C., and Epstein, L.H. (1991). Vulnerability and risk for anxiety disorders. *Journal of Anxiety Disorders*, **5**, 151–166.

Velez, C.N., Johnson, J., and Cohen, P. (1989). A longitudinal analysis of selected risk factors for childhood psychopathology. *Journal of the American Academy of Child and Adolescent Psychiatry*, **28**, 861–864.

Watson, J. and Rayner, R. (1920). Conditioned emotional reactions. *Journal of Experimental Psychology*, **3**, 1–22.

Warren, R. and Zgourides, G. (1988). Panic attacks in high school students: Implications for prevention and intervention. *Phobia Practice and Research Journal*, **1**, 97–113.

Weissman, M.M. (1988). The epidemiology of anxiety disorders: Rates, risks and familial patterns. *Journal of Psychiatric Research*, **22**, 99–114.

Weisz, J.R., Weiss, B, Alicke, M.D., and Klotz, M.L. (1987). Effectiveness of psychotherapy with children and adolescents. A meta-analysis for clinicians. *Journal of Consulting and Clinical Psychology*, **55**, 542–549.

Weisz, J.R., Weiss, B., Han, S.S., Granger, D.A. and Morton, T. (1995). Effects of psychotherapy with children and adolescents revisited: A meta-analysis of treatment outcome studies. *Psychological Bulletin*, **17**, 450–468.

Werry, J.S., Reeves, J.C., Elkind, G.S. (1987). Attention deficit, conduct, oppositional, and anxiety disorders in children: I: A review of research on differentiating characteristics. *Journal of the American Academy of Child and Adolescent Psychiatry*, **26**, 133–143.

Whitaker, A., Johnson, J., Shaffer, D., Rapoport, J.L., Kalikow, W., Walsh, T.B., Davies, M., Braiman, S., and Dolinsky, A. (1990). Uncommon troubles in young people: Prevalence estimate of selected psychiatric disorders in a nonreferred adolescent population. *Archives of General Psychiatry*, **47**, 487–496.

Windheuser, H.J. (1977). Anxious mothers as models for coping with anxiety. *Behavioural Analysis and Modification*, **1**, 39–58.

Woolston, J., Rosenthal, S.L., Riddle, M.A., Sparrow, S.S., Cicchetti, D., and Zimmerman, I. (1989). Childhood comorbidity of anxiety/affective disorders and behavior disorders. *Journal of the American Academy of Child and Adolescent Psychiatry*, **30**, 973–981.

World Health Organization (1993). *The ICD-10 classification of mental and behavioural disorders*. Geneva: World Health Organization.

Zoccolillo, M. (1992). Co-occurrence of conduct disorder and its adult outcomes with depressive and anxiety disorders: A review. *Journal of the American Academy of Child and Adolescent Psychiatry*, **31**, 547–556.

CHAPTER 8
MOOD DISORDERS

Cecilia Ahmoi Essau and
Ulrike Petermann

Until about three decades ago, there was a prevailing assumption that mood disorders rarely occurred in children and adolescents, although descriptions of melancholia in children can be traced back to the mid-eighteenth century (see Merikangas and Angst, in press for a review). This view stems from the theoretical notion that children do not have sufficient cognitive maturity to be depressed, and the concept that psychopathological manifestations and difficulties represent normal developmental processes of childhood and adolescence (Rie, 1966).

In considering the possibility of mood disorders in children and adolescents, some authors proposed the concept of "masked depression" during the late 1960s and early 1970s. According to this concept, mood disorders do occur in children, but depressive symptoms are manifested primarily as somatic symptoms, conduct disturbances, enuresis, and encopresis (Cytryn and McKnew, 1972). Despite these early assumptions, there has been an increasing recognition that children and adolescents exhibit the essential features of adult depression. This change in viewpoints is reflected in the use of the same adult criteria for mood disorders in children and adolescents in the third edition of the Diagnostic and Statistical Manual of Mental Disorders (DSM-III; American Psychiatric Association; APA, 1980), and in its revised (DSM-III-R; APA, 1987) and most recent versions (DSM-IV; APA, 1994). In the DSM-IV, mood disorders are divided into the depressive disorders, the bipolar disorders, and two disorders which are based on their etiology (mood disorder due to a general medical condition and substance-induced mood disorders). Both DSM-IV and ICD-10 systems contain categories for single episodes of mood disorders and for recurrent episodes. They both recognize mild but persisted mood disturbance; in the DSM-IV, there is a sustained depressed mood (dysthymic disorder) whereas in ICD-10, this is shown in a repeated alternatives high and low mood (cyclothymic disorder).

Definition and Classification

Depressive Disorders

Depressive disorders are characterized by the presence of depressed moods along with a set of additional symptoms, persisting over time, and causing disruption and impairment of function. In DSM-IV (APA, 1994), depressive disorders fall under the category of major depressive disorder, dysthymic disorder, and depressive disorder not otherwise specified. While all adult depressive disorders can be diagnosed in childhood and adolescence, minor criterion changes may be made for children and adolescents. These include the substitution of "irritability" for "depressed mood", and the substitution of "failure to make expected weight gains" for "weight loss" in the diagnosis of major depressive disorder. One year's duration, instead of two, will suffice for the diagnosis of dysthymic disorder in children and adolescents.

Major Depressive Disorder

Major depressive disorder denotes a severe, acute form of depressive disorder (DSM-IV; APA, 1994). The disorder is diagnosed when the child or adolescent has experienced at least five of the following nine symptoms nearly every day for at least a two-week period at a level that represents a change from previous functioning: depressed mood (or can be irritable mood in children and adolescents); markedly diminished interest or pleasure in all, or almost all activities; significant weight loss or weight gain, or decrease or increase in appetite (in children, consider failure to make expected weight gains); insomnia or hypersomnia; psychomotor agitation or retardation; fatigue or loss of energy; feelings of worthlessness or excessive or inappropriate guilt; diminished ability to think or concentrate, or indecisiveness; and recurrent thoughts of death, recurrent suicidal ideation without a specific plan, or a suicide attempt or a specific plan for committing suicide (Table 8.1).

At least one of the two cardinal symptoms, *depressed mood* (or irritable mood in children and adolescents) or *loss of interest or pleasure* must be present for the diagnosis to be made (APA, 1994). The diagnosis may not be made if (a) symptoms meet criteria for a mixed episode (i.e., symptoms of a manic and major depressive episode) that occur almost daily for a period of at least one week; (b) symptoms are a result of direct physiological effects of a substance or a general medical condition; or (c) symptoms are accounted for by a normal reaction to the loss of a loved one (bereavement).

Table 8.1 Criteria for major depressive episode

A) Five (or more) of the following symptoms have been present during the same 2-week period and represent a change from previous functioning: at least one of the symptoms is either (1) depressed mood or (2) loss of interest or pleasure.

 Note: Do not include symptoms that are clearly due to a general medical condition, or mood-incongruent delusions or hallucinations.

1) depressed mood most of the day, nearly every day, as indicated by either subjective report (e.g., feels sad or empty) or observation made by others (e.g., appears tearful). **Note**: In children and adolescents, can be irritable mood.
2) markedly diminished interest or pleasure in all, or almost all, activities most of the day, nearly every day (as indicated by either subjective account or observation made by others)
3) significant weight loss when not dieting or weight gain (e.g., a change of more than 5% of body weight in a month), or decrease or increase in appetite nearly every day. **Note**: In children, consider failure to make expected weight gains
4) insomnia or hypersomnia nearly every day
5) psychomotor agitation or retardation nearly every day (observable by others, not merely subjective feelings of restlessness or being slowed down)
6) fatigue or loss of energy nearly every day
7) feelings of worthlessness or excessive or inappropriate guilt (which may be delusional) nearly every day (not merely self-reproach or guilt about being sick)
8) diminished ability to think or concentrate, or indecisiveness nearly every day (either by subjective account or as observed by others)
9) recurrent thoughts of death (not just fear of dying), recurrent suicidal ideation without specific plan, or a suicide attempt or a specific plan for committing suicide

B) The symptoms do not meet criteria for a mixed episode

C) The symptoms cause clinically significant distress or impairment in social, occupational, or other important areas of functioning

D) The symptoms are not better account for by bereavement, i.e., after the loss of a loved one, the symptoms persist for longer than 2 months or are characterized by marked functional impairment, morbid preoccupation with worthlessness, suicidal ideation, psychotic symptoms, or psychomotor retardation

Reprinted with permission from the Diagnostic and Statistical Manual of Mental Disorders, Fourth Edition. Copyright 1994 American Psychiatric Association.

Major depressive disorder may be specified as a single episode or as recurrent, the former indicates the presence of a single and the latter the presence of two or more major depressive episodes. Major depressive episodes can be classified as mild, moderate, severe without psychotic features, or severe with psychotic features. If the episode fails to meet these severity criteria, it is described as either being in partial or in full remission. Additionally, major depressive episodes can be specified as chronic, with catatonic features, with melancholic features, with atypical features, and postpartum onset.

Dysthymic Disorder

Dysthymic disorder is a chronic, but a less severe form of depressive disorder (DSM-IV; APA, 1994). Children and adolescents are diagnosed with this disorder when they have had a period of at least one year in which they have shown depressed or irritable moods every day without more than two symptom-free months. Together with irritable or depressed mood, at least two of the following symptoms must be present: poor appetite or overeating, insomnia or hypersomnia, low energy or fatigue, low self-esteem, poor concentration or difficulty making decisions, and feelings of hopelessness. The diagnosis of dysthymic disorder is made if (a) a major depressive episode has never been present during the initial year of the disorder; (b) neither manic, mixed, or a hypomanic episodes, or cyclothymic disorder have ever been present; (c) the disorder did not occur during the course of a chronic psychotic disorder; and (d) the symptoms are not due to physiological effects of a substance or a general medical factor. Dysthymic disorder can be specified as having an early onset (i.e., onset of the dysthymic symptoms before age 21 years), late onset (i.e., onset of the dysthymic symptoms at age 21 years or older), and with atypical features.

Bipolar Disorders

Bipolar disorders are divided into bipolar I disorder, bipolar II disorder, cyclothymic disorder, and bipolar disorder not otherwise specified (DSM-IV; APA, 1994). Bipolar in children and adolescents include the same core components present in the adult which clinical manifestations involve the presence of manic, mixed or hypomanic episodes, as well as major depressive episodes.

Bipolar I Disorder

Bipolar I disorder is characterized by the presence of at least one manic or mixed episode (DSM-IV; APA, 1994). Additionally, individuals often have had at least one major depressive episodes. As shown in Table 8.2, manic episode is described as a notable period of abnormally and persistently elevated, expansive, or irritable mood that last for one week or more. Additionally, three of seven (four if evidence of the essential symptom is

Table 8.2   Criteria for manic episode

A)   A distinct period of abnormally and persistently elevated, expansive, or irritable mood, lasting at least 1 week (or any duration if hospitalization is necessary)

B)   During the period of mood disturbance, three (or more) of the following symptoms have persisted (four if the mood is only irritable) and have been present to a significant degree:

   1) inflated self-esteem or grandiosity
   2) decreased need for sleep (e.g., feels rested after only 3 hours of sleep)
   3) more talkative than usual or pressure to keep talking
   4) flight of ideas or subjective experience that thoughts are racing
   5) distractibility (i.e., attention too easily drawn to unimportant or irrelevant external stimuli)
   6) increase in goal-directed activity (either socially, at work or school, or sexually) or psychomotor agitation
   7) excessive involvement in pleasurable activities that have a high potential for painful consequences (e.g., engaging in unrestrained buying sprees, sexual indiscretions, or foolish business investments)

C)   The symptoms do not meet criteria for a mixed episode

D)   The mood disturbance is sufficiently severe to cause marked impairment in occupational functioning or in usual social activities or relationships with others, or to necessitate hospitalization to prevent harm to self or others, or there are psychotic features

E)   The symptoms are not due to the direct physiological effects of a substance (e.g., a drug of abuse, a medication, or other treatment) or a general medical condition (e.g., hyperthyroidism)

   Note: Manic-like episodes that are clearly caused by somatic antidepressant treatment (e.g., medication, electroconvulsive therapy, light therapy) should not count toward a diagnosis of biploar disorder

---

Reprinted with permission from the Diagnostic and Statistical Manual of Mental Disorders, Fourth Edition. Copyright 1994 American Psychiatric Association.

irritability) symptoms must also be present including grandiosity, decreased need for sleep, increased talkativeness, flight of ideas, distractibility, increased goal-directed activity, and excessive involvement in pleasurable activities which have a high potential for painful consequence. A mixed episode is characterized by a period of at least one week in which the criteria of manic and major depressive episodes are met nearly everyday.

A diagnosis of bipolar I disorder is not met if the symptoms are due to episodes of substance-induced mood disorder or of mood disorder due to a general medical condition, or of mood disorder due to a general medical condition. The episodes are not accounted for by schizo-affective disorder and are not superimposed on schizophrenia, schizo-phreniform disorder, delusional disorder, or psychotic disorder not otherwise specified.

Bipolar II Disorder

The bipolar II disorder is characterized by the occurrence of one or more major depressive episodes which are accompanied by at least one hypo-manic episode (DSM-IV; APA, 1994). Hypomanic episode is defined as a period of elevated, expansive or irritable mood that persistently last for at least four days. This period is accompanied by three or more of the following symptoms: inflated self-esteem, decreased need for sleep, pressure of speech, flight of ideas, distractibility, increased involvement in goal-directed activities, and excessive involvement in pleasurable activities with high potential for painful consequences. Although the disturbances in mood is noticed by others, the episode is not severe enough to cause marked impairment in social or occupational functioning, or to require hospitalization. The diagnosis of bipolar II disorder is precluded if a manic or mixed episode is present. Episodes of substance-induced mood disorder or of mood disorder due to a general medical condition do not count toward a diagnosis of bipolar II disorder.

Cyclothymic Disorder

This disorder refers to chronic, fluctuating mood disturbance that involve numerous periods of depressive and hypomanic symptoms that last at least one year for children and adolescents, compared to two years for adults (DSM-IV; APA, 1994). However, the number, severity, pervasiveness or duration of hypomanic symptoms are not sufficient to meet the full criteria for a manic episode. Similarly, depressive symptoms are not enough in number, severity, pervasiveness, or duration to meet the full criteria for a major depressive episode. The diagnosis of cyclothymic disorder is not met if the mood swing is accounted for by schizoaffective disorder or is superimposed on a psychiatric disorder. The mood disturbance must not be the consequence of direct physiological effects of a substance or a general medical condition. The symptoms cause significant impairments in important areas of functioning such as in social and occupational areas.

Other Mood Disorders

Mood Disorder due to a General Medical Condition

This disorder is characterized by the persistent disturbance in mood due to a direct physiological effects of a general medical condition as evidenced from history, physical examination, or laboratory findings (DSM-IV; APA, 1994). The mood disturbance can involve depressed mood or markedly diminished interest or pleasure, or elevated, expansive, or irritable mood. The disturbance is not due to another mental disorders, and that it does not occur exclusively during the course of a delirium. The mood disturbance cause marked impairment in social, occupational, or other important areas of functioning.

Substance-induced Mood Disorder

The core feature of substance-induced mood disorder is a prominent and persistent disturbance in mood (depressed mood, diminished interest or pleasure; elevated, expansive or irritable mood) due to the direct physiological effects of a substance (DSM-IV; APA, 1994). As evidenced from history, physical examination, or laboratory findings, the symptoms develop during, or within a month of substance-intoxication or withdrawal. The diagnosis is not made if the mood disturbance is accounted for a mood disorder that is not substance induced, or if it occurs only during the course of delirium. The symptoms cause marked impairment in social, occupational, or other important areas of functioning.

EPIDEMIOLOGY

Numerous studies have assessed the prevalence of depressive disorders in children and adolescents in the general population, with prevalences varying across studies (Table 8.3). The rates of major depressive disorder

Table 8.3 Prevalence of major depressive disorder and dysthymic disorder in children and adolescents

Authors/years	Age (years)	Diagnostic Instrument/ (diagnostic criteria)	Major depressive disorder (%)				Dysthymic disorder (%)
			LT	1-year	6-month	Point	
Deykin et al. (1987)	16–19	DIS (DSM-III)	6.8	–	–	–	–
Kashani et al. (1987)	14–16	DICA (DSM-III)	–	–	–	4.7	8.0
McGee and Williams (1988)	15	DISC (DSM-III)	1.9	–	–	1.2	1.1
Velez et al. (1989)	13–18	DISC (DSM-III-R)	–	–	–	3.7	–
Fleming et al. (1989)	12–16	SDI (DSM-III)	–	–	9.8	–	–
Whitaker et al. (1991)	14–17	Clinical Interview (DSM-III)	4.0	–	–	–	4.9
Lewinsohn et al. (1993)	14–18	K-SADS-E (DSM-III-R)	18.4	–	–	2.9	0.5
Reinherz et al. (1993)	18	DIS-III-R (DSM-III-R)	9.4	–	6.0	–	–
Fergusson et al. (1993)	15	DISC (DSM-III-R)	–	4.2	–	0.7	0.4
Cooper and Goodyer (1993)	11–16	DISC (DSM-III-R)	–	6.0	3.6	–	–
Feehan et al. (1994)	18	DIS-III-R (DSM-III-R)	–	16.7	–	–	–

% = Prevalence rates; LT = lifetime prevalence rates; 1-year = 1-year prevalence rates; 6-month = 6-month prevalence rates; point = point prevalence rates; DIS = Diagnostic Interview Schedule; DISC = Diagnostic Interview Schedule for Children; DICA = Diagnostic Interview for Children and Adolescents; K-SADS-E = Schedule for Affective Disorders and Schizophrenia for School-age Children (Epidemiologic version); DIS-III-R = Diagnostic Interview Schedule, revised version; SDI = Survey Diagnostic Instrument; – = Not reported in preschool children are less than 1% (Kashani *et al.*, 1986; Kashani and Carlson, 1987). Major depressive disorder is more common in school-age children, with a point prevalence of about 2% (Anderson *et al.*, 1987; Kashani and Simonds, 1979). It is even more common in adolescents, with a point prevalence of about 5%, and a lifetime rate of about 10% (range from 6.8 to 18.4%) (Feehan *et al.*, 1994; Fergusson *et al.*, 1993; Kashani *et al.*, 1987; Lewinsohn *et al.*, 1993; McGee and Williams, 1988). Prevalences of dysthymic disorder also vary widely across studies, with values ranging from 0.1 to 8% (Fergusson *et al.*, 1993; Lewinsohn *et al.*, 1993; McGee and Williams, 1988; Whitaker *et al.*, 1990). Compared with major depressive disorder, bipolar disorder is much rarer in the general population, with lifetime rates ranging from 0.4–1.2% (Carlson and Kashani, 1988; Lewinsohn *et al.*, 1993). Based on the ECA data, the lifetime prevalence of bipolar disorder in the 18–24 years was 1.3%, and among the 14–16 year olds 0.7% (Robins *et al.*, 1984).

Depressive symptoms that do not meet full criteria for major depressive disorder are relatively common. On the basis of self-report questionnaires such as the Beck Depression Inventory and the Centre for Epidemiologic Studies-Depression Scale, about 34% of the adolescents in the general population ages 11–19 years have experienced depressive symptoms sometimes in their life (see Merikangas and Angst, in press for review). Based on the modified form of the Diagnostic Interview Schedule for Children, Cooper and Goodyer (1993) found the most common depressive symptoms among girls attending secondary school were depressed mood, social withdrawal and insomnia; depressive thoughts such as guilt and feelings of worthlessness occurred less often. In a large community survey of adolescents aged 12–16 years using the Revised Ontario Child Health Study Scales which operationalizes depressive symptoms according to DSM-III-R, Boyle *et al.* (1993) found "diminished ability to think or concentrate or indecisiveness" and "depressive mood" as the most common depressive symptoms. High rates of suicidal behaviour were also found, with about 14.6% of the adolescents reported having had suicidal ideation, and 6% had actually attempted suicide (Boyle *et al.*, 1993). In a study that used the German translation of the Revised Ontario Child Health Study Scales, Essau *et al.* (1995b, 1995b, 1996) reported the most common depressive symptoms among German high school adolescents aged 12–18 years to be "diminished ability to think or concentrate or indecisiveness" and being "overtired". About 15.9% of the adolescents have had suicidal ideation and 5.6% had attempted suicide.

Since little research has been done on bipolar disorder and other mood disorders (mood disorder due to a general medical condition, and substance-induced mood disorder), our review will concentrate on major depressive disorder.

RISK FACTORS

Sociodemographic Factors

Sex

Whereas no significant sex differences (Anderson *et al.*, 1987; Fleming *et al.*, 1989) have been reported among preadolescents, studies of adolescents have reported 2 to 3 times higher rates of depressive disorders in girls than in boys (Aro, 1994; Cohen *et al.*, 1993; Fleming *et al.*, 1989; Kashani *et al.*, 1987; Lewinsohn *et al.*, 1993; Rutter, 1986, 1989; Reinherz *et al.*, 1993). A tendency toward a change in the sex ratio usually occurs around puberty (Cohen *et al.*, 1993; Harrington *et al.*, 1990; Petersen *et al.*, 1991). Petersen *et al.* (1991), for example, showed that girls were significantly more depressed than boys by grade 12, with sex differences emerging around grade 8, increasing over time. Using data from the Dunedin Study, McGee *et al.* (1992) found a male to female sex ratio of 4.3:1 at age 11, and 0.4:1 at age 15.

Most authors consider this sex difference in adolescence to be a true difference rather than simply an artifact of differences in styles of responding to questions or differences in openness (Nolen-Hoeksema, 1987; Nolen-Hoeksema *et al.*, 1991). Explanations given for this sex difference include divergent socialization practices concerning power and control, management of feelings and sex role orientation, as well as differences in the biological changes of puberty (Petersen *et al.*, 1991; Simmons and Blyth, 1987). Another explanation is that girls experience more challenges in early adolescence (Petersen *et al.*, 1991), and that they are more affected than boys by stressful life events such as parental divorce (Block *et al.*, 1986; Petersen *et al.*, 1991). Others (Aro, 1994) suggested that the coping styles of girls are less effective and more dysfunctional compared to boys.

Female adolescents do not only have a higher prevalence of major depressive disorder when compared to boys, but they also experience more severe depressive episodes (Reinherz *et al.*, 1993). Specifically, about three-quarters of the females with major depressive disorder experienced either moderate or severe depressive episodes. Among males, only one-third of the depressed cases experienced moderate depressive episodes, and none had experienced a severe episode (Reinherz *et al.*, 1993).

Age

In both clinical and epidemiological studies, the prevalence of major depressive disorder has been found to increase with age (Fleming *et al.*, 1989; Harrington *et al.*, 1990; Kashani, Rosenberg and Reid, 1989), with most studies reporting higher rates of major depressive disorder in adolescents than in children. For example, re-interviews of the 10-year olds in the Isle of Wright Study four years later showed a ten-fold increase in depression (Rutter, 1986).

Certain types of depressive symptoms are more common in one age group than in the other. Compared to depressed cases in the other age groups, the 11–12 year-old girls reported more hopelessness, the 12–14 year-old girls reported more weight loss and guilt, and the 15–16 year-old girls more irritability and agitation (Goodyer and Cooper, 1993). Depressive symptoms such as depressed mood, social withdrawal, agitation, early insomnia, and nihilistic ideas were unaffected by age. Other authors have reported depressed appearance, somatic complaints and psychomotor agitation as being more predominant in children, whereas in adolescents the most common depressive symptoms include anhedonia, hopelessness, weight-change, and drug/alcohol use (Carlson and Kashani, 1988). Recently, Essau *et al.* (1996) reported that the depressive symptoms "overtired" and "depressed mood" increased with age, whereas "deliberately harms self or attempt suicide" and "feels worthless or inferior" decreased with age. Their data also showed an increase in suicidal ideation with age in girls, but not in boys. In boys, the highest rate of suicidal ideation and attempted suicide was observed in the youngest group. Variations in the type of depressive symptoms in certain age groups may be related to the qualitative and quantitative changes in cognitive development in children.

Socioeconomic Status

Higher rates of depressive disorders have been reported for adolescents from lower socioeconomic status (Kaplan *et al.*, 1984; Reinherz *et al.*, 1993). However, a study by Kandel and Davies (1982) failed to find any association between family income or father's education on the number of depressive symptoms in high school children. A study by Berney *et al.* (1991) even indicated that the depressed children come from a higher social class. As with life events, social class seems to be a non-specific risk factors for depressive disorders.

Biological Factors

According to the *catecholamine hypothesis*, depression is associated with deficiency of catecholamines, particularly noradrenaline (Schildkraut, 1965). The hypothesis was derived from the observation that antidepressants such as monoamine oxidase inhibitors (MAOI) and the tricyclic compounds, tend to increase the availability of norepinephrine at brain synapses. Additional support comes from the observation that the antihypertensive medication reserpine depletes norepinephrine from synaptic storage vesicles and causes depressive reactions in patients receiving treatment for high blood pressure. The *indoleamine hypothesis* postulates that a deficiency in central serotonin could lead to depression (Coppen, 1967). Support for this hypothesis comes from observation that MAOI and the tricyclic reuptake inhibitor imipramine increased the availability of serotonin and norepinephrine in the brain. Effectiveness of the MAOI in depressive disorders increased with the addition of tryptophan which is the amino acid precursor for serotonin formation (Coppen, 1967).

Research has also focused on various psychobiological correlates of depressive disorders including plasma cortisol secretion, growth hormone secretion, and sleep EEG. *Plasma cortisol*, a hormone secreted by the adrenal cortex, has been shown to be hypersecreted in depressed prepubertal children (Puig-Antich *et al.*,1978), although their subsequent study failed to confirm this, since no significant differences in plasma cortisol concentration could be noted among depressed prepubertal children and controls (see Burke and Puig-Antich, 1990 for review). Atypical *growth hormone secretion* has been detected in depressed children. Puig-Antich *et al.* (1984) reported significantly greater growth hormone during sleep in depressed prepubertal children than in controls. According to several *EEG sleep studies*, unlike depressed adults, depressed prepubertal children showed no decrease in slow wave sleep, no decrease in sleep efficency, no shortening of latency to the first REM episode, no increase in REM density, and no abnormality in the temporal distribution of REM sleep during the night (Puig-Antich *et al.*, 1982; Young *et al.*, 1982). Lahmeyer and colleagues (1983), by contrast, reported decreased REM latency in depressed adolescents in comparison to controls, and in Goetz *et al.*'s study (1987), the REM latency becomes abnormal as the depressed patients enter late adolescence (see Burke and Puig-Antich, 1990 for review). These findings suggest that children and adolescents with depressive disorders show a normal age-related change of EEG sleep (Cicchetti and Toth, 1995).

Children of depressed parents have been shown to have about six times higher rates of depressive disorders than control children (Keller *et al.*, 1986; Orvaschel *et al.*, 1988; Weissman *et al.*, 1987; see review by Downey and Coyne, 1990; Hammen, 1991; Merikangas *et al.*, 1988; Weissman, 1990). As for bipolar disorder, studies have similarly shown that offspring of bipolar parents are at a greater risk for having bipolar disorder and various types of psychopathology (Beardslee *et al.*, 1992; Klein *et al.*, 1985, 1986; Weintraub, 1987).

The most common explanation for this finding is that of direct genetic transmission of the disorder. However, there is no direct evidence of a genetically transmitted disease so that it is not known what it is that may be transmitted, or how biological vulnerability may be activated.

Family and Psychological Factors

Family factors

Based on the findings of several studies, a number of psychosocial factors may be involved in the transmission of depression from parents to children. These include dysfunctional parent-child interaction, marital conflict, and emotional unavailability of parents. Parents exert influence over their child's development through dyadic interaction, coaching and teaching, and managing of social activities (Dodge, 1990; Parke *et al.*, 1988). These parenting functions may be interfered with by depression due to hospitalization, lack of interest, or lack of attention to or skill in structuring social activities for the child. Indeed, compared to non-depressed mothers, depressed mothers express negativity toward the demands of parenthood and view their role as parents less positively, and they also perceive themselves to be less competent and less adequate (Colletta, 1983; Davenport *et al.*, 1984; Webster-Stratton and Hammond, 1988).

The parent-child relationship of depressed children has been characterized by hostility, rejection, less secure attachment, anger, detachment, punitiveness or even abuse and neglect (Armsden *et al.*, 1990; Puig-Antich *et al.*, 1985). Verbal interchanges between depressed mothers and their adolescents has been described as being dominated by irritability (Tarullo *et al.*, 1994). Based on observed parent-child interaction, depressed mothers are less active, less playful and less contingently responsive, and show less reciprocal vocalization and affectionate contact in interactions with their infants (Field, 1984; Field *et al.*, 1990). Depressed mothers tend to be the most negative and critical, and the least positive and affirming to their children (Gordon *et al.*, 1989). Such linkages may mean that parents act these ways toward children, which in turn causes the children to become depressed (Weisz *et al.*,1992). However, other plausible interpretations may include the notion that the child's depression causes these reactions in the parents (Weisz *et al.*, 1992).

Maternal depression may lead to marital discord or to divorce, which may expose the child to negative socialization experiences. As reported by several authors, children of depressed parents have high rates of adverse parenting experiences and stressful family conditions such as parental divorce or separation (Fendrich *et al.*, 1990; Kovacs *et al.*, 1984), and have higher than normal rates of abuse and neglect (Kashani and Carlson, 1987). Furthermore, depressed adolescents have reported low family cohesion and exposure to "affectionless control" (i.e., having non-caring and overprotective parents) (Fendrich *et al.*, 1990). It is important to be cautious in interpreting the relationship between family factors and depressive disorders because many of these findings are correlational in nature.

Behavioural Model

Depression is viewed as a consequence of a loss or a lack of response-contingent positive reinforcement in major life areas (Lewinsohn and Arconad, 1981). The decrease in response-contingent positive reinforcement may be a function of three factors: (i) the person does not possess adequate skills to achieve the reinforcers or to cope with aversive situations; (ii) there may be a lack of positive reinforcers in the environment or surplus of aversive experiences or punishment; and (iii) the person may have a decreased capacity to enjoy positive experiences, or an increase in their sensitivity to negative events.

Lewinsohn also posited that depressed individuals may have social skills which make it difficult for them to obtain reinforcement from their social environment, leading them to experience a decreased rate of positive reinforcement. Depression is maintained when depressed adolescents withdraw from others, thereby reducing the opportunity for developing rewarding and pleasurable activities.

Self-control Model

This model considers depression as a consequence of deficits in self-control (Rehm, 1981), namely in self-monitoring, self-evaluation, and self-reinforcement. With respect to self-monitoring, depressed individuals may selectively attend to negative rather than to positive events or outcomes. Such a cognitive style may account for the pessimism and gloomy outlook of depressed individuals. In self-evaluation, depressed persons may set unrealistic, perfectionistic and high internal standards for themselves which make attainment of goals unlikely. This may lead them to evaluate themselves negatively and in a global and generalized way. The final deficit is related to self-reinforcement, whereby depressed persons fail to administer sufficient contingent reward to maintain their adaptive behaviour. Furthermore, depressed persons tend to administer excessive self-punishment, which may suppress potentially productive behaviour.

Learned Helplessness Model

The learned helplessness theory of depression has been reformulated to include cognitive attributions for success or failure (Abramson *et al.*, 1978), and has been applied to the study of depression in children (Seligman and Peterson, 1986). The reformulated theory considers depression as a result of beliefs that a negative outcome will occur, along with the expectation that the event or outcome is uncontrollable. The causal attribution made determines the generality and chronicity of helplessness deficits and self-esteem. Accordingly, causal attributions that produce depression following negative events include: (i) the cause is considered internal instead of external; (ii) the cause is a stable factor rather than an unstable factor; and (iii) the cause is global instead of specific.

Problem-solving Model

This model considers ineffective problem-solving skills as an important factor in the onset and maintenance of depression (Nezu *et al.*, 1989). Specifically, depression can occur due to deficits in any or all of five components of problem-solving: orientation definition and formulation, generation of alternatives, decision making and solution implementation and verification. The problem-orientation component is a motivation process, whereas the other components consist of specific skills and abilities which enable a person to effectively solve a particular problem.

Social problem-solving is regarded as a set of skills that is learned through direct and vicarious experience with other people, especially significant others. Some people are ineffective problem solvers because they have not learned the necessary skills, or they may have acquired the skills but fail to demonstrate effective problem-solving due to negative emotions (e.g., anxiety).

Regardless of the specific problem-solving deficiency, depression is believed to occur when the individual is confronted with some problems which could not be resolved. This unresolved problem could lead to negative consequence and a decrease in the individual's reinforcement. Deficits in problem-solving ability could result in a depressive episode being severe and long-lasting, and could increase relapse rates.

Integrative Model

This model views depression as a product of both environmental and dispositional factors (Lewinsohn *et al.*, 1985). Situational factors are important "triggers" of the depressogenic process, and cognitive factors are "moderators" of the effects of the environment. That is, depressogenic process is initiated by the occurrence of antecedent risk factors (e.g., negative life events) which may disrupt personal relationships. Such disruption may lead to a reduction of positive experiences and/or to an elevated rate of aversive experience, leading to a heightened state of self-awareness. This increase in self-awareness makes salient the individual's sense of failure to meet internal standards and consequently leads to increased dysphoria and other depressed symptoms. The model considers depressive episodes as the outcome of multiple events and processes, and that it is the product of the transformation of behaviour, affect, and cognition in the face of challenging interactions between individuals and their environments.

Cognitive Model

Beck's cognitive theory (1976) considers irrational cognitions and cognitive distortions as the cause of the disorder, or of its exacerbation and maintenance. In conceptualizing depression, Beck uses three concepts: cognitive triad, negative schemas, and cognitive errors. The cognitive triad consists of negative ideas and attitudes the person has towards self, the world, and the future. The negative cognitive triad is therefore responsible for many depressive symptom patterns, including deficits in affective, motivational, behavioural, and physiological functioning. Due to gross errors in logical thinking, depressed adolescents erroneously conclude that they are worthless or unlovable. The second element is the schema, a stable thought pattern that represents a person's generalizations about past experiences. As such, the schemas influence the selection, encoding, organization, and evaluation of the situation. According to Beck, the schemas that produce depression often involve the perception of a personal loss or damage to one's self-worth. The third component consists of cognitive errors made in the processing of information. These include: (i) arbitary inferences — tendency to draw conclusion in the absence of or contrary to evidence; (ii) selective abstraction — focus on elements of a situation that are consistent with the person's negative view of the self and the world; (iii) over-generalization — conclusions are based on simple, minor experiences or incidents; (iv) magnification or minimization — tendency to magnify negative events or faults and to minimize positive events and accomplishments. Because of these errors in logic, thoughts of depressed adolescents are characterized by extreme, negative, categorical, absolute and judgmental cognitions. These distorted perceptions serve to maintain depressed individuals' negative views of themselves, the world, and the future.

Consistent with Beck's cognitive theory, depressed children and adolescents have been reported to have low self-esteem, negative self-perceptions, and negative views of their competence in social, academic, and conduct domains (Allgood-Merten *et al.*, 1990; Harter, 1990; Kazdin *et al.*, 1986; King *et al.*, 1993; Reinherz *et al.*, 1989; Renouf and Harter, 1990; Weisz *et al.*, 1992; see Fleming and Offord, 1990; Hammen, 1990 for review). According to Weisz *et al.*'s review (1992), these beliefs tend to be more veridical in some areas (e.g., social and academic competence) than in others (e.g., conduct problems). In a longitudinal study by Reinherz *et al.* (1993), depressed girls who subsequently develop major depressive disorder tend to have low self-esteem. That is, many adolescents who subsequently develop major depressive disorder in late adolescence already had feelings of low self-worth as early as 9 years of age.

Other cognitive factors such as hopelessness cognitions, depressive attribution styles, external locus of control, and perceived lack of control are also common in depressed children and adolescents (Asarnow *et al.*, 1987; Benfield *et al.*, 1988; McCauley *et al.*, 1988; McGee *et al.*, 1986; Weisz *et al.*, 1987). Weisz *et al.* (1989) found depressive symptoms among inpatient children and adolescents to be more related to "personal helplessness" (i.e., a belief that one cannot produce responses which will cause personally valued outcomes, but that relevant others can do so) as compared to "universal helplessness" (i.e., a belief that desired outcomes are not contingent on behaviour that either the individual or relevant others may produce). Their result also showed depressive symptoms to be associated to uncertainty about the causes of significant events than to firm beliefs in noncontingency. In a similar study, Weisz *et al.* (1993) found a strong association between depressive symptoms and perceived incompetence and perceived noncontingency in a group of general population school children. The authors speculated that such an inability would be pronounced to the extent that the children believed their personal outcomes as not being contingent on their behaviour and that they are not competent in producing good outcomes.

Social Factors

Life Events

Depressed adolescents tend to have been exposed to negative life events prior to the onset of the depressive episode (Berney *et al.*, 1991; Goodyer *et al.*, 1993; Kashani *et al.*, 1986; Kovacs *et al.*, 1984; Nolen-Hoeksema *et al.*, 1986; Reinherz *et al.*, 1989). Life events predict subsequent depressive disorder (Garrison *et al.*,1990; Siegel and Brown, 1988), and those which are chronic in nature (e.g., chronic family turmoil) also influence the persistence of depressive symptoms, and intensify the distancing from family and low investment in peer relations (Aseltin *et al.*, 1994). The types of life events which act as risk factors for major depressive disorder seem to differ in boys and girls. In Reinherz *et al.*'s study (1993), for example, the death of a parent before age 15, pregnancy, and an early onset of health problems (e.g., respiratory disorders, mononucleosis, arthristis and headaches) which interfered with daily functioning were antecedent risks for major depressive disorder in females; in males it was the remarriage of a parent (Reinherz *et al.*, 1993).

In a study by Adams and Adams (1991), depressed adolescents tended to use more negative alternatives (e.g., becoming intoxicated, isolating themselves, or running away from home), whereas the nondepressed adolescents generally used positive alternatives (e.g., minimizing the importance of the events) in dealing with the life events experienced. According to several other authors, major depressive disorder was generally positively correlated with emotion-focused strategies (Compas *et al.*, 1988) and cognitive avoidance (Ebata and Moos, 1991), and negatively correlated with problem-focused coping (Compas *et al.*, 1988). In Nolen-Hoeksema *et al.*'s study (1992), the association between life events and depressive disorders was related to chronic disruption in the child's environment; among older children, the impact of life events on depressive disorders was mediated by pessimistic explanatory style, and among girls by self-perceived body image, self-esteem, and self-efficacy.

Children who were exposed to high stress levels were especially likely to become depressed if the mothers were currently symptomatic (Hammen and Goodman-Brown, 1990). Thus, the presence of the mother to help buffer the ill effects of stress may moderate the impact of stressors on children's probability to develop depressive disorders. In Goodyer *et al.*'s study (1993), adolescents whose mothers had a history of psychiatric disorder were exposed to more negative events than those whose mothers had no such history. Thus, both lifetime maternal psychiatric disorder and increased exposure to undesirable life events significantly exerted an increased risk for major depressive disorder in adolescents.

It should, however, be stated that life events appear to be a non-specific risk factor for major depressive disorder; that is, negative life events increase the risk of both depression and a number of other psychiatric disorders. As shown by Kendler *et al.* (1992), parental loss before the age of 17 years was significantly related to the presence of five major psychiatric disorders. Others concluded that life events may lead to depression when they are disruptive, chronic, and have a severe impact on the person's life (Merikangas and Angst, in press).

Peer Relationship

Depressed preadolescents have significant problems in social relations with siblings and friends, have less friend contact, more experiences of rejection, and low peer popularity (Jacobsen *et al.*, 1983; Vernberg, 1990). One interpretation of these findings is the presence of distorted social information-processing mechanisms in depressed children and adolescents (see Weisz *et al.*, 1992 for a review). Another interpretation is that depressed children and adolescents really have social difficulties (see Weisz *et al.*, 1992 for a review). As reported by Proffitt and Weisz (1992, cited in Weisz *et al.*, 1992), both self-rated social competence and teacher-rated sociometric status in children similarly indicated a significant relationship between depression and social incompetence. It could be that these deficits in social competence cause the children to feel depressed.

Whereas poor peer relationships constitute a risk factor for depressive disorders in early adolescence, good peer relationships at this age do not provide a protective influence. However, later in adolescence, close peer relationships tend to be protective, particularly when the parent-child relationship is impaired (Petersen *et al.*, 1991; Sarigiani *et al.*, 1990).

COMORBIDITY

Depressive disorders in children and adolescents are frequently comorbid with other psychiatric disorders (Essau and Petermann, 1995a, b; Kusch and Petermann, 1994). Between 25 to 75% of the depressed cases had anxiety disorders, 21 to 50% had comorbid conduct disorder, and about 25% had comorbid alcohol and drug abuse (Cohen *et al.*, 1993; Goodyer and Cooper, 1993; Kashani *et al.*, 1987). There seems to be developmental and sex differences in the type of comorbid disorders with major depressive disorder. In children, major depressive disorder usually occurs with conduct disorder and anxiety disorders (Ryan *et al.*, 1987), and in adolescence with eating disorders and drug or alcohol abuse. Antisocial behaviour and conduct disorder are more likely to be comorbid with major depressive disorder in boys than in girls (McGee and Williams, 1988; Mitchell *et al.*, 1988).

Major depressive disorder which is comorbid with other disorders tends to be chronic and severe (Kovacs *et al.*, 1989). Among community adolescents, Rohde *et al.* (1991) found comorbidity to be associated with high frequency of treatment-seeking and suicidal behaviour, with about one-quarter of the comorbid depressed adolescents reported having made a suicide attempt. In both community (Reinherz *et al.*, 1989; Rohde *et al.*, 1991) and clinical (Kovacs *et al.*, 1989) settings, most depressed cases with a comorbid anxiety disorder reported that anxiety preceded the onset of depressive disorder. Reinherz *et al.* (1989) also reported that the presence of anxiety disorders in childhood predicted the occurrence of major depressive disorder in adolescence. Anxiety that antedated major depressive disorder tended to persist beyond major depressive episode.The finding that depressive disorder generally follows the occurrence of another psychiatric disorder fits a theoretical formulation that considers depressive episodes as being evoked by the presence of stressful events (Lewinsohn *et al.*, 1985). The development of a psychiatric disorder is assumed to disrupt person-environment interactions, which consequently lead the person to have an increased likelihood of being depressed (Rohde *et al.*, 1991).

Despite the high comorbidity rates of depressive disorders with other psychiatric disorders, the meaning of comorbidity for psychopathology and classification issues remains unclear (Wittchen and Essau, 1993a,b). According to some authors (Merikangas and Angst, in press), comorbidity is not an artifact of sampling bias since findings across studies consistently reported high comorbidity rate despite different methodological procedures. Comorbidity may have arisen from a lack of nosologic precision or from the lack of specificity of the symptoms of these conditions during the early stages of their inception (Merikangas and Angst, in press). In a review of the possible cause of comorbidity in children and adolescents, Caron and Rutter (1991) concluded that the two disorders (i) could have resulted from shared and overlapping risk factors; or (ii) that the co-occurring of conditions could have consisted of a single condition with multiple manifestations; or (iii) that the disorder causes or lowers the threshold for the expression of the other; or (iv) one disorder represents an early manifestation of the other; or (v) the comorbidity could be due to overlapping diagnostic criteria.

LONG-TERM COURSE AND OUTCOME

Age of Onset

The first episode of major depressive disorder among depressed cases generally occurs during late childhood or early adolescence. As reported by Lewinsohn *et al.* (1994) and Giaconia *et al.* (1994), the mean age of onset of major depressive episodes was about 15 years. Earlier age of onset has been reported in clinical samples, the mean age of onset being 11 years (Kovacs *et al.*, 1984). Children of depressed parents have an earlier onset of depressive disorders than children with non-depressed parents (Weissman *et al.*, 1984). An early onset was associated with suicidal ideation (Lewinsohn *et al.*, 1994) and with female gender (Giaconia *et al.*, 1994; Lewinsohn *et al.*, 1993, 1994; Reinherz *et al.*, 1993); on average, females experienced onset of major depressive disorder about two years earlier than males (Giaconia *et al.*, 1994). Parallel to those found in adults, recent studies have also reported a secular increase in depressive disorders (Ryan *et al.*, 1992). That is, those born later had a higher risk for depressive disorders than those born earlier. The ages of onset for dysthymic disorder among school-age children have been reported to range from 6 to 13 years (Kovacs *et al.*, 1984). The onset of cyclothymic disorders have been reported to range from 7 to 15 (Klein *et al.*, 1985), and rarely later than early adulthood (Akiskal *et al.*, 1977; Klein *et al.*, 1986).

Children and adolescents who have an earlier onset of depressive disorders have a more protracted course of the disorder than those with a later onset (Kovacs *et al.*, 1984). In both epidemiological (Giaconia *et al.*, 1994) and clinical (Kovacs *et al.*, 1984) studies, adolescents with an early onset of major depressive episode reported significantly more major depressive episodes than adolescents with later onset. Early onset of major depressive disorder was also associated with suicide (Harrington *et al.*, 1990; Rao *et al.*, 1993) and psychosocial impairment including interpersonal problems and having high emotional and behavioural problems. The reason for this association is unclear, although some authors claimed that an early onset of major depressive disorder may represent severe forms of this disorder (Weissman *et al.*, 1988). Other authors stated that adolescents with an early onset had more time to experience additional episodes (Sorenson *et al.*, 1991). Yet others argued that early onset may signal a strong vulnerability that could be genetically, perinatally, and/or constitutionally determined and/or precipitated by environmental adversity (Kovacs *et al.*, 1984). Another argument is that the younger the child, the less likely that he or she has the repertoire of personal coping responses and external coping resources to ameloriate depression. Thus, the child's emotional and intellectual immaturity could prolong the course of depression (Kovacs *et al.*, 1984). Regardless of the validity of these explanations, an early onset of depression may signal the beginning of multiple occurrences of major depressive episodes, and not simply a single episode with little developmental significance (Giaconia *et al.*, 1994). In this respect, it is appropriate to consider Kutcher and Marton's argument (1989) that the previous assumption that the presence of major depressive disorder in adolescents was a mere reflection of transient difficulties is no longer valid.

Later onset was associated with shorter duration and quicker recurrence (Lewinsohn *et al.*, 1994). Based on this finding, it was suggested that within the child-adolescent age span, later and earlier onset major depressive disorder may represent different subtypes. Furthermore, there seems to be an increase in the so-called "rapid cycling" depressions (Angst *et al.*, 1990) among adolescents with a later onset.

Duration of Episodes

As in adults, the most frequent course for depressive disorders in adolescents is chronic and persistent. The mean length of major depressive episode in community samples is about 30 weeks (ranging from 23 to 36 weeks), and for dysthymic disorder 134 weeks (Lewinsohn *et al.*,

1993); the average length of dysthymic disorder in clinical sample is about 3 years (Kovacs *et al.*, 1984).The average duration for bipolar episodes is 4–6 months if untreated. In both epidemiological and clinical settings, between 21% and 41% of the depressed children and adolescents were still depressed after one year, and between 8% and 10% after 2 years (Kovacs *et al.*, 1984; Lewinsohn *et al.*, 1988, 1994; McCauley *et al.*, 1993). A study by McGee and Williams (1988) even showed that 31% of depressed children had persistent major depressive disorder when interviewed 2 to 4 years later. Over a period of about 8 years, adolescents with bipolar disorder spent 12.6% of their time in hospital (Coryell and Norten, 1980).

Longer duration of initial depressive episode was related to female gender, greater severity of initial depression, more dysfunctional family environment, high expressed emotion by parents, and more intervention received (Kovacs *et al.*, 1984; Garber *et al.*, 1988; McCauley *et al.*, 1993). Lewinsohn *et al.* (1994) reported longer major depressive episodes to be associated with an early onset, receipt of treatment for depression, and the presence of suicidal ideation. As for dysthymic disorder, the duration was significantly longer for females than males (Lewinsohn *et al.*, 1993). Among child patients, those who were older at first onset of major depressive episode recovered more quickly than children with an earlier onset (Kovacs *et al.*, 1984). However, McCauley *et al.* (1993), did not find age to be a significant factor in the duration of major depressive episode.

Relapse

Relapse occurs at a high frequency after recovery for children and adolescents with depressive disorders. Within one year of recovery, 26% of the treated depressed patients had a new depressive episode, which in most cases resulted in rehospitalization (Kovacs *et al.*, 1984). In Lewinsohn *et al.*'s study (1994), 50% of those who recovered had relapsed within 6 months, 12% developed a recurrent/depressive epsiode within a year, and about one-third become depressed within 4 years. Higher relapse rates have been reported in studies that used longer observation periods: within an observation period of two to five years, there was 40 to 72% risk of recurrence of major depressive disorder (Garber *et al.*, 1988; Hammen and Goodman-Brown, 1990; Kovacs *et al.*, 1984; McCauley *et al.*, 1993; Ryan *et al.*, 1987). In Harrington *et al.*'s study (1990), 60% of the depressed adolescents experienced at least one recurrence of major depressive disorder during adulthood. More than half of the children continued to have some psychiatric difficulties, mostly anxiety disorders followed by conduct disorder and dysthymic disorder (McCauley *et al.*, 1993).

Shorter time to relapse with major depressive disorder was associated with a history of suicide ideation and attempt during the first major depressive episode, greater severity of first major depressive episode, later age of first onset, and shorter first episode duration (Lewinsohn *et al.*, 1994), as well as the presence of comorbid dysthymic disorder (Kovacs *et al.*, 1984).

Psychosocial Impairment

Depressive disorders are associated with substantial psychosocial impairment including school functioning difficulties (Hammen *et al.*, 1987; Puig-Antich *et al.*, 1985, 1993), low grade point averages (Forehard *et al.*, 1988), and impairment in the teacher-child relationship. These evidences are based on correlational studies, and therefore should be interpreted with cautious. Furthermore, a study by Puig-Antich *et al.* (1985) indicated that depressed children and children with other psychiatric disorders were significantly impaired in school behaviour and academic achievement, suggesting that academic deficiencies may not be specific to those with depressive disorders.

According to several longitudinal studies, depressed adolescents showed impaired psychosocial functioning at follow-up investigations (Fleming *et al.*, 1993; Harrington *et al.*, 1990; Kandel and Davies, 1986; Puig-Antich *et al.*, 1993). Data from the Ontario Child Health Study showed that about one quarter of the depressed adolescents had problems with their family and friends, half had dropped out of school, and one third had been involved with the police or court at a 4-year follow-up investigation (Fleming *et al.*, 1993). In a study by Kandel and Davies (1986), "highly depressed" adolescents were more likely than "not highly depressed" adolescents to experience various types of adverse psychological and social outcomes nine years later. Puig-Antich *et al.* (1985) reported that after the depressive episodes, the formerly depressed children as compared to normal controls remained significantly inferior in their communication skills with mothers, tension in relationship with fathers, and being teased by peers. These findings seem to suggest that some social deficits related to child depression may be a reflection of enduring characteristics of children who are prone to be depressed.

As for bipolar disorder, little data is available on the social, academic, and psychological effects of this disorder in children and adolescents in the community setting. However, among adolescents in clinical setting, the best predictors of the course of bipolar disorder were acute onset, hypomanic response to an antidepressant medication, a family history of major depression or bipolar disorder, and psychotic symptoms (Strober and Carlson, 1982).

Health Services Utilization

Depressed adolescents were significantly more likely to have sought treatment for an emotional or behavioural problem in mental health settings or in social services than were controls (Fleming *et al.*, 1989, 1993), especially when the depressive episode was of long duration (Kovacs *et al.*, 1984). Using data from the Dunedin Multidisciplinary Health Development Study, Feehan *et al.* (1994) reported strong association between depression and self-medication. On a symptom level, Essau *et al.* (1995c, 1996), reported a significant positive correlation between depressive symptoms and doctor's visit in girls, but not in boys. The reason girls with high depressive symptoms made more doctor's visits than depressed boys was not clear, however, perhaps boys and girls differed in major concerns in their perceptions of health. For example, girls have been known to be more concerned with body image and weight, and they frequently report physical problems; boys, by contrast, are more concerned about drug and alcohol use (Dubow *et al.*, 1990).

In a follow-up investigation, depressed adolescents showed an increased likelihood of seeking professional help (Kashani *et al.*, 1987), being prescribed psychotropic medication, attending psychiatric services, and being hospitalized for mental illness (Harrington *et al.*, 1990).

ASSESSMENT

Numerous procedures have been developed for the assessment of mood disorders in children and adolescents, including self-report questionnaires (Table 8.4), report by significant others (e.g., parents, teachers, and peers), and clinical interviews. Various characteristics of depression support the use of and the need for self-report assessment procedures. Many symptoms reflect subjective feelings and self-perceptions are difficult to observe (e.g., suicidal ideation, hopelessness, feelings of worthlessness) and may be undetectable by others (e.g., insomnia and loss of appetite) (Table 8.5). However, in using self-report questionnaires one needs to determine the extend to which the measure fit the children´s metacognitive, and their reading and language ability. Furthermore, self-report questionnaires do not contain the required information to make

Table 8.4 Questionnaires used to measure depression in children and adolescents

Instruments/Authors	Items	Description
Children's Depression Inventory (Kovacs, 1981)	27	The items reflect the cognitive, affective, and behavioral signs of depression. Each item presents three choices, scored 0, 1, or 2 in severity level. Instructions to the child specify that he/she rate each item on the basis of feelings and thoughts during the past two weeks.
Children's Depression Scale (Lang and Tischer, 1978)	66	Comprise of 2 scales: depression and positive-affective experience. The depression scale has been subdivided into: affective response, social problems, self-esteem, guilt, and miscellaneous depression items. The positive experience scale includes a pleasure and enjoyment scale and miscellaneous positive scale.
Reynolds Child Depression Scale (Reynolds, 1989)	30	Measure of depressive symptoms. The child responds by endorsing how often they have experienced the specific symptom status. The last item consists of five "smiley-type" faces ranging from sad to happy, to which the child responds by placing an X over the face that indicates how he feels.
Beck Depression Inventory (Beck et al., 1961)	21	The rating of each item relies on the endorsement of one or more of four statements listed in order of symptom severity. Item categories are: mood pessimism, crying, spells, guilt, self-hate and accusations, irritability, social disturbance and loss of libido.

Table 8.5 Examples of questions in the selected self-report questionnaires

Instruments/Authors	Examples of questions	Responses
Children's Depression Scale (Lang and Tisher, 1978)	I feel life is not worth living I feel tired most of the time when I'm at school Often I feel like I'm letting my mother/father down	ranging from "very wrong" to "very right"
Revised Ontario Child Health Study Scales (Boyle *et al.*, 1993)	I am unhappy, sad, or depressed I feel hopeless I deliberately try to hurt or kill myself	ranging from "never or not true" to "often or very true"
Children's Depression Inventory (Kovacs, 1981)	0 I am sad once in a while 1 I am sad many times 2 I am sad most of the time	
Beck Depression Inventory (Beck *et al.*, 1961)	0 I do not feel sad 1 I feel sad 2 I am sad all the time and I can't snap out of it 3 I am so sad or unhappy	

Table 8.6 Clinician Rating Scales for Depression

Instruments	Items	Description
Bellevue Index of Depression (Petti, 1978)	40	The items can be evaluated across 10 symptoms domains: dysphoric mood, self-deprecation, aggression, sleep disturbance, diminished school performance, diminished socialization, changing attitude toward school, somatic complaints, loss of energy, and weight loss or appetite change. Each item is scored on a 4-point symptom severity scale from 0 (absent) to 3 (severe). To be classified as depressed the child must obtain at least one positive symptom rating from the categories dysphoric mood and self-deprecation, and receive a minimum total score of 20.
Children's Depression Rating Scale-Revised (Poznanski *et al.*, 1979)	17	A semistructured clinical interview measure of the severity of depressive symptoms in children ages 8 to 12. 14 of the items are presented in an interview format, whereas 3 items (depressed affect, tempo of language, hyperactivity) are observational.
Hamilton Depression Rating Scale (Hamilton, 1967)	17	Measure severity of depressive symptoms. Items are rated on the basis of their severity, with higher scores indicative of greater pathology. Two of the items (psychomotor retardation and agitation) are observational in nature.

Table 8.7 Examples of questions from some selected diagnostic interview schedule in children and adolescents

Instruments	Examples of questions	Coding options
DISC (Costello et al., 1984)	In the past 6 months, were there times when you were **very sad**?	0 1 2 9
	IF YES, A) When you feel sad this way, does it last most of the day?	0 1 2 9
	B) Would you say you have been very sad a *lot* of the time for as long as a year?	0 2 9
	IF YES, C) Would you say most of the time?	0 [2*] 9
	IF YES, D) Were you very sad *most* of the time for as long as 2 years?	0 2 9
	E) Now thinking about just the last 6 months … Was there a time when you were sad almost every day?	0 2 9
	IF YES, F) Did this go on for 2 weeks or more?	0 2 9
	During the last 6 months, have you had more trouble sleeping than usual, that is, more trouble than usual falling asleep or staying asleep or waking up too early?	0 1 2 9
	IF YES, A) Did you have trouble sleeping during the time you were [VERY SAD/ GROUCHY HAVING NO FUN/NOT INTERESTED IN THINGS]	[1] [2]
	B) Did you have trouble sleeping most nights for two weeks or more?	0 2 9
DICA-R (Reich and Welner, 1988)	In the past year, have you felt sad, blue, down in the dumps, or low for long periods of time, for example, weeks or months?	1 2 4 9
	IF YES or SOMETIMES, A) Could you tell me about that? ( )1 Yes ( )4 No ( )9 Don't know RECORD _____	
	Some kids have trouble falling asleep, but other kids sleep more than they really need to. For example, they take naps during the day, go to bed early at night, and sometimes they even sleep in class. Have you been like that at all during the past year?	1 2 4 9

Table 8.7 *continued*

Instruments	Examples of questions	Coding options
K-SADS (Puig-Antich and Chambers, 1978)	How have you been feeling? Are you a happy child or a sad child? Mostly happy or mostly sad? Have you felt sad, blue, moody, down in the dumps, very unhappy, empty, like crying? (ASK EACH ONE). Is this a good feeling or a bad feeling? Have you had any other bad feelings? Do you have a bad feeling all the time that you can't get rid of? Have you cried or been tearful? Do you feel (....) all the time, most of the time, some of the time? (Percent of awake time: summation of % of all labels if they do not occur simultaneously.) (ASSESSMENT OF DIURNAL VARIATION CAN SECONDARILY CLARIFY DAILY DURATION OF DEPRESSIVE MOOD.) Does it come and go? How often? Every day? How long does it last? All day? How bad is the feeling? Can you stand it? What do you do when you can't stand it? Do you feel sad when mother is away? IF SEPARATION FROM MOTHER IS GIVEN AS A CAUSE: Do you feel (...) when mother is with you? Do you feel a little better or is the feeling totally gone? Can other people tell when you are sad? How can they tell? Do you look different?	0 1 3 4 5 6 7
	WHAT ABOUT DURING THE LAST WEEK?	LAST WK: 0 1 2 3 4 5 6 7

Coding used: (1) DISC: 0 = No , 1 = Sometimes/Somewhat , 2 = Yes, 9 = Don't know; (2) DICA-R: 1 = Yes, 2 = Sometimes , 4 = No, 9 = Don't know; (2) K-SADS: 0 = No information; 1 = not at all less than once a week; 2 = slight: occasionally has dysphoric mood at least once a week for more than one hour; 3 = mild: sometimes experiences dysphoric mood at least 3 times a week for at least 3 hours total time each day; 4 = moderate: often feels "depressed" (including weekends) or over 50% of awake time; 5 = severe: most of the time feels depressed, and it is almost painful, feels wretched; 6 = extreme: almost all of the time feels extreme depression which "I can't stand"; 7 = pervasive: constant unrelieved, extremely painful feelings of depression.

the diagnosis of depression, but to assess the severity of depressive symptomatology. The most commonly used self-report measures include the Children's Depression Inventory (Kovacs and Beck, 1977), the Children's Depression Scale (Long and Tiser, 1978), and the Children's Depression Adjective Checklist (Sokoloff and Lubin, 1983).

A number of scales have been developed to measure general psychopathology including the depression subscales. These scales include the Behavior Disorders Identification Scale (Wright, 1988) and the Child Behavior Checklist (Achenbach and Edelbrock, 1983). Report by significant others allow parents, teachers, or peers to observe depressive symptoms during social interaction, and in various settings in the neighbourhood and school. The most commonly used rating scale is the Peer Nomination Inventory of Depression (Lefkowitz and Tesiny, 1980). Clinical rating scale is another type of assessment instrument used to assess depression, especially in the clinical settings (Table 8.6). Some examples include the Bellevue Index of Depression (Petti, 1978), Children's Depression Rating Scale-Revised (Poznanski *et al.*, 1979), and the Hamilton Depression Rating Scale (Hamilton, 1967). Ratings by significant others or clinicians have however some disadvantages, including an inability to rate the unobservable nature of depressive symptoms (e.g., excessive guilt feelings), and individual differences among raters (stringency).

In contrast to self-report questionnaires, diagnostic interview schedules allow the generation of a diagnosis of mood disorders via algorithms. Some examples of diagnostic interview schedules that contain a section to assess depressive disorders include the Diagnostic Interview Schedule for Children (DISC; Costello *et al.*, 1984), the Schedule for Affective Disorders and Schizophrenia for school-age Children (K-SADS; Puig-Antich and Chambers, 1978), and the Diagnostic Interview for Children and Adolescents (DICA-R; Reich and Welner, 1988) (Table 8.7).

TREATMENT

Pharmacotherapy

Tricyclic Antidepressants

Most of the psychopharmacological research on the treatment of depression in children and adolescents has focused on the tricyclic antidepressant (TCAs) such as imipramine, amitriptyline, nortriptyline and desipramine (see Ambrosini *et al.*, 1993; Reynolds, 1993, for review).

The Ambrosini *et al.* (1993) review showed that prepubertal child recovery rates ranged from 31 to 75% with tricyclic antidepressants, and from 0 to 68% with placebo. Among adolescents, the recovery rates ranged from 8 to 71% in double-blind studies, and between 21 to 63% with placebo. These findings seem to suggest no reliable effects of medication.

Monoamine Oxidase Inhibitors (MAOI)

Few studies have used MAOI in the treatment of depression in children and adolescents because of the possible side effects such as dry mouth, constipation, tremor, and mild weight loss. In a study by Ryan *et al.* (1988), 74% of depressed adolescents showed good to fair treatment improvement, most of whom had previously failed to respond to a tricyclic antidepressant (see Ambrosini *et al.*, 1993; Reynolds, 1993, for review). This finding should, however, be interpreted with caution because it was based on a chart review. Therefore, it is not clear that these findings are true medication effects.

Lithium and Carbamazepine

Two types of pharmacotherapy which may be used to treat children and adolescents with bipolar disorders are lithium and carbamazepine. Lithium is generally used for the acute or maintenance treatment of bipolar disorders (Puig-Antich *et al.*, 1985). However, lithium has a number of side effects including polyuria, polydipsia, diarrehea and weight gain, nausea, vomitting, sedation, slurred speech, ataxia and change in sensorium. Furthermore, the relapse rate of those who take lithium prophylactically tend to be quite high. As reported by Strober *et al.* (1990), the relapse rate of 38% was found among those who received lithium prophylactically for 18 months compared to a relapse rate of 92% in those who discontinued the medication prior to the end of the 18-month period.

Carbamazepine is an anticonvulsant used to improve attention, social behavior, and mood in epileptic patients. Although no systematic studies have been carried out to delineate the efficacy of carbamazepine for the treatment of bipolar disorder in adolescents, a number of case reports are available documenting it´s efficacy (Hsu, 1986). However, the use of carbamazepine in children and adolescents should be kept to a minimal because of its side effects including nausea, drowsiness, and blurred vision (Evans *et al.*, 1987).

Psychological Interventions

Behaviour Therapy

Behavioural approaches use the principle of classical and operant conditioning. The approaches generally consist of functional analysis of behaviour, use of specific techniques, and monitoring or record keeping. Functional analysis of behaviour involves defining and determining both the frequency of behaviour that is to be changed and identifying the environmental contingencies that maintain it. Assessment techniques used for these purposes may include interview and home observation by the therapist or self-observation by the clients themselves. When the problems are identified, specific techniques may be used, including: (i) relaxation training for reducing aversiveness of unpleasant stimuli; (ii) assertive training, role playing, and modeling as a way for increasing social skills and positive thinking; (iii) time management and behaviour-mood monitoring for increasing activity level and participating in pleasurable activities; and (iv) thought-stopping for decreasing negative thinking. To determine progress and the effectiveness of the program, behaviour change needs to be monitored.

Self-control Therapy

The main emphasis of the self-control therapy is on progressive goal attainment, self-reinforcement and contingency management strategies, and behavioural productivity (Antonucci *et al.*, 1989); it is primarily a treatment of adults but has been used in adolescents (Stark *et al.*, 1987). The therapy is a structured and group-format treatment approach, which is divided into three parts. Each part focuses on one of the three deficits: self-monitoring, self-evaluative, and self-reinforcement.

In the self-monitoring phase, patients are asked to keep a daily record of positive experiences and their associated mood. In the self-evaluative phase, patients are taught to develop specific goals in terms of positive activities and behavioural productivity. In the self-reinforcement phase, patients are taught to identify reinforcers and to reward themselves when their specific goals are accomplished.

Problem-solving Therapy

The main goals of problem-solving therapy are to (i) help depressed persons identify past and present life situations that may have precipitated a depressive episode; (ii) minimize the negative impact of depressed symptoms on present and future coping attempts; (iii) increase the effectiveness of their problem-solving efforts in coping with present life situations; and finally (iv) teach depressed subjects general skills so that they can deal with future problems more effectively, and thereby prevent future depressive reactions (Nezu *et al.*, 1989).

In order to achieve these goals, patients are given training in the major problem-solving components, namely, problem orientation, problem definition and formation, generation of alternatives, decision making, as well as solution implementation and verification. This treatment program uses such therapeutic techniques as instruction, prompting, modeling, behavioural rehearsal, homework assignments, shaping, reinforcement, and feedback.

Social Skills Therapy

The main assumption of social skills therapy is that the depressed patient has either lost socially skillful responses, or that the patient never possessed social skills in his or her behaviour repertoire (Bellack *et al.*, 1983; Petermann and Petermann, 1996; Ross and Petermann, 1987). Treatment occurs over 12 weekly one-hour sessions, followed by 6 to 8 maintenance sessions spread over a period of six months.

The primary focus of the training program is on three types of behaviour repertoires: (i) negative assertion that involves teaching patients how to refuse unreasonable requests and how to compromise and negotiate; (ii) positive assertion that involves training patients to express positive feelings about others; (iii) conversational skills that involve learning to initiate, maintain, and end conversations, and on how to ask questions and make appropriate self-disclosures.

Since social skills are situation-specific, training is given in how to interact with different types of people (e.g., strangers, family members, friends) and under different situations (e.g., at work or school). For each social context, the training is composed of four components: (i) social skills training that involves learning specific response skills; (ii) social perception training. This includes instruction in the social meaning of various response cues, attention to the relevant aspects of interaction context, and an ability to accurately predict interpersonal consequences; (iii) practicing the newly learned skills and behaviour across different situations; and (iv) self-evaluation and self-reinforcement that involve training the patients to evaluate their responses more objectively and to employ self-reinforcements.

Cognitive Therapy

A major premise of cognitive therapy is that an individual's affective state is highly influenced by the way in which he or she perceives his or her experience (Beck, 1976). Thus, the main task of this therapy is to teach patients that: (i) their emotional distress is mediated by the content and the process of their thinking styles; (ii) they can learn to monitor and identify such cognitive patterns; and (iii) modification of their thoughts to make them more objective and systematic.

The main components of Beck's cognitive therapy are thought-catching and cognitive restructuring, as well as identification and challenging of underlying maladaptive beliefs. For thought-catching of "automatic negative thoughts", patients are taught to observe the link between thoughts and feelings, and to clarify their emotion-related thoughts. Patients are asked to keep records of emotion-arousing experience, the automatic negative thoughts associated with them, and challenges to the maladaptive thoughts. Patients are taught to challenge each negative thought using several techniques such as "Is there a distortion?", "What is the evidence?", "Is there another way to look at it?", and "So what?", and to replace the dysfunction of thought with more realistic ones.

Studies that compare the efficacy of these various types of psychological interventions are rare (see Weisz *et al.*, 1992 for a review). However, the few studies that have used these psychological interventions such as cognitive-behavioural methods (Kahn *et al.*, 1990; Reynolds and Coats, 1986), social competence training (Liddle and Spence, 1990), and coping with depression course (Lewinsohn *et al.*, 1990) have a positive and a significant effect in ameliorating depression among depressed children and adolescents (Fine *et al.*, 1991; Petermann and Petermann, 1996; Stark *et al.*, 1987; see Reynolds, 1993 for review). A meta-analysis of treatment outcome studies by Weisz and his colleagues (Weisz *et al.*, 1995) has shown effects to be more positive for behavioural than for nonbehavioural treatments, and among adolescents girls than other Age X Gender group. The benefical of therapy was maintained over a period of five weeks to six months (Petersen *et al.*, 1993). Most studies used number of depressive symptoms as the outcome measures; others used related constructs such as self-concept, anxiety, social skills deficits, somatic complaints, and social withdrawal (see Weisz *et al.*, 1992 for a review).

Preventive Programs

In addition to the various types of psychological interventions, several authors have proposed the importance of prevention programs (Petersen *et al.*, 1993). One form involves delivering preventive services to the whole population of adolescents and teaching the problem-solving skills and social competence. This program is based on the assumption that adolescents are at some risks of experiencing depressive symptoms and/or in developing depressive disorders, and that teaching the adolescents to appropriately respond to the risk factors will help reduce the frequent occurrence of depressive disorders. Another form of preventive program is to deliver services to adolescents who are at greatest risk (e.g., having depressed parent) (Beardslee *et al.*, 1992). Such program may involve helping adolescents cope with the stressors encountered, or in having adolescents and their parents participate in a psychoeducational intervention where they will be informed about the nature of depressive disorders, and on how to deal with it effectively.

Clark and colleagues (1995) recently presented some findings on the impact of a prevention program of depressive disorders in an at-risk sample of highschool adolescents. Adolescents at risk for depressive disorders (i.e., those having elevated depressive symptomatology) were randomized to a 15-session cognitive group prevention intervention or a "usual care" control condition. Adolescents in the active intervention participated in the "coping with stress course," where they were taught cognitive techniques to identify and challenge negative or irrational thoughts which may lead to the development of depressive disorders. The intervention was based on the notion that teaching individuals new coping mechanisms and strengthening their repertoire of current coping strategies could help with some measure of "immunity" (e.g., high self-esteem) or resistance against having depressive disorder. Adolescents in the "usual care" can continue with any preexisting intervention or to have any new assistance. The results showed a significant advantage for the prevention program across the 12-month period; the incidence rates of depressive disorders in the active intervention group was 14.5%, and in the "usual care" group 25.7%. It was concluded that it is possible to prevent depressive disorders among adolescents at high risk for the disorder.

CONCLUDING REMARKS

Major depressive disorder is a common disorder that affects about 10% of the adolescents in the general population. The prevalence of dysthymic disorder vary from 0.1 to 8%. Bipolar disorder is a much rarer in the general population, with the rates ranging from 0.4 to 1.2%. The course of depressive disorder is chronic and persistent, the average length of depressive episodes among adolescents in the community setting being about 30 weeks and for dysthymic disorder 134 weeks. Relapse occurs frequently, with a high percentage of the depressed patients experiencing a new depressive episode a year after recovery. Given the frequency, chronicity and severity of depressive disorders experienced by children and adolescents, these disorders should not be viewed as a normal part of development. However, a major challenge is the question of whether our current classification system of depressive disorders, designed for adults is valid for use with children and adolescents. Another challenge involves defining a threshold to discriminate between normal expression of depressive symptoms and depressive disorders. To solve the issues of diagnostic specificity and etiologic mechanisms in depressive disorders, future studies need to explore the temporal relationship of the disorders by examining their age of onset. Longitudinal studies are also needed to examine specific risk factors and their interactions that are involved in the development and maintenance of depressive disorders. A number of such studies are currently taking place, like the one which are being undertaken by our working group-the "Bremer Jugendstudie" (i.e., Bremen Adolescent Study; Essau and Petermann, in preparation). Furthermore, there is a real need for more developmental research that will help clarify our understanding of how children and adolescents at different developmental levels may differ in: (a) the nature and symptomatology of depressive disorders; (b) precursors, precipitators, and correlates of depressive disorders; (c) typical course and episode duration; and (d) treatment effects, with drugs and psychological interventions.

REFERENCES

Achenbach, T.M. and Edelbrock, C. (1983). *Manual for the Child Behavior Checklist und Revised Child Behavior Profile*. Burlington: Department of Psychiatry, University of Vermont.

Abramson, L.Y., Seligman, M.E.P., and Teasdale, J.D. (1978). Learned helplessness in humans: Critique and reformulation. *Journal of Abnormal Psychology, 87*, 49–74.

Adams, M. and Adams, J. (1991). Life events, depression, and perceived problem solving alternatives in adolescents. *Journal of Child Psychology and Psychiatry*, **32**, 811–820.

Allgood-Merten, B., Lewinsohn, P.M., and Hops, H. (1990). Sex differences and adolescent depression. *Journal of Abnormal Psychology*, **99**, 55–63.

Akiskal, H.S., Djenderedjian, A.H., Rosenthal, R.H., and Khani, M. (1977). Cyclothymic disorder: Validating criteria for inclusion in the bipolar affective group. *American Journal of Psychiatry*, **134**, 1227–1233.

Ambrosini, P.J., Bianchi, M.D., Rabinovich, H., and Elia, J. (1993). Antidepressant treatments in children and adolescents. I. Affective disorders. *Journal of the American Academy of Child and Adolescent Psychiatry*, **32**, 1–6.

American Psychiatric Association (1980). *Diagnostic and statistical manual of mental disorders (3rd ed.)*. Washington, DC: American Psychiatric Association.

American Psychiatric Association (1987). *Diagnostic and statistical manual of mental disorders (3rd ed. rev.)*. Washington, DC: American Psychiatric Association.

American Psychiatric Association (1994). *Diagnostic and statistical manual of mental disorders (4th ed.)*. Washington, DC: American Psychiatric Association.

Anderson, J.C., Williams, S., McGee, R., and Silva, P.A. (1987). DSM-III disorders in preadolescent children. Prevalence in a large sample from the general population. *Archives of General Psychiatry*, **44**, 69–76.

Angst, J., Merikangas, K.R., Scheidegger, P., and Wicki, W. (1990). Recurrent brief depression: A new subtype of affective disorder. *Journal of Affective Disorders*, **19**, 37–38.

Antonucci, D.O., Ward, C.H., and Tearnan, B.H. (1989). The behavioral treatment of unipolar depression in adult outpatients. In M. Hersen, R.M. Eisler, and P.M. Miller (Eds.), *Progress in behavior modification* (Vol. 24, pp. 152–191). New York: Sage.

Armsden, G., McCauley, E., Greenberg, M., Burke, P., and Mitchell, J. (1990). Parent and peer attachment in early adolescent depression. *Journal of Abnormal Child Psychology*, **18**, 683–697.

Aro, H. (1994). Risk und protective factors in depression: A developmental perspective. *Acta Psychiatrica Scandinavica*, **(Suppl. 377)**, 59–64.

Asarnow, J.R., Carlson, G.A., and Guthrie, D. (1987). Coping strategies, self-perceptions, hopelessness, and perceived family environments in depressed and suicidal children. *Journal of Consulting and Clinical Psychology*, **55**, 361–366.

Aseltin, R.H., Gore, S., and Colten, M.E. (1994). Depression and the social developmental context of adolescence. *Journal of Personality and Social Psychology*, **67**, 252–263.

Beardslee, W.R., Hoke, L., Wheelock, I., Rothberg, P.C., van de Velde, P., and Swatling, S. (1992). Initial findings on preventive intervention for families with parental affective disorders. *American Journal of Psychiatry*, **149**, 1335–1340.

Beck, A.T. (1976). *Cognitive therapy and the emotional disorders*. New York: International Universities Press.

Bellack, A.S., Hersen, M., and Himmelhoch, J. (1983). A comparison of social skills training, pharmacotherapy, and psychotherapy for depression. *Behavior Research and Therapy*, **21**, 101–107.

Benfield, C.Y., Palmer, D.J., Pfefferbaum, B., and Stowe, M.L. (1988). A comparison of depressed and nondepressed disturbed children on measures of attributional style, hopelessness, life stress, and temperament. *Journal of Abnormal Child Psychology*, **16**, 397–410.

Berney, T.P., Bhate, S.R., Kolvin, I., Famuyima, M.L., Barrett, T., Fundudis, T. *et al.* (1991). The context of childhood depression. *British Journal of Psychiatry*, **11**, 28–35.

Block, J.H., Block, J., and Gjerde, P.F. (1986). The personality of children prior to divorce: A prospective study. *Child Development*, **57**, 827–840.

Boyle, M.H., Offord, D.R., Racine, Y., Fleming, J.E., Szatmari, P., and Sanford, M. (1993). Evaluation of the revised Ontario Child Health Study scales. *Journal of Child Psychology and Psychiatry*, **34**, 189–213.

Burke, P. and Puig-Antich, J. (1990). Psychobiology of childhood depression. In M. Lewis and S.M. Miller (Eds.), *Handbook of developmental psychopathology* (pp. 327–339). New York: Plenum Press.

Carlson, G.A. and Kashani, J.H. (1988). Phenomenology of major depression from child hood through adulthood: Analysis of three studies. *American Journal of Psychiatry*, **145**, 1222–1225.

Caron, C. and Rutter, M. (1991). Comorbidity in child psychopathology: Concepts, issues and research strategies. *Journal of Child Psychology and Psychiatry*, **32**, 1063–1080.

Cicchetti, D. and Toth, S.L. (1995). Developmental psychopathology and disorders of affect. In D. Cicchetti and D. Cohen (Eds.), *Developmental psychopathology. Vol. 2: Risk, disorder, and adaptation* (pp. 369–420). New York: Wiley.

Clark, G.N., Hawkins, W., Murphy, M., Sheeber, L.B., Lewinsohn, P.M., and Seeley, J.R. (1995). Targeted prevention of unipolar depressive disorder in an at risk sample of high school adolescents: A randomized trial of a group cognitive intervention. *Journal of the American Academy of Child and Adolescent Psychiatry*, **34**, 312–321.

Colletta, N.D. (1983). At risk for depression: A study of young mothers. *Journal of Genetic Psychology*, **142**, 301–310.

Cohen, P., Cohen, J., Kasen, S., Velez, C.N., Hartmark, C., Johnson, J., Rojas, M., Brook, J., and Streuning, E.L. (1993). An epidemiological study of disorders in late child-hood and adolescence-I: Age-and gender-specific prevalence. *Journal Child Psychology and Psychiatry*, **34**, 851–866.

Compas, B., Malcarne, V.L., and Fondacara, K.M. (1988). Coping with stressful events in older children and young adolescents. *Journal of Consulting and Clinical Psychology*, **56**, 405–411.

Coppen, A. (1967). The biochemistry of affective disorder. *British Journal of Psychiatry*, **113**, 1237–1243.

Cooper, P.J. and Goodyer, I. (1993). A community study of depression in adolescent girls. I: Estimates of symptom and syndrome prevalence. *British Journal of Psychiatry*, **163**, 369–374.

Costello, A.J., Edelbrock, C., Dulcan, R.K., Kalas, R., and Klaric, S.H. (1984). *Development and testing of the NIMH Diagnostic Interview Schedule for Children.* Rockville, MD: National Institute of Mental Health.

Coryell, W. and Norten, S.G. (1980). Mania during adolescence. *Journal of Nervous and Mental Disease*, **168**, 611–613.

Cytryn, L. and McKnew, D.H. (1972). Proposed classification of childhood depression. *American Journal of Psychiatry*, **129**, 149–155.

Davenport, Y.B., Zahn-Waxler, C., Adland, M.L., and Mayfield, A. (1984). Early child-rearing practices in families with a manic-depressive parent. *American Journal of Psychiatry*, **141**, 230–235.

Deykin, E.Y., Levy, J.C., and Wells, V. (1987). Adolescent depression, alcohol and drug abuse. *American Journal of Public Health*, **77**, 178–182.

Dodge, K.A. (1990). Developmental psychopathology in children of depressed mothers. *Developmental Psychology*, **26**, 3–6.

Downey, G. and Coyne, J.C. (1990). Children of depressed parents: An integrative review. *Psychological Bulletin*, **108**, 50–76.

Dubow, E.F., Lovko, J.R., and Kausch, D.F. (1990). Demographic differences in adolescents' health concerns and perceptions of helping agents. *Journal of Clinical Child Psychology*, **19**, 44–54.

Ebata, A.T. and Moos, R.H. (1991). Coping and adjustment in distressed and healthy adolescents. *Journal of Applied Developmental Psychology*, **12**, 33–54.

Essau, C.A. and Petermann, U. (1995a). Depression. In F. Petermann (Ed.), *Lehrbuch der Klinischen Kinderpsychologie* (pp. 241–264). Göttingen: Hogrefe.

Essau, C.A. and Petermann, U. (1995b). Depression bei Kindern und Jugendlichen. *Zeitschrift für Klinische Psychologie, Psychopathologie und Psychotherapie*, **43**, 18–33.

Essau, C.A., Petermann, F., and Conradt, J. (1995c). Symptomen von Angst und Depression bei Jugendlichen. *Praxis der Kinderpsychologie und Kinderpsychiatrie,* **44**, 322–328.

Essau, C.A., Petermann, F., and Conradt, J. (1996). Depressive Symptome und Syndrome bei Jugendlichen. *Zeitschrift für Psychologie, Psychiatrie und Psychotherapie,* **44**, 150–157.

Evans, R.W., Clay, T.H., and Gualtieri, C.T. (1987). Carbamazepine in pediatric psychiatry. *Journal of the American Academy of Child and Adolescent Psychiatry,* **26**, 2–8.

Feehan, M., McGee, R., Nada-Raja, S., and Williams, S.M. (1994). DSM-III-R disorders in New Zealand 18-year-olds. *Australian and New Zealand Journal of Psychiatry,* **28**, 87–99.

Feindrich, M., Warner, V., and Weissman, M.M. (1990). Family risk factors, parental depression, and psychopathology in offspring. *Developmental Psychology,* **26**, 40–50.

Fergusson, D.M., Horwood, L.J., and Lynskey, M.T. (1993). Prevalence and comorbidity of DSM-III-R diagnoses in a birth cohort of 15 year olds. *Journal of the American Academy of Child and Adolescent Psychiatry,* **32**, 1127–1134.

Field, T. (1984). Early interactions between infants and their postpartum depressed mothers. *Infant Behavior and Development,* **7**, 517–522.

Field, T., Healy, B., Goldstein, S., and Guthertz, M. (1990). Developmental psychopathology in children of depressed mothers. *Developmental Psychology,* **26**, 7–14.

Fine, S., Forth, A., Gilbert, M., and Haley, G. (1991). Group therapy for adolescent depressive disorder: A comparison of social skills and therapeutic support. *Journal of the American Academy of Child and Adolescent Psychiatry,* **30**, 79–85.

Fleming, J.E., Boyle, M.H., and Offord, D.R. (1993). The outcome of adolescent depression in the Ontario Child Health Study follow-up. *Journal of the American Academy of Child and Adolescent Psychiatry,* **32**, 28–33.

Fleming, J.E. and Offord, D.R. (1990). Epidemiology of childhood depressive disorders: A critical review. *Journal of the American Academy of Child and Adolescent Psychiatry,* **29**, 571–580.

Fleming, J.E., Offord, D.R., and Boyle, M.H. (1989). Prevalence of childhood and adolescent depression in the community: Ontario Child Health Study. *British Journal of Psychiatry,* **155**, 647–654.

Forehand, R., Brody, G.H., Long, N., and Fauber, R. (1988). The interactive influence of adolescent and maternal depression on adolescent social and cognitive functioning. *Cognitive Therapy and Research,* **12**, 341–350.

Garber, J., Kriss, M.R., Koch, M., and Lindholm, L. (1988). Recurrent depression in adolescents: A follow-up study. *Journal of the American Academy of Child and Adolescent Psychiatry,* **27**, 49–54.

Garrison, C.Z., Jackson, K.L., Marsteller, F., McKeown, R., and Addy, C. (1990). A longitudinal study of depressive symptomatology in young adolescents. *Journal of the American Academy of Child and Adolescent Psychiatry,* **29**, 581–585.

Giaconia, R., Reinherz, H.Z., Silverman, A.B., Pakiz, B., Frost, A.K., and Cohen, E. (1994). Ages of onset of psychiatric disorders in a community population of older adolescents. *Journal of the American Academy of Child and Adolescent Psychiatry,* **33**, 706–717.

Goetz, R.R., Puig-Antich, J., Ryan, N., Rabinovich, H., Ambrosini, P.J., Nelson, B. and Krawiec, V. (1987). Electroencephalographic sleep of adolescents with major depression and normal controls. *Archives of General Psychiatry,* **44**, 61–68.

Goodyer, I. and Cooper, P.J. (1993). A community study of depression in adolescent girls. II: The clinical features of identified disorder. *British Journal of Psychiatry,* **163**, 374–380.

Goodyer, I.M., Cooper, P.J., Vize, C.M., and Ashby, L. (1993). Depression in 11–16-year-old girls: The role of past parental psychopathology and exposure to recent life events. *Journal of Child Psychology and Psychiatry,* **34**, 1103–1115.

Gordon, D., Burge, D., Hammen, C., Adrian, C., Jaenicke, C., and Hiroto, D. (1989). Observations of interactions of depressed women with their children. *American Journal of Psychiatry*, **146**, 50–55.

Hammen, C. (1990). Cognitive approaches to depression in children: Current findings and new directions. In B.B. Lahey and A.E. Kazdin (Eds.), *Advances in clinical psychology* (Vol. 13, pp. 139–173). New York: Plenum Press.

Hammen, C. (1991). *Depression runs in families: The social context of risk and resilience in children of depressed mothers.* New York: Springer.

Hammen, C., Adrian, C., Gordon, D., Burge, D., Jaenicke, C., and Hiroto, D. (1987). Children of depressed mothers: Maternal strain and symptom predictors of dysfunction. *Journal of Abnormal Psychology*, **96**, 190–198.

Hammen, C. and Goodman-Brown, T. (1990). Self-schemas and vulnerability to specific life stress in children at risk for depression. *Cognitive Therapy and Research*, **14**, 215–227.

Harrington, R., Fudge, H., Rutter, M., Pickles, A., and Hill, J. (1990). Adult outcomes of childhood and adolescent depression: I. Psychiatric status. *Archives of General Psychiatry*, **47**, 465–473.

Harter, S. (1990). Causes, correlates and the functional role of global self-worth: A life span perspective. In R. Sternberg and J. Kolligian (Eds.), *Competence considered* (pp. 68–97). New Haven, CT: Yale University Press.

Jacobsen, R.H., Lahey, B.B., and Strauss, C.C. (1983). Correlates of depressed mood in normal children. *Journal of Abnormal Child Psychology*, **11**, 29–39.

Kahn, J.S., Kehle, T.J., Jenson, W.R., and Clark, E. (1990). Comparison of cognitive-behavioral, relaxation, and self-modeling interventions for depression among middle-school students. *School Psychology Review*, **19**, 196–211.

Kandel, D.B. and Davies, M. (1982). Epidemiology of depressive mood in adolescents: An empirical study. *Archives of General Psychiatry*, **39**, 1205–1212.

Kandel, D.B. and Davies, M. (1986). Suicidality, depression, and substance abuse in adolescence. *American Journal of Psychiatry*, **43**, 255–262.

Kaplan, S.L., Hong, G.K., and Weinhold, C. (1984). Epidemiology of depressive symptomatology in adolescents. *Journal of the American Academy of Child Psychiatry*, **23**, 91–98.

Kashani, J.H. and Carlson, G.A. (1987). Seriously depressed pre-schoolers. *American Journal of Psychiatry*, **144**, 348–350.

Kashani, J.H., Carlson, G.A., Beck, N.C., Hoeper, E.W., Corcoran, C.M., McAllister, J.A., Fallahi, C., Rosenberg, T.K., and Reid, J.C. (1987). Depression, depressive symptoms, and depressed mood among a community sample of adolescents. *American Journal of Psychiatry*, **144**, 931–934.

Kashani, J.H., Holcomb, W.R., and Orvaschel, H. (1986). Depression and depressive symptoms in preschool children from the general population. *American Journal of Psychiatry*, **143**, 1138–1143.

Kashani, J.H., Rosenberg, T.K., and Reid, J.C. (1989). Developmental perspectives in child and adolescent depressive symptoms in a community sample. *American Journal of Psychiatry*, **146**, 871–875.

Kashani, J.H. and Simonds, J.F. (1979). The incidence of depression in children. *American Journal of Psychiatry*, **136**, 1203–1205.

Kazdin, A.E., Rodgers, A., and Colbus, D. (1986). The hopelessness scale for children: Psychometric characteristics and concurrent validity. *Journal of Consulting and Clinical Psychology*, **54**, 241–245.

Keller, M.B., Beardslee, W.R., Dorer, D.J., Lavori, P.W., Samuelson, H., and Klerman, G.L. (1986). Impact of severity and chronicity of parental affective illness on adaptive functioning and psychopathology in children. *Archives of General Psychiatry*, **43**, 930–937.

Kendler, K.S., Neale, M.C., Kessler, R.C., Heath, A.C., and Eaves, L.J. (1992). Childhood parental loss and adult psychopathology in women. *Archives of General Psychiatry*, **49**, 109–116.

King, C.A., Naylor, M.W., Segal, H.G., Evan T., and Shain, B.N. (1993). Global self-worth, specific self-perceptions of comptence, and depression in adolescents. *Journal of the American Academy of Child and Adolescent Psychiatry*, **32**, 745–752.

Klein, D.N., Depue, R.A., and Slater, J.F. (1985). Cyclothymia in the adolescent offspring of parents with bipolar affective disorder. *Journal of Abnormal Psychology*, **94**, 115–127.

Klein, D.N., Depue, R.A., and Slater, J.F. (1986). Inventory identification of cyclothymia. IX. Validation in offspring of bipolar patients. *Archives of General Psychiatry*, **43**, 441–445.

Kovacs, M. (1981). Rating scales to assess depression in school aged children. *Acta Paedopsychiatrica*, **46**, 305–315.

Kovacs, M. and Beck, A.T. (1977). An empirical-clinical approach toward a definition of childhood depression. In J.G. Schulterbrandt and A. Raskin (Eds.), *Depression in childhood: Diagnosis, treatment and conceptual models* (pp. 1–25). New York: Raven Press.

Kovacs, M., Feinberg, T.L., Crouse-Novak, M., Paulauskas, S.L., and Finkelstein, R. (1984). Depressive disorders in childhood: I. A longitudinal prospective study of characteristics and recovery. *Archives of General Psychiatry*, **41**, 229–237.

Kovacs, M., Gatsonis, C., Paulauskas, S.L., and Richards, C. (1989). Depressive disorders in childhood: IV. A longitudinal study of comorbidity with and risk for anxiety disorders. *Archives of General Psychiatry*, **46**, 776–782.

Kusch, M. and Petermann, F. (1994). Entwicklungspsychopathologie depressiver Störungen im Kindes-und Jugendalter. *Kindheit und Entwicklung*, **3**, 142–156.

Kutcher, S.P. and Marton, P. (1989). Parameters of adolescents depression: A review. *Psychiatric Clinics of North America*, **12**, 895–918.

Lahmeyer, H.W., Poznanski, E.O., and Bellur, S.N. (1983). EEG sleep in depressed adolescents. *American Journal of Psychiatry*, **19**, 239–240.

Lang, M. and Tisher, M. (1978). *Children´s Depression Scale*. Victoria: Australian Council for Educational Research.

Lefkowitz, M.M. and Tesiny, E.P. (1980). Assessment of childhood depression. *Journal of Consulting and Clinical Psychology*, **48**, 43–50.

Lewinsohn, P.M. and Arconad, M. (1981). Behavioral treatment of depression: Social learning approach. In J.F. Clarkin and A.I. Glazer (Eds.), Depression: *Behavioral and directive intervention strategies* (pp. 33–67). New York: Garland STPM Press.

Lewinsohn, P.M., Clark, G.N., Hops, H., and Andrews, J. (1990). Cognitive-behavioral treatment for depressed adolescents. *Behavioral Therapy*, **21**, 385–401.

Lewinsohn, P.M., Hoberman, H.M., and Rosenbaum, M. (1988). A prospective study of risk factors for unipolar depression. *Journal of Abnormal Psychology*, **97**, 251–264.

Lewinsohn, P.M., Hoberman, H., Teri, L., and Hautzinger, M. (1985). An integrative theory of depression. In S. Reiss and R. Bootzin (Eds.), *Theoretical issues in behavior therapy* (pp. 331–359). New York: Academic Press.

Lewinsohn, P.M., Hops, H., Roberts, R.E., Seeley, J.R., and Andrews, J.A. (1993). Adolescent psychopathology: I. Prevalence and incidence of depression and other DSM-II-IR disorders in high school students. *Journal of Abnormal Psychology*, **102**, 133–144.

Lewinsohn, P.M., Clarke, G.N., Seeley, J.R., and Rohde, P. (1994). Major depression in community adolescents: Age of onset, episode duration, and time to recurrence. *Journal of the American Academy of Child and Adolescent Psychiatry*, **33**, 809–819.

Liddle, B. and Spence, S.H. (1990). Cognitive-behavior therapy with depressed primary school children: A cautionary note. *Behavioral Psychotherapy*, **18**, 85–102.

McCauley, E., Myers, K., Mitchell, J., Calderon, R., Schloredt, K., and Treder, R. (19–93). Depression in young people: Initial presentation and clinical course. *Journal of the American Academy of Child and Adolescent Psychiatry*, **32**, 714–722.

McCauley, E., Mitchell, J.R., Burke, P., and Moss, S. (1988). Cognitive attributes of depression in children and adolescents. *Journal of Consulting and Clinical Psychology*, **56**, 903–908.

McGee, R. and Williams, S. (1988). A longitudinal study of depression in nine-year-old children. *Journal of the American Academy of Child Psychiatry*, **27**, 342–348.

McGee, R., Feehan, M., Williams, S., and Anderson, J. (1992). DSM-III disorders from age 11 to age 15 years. *Journal of the American Academy of Child and Adolescent Psychiatry*, **31**, 50–59.

McGee, R., Anderson, J., Williams, S., and Silva, P.A. (1986). Cognitive correlates of depressive symptoms in 11-year-old children. *Journal of Abnormal Child Psychology*, **14**, 517–524.

Merikangas, K.R. and Angst, J. (in press). The challenge of depressive disorders in adolescence. In M. Rutter (Ed.), *Psychosocial disturbances in young people*. Cambridge: Cambridge University Press.

Merikangas, K.P., Prusoff, B.A., and Weissman, M.M. (1988). Parental concordance for affective disorders: Psychopathology in offspring. *Journal of Affective Disorders*, **15**, 279–290.

Mitchell, J., McCauley, E., Burke, P.M., and Moss, S. (1988). Phenomenology of depression in children and adolescents. *Journal of the American Academy of Child and Adolescent Psychiatry*, **27**, 12–20.

Nezu, A.M., Nezu, C.M., and Perri, M.G. (1989). *Problem-solving therapy for depression: Theory, research, and clinical guidelines*. New York: Wiley.

Nolen-Hoeksema, S. (1987). Sex differences in unipolar depression: Evidence and theory. *Psychological Bulletin*, **101**, 259–282.

Nolen-Hoeksema, S., Girgus, J.S., and Seligman, M.E.P. (1986). Learned helplessness in children: A longitudinal study of depression, achievement, and explanatory style. *Journal of Personality and Social Psychology*, **51**, 435–442.

Nolen-Hoeksema, S., Girgus, J.S., and Seligman, M.E.P. (1991). Sex differences in depression and explanatory style in children. *Journal of Youth and Adolescence*, **20**, 233–246.

Nolen-Hoeksema, S., Girgus, J.S., and Seligman, M.E.P. (1992). Predictors and consequences of childhood depressive symptoms: A 5-year longitudinal study. *Journal of Abnormal Psychology*, **101**, 405–422.

Orvaschel, H., Walsh-Allis, G., and Ye, W. (1988). Psychopathology in children of parents with recurrent depression. *Journal of Abnormal Child Psychology*, **16**, 17–28.

Parke, R.D., MacDonald, K.B., Beitel, A., and Bhavnagri, N. (1988). The role of the family in the development of peer relationships. In R. Peters and R.J. McMahan (Eds.), *Social learning systems: Approaches to marriage and the family* (pp. 17–44). New York: Brunner-Mazel.

Petermann, U. and Petermann, F. (1996). *Training mit sozial unsicheren Kindern*. Weinheim: Psychologie Verlags Union 6th Edition.

Petersen, A.C., Sarigiani, P.A., and Kennedy, R.E. (1991). Adolescent depression: Why more girls? *Journal of Youth and Adolescence*, **20**, 247–271.

Petersen, A.C., Compas, B.E., Brooks-Gunn, J., Stemmler, M., Ey, S., and Grant, K.E. (1993). Depression in adolescence. *American Psychologist*, **48**, 155–168.

Puig-Antich, J. (1986). Possible prevention strategies for depression in children and adolescents. In J.T. Barter and S.W. Talbott (Eds.), *Primary prevention in psychiatry: State of the art* (pp. 69–84). Washington, DC: American Psychiatric Press.

Puig-Antich, J., Blau, S., Marx, N., Greenhill, L.L., and Chambers, W. (1978). Prepubertal major depressive disorder: A pilot study. *Journal of the American Academy of Child and Adolescent Psychiatry*, **17**, 695–707.

Puig-Antich, J. and Chambers, W. (1978). *The Schedule for Affective Disorders and Schizophrenia for School-aged children*. New York: State Psychiatric Institute, NY.

Puig-Antich, J., Kaufman, J., Ryan, N.D., Williamson, D.E., Dahl, R.E., Lukens, E., Todak, G., Ambrosini, P., Rabinovich, H., and Nelson, B. (1993). The psychosocial functioning and family environment of depressed adolescents. *Journal of American Academy of Child and Adolescent Psychiatry*, **32**, 244–253.

Puig-Antich, J., Goetz, R., Hanlon, C., Tabrizi, M.A., Davies, M., and Weitzman, E. (1982). Sleep architecture and REM sleep measures in prepubertal major depressives during an episode. *Archives of General Psychiatry*, **39**, 932–939.

Puig-Antich, J., Lukens, E., Davies, M., Goetz, D., Brennan-Quattrock, J. and Todak, G. (1985). Psychosocial functioning in prepubertal children with major depressive disorders: I. Interpersonal relationships during the depressive episode. *Archives of General Psychiatry*, **42**, 500–507.

Puig-Antich, J., Novacenko, H., Davies, M., Chambers, W.J., Tabrizi, M.A., Krawiec, V., Ambrosini, P.J., and Sachar, E.J. (1984). Growth hormone secretion in prepubertal major depressive children: I. Sleep related plasma concentrations during a depressive episode. *Archives of General Psychiatry*, **41**, 455–460.

Puig-Antich, J., Ryan, N.D., and Rabinovich, H. (1985). Affective disorders in childhood and adolescence. In J.M. Wiener (Ed.), *Diagnosis and psychopharmacology of childhood and adolescent disorders* (pp. 151–178). New York: John Wiley.

Rao, U., Weissman, M.M., Martin, J.A., and Hammond, R.W. (1993). Childhood depression and risk of suicide: A preliminary report of a longitudinal study. *Journal of the American Academy of Child and Adolescent Psychiatry*, **32**, 21–27.

Rehm, L.P. (1981). A self-control therapy program for treatment of depression. In J.F. Clarkin and A.I. Glazer (Eds.), Depression: Behavioral and directive intervention strategies (pp. 68–109). New York: Garland STPM Press.

Reich, W. and Welner, Z. (1988). *Revised version of the Diagnostic Interview for Children and Adolescents (DICA-R)*. St. Louis, MO: Department of Psychiatry, Washington University School of Medicine.

Reinherz, H.Z., Giaconia, R.M., Pakiz, B., Silverman, A.B., Frost, A.K., and Lefkowitz, E.S. (1993). Psychosocial risks for major depression in late adolescence: A longitudinal community study. *Journal of the American Academy of Child and Adolescent Psychiatry*, **32**, 1155–1163.

Reinherz, H.Z., Stewart-Berghauer, G., Pakiz, B., Frost, A.K., Moeykens, B.A., and Holmes, W.M. (1989). The relationship of early risk and current mediators to depressive symptomatology in adolescence. *Journal of the American Academy of Child and Adolescent Psychiatry*, **28**, 942–947.

Renouf, A.G. and Harter, S. (1990). Low self-worth and anger as components of the depressive experience in young adolescents. *Development and Psychopathology*, **2**, 293–310.

Reynolds, W.M. (1993). Depression in children and adolescents. In W.M. Reynolds (Ed.), *Internalizing disorders in children and adolescents* (pp. 149–254). New York: Wiley.

Reynolds, W.M. and Coats, K.J. (1986). A comparison of cognitive-behavioral therapy and relaxation training for the treatment of depression in adolescents. *Journal of Consulting and Clinical Psychology*, **54**, 653–660.

Rie, H.E. (1966). Depression in childhood: A survey of some pertinent contributions. *Journal of the American Academy of Child Psychiatry*, **5**, 653–685.

Robins, L.N., Helzer, J.E., Weissman, M.M., Orvaschel, H., Gruenberg, E., Burke, J.D., and Regier, D.A. (1984). Lifetime prevalence of specific psychiatric disorders in three sites. *Archives of General Psychiatry*, **41**, 949–958.

Rohde, P., Lewinsohn, P., and Seeley, J. (1991). Comorbidity of unipolar depression: II. Comorbidity with other mental disorders in adolescents and adults. *Journal of Abnormal Psychology*, **100**, 214–222.

Ross, A.O. and Petermann, F. (1987). *Verhaltenstherapie mit Kindern und Jugendlichen*. Stuttgart: Hippokrates.

Rutter, M. (1986). The developmental psychopathology of depression: Issues and perspectives. In M. Rutter, C.E. Izard, and P.B. Read (Eds.), *Depression in young people* (pp. 3–30). New York: Guilford Press.

Rutter, M. (1989). Isle of Wright revisited: Twenty-five years of child psychiatric epidemiology. *Journal of the American Academy of Child and Adolescent Psychiatry*, **28**, 633–653.

Ryan, N.D., Puig-Antich, J., Cooper, T.B., Rabinovich, H., Ambrosini, P., Fried, J., Davies, M., Torres, D., and Suckow, R.F. (1987). Relative safety of single versus divided dose imipramine in adolescent major depression. *Journal of the American Academy of Child and Adolescent Psychiatry*, **26**, 400–406.

Ryan, N.D., Puig-Antich, J., Rabinovich, H., Fried, J., Ambrosini, P., Meyer, V., Torres, D., Dachille, S., and Mazzie, D. (1988). MAOIs in adolescent major depression unresponsive to tricyclic antidepressants. *Journal of the American Academy of Child and Adolescent Psychiatry*, **27**, 755–758.

Ryan, N.D., Williamson, D.E., Iyengar, S., Orvaschel, H., Reich, T., Dahl, R.E., and Puig-Antich, J.A. (1992). A secular increase in child and adolescent onset affective disorder. *Journal of the American Academy of Child and Adolescent Psychiatry*, **31**, 600–605.

Sarigiani, P.A., Wilson, J.L., Petersen, A.C., and Vicary, J.R. (1990). Self-image and educational plans for adolescence from two contrasting communities. *Journal of Early Adolescence*, **10**, 37–55.

Schildkraut, J.J. (1965). The catecholamine hypothesis of affective disorders: A review of supporting evidence. *American Journal of Psychiatry*, **122**, 509–522.

Seligman, M.E.P. and Peterson, C. (1986). A learned helplessness perspective on childhood depression: Theory and research. In M. Rutter, C.E. Izard, and P.B. Read (Eds.), *Depression in young people: Developmental and clinical perspectives* (pp. 223–249). New York: Guilford.

Siegel, J.M. and Brown, J.D. (1988). A prospective study of stressful circumstances, illness symptoms, and depressed mood among adolescents. *Developmental Psychology*, **24**, 715–721.

Simmons, R.G. and Blyth, D.A. (1987). *Moving into adolescence: The impact of pubertal change and school context.* Hawthorne, NY: Aldine de Gruyter.

Sokoloff, R.M. and Lubin, B. (1983). Depressive mood in adolescent, emotionally disturbed females: Reliability and validity of an adjective checklist (C-DACL). *Journal of Abnormal Child Psychology*, **11**, 531–536.

Sorenson, S.B., Rutter, C.M., and Aneshensel, C.S. (1991). Depression in the community: An investigation into age of onset. *Journal of Consulting Clinical Psychology*, **59**, 541–546.

Stark, K.D., Reynolds, W.M., and Kaslow, N. (1987). A comparison of the relative efficacy of self-control therapy and a behavioral problem-solving therapy for depression in children. *Journal of Abnormal Child Psychology*, **15**, 91–113.

Strober, M. and Carlson, G. (1982). Bipolar illness in adolescents: Clinical, genetic and pharmacologic predictors in a three- to four-year prospective follow-up. *Archives of General Psychiatry*, **39**, 549–555.

Tarullo, L., DeMulder, E., Martinez, P., and Radke-Yarrow, M. (1994). Dialogues with preadolescents and adolescents: Mother-child interaction patterns in affectively ill and well dyads. *Journal of Abnormal Psychology*, **22**, 33–51.

Velez, C.N., Johnson, J., and Cohen, P. (1989). A longitudinal analysis of selected risk factors for childhood psychopathology. *Journal of the American Academy of Child and Adolescent Psychiatry*, **28**, 851–864.

Vernberg, E.M. (1990). Psychological adjustment and experiences with peers during early adolescence: Reciprocal, incidental, or unidirectional relationships? *Journal of Abnormal Child Psychology*, **18**, 187–198.

Webster-Stratton, C. and Hammond, M. (1988). Maternal depression and its relationship to life stress, perceptions of child behavior problems, parenting behaviors, and child conduct problems. *Journal of Abnormal Child Psychology*, **16**, 299–315.

Weintraub, S. (1987). Risk factors in schizophrenia: The Stony Brook high-risk project. *Schizophrenia Bulletin*, **13**, 439–450.

Weissman, M.M. (1990). Evidence for comorbidity of anxiety and depression: Family and genetic studies of children. In J.D. Maser and C.R. Cloninger (Eds.), *Comorbidity of mood and anxiety disorders* (pp. 349–368). Washington, DC: American Psychiatric Press.

Weissman, M.M., Gammon, G.D., John, K., Merikangas, K.R., Prusoff, B.A., and Scholomskas, D. (1987). Children of depressed parents: Increased psychopathology and early onset of major depression. *Archives of General Psychiatry*, **44**, 847–853.

Weissman, M.M., Prusoff, B.A., Gammon, G.D., Merikangas, K.R., Leckman, J.F., and Kidd, K.K. (1984). Psychopathology in the children (ages 6–18) of depressed and normal parents. *Journal of the American Academy of Child Psychiatry*, **23**, 78–84.

Weissman, M.M., Warner, V., Wickramaratne, P., and Prusoff, B.A. (1988). Early onset major depression in parents and their children. *Journal of Affective Disorder*, **15**, 269–277.

Weisz, J.R., Rudolph, K.D., Granger, D.A., and Sweeney, L. (1992). Cognition, competence, and coping in child and adolescent depression: Research findings, developmental concerns, therapeutic implications. *Development and Psychopathology*, **4**, 627–653.

Weisz, J.R., Stevens, J.S., Curry, J.F., Cohen, R., Craighead, E., Burlingame, W.V., Smith, A., Weiss, B., and Parmelee, D.X. (1989). Control-related cognitions and depression among inpatient children and adolescents. *Journal of the American Academy of Child and Adolescent Psychiatry*, **28**, 358–363.

Weisz, J.R., Sweeney, L., Proffitt, V., and Carr, T. (1993). Control-related beliefs and self-reported depressive symptoms in late childhood. *Journal of Abnormal Psychology*, **102**, 411–418.

Weisz, J.R., Weiss, B., Han, S.S., Granger, D.A., and Morton, T. (1995). Effects of psychotherapy with children and adolescents revisited: A meta-analysis of treatment outcome studies. *Psychological Bulletin*, **117**, 450–468.

Weisz, J.R., Weiss, B., Wasserman, A.A., and Rintoul, B. (1987). Control-related belief and depression among clinic-referred children and adolescents. *Journal of Abnormal Psychology*, **96**, 149–158.

Whitaker, A., Johnson, J., Shaffer, D., Rapoport, J.L., Kalikow, K., Walsh, B.T., Davies, M., Braiman, S., and Dolinsky, A. (1990). Uncommon troubles in young people: Prevalence estimates of selected psychiatric disorders in a nonreferred population. *Archives of General Psychiatry*, **47**, 487–496.

Wittchen, H.-U. and Essau, C.A. (1993a). Epidemiology of panic disorder: Progress and unresolved issues. *Journal of Psychiatric Research*, **27**, 47–68.

Wittchen, H.-U. and Essau, C.A. (1993b). Epidemiology of anxiety disorders. In P.J. Willner (Ed.), *Psychiatry*. Philadelphia: J.B. Lippincott Company.

Wright, E. (1988). *Behavior Disorders Identification Scale*. Columbia, MO: Hawthorne.

Young, W., Knowles, J.B., MacLean, A.W., Boag, L., and McConville, B.J. (1982). The sleep of childhood depressives. *Biological Psychiatry*, **17**, 1163–1168.

CHAPTER 9

SUBSTANCE USE DISORDERS

Lisa Dierker, Kathleen R. Merikangas and Cecilia Ahmoi Essau

Beginning in the early 1970s, substance abuse in adolescents and young adults was identified as an important public health problem. As reported by Bean-Bayog (1987), substance abuse is involved in about 50% of the suicides among college students in the US, and drinking is involved in 80 to 90% of traffic accidents. Less dramatic but more insidious consequences of substance dependence in adolescence include their developmental, emotional, and social costs.

This chapter presents a summary of current research relating to the epidemiology, risk factors, course, and prevention and treatment of substance use disorders in adolescents. Substance use disorders, that include substance abuse and substance dependence, refer to maladaptive behaviour associated with regular use of substances including alcohol, amphetamine, caffeine, cannabis, cocaine, hallucinogens, inhalants, nicotine, opioids, phencyclidine (PCP), and sedatives, hypnotics or anxiolytics (American Psychiatric Association; APA, 1994).

DEFINITION AND CLASSIFICATION

Issues Surrounding Adolescent Classification

Substance use refers to more than use of one or two occasions, but is below the threshold of abuse. Since experimental and recreational use of substance is both occasional and limited in the amount taken, it is not likely to lead to any impairment (Silbereisen *et al.*, 1995). Also, experimentation with various substances is so common during adolescence that the detection and subsequent treatment of actual substance disorders in the adolescent population is relatively low. MacDonald (1984) identified alcohol and drug misuse as the most commonly missed pediatric diagnoses. However, the phase of substance use may proceed to regular or heavy use which may put the adolescents at the risk of developing substance use disorders.

Classification Systems

The International Classification of Diseases (ICD; World Health Organization; WHO, 1993) now in its tenth edition and the Diagnostic and Statistical Manual of Mental Disorders (APA, 1994) now in its fourth edition, have long been considered the diagnostic standard for substance related disorders. Due to an interest in consensus between the authors of the most recent editions, DSM-IV and ICD-10 have become more highly compatible in classifying substance use disorders than earlier editions of these systems. In ICD-10, the particular type of psychoactive substance is first identified, followed by the subsequent classification of the behaviour as hazardous, harmful or including dependence symptoms. DSM-IV similarly separates abuse (Table 9.1) and dependence (Table 9.2) on the basis of the consequences of substance use, including tolerance and withdrawal. The major differences that remain between these two systems include the number of diagnostic criteria and specific definitions of symptoms. ICD-10, for example, has fewer dependence criteria than DSM-IV, and has defined symptoms more broadly.

Table 9.1   DSM-IV criteria for substance abuse .

A.   A maladaptive pattern of substance use leading to clinically significant impairment or distress, as manifested by one (or more) of the following occurring within a 12-month period:

   1) recurrent substance use resulting in a failure to fulfill major role obligations at work, school, or home (e.g., repeated absences or poor work performance related to substance use; substances-related absences, suspensions, or expulsions from school; neglect of children or household)

   2) recurrent substance use in situations in which it is physically hazardous (e.g., driving an automobile or operating a machine when impaired by substance use)

   3) recurrent substance-related legal problems (e.g., arrests for substance-related disorderly conduct)

   4) continued substance use despite having persistent or recurrent social or interpersonal problems caused or exacerbated by the effects of the substance (e.g., arguments with spouse about consequences of intoxication, physical fights)

B.   The symptoms have never met the criteria for substance dependence for the class of substance.

Reprinted with permission from the Diagnostic and Statistical Manual of Mental Disorders, Fourth Edition. Copyright 1994 American Psychiatric Association.

Table 9.2 DSM-IV criteria for substance dependence

A maladaptive pattern of substance use, leading to clinically significant impairment or distress, as manifested by three (or more) of the following, occurring at any time in the same 12-month period:

1) tolerance, as defined by either of the following:
   a) a need for markedly increased amounts of the substance to achieve intoxication or desired effect
   b) markedly diminished effect with continued use of the same amount of the substance

2) withdrawal, as manifested by either of the following:
   a) the characteristic withdrawal syndrome for the substance (refer to Criteria A and B of the criteria sets for withdrawal from the specific substances)
   b) the same (or a closely related) substance is taken to relieve or avoid withdrawal symptoms

3) the substance is often taken in larger amounts or over a longer period than was intended

4) there is a persistent desire or unsuccessful efforts to cut down or control substance use

5) a great deal of time is spent in activities necessary to obtain the substance (e.g., visiting multiple doctors or driving long distances), use the substance (e.g., chain-smoking), or recover from its effects

6) important social, occupational, or recreational activities are given up or reduced because of substance use

7) the substance use is continued despite knowledge of having a persistent or recurrent physical or psychological problem that is likely to have been caused or exacerbated by the substance (e.g., current cocaine use despite recognition of cocaine-induced depression, or continued drinking despite recognition that an ulcer was made worse by alcohol consumption)

Reprinted with permission from the Diagnostic and Statistical Manual of Mental Disorders, Fourth Edition. Copyright 1994 American Psychiatric Association.

While etiological factors associated with substances have often been separated by the type of substance use, many studies have supported the usefulness of conceptualizing adolescent substance abuse as a unitary phenomenon. Hansen and colleagues (1987), for example, found striking similarity for predictive relationships among environmental factors found to be associated with substance use. Using structural equation modeling, the same constellation of environmental variables including parental care, parental use, and peer use were found to be equal contributors to a single substance use construct.

Methodological Issues in Substance Research

Although a good deal has been learned in recent years about the prevalence of substance use and the factors that play a role in the development of substance abuse and dependence, much of the research has been limited interpretively by methodological problems. First, much research has been conducted on samples that may not be representative of the general population. School and treatment based samples may lead to an underestimation of substance use because they fail to include school dropouts and youths residing in institutional settings. Epidemiological studies focusing on prevalence rates most commonly solicit participation from a cross-section of school districts. Given the evidence that school dropouts and absentees are at higher risk for substance use than those who remain in school, a sample selected in this way may produce a substantial underestimation of substance use among youth.

A second major methodological consideration in the substance literature is cross-sectional design employed in most research on substance use disorders in youth. While these studies have been a useful way to demonstrate risk factors associated with substance use, they have been unable to establish causal relations among those variables, and therefore cannot lead to a clear developmental understanding of substance use and misuse. Only prospective longitudinal investigations create an opportunity for identifying developmental continuities that definitively precede and possibly cause progression toward a substance use disorder. Relatively few studies focusing on adolescent substance use have collected data in this way.

Another important methodological issue involves the lack of cross-cultural comparative data. The vast majority of data on substance use and abuse in youth has been collected in the United States. Unfortunately, there is sparse information on cross-cultural patterns of substance abuse. Finally, the reliability and validity of the measures of substance abuse among youth have not been well established. Most existing studies have used surveys or checklists to determine prevalence rates. In that substance use is illegal (including alcohol for adolescents), social desirability strongly affects the assessment of substance use and associated problems. Response bias may play a large role in survey assessment.

EPIDEMIOLOGY

Within the past two decades, epidemiological data on substance abuse and dependence has been collected by governmental agencies and private organizations in countries throughout the world. While recent prevalence rates have occasionally represented a decline from the previous years, early exposure to a variety of substances remains the norm. Although there is substantial data on the patterns of substance use in the United States, there is sparse information regarding the prevalence rates of abuse and/or dependence among adolescents either in the United States or in other countries. Aggregation of available data reviewed below is precluded by variations in definitions, age composition of the samples, and the prevalence periods which ranged from current to lifetime.

Prevalence of Substance Use

United States

Within the United States, several epidemiologic surveys have been monitoring trends in substance use among youth since the early 1970s. The largest research and reporting program is conducted by the University of Michigan Institute for Social Research. This survey collects information from senior high school students (age 17 and 18) from 130 high schools across the United States, and more recently has also included annual surveys of eighth grade (age 13 and 14) and tenth grade (age 15 and 16) students. This study surveys approximately 17,000 students from each age group in order to identify prevalence rates as well as changes in beliefs and attitudes surrounding the use of substances (Johnson *et al.*, 1994).

According to the 1993 survey, 32.3% of the eighth grade students, the youngest group in the sample, reported having some experience with illicit substances including marijuana, inhalants, hallucinogens, cocaine and heroin. Inhalants were the most frequent class of substances (i.e., 19.4%) followed by marijuana (12%), cocaine (2.9%), hallucinogens (1.7%), and heroin (1.4%). The lifetime prevalence of alcohol use was 67.1% among eighth graders, a rate that has remained relatively stable in this age group over the past few years. Well over one-third of the students who had used alcohol in the past, reported having experienced alcohol intoxication (i.e., "drunkenness").

Among tenth grade students, 38.7% reported some experience with illicit substances. While rates were higher, the pattern of specific use was found to be similar to the patterns of eighth grade students with marijuana (24.4%) and inhalants (17.5%) representing the most commonly used illicit substances, followed by the relatively less prevalent lifetime use of hallucinogens (6.8%), cocaine (3.6%), and heroin (1.3%). The lifetime rate of alcohol use among tenth graders was 80.8% in 1993. Over half of whom reported having been drunk.

Senior high school students reported even higher lifetime rates of illicit drug and alcohol use, but again demonstrated similar prevalence patterns to those of the younger adolescents. Marijuana use (35.3%) and inhalant use (17.4%) showed the highest prevalence rates, followed by hallucinogens (10.9%), cocaine (6.1%), and heroin (1.1%). The lifetime rate of alcohol use among seniors was a striking 91.2%, showing that by age 18 exposure to alcohol is universal. Moreover, among high school seniors, almost half reported having been drunk at some time in their life.

Substantial sex differences were found among high school seniors, particularly in the heavy use of alcohol and illicit drugs. Twenty-one percent of the females versus 35% of the males in the 1993 survey reported occasions of heavy drinking. (This sex difference has slowly been diminishing since the first survey was conducted in the early 1970s). Similarly, sex differences in illicit drug use also show an excess of males. Daily marijuana use, for example, is reported by 3.3% of the males and 1.3% of the females. Sex differences in illicit drug use was not found among the groups of younger adolescents.

These rates generally represent upward trends in illicit drug use during the 1990s which has been particularly pronounced in the use of marijuana. Use of this substance has doubled among eighth-graders (to 13%), has grown by two-thirds among tenth-graders (to 25%), and has grown by two-fifths among 12th-graders (to 31%). Other illicit drugs, such as lysergic acid diethylamide (LSD), other hallucinogens, inhalants, stimulants, barbiturates and cocaine and crack have exhibited smaller upward trends that may not have reached significance within the past year, but show gradual increases that represent a significant long-term trend. While alcohol use has not shown a statistically significant increase during 1994, the stable rates show that drinking remains common among American adolescents Johnson *et al.*, 1994.

Another large-scale survey conducted within the United States is the "National Parents' Resource Institute for Drug Education" (PRIDE). This survey polls over 200,000 adolescents ages 12 to age 18 attending high schools from 34 states across the U.S. Findings from the 1993-94 survey also revealed substantial past year prevalence for substance use among youth. Among those age 15 to 18 years, use of alcohol was reported by 65.9% of the sample; use of marijuana was reported by 24.6%; use of inhalants, 6.9%; use of hallucinogens, 6.6%; and use of cocaine, 4.0%. A sample of children age 12 to 14 had past year prevalence rates of 39.3% for alcohol; 8.2% for marijuana; 5.9% for inhalants, 2.1% for hallucinogens and 1.9% for cocaine.

Greece

A large-scale study of licit and illicit substance use conducted in Greece sampled over 11,000 adolescents age 14-18 (Kokkevi and Stefanis, 1991). The prevalence of alcohol use among Greek adolescents was 94.8% for the past year and 82.4% for the past month. The past year prevalence of marijuana use was 2.7%, cocaine, 1.1%, opiates, 2.1% and hallucinogens, less than 1%. Lifetime prevalence of illicit drug use was reported by 6% of the sample. Approximately half of the adolescents who used illicit substances reported having used them more than twice. As in similar surveys, use of substances was found to increase significantly with age. Lifetime drug use for illicit substances, for example, was reported by: less than 1% of the 13 and 14 year-olds; 4.3% of the 15 and 16 year-olds; and 10.9% of the 17 and 18 year-olds.

Germany

According to a representative study done between 1990 and 1991, 14.4% of the 12–39 year-olds in the former East Germany and 7.9% in the former West Germany have reported daily consumption of alcohol (DFG, 1991; cited in Perkonigg, Wittchen, and Lachner, in press). The lifetime frequency in the use of illegal drugs was 16.3% in the former West Germany as compared to only 1.5% in the former East Germany. The most commonly used drug was marijuana (3.9%), followed by cocaine (0.3%) and opiates (0.2%). In Nordlohne's 1992 study, 50% of the 12-17 year-olds have indicated having drunk "soft" (e.g., wine, beer) and 25% "hard" alcoholic beverages (e.g. liquor) at sometime in their lives.

A recent report by Silbereisen *et al.* (1995) has shown that the drinking pattern in Germany among adolescents seem to be affected by the German reunification. As the consequence of the open market that follow unification, the East German´s data showed a twofold increase in alcohol consumption from 1989 to 1990. As for the use of drugs, the West German adolescents showed the highest use in the early 1970s, but then significantly decline thereafter (Reuband, 1988). Among the 12 to 25 year olds, 5% reported current use in 1990, and at the beginning of the 1980s this rate dropped by one half.

France and Israel

One of the only examples of comparative cross-cultural epidemiologic surveys to be conducted on adolescent substance use is a study of substance trends in France and Israel (Kandel *et al.*, 1981). Overall, France was found to have higher lifetime and current rates of adolescent substance use than Israel. The lifetime prevalence rate in French adolescents were 80% for alcohol and 26% for any illicit substance. As in the studies previously mentioned, the illicit drug with the highest lifetime prevalence rate was marijuana at 23%. Although the rate of a lifetime alcohol use was similar in the Israeli sample (i.e., 70%), the lifetime prevalence of an illicit drug use of 8% was far lower than that of the French sample. Marijuana was reported to have been used by only 3% of the Israeli sample, nearly eight times lower than that of French youth.

Prevalence of Substance Abuse and Dependence

United States

In a community-based study of 386 adolescents living in the United States, Reinherz *et al.* (1993) found high prevalence rates of substance related disorders. Alcohol abuse/dependence had the highest lifetime prevalence rate at 32.4% while drug abuse/dependence were found among 9.8% of the sample. Similarly, in Lewinsohn *et al.*'s (1993) community adolescent sample, the lifetime prevalence rate of alcohol disorders was 4.6% and that of hard drug disorders (i.e., cocaine, amphetamine, hallucinogen, inhalant, opioid, phencyclindine and sedative abuse/dependence) was 2.6%. Cohen *et al.* (1993) focused particularly on sex differences in substance related disorders and found similar rates of alcohol abuse for 14-16 year-old males and females. Among 17–20 year-olds, however, prevalence rate for males was 20%, more than twice that of females (8.9%). By comparison marijuana abuse was found to be relatively rare in both males (4.1%) and females (1.8%). This was not a significant difference.

New Zealand

Data from the Dunedin Multidisciplinary Health and Developmental Study showed a 1-year prevalence of alcohol dependence to be 10.4% and of marijuana dependence 5.2% among 18 year-olds (Feehan *et al.*, 1994). In the Christchurch Health and Development Study, the rates of substance use disorder ranged from 5.2 to 7.7%; the rate of alcohol abuse/dependence based on maternal report was 1.9% and on self-report was 3.5% (Fergusson *et al.*, 1993). The differences in prevalence rates between these two studies maybe accounted for by differences in age: the sample in the Dunedin study was 18 years old, and in the Christchurch study 15 years old.

RISK FACTORS

While exposure to alcohol and drugs is a common phenomenon among adolescents, a relatively small proportion of adolescents who experiment with these substances go on to develop substance problems. Therefore, a large amount of research has been devoted to the identification of factors that increase an individual's risk for substance related

Table 9.3 Factors associated with increased risk for substance use disorders

Factors	Consequences
Genetic/Biological factors	Abnormal brain functioning; Pre-natal environmental experiences.
Individual vulnerability factors	Aggressive behaviors; Difficult to manage temperament; Impulsivity; Attention and conduct problems; Decreased religiosity; Relaxed attitudes towards substance use.
Low valuation of academic achievement	Low expectations for academic success; Low self esteem; Low frustration tolerance.
Psychopathology	Anxiety and affective disorders; Conduct problems and antisocial personality.
Familial vulnerability factors	Modeling of substance use by parental figures; Disrupted environment (e.g., marital discord, family conflict and violence); Older siblings drug modelling and advocacy; Highly interdependent relationships; High direct expression of conflict.
Non-familial environmental factors	Peer substance modeling and advocacy; Availablility of substances in school; Availability of sustances in neighbourhood.

disorders (Table 9.3). Specific risk factors (i.e., determinants that occur before substance abuse and are statistically associated with an increased probability of abuse) include environmental, behavioural, psychological, and social attributes (Hawkins *et al.*, 1992).

Although identified risk factors are plentiful, there is little evidence regarding their relative importance and interactions in the etiology of substance abuse. Current research is just beginning to examine a broad range of risk factors through multidisciplinary means and take into consideration developmental stages. Many studies emphasize a multicausal model of youthful substance use that does not attempt to identify one pathway to abuse. Risk factors are not considered definitive causes of drug use, but rather each is one factor in an array of influences that are associated with increased substance use (Newcomb *et al.*, 1987).

Newcomb and colleagues (1986), for example, examined longitudinal associations between risk factors and substance use for a sample of high school students and found that the number of different risk factors was predictive of use, frequency, and increases in substance use over a one year period.

Biological Factors

Genetic Factors

Although the familial nature of substance abuse has been known for centuries, the specific mode of transmission involved in familial aggregation remains unknown (Merikangas, 1990). Recent twin studies suggest that significant portions of the variance in both alcohol and drug dependence can be attributed to genetic factors (Pickens *et al.*, 1991). There are, however, several possible mechanisms through which genes exert their influence on the development of substance problems. Children may inherit in their biological make-up certain factors which may predispose them directly (e.g., drug metabolism, brain reward systems) or indirectly (temperament, psychiatric disorders) to substance abuse. The most consistent vulnerability factors for alcoholism identified from longitudinal high risk studies include abnormal brain functioning (as assessed in the event-related potential and Electroencephalogram), impulsivity, hyperactivity, and increased ability to tolerate the effects of alcohol (Alterman and Tarter, 1983; Schuckit, 1985), which suggest the importance of genetic/biological factors in the etiology of the condition. Non-genetic biological factors, such as pre-natal environmental experiences (e.g., pre-natal exposure to drugs due to maternal use) may also enhance vulnerability to substance abuse and dependence. Genetic make-up and pre-natal history are examples of factors which may make youths vulnerable to the development of substance use disorders.

Genetic factors may also operate through indirect mechanisms which enhance vulnerability to substance abuse through individual factors such as psychiatric disorders, temperament, or neurophysiologic phenomena. Non-genetic biologic factors may also increase vulnerability through such mechanisms as sensitization to drugs resulting from pre-natal exposure to drugs. While genes may be neither necessary nor sufficient to cause substance problems, they may predispose certain individuals to the development of abuse only at a particular level of environmental exposure. It is therefore critical to identify the joint role of environmental and genetic factors in the etiology of substance abuse. Rutter *et al.* (1986) have shown that environmental risk factors tend to operate most strongly in children with genetic vulnerability. Identification of such risk factors is critical to effective prevention of substance abuse and its sequelae.

Individual Vulnerability Factors for Substance Abuse

There are several factors related to the individual that have been shown to increase vulnerability to substance disorders. These factors include disposition (e.g., temperament and personality), behaviour patterns (e.g., nonconformity and antisocial behaviours), capabilities (e.g., cognitive, social and physical), preexisting psychopathology (e.g., anxiety and depression), as well as attitudes and beliefs. These factors have been identified in research focusing on individuals from early childhood through late adolescence.

There is evidence that a number of early childhood characteristics such as aggressive behaviours, difficult to manage temperament, impulsivity, attention, and conduct problems are associated with early adolescence deviance including substance use. Block *et al.* (1988) found that drug usage in early adolescence was related to preschool personality characteristics for a sample of 54 girls and 51 boys studied prospectively from age 3. In this sample, frequent substance users in adolescence appeared to be relatively maladjusted as children. As early as age 7, these children were unable to form good relationships, were insecure, and showed numerous signs of emotional distress. In a similar longitudinal study,

Kellam *et al.* (1983) reported that aggressiveness measured in the first grade was a strong predictor of teenage substance use for males, but was not associated with other forms of teenage psychopathology. Early adolescents are in the process of developing beliefs and attitudes which influence the way they cope with their environments in leading to substance use. Longitudinal studies have observed that, prior to the onset of drug abuse, adolescents tend to show decreased religiosity; relaxed attitudes towards substance use, low valuation of academic achievement and low expectations for academic success, low self esteem; low frustration tolerance; early aggressive behaviours; and favourable attitudes toward social deviance (e.g., Jessor, 1973; Kandel, 1985; Robins and McEvoy, 1990).

Psychopathology

The presence of a pre-existing psychiatric disorder, is also an important predictor of substance abuse. Substance abuse has been found to be associated with the major psychiatric disorders — particularly anxiety and affective disorders — both in clinical samples and in the general population (Anthony and Helzer, 1991; Bukstein *et al.*, 1989; Deykin *et al.*, 1987). Persons with major psychiatric disorders may have increased vulnerability to substance abuse, because the substance may ameliorate the symptoms of the underlying psychiatric condition. A cross-sectional study of high school students found that children above the 85th percentile in anxiety were four times more likely to have used alcohol than those below this percentile (Walter *et al.*, 1991). Moreover, Knop (1991) recently demonstrated a specific association between anxiety in childhood and the subsequent development of alcoholism in a 30 year prospective longitudinal study of a large birth cohort in Copenhagen, Denmark.

The evidence also indicates that deviant behaviours, conduct problems and antisocial personality are strongly associated with both alcohol and illicit drug use/abuse (Kandel, 1980; Robins and McEvoy, 1990). A prospective study of a cohort of 8–12 year-olds by Boyle *et al.*, (1993) showed that teacher-rated conduct disorder predicted the use of alcohol and hard drugs 4 years later. Although attention deficit disorder and hyperactivity have been considered to be etiologically related to substance abuse, more recent evidence has suggested that the majority of hyperactive children who later abused drugs had conduct/oppositional disorder either before or coincident with the onset of substance abuse (Alterman and Tarter, 1983; Gittelman *et al.*, 1985).

Familial Vulnerability Factors for Substance Abuse

The family environment can influence the unfolding of this behaviour either directly (e.g., modelling of substance use by parental figures or siblings) or indirectly by promoting a disrupted environment (e.g., marital discord, family conflict and violence). Familial factors may enhance vulnerability to substance abuse by exposure to siblings and parents engaged in drug abuse or through the disrupted home environments which characterize the family background of substance abusers. Whereas peer groups and other non-familial factors may be involved in exposure to substances, the transition from substance use to abuse may be attributable to familial factors.

Siblings

In a cross-sectional study, Needle *et al.* (1986) found that older siblings played an important role in supplying younger siblings with various drugs. Drug modelling and advocacy among older siblings was found to have a stronger influence on younger siblings drug use than parental drug modelling and advocacy. Needle *et al.* (1986) also suggested a possible indirect pathway in that older siblings may influence younger siblings to choose friends who are themselves substance users. For example, in a recent study of the relatives of opioid probands with opioid abuse, it was found that any experimentation with illicit substances ultimately led to abuse among the majority of siblings of drug abusers (Merikangas *et al.*, 1991). For all substances, over 90% of the siblings of abusers who tried the substance eventually proceeded to develop abuse.

Disease and Biological Models

According to the disease model, the etiology of substance dependence involves an interaction of the biological, psychological, and social factors (Milhorn, 1990). Substance dependence is therefore considered as a biopsychosocial disorder with the following features: compulsion to use the substance, loss of control over its use, and continued use despite negative consequences (Milhorn, 1990). In the biological model, findings from family genetic studies that involved twins and adopted children have provided strong support for the genetic predisposition to substance use disorders.

Social Factors

Family Interaction

The importance of family relationships in the development of adolescent substance abuse has been repeatedly documented (Barnes and Windle, 1987; Climent *et al.*, 1990; Crowley, 1988; Jacob *et al.*, 1983; McCord, 1988; Schweitzer and Lawton, 1989; Stoker and Swadi, 1990). Based on the available evidence, specific dimensions of family interactions appear to be strongly linked with substance abuse. Families of substance abusers have been discriminated from those of schizophrenics, psychosomatic youngsters and controls on separation and degree of individuation of the subjects, highly interdependent relationships with the mother; high direct expression of conflict, and more primitive and direct in their expression of conflict (Alexander and Dibb, 1975; D'Agnone and Basyk, 1989; Huberty, 1975; Reilly, 1976; Stanton, 1985; Stanton and Todd, 1982). Moreover, the quality of parenting measured with behavioural observation of parent and child in early childhood has been found to distinguish frequent substance users from other children (Shedler and Block, 1990). Shedler and Block (1990) found that mothers of the frequent substance users were perceived as relatively unresponsive and unprotective of these children in early childhood.

Peer Factors

Other non-familial environments also exert great influence in the development of substance use in adolescence. An increased desire for autonomy and self-determination, as well as increased peer orientation are characteristics of this developmental stage (Simmons and Blyth, 1987 cited in Eccles *et al.*, 1993). The importance of peers in the initiation and maintenance of substance use and abuse has been demonstrated both clinically and in the research literature (Brook *et al.*, 1983). Peers provide emotional support, information, assistance, but can also provide the context for socialization into deviance and drug use (Kandel, 1980). The association with drug using peers has been consistently found to be one of the strongest predictors of drug use (Kandel, 1980; Swaim, 1991).

However, few studies have examined the factors which may predict whether a child will choose a positive or negative peer environment. Kandel (1980) has reported that adolescents with poor parental bonds and relationships are more likely to choose deviant friends. Brooks *et al.* (1983) found that parental peer's use of drugs as well as the child's characteristics and the familial environment were important to determine the risk for drug use in the adolescent. For example, they found that lack of maternal positive reinforcement interacted with friends' drug use, resulting in higher stages of drug use. Adolescent unconventionality also interacted with maternal and peer marijuana use to increase the risk of adolescent use.

School Environment

Schools may also influence substance use behaviour if they provide an environment conducive to school failure. There is ample evidence that low achievement motivation and bonding, poor school performance, school desertion, failure and suspension are strongly associated with both deviant behaviour and the onset of substance use (Kandel, 1980; Kumpfer and Turner, 1990–1991). Some recent literature has identified a number of factors which have deleterious effects on early adolescents. Some of these are poor or few personal and positive teacher-student relationships, violence and availability of drugs in the school (Eccles *et al.*, 1993; Kumpfer and Turner, 1990–1991). Eccles *et al.* (1993) provide evidences that the mismatch between the adolescents, personal and educational needs and the school environment, tend to evoke in some youths a downward academic spiral which eventually leads to school drop out and conduct problems, both precursors of substance use.

Neighbourhood Environment

Dembo *et al.* (1985) examined the impact of a variety of environmental influences on the early drug involvement of inner city youth, a setting where the risk of substance abuse is greatest. Their assessment of availability of drugs and peer/neighbourhood influences revealed that availability is not sufficient to predict substance use; the influence of availability is dependent on other environmental variables, especially friends' substance use.

Communities also present opportunities and challenges to adolescents which can influence their behaviour (Jessor, 1993). For example, disadvantaged neighbourhoods (e.g., poverty areas) characteristically present risks and dangers, like deviant models and witnessing and being victims of violence, which may lead to anti-social behaviour and substance use. The effect that exposure to violence may have in increasing the risk for substance use is not known. However, there is ample evidence that children exposed to violence are at increased risk for some of the precursors of drug use, such as aggressive or delinquent behaviour (Browne and Finkelhor, 1986; Gelles and Conte, 1990), depressive, anxiety and/or PTSD symptoms and suicidal behaviour and ideation (Kiser *et al.*, 1988; Spatz-Windom, 1989).

Psychological Factors

Social Learning Theory

According to the social learning theory (Akers and Cochran, 1985), substance use originates in the substance-specific attitudes and behaviour of the adolescent's role models. The substance-using role models affect an adolescent's involvement with substances through the observation and imitation of substance-specific behaviour, receiving of social reinforcement mostly in the form of encouragement and support, culminating in the adolescent's expectation of positive social (e.g., acceptance by peer) and physiological consequences (e.g., positive physiological reaction to the subjects) for substance use. Social learning theory has been modified so that "distal" factors (e.g., personal characteristics, cognitive factors, and deficits in psychosocial coping skills) are given more importance than previously (Abrams and Niaura, 1987).

Social Cognitive/Learning Theory

Adolescents acquire beliefs about the substance use through their exposure to role models (e.g., close friends and parents) who use substances (Bandura, 1986). Such exposure helps shape the adolescent's belief related to the social, personal, and physiological consequences of substance use. Role models can also shape use of self-efficacy such as giving knowledge and skills for obtaining and using a substance, as well as refusal self-efficacy (e.g., learning skills to avoid substance use).

Multistage Social Learning Model

Multistage social learning theory is an integration of social learning process, intrapersonal characteristics, inadequate coping and social interaction skills, and a personal value system which stresses present-oriented goals (Simons *et al.*, 1988). The use of substances is considered to occur in three sequential stages: (i) The first stage deals with the adolescent's reason for their initial contact with subjects. Major factors that influence the adolescent's initial contact include parental failure to provide them with warmth, support, and discipline or the adolescent's personal value system that emphasizes present-oriented goals; (ii) the second stage concerns the well-established tendency for adolescents who have used substances to be friends with substance-using peers; and (iii) the third stage describes an adolescent's escalation to regular use and abuse of a substance. Factors which may influence this behaviour include having parents and peers with regular substance use, being emotionally disturbed, and having inadequate coping skills.

Problem-behaviour Theory

Problem-behaviour theory is generally used to describe the cause of substance use and also other behavioural problems in adolescents (Jessor *et al.*, 1991). The main assumption of problem-behaviour theory is that adolescents who have one problem (e.g., conduct disorder) also have another problem (e.g., substance use disorder). That is, problem behaviours tend to be correlated, whereas they are negatively correlated with conventional and conforming behaviour. Some characteristics of adolescents who are at risk for substance use include: being socially critical and culturally aliented; having low self-esteem; having an external locus of control; seeking independence from parents and valuing their involvement with peers; having low expectations for academic achievement; and being tolerant of any deviant behaviour.

Peer Cluster Theory

This theory stems from the findings that peer involvement consistently and significantly correlated with adolescent substance use. That is, an adolescent's influence in substance use is provided by the peers he chooses (Oetting and Beauvais, 1987). An adolescent's involvement with substance-using peers is determined by the: (i) social structure variables (e.g., parental divorce, socioeconomic status); (ii) psychological characteristics (e.g., personality trait); (iii) attitudes and beliefs; and (iv) socialization link.

Domain Model

This model considers substance use as one of a larger set of behavioural tendencies or adolescent life styles. The causes of substance use are divided into four domains: (i) biological influences on the adolescent's physiological reactions to substances and general health; (ii) intrapersonal influence which includes the adolescent's subjective belief about the negative consequences of substance use, personal values (e.g., wish for independence), and personality characteristics (e.g., sensation seeking); (iii) interpersonal influence such as the characteristics of people who are emotionally attached to the adolescent; and (iv) sociocultural influences including the availability of substance and social sanctions against their use (Huba and Bentler, 1982). Thus, this domain seems to consider substance use as being influenced by both environmental and biological factors.

Summary of Factors

The contribution of genetic and biologic factors to the individual vulnerability for substance abuse, both transmitted and non-transmitted familial factors, as well as unique environmental factors (e.g., peer relationships and life events) may be equally involved in the complex pathway of the development of substance abuse. It is therefore critical to identify the joint role of environmental and genetic factors in the etiology of substance abuse.

Risk factors should not be viewed as isolated phenomena. Risk factors do not always have a simple effect on substance use, but rather may interact with each other. Parental attitudes and behaviours, for example, may be predictive of drug use in peers, which in turn influences an individual's use of substances (Hansen *et al.*, 1987). Despite the substantial progress that has occurred in the identification of risk factors for drug abuse, particularly those associated with exposure to substances (Kandel, 1985; Brook *et al.*, 1988), the complex pathways in the etiology of substance abuse remain elusive.

PROTECTIVE FACTORS

Early studies on high-risk samples were concerned chiefly with identifying the prevalence of disorders among the children, as well as the factors predicting their onset. Protective factors which inhibit pathogenic processes among children at high risk have been largely neglected until recently (Garmezy, 1985; Rutter, 1979). As noted by Rutter (1979), these factors constitute an important issue to investigate because the potential for prevention lies precisely in understanding those factors which render some children resilient against the high-risk conditions they face. While many protective factors that have been identified are of a more general or nonspecific nature, this line of research has important implication for preventive efforts in cases where risk factors are found to be relatively high. Previous research indicates three categories of factors that protect against stress: dispositional attributes of the child; family cohesion and warmth; and the availability and use of external support systems by parents and children (Garmezy, 1985; Luthar and Zigler, 1991).

As reviewed by Luthar and Zigler (1991), factors which constitute protective effects against vulnerability in each of these three areas are as follows: (i) dispositional attributes of the child — intelligence, internal locus of control (beliefs in the controllability of events in life), and constitutional and temperamental factors; (ii) familial factors — a warm relationship with at least one parental figure, and quality of the marital relationship; and (iii) the use of support systems — positive school experiences, support for parents, and both intra-familial and extra-familial supports for parents such as church attendance, quality of housing and the presence of a telephone.

OUTCOME

Generally, the earlier the onset of regular substance use, the more likely it is that the substance will be abused. Thus, regular substance use in childhood or adolescence should be regarded as a serious matter. For example, in the study by Schuckit and Russell (1983), male university students with an early onset of drinking had a poorer outcome. As indicated by Kandel´s longitudinal study (1975), there seem to be a consistent sequential pattern of substance use. Adolescents generally start first with beer and wine, followed with hard liquor or spirits, then marijuana and other hand drugs such as opiates. What seems to be variable is the age of entry into the sequence and the time of progression or time spent in each stage. Both the age of onset into a particular stage of the substance use and the frequency of use at an earlier stage strongly predict further progression to later stage (Kandel *et al.*, 1992).

According to longitudinal studies, the use of substances drug during adolescence may lead to delinquent behaviour, physical and psychological problem and high rates of divorce in young adulthood (Kandel *et al.*, 1986; Newcomb and Bentler, 1988). In Holmberg's study (1985), Swedish children and adolescents who abused drugs had a high rate of problems continuing into young adulthood. When reinterviewed after

5 years, drug abuse was reported in 70 to 90% of males, and in 50 to 60% of the females who had admitted frequent drug use (Holmberg, 1985). Over the 11-year follow-up, early drug users appeared more often in social and child psychiatric case registers, were more often reported to be sick, and had no income as compared to controls.

In Kandel and Logan's study (1984), continued use of marijuana into young adulthood was associated with a higher use of other substances, lower involvement in conventional roles of adulthood, history of psychiatric hospitalization, lower psychological well-being, and participation in deviant activities. Heavy drug use has also been associated with early involvement in marriage, family, and the work force, as well as in forsaking educational pursuits (Newcomb and Bentler, 1988). Drug use also interferes with the developmental tasks of adolescents, leading to poor role acquisition as young adults such as failure in marriage (Newcomb and Bentler, 1989).

ASSESSMENT

Since substance use disorders are related to multiple risk factors and have numerous impairment, it is important to conduct a comprehensive assessment of the disorders. Tarter (1990) suggested that adolescents with substance use disorders be assessed along the domains of (i) substance use disorders, (ii) comorbid disorders, (iii) school and/or vocational functioning, family functioning, social competency and peer relations, leisure and recreation. Others have suggested that assessment of substance use should cover (i) the patterns of use (e.g., quantity, frequency), (ii) negative consequences for various life areas, (iii) context of use (e.g., time and place of use, peer pressure), and (iv) control of use (e.g., attempt to decrease or stop use).

A number of instruments have been developed to assess adolescent's substance use, and the functioning which may be affected by their use. Some examples of such instruments include the Drug Abuse Screening Test (Skinner, 1982), Drug Use Screening Inventory (Tarter, 1990), the Adolescent Alcohol Involvement Scale (Mayer and Filstead, 1979) (Table 9.4). Questionnaires that have been developed for assessing various symptoms of psychopathology also contain a scale to measure the use of alcohol and/or drug. Such instruments include the Child Behavior Checklist (Achenbach and Edelbrock, 1983) and the Ontario Child Health Study Scales (Boyle *et al.*, 1993). Other types of

Table 9.4 Examples of questions in the selected self-report questionnaires to measure alcohol and drug use

Instruments/Authors	Examples of questions	Responses
Drug Abuse Screening Test (Skinner, 1982)	Have you used drugs other than those required for medical reasons? Have you abused prescription drugs? Has any family member ever sought help for problems related to your drug use?	Yes / No
Drug Use Screening Inventory (Tarter, 1990)	Have you ever had a craving or very strong desire for alcohol or drugs? Have you ever felt that you could not control your alcohol or drug use? Have you ever had trouble getting along with any of your friends because of alcohol or drug use?	Yes / No
The Michigan Alcoholism Screening Test (Selzer, 1971)	Do you feel bad about your drinking? Have you gotten into fights when drinking? Do you ever drink before noon?	Yes / No
Child Behavior Checklist (Achenbach and Edelbrock, 1983)	Drinks liquor or an alcoholic beverage without parents' permission Uses medicine or drug without reason of illness	ranging from "not at all true" to "very frequent"

Table 9.4 *continued*

Instruments/Authors	Examples of questions	Responses
Ontario Child Health Study Scales (Boyle *et al.*, 1993)	In the past 6 months did you have three or more drinks of beer, wine or other alcoholic beverages at one time? Have you been drunk at any time in the last 6 months?	Yes / No
	From the following list, mark "Yes" for those drugs you have used without prescription, in the last 6 months and "No" for those drugs you have not used in the past 6 months: (a) marijuana, hashish, pot, grass; (b) amphetamines, stimulants, uppers, speed; (c) barbiturates, sedatives, downers, sleeping pills, seconal, quaaludes; (d) tranquilizers, valium, librium; (e) cocaine, crack, snow; (f) heroin; (g) opiates other than heroin (demerol, morphine, methadone, darvon, opium); (h) psychedelics, hallucinogens; (i) sniffed or inhaled glue, gasoline or other fumes; (j) something else _____	Yes / No

assessment methods are available in an interview format such as the Adolescent Problem Severity Index (Metzger *et al.*, 1991), the Adolescent Drug Abuse Diagnosis Instrument (Friedman and Utada, 1989), and the Teen Addiction Severity Index (Kamier *et al.*, 1993).

Some structured and semi-structured diagnostic interviews developed for the assessment of various psychiatric disorders also contain a section for assessing substance use disorders (Table 9.5 and 9.6). These include the Diagnostic Interview Schedule for Children (Costello *et al.*, 1984), the revised version of the Diagnostic Interview for Children and Adolescents (Reich and Welner, 1988), and the Childhood Schedule for Schizophrenia and Affective Disorders (K-SADS) (Puig-Antich and Chambers, 1978).

INTERVENTION

A number of treatment programs for adolescent's substance use disorders have been developed that combine behavioural, medical, cognitive, and psychoeducational approaches which may be integrated within a context of individual, group, and family therapy. Most treatment programs focus on sociocultural, family, peer, and personal factors which contribute to substance use (Bukstein, 1995). Hospital-based programs should be considered after unsuccessful treatment in outpatient programs, or to manage an overdose, severe discomfort or psychological and physical effects of withdrawal, or serious behaviour problems such as truancy or stealing.

The major aims of substance use treatments are to (i) significantly reduce the frequency and amount of substances consumed, or to eliminate their use altogether; and (ii) to assist the adolescent in developing psychosocial competencies and master experiences that may lead to an alcohol- and drug-free life style. By improving psychosocial competency, adolescents are equipped with the resources that enable them to feel good about themselves and to seek positive solutions to interpersonal and intrapersonal conflicts which will lead to a decreased likelihood of engaging in future alcohol and drug abuse.

According to Jarvis *et al.* (1995), treatment of substance use can be divided into three phases: (a) The *first phase* involves establishing motivation and setting goals for personal growth and future substance use; (b) The *second phase* involves dealing with intrapersonal and interpersonal conflicts which can be both a cause and a consequence of

Table 9.5 Examples of questions in selected diagnostic interviews to assess alcohol use disorder

Interviews	Examples of questions	Coding options
DISC (Costello et al., 1984)	For the following questions, please think about the time during the past 6 months when you were drinking most.	
	• Did you often drink more than you thought you would?	0 1* 2* 9
	• ...... or spend more time drinking than you planned?	0 1* 2* 9
	• Was drinking something you couldn't stop thinking about ..... that you couldn't put out of your head?	0 1* 2* 9
	• Did your grades go down (Did you have problems doing your jobs) because of drinking?	0 1* 2* 9
	You told me that you [NAME "*" ITEMS CODED IN Q2-25]. Was this going on for as long as a month?	0 2 9
	IF YES, A. Did this go on for as long as six months?	0 2 9
	How old were you when [this/any of these things] began to happen? SPECIFY AGE _____	____ YRS.
DICA-R (Reich and Welner, 1988)	In the last 6 months have you had at least one drink of beer, wine or other alcoholic beverage 4 or more weeks in a row?	1 4 8 9
	Have you been drunk at any time in the last 6 months?	1 4 8 9
	Have you ever worried that you drink too much?	1 4 8 9

Table 9.5 *continued*

Interviews	Examples of questions	Coding options
K-SADS (Puig-Antich and Chambers, 1978)	Have you tried any alcohol or beer? What do you drink? How often do you have a drink? Do you drink in the morning? Have you ever gotten drunk in the morning? Have you ever gotten drunk or gotten into difficulty (trouble) from drinking? Have you found that you need to drink more now to get the same high feeling? If you don't have a drink, do you feel nervous and notice you're shaking? Were you ever addicted to alcohol drugs? (Ask similar types of questions regarding drugs e.g., reefer, coke, uppers, smack, ludes, etc) WHAT ABOUT DURING THE LAST WEEK? SUBSTANCE(S) USED Specify: 0 = no information _____ 1 = none _____ 2 = yes	0 = no information; 1 = not at all; 2 = slight; 3 = mild; 4 = moderate, 5 = severe; 6 = extreme, 0 1 2 3 4 5 6 LAST WK: 0 1 2 DURATION 0 = no information 1 = less than 1 month 2 = more than 1 month

Coding used: (1) DISC: 0 = No , 1 = Sometimes/Somewhat , 2 = Yes, 9 = Don't know; (2) DICA-R: 1 = Yes, 2 = Sometimes, 4 = No, 9 = Don't know, 8 = Respondent refuses to answer the questions

Table 9.6 Examples of questions in diagnostic interviews to assess drug use disorders

Interviews		Coding options
DISC (Costello et al., 1984)	For the following questions, please think about the time during the past 6 months when you were using marijuana the most.	
	• Did you often smoke more marijuana than you thought you would?	0 1* 2* 9
	• Did it seem you could smoke more and more marijuana as time went on?	0 1* 2* 9
	• Were you often sick after using marijuana?	0 1* 2* 9
	• Did using marijuana cause any problems with how you got along with other people?	0 1* 2* 9
	IF YES, A. Did you have problems with family members because you used marijuana?	0 1 2 9
	B. Did you lose friends because you used it?	0 1 2 9
DICA-R (Reich and Welner, 1988)	In the last 6 months have you ever sniffed or inhaled glue, gasoline or other fumes to get high?	1 4 8 9
	In the last 6 months have you ever smoke marijuana?	1 4 8 9
	In the last 6 months have you ever taken any street drugs? (PROBE: COCAINE, CRACK, SPEED — UPPERS, DOWNERS — THAT SORT OF THINGS)	1 4 8
	IF YES, A. Could you tell me what they were?	1 4 8

substance abuse. This is facilitated by exposing the adolescent to a planned sequence of psychoeducational experiences, designed to improve communication, coping, and problem-solving skills, to establish goals and a sense of direction, to increase awareness of cues that trigger drinking and drug use, and to develop stress-reduction methods; and (c) The *aftercare phase* consists of developing and carrying out a plan to maintain treatment gains and to prevent relapse into alcohol and drug abuse. These include maintenance of a support system, recognition of relapse warning signs, and the development of a relationship with a primary resource person.

Pharmacotherapy

Pharmacotherapy for the treatment of adolescents with substance use disorders has been rarely been used. A major objection to it´s use is the fear of abuse of that medication or the promotion of future substance use or abuse (Bukstein, 1995). Three areas in which pharmacotherapy can be used include the: (i) treatment of withdrawal effects or syndrome; (ii) treatment of the substance use behaviour by using drug substitution (e.g., methadone maintenance), antagonist therapy (e.g., naltrexone), and aversion agents (e.g., disulfiram) (Bukstein, 1995); and (iii) the treatment of comorbid disorders. To prevent adolescents with substance use disorders from abusing the medication used to treat any of these areas would require a careful supervision by their significant others.

Psychological Intervention Programs

Problem-solving Skills Training

In problem-solving skills training, adolescents are trained to develop a general skill for resolving life problems which may threaten their comittment to change their drinking or drug use. The main aims of the training are to: help the adolescent to recognize when a problem is present; generate potential solutions to the problems; choose the best option and generate a plan for carrying it out; and evaluate the effectiveness of the chosen approach (Jarvis *et al.*, 1995). For the problem-solving to be effective, the following stages need to be carried out: (a) *Problem definition.* This exercise involves having the adolescents select a problem situation, which is defined in terms of concrete behaviour that can be changed. Some adolescents who may have difficulties in recognizing the existence of the problems, need to be given clues (e.g., unpleasant physical signs, negative feelings, negative reactions from other people, and negative reactions to other people) to identify situations when the problem arises; (b) *Brainstorming options in dealing with the problem*. Adolescents are encouraged to develop as many alternatives as possible; (c) *Choosing the best options*. Adolescents are asked to select the alternatives which are believed to be the most realistic to carry out and most likely to be effective; (d) *Generating a plan of action*. This involves making a plan for carrying out the selected option; (e) *Carrying out the planned action*. Involves practicing the plan by using a role-play or mental rehearsal, followed by home practice exercises; and (f) *Evaluating the results*. The options chosen to resolve the problem need to be evaluated. If the chosen solution does not work, the action plan and strategy need to be evaluated.

Life Skills Training

The life skills training (Holden *et al.*, 1990) encompasses problem-solving, personal coping, and interpersonal communication skills which emphasize health and life-style promoting strategies. Such strategies enable adolescents to advance their lives educationally, vocationally, and socially while avoiding substance abuse. The training comprises six issues: (a) *Information giving*. This stage involves discussing the adverse health, social, and legal consequences of substances; (b) *Problem solving*. Adolescents review chronic problem situations in their lives and brainstorm potential solutions which are ranked according to their attractiveness and feasibility. It focuses on the cognitive process of generating solution, weighting the consequences of each and deciding on the most appropriate course. Adolescents are taught skills needed to delay impulsive behaviour through modelling, role play and homework assignments; (c) *Self-instruction counselling*. Inner dialogues that are appropriate for the decisions made are chosen and practiced by adolescents; (d) *Coping*. Adolescents are taught coping skills training to deal with stressful and unpleasant situations. Coping skills include cognitive and behavioural strategies of self-instruction and progressive relaxation techniques; (e) *Communication*. Adolescents learn both non-verbal and verbal behaviours that are associated with assertiveness training. Communication skills included role-playing of refusal skills with other subjects, emphasizing how eye contact, verbal voice intonation, affect and word choice can be effective in making a point; (f) *Support system*. Adolescents are trained to enhance and expand their competence in building, negotiating, and maintaining positive, supportive familial, peer, and community social networks (Schinke and Gilchrist, 1985).

Cognitive Restructuring

In cognitive restructuring, adolescents are taught to identify and challenge thoughts or feelings which may lead to substance use. The main aims of cognitive restructuring are to help adolescents: (i) become aware of negative thinking or the way in which negative thinking leads to substance use through identification of situations in which negative emotions are experienced, or where they ended up drinking or taking drugs; (ii) challenge negative thoughts and replace them with positive ones; and (iii) review their automatic thoughts by considering the evidence that supports this automatic thought, the advantages/disadvantages of thinking this way, the presence of thinking errors, and alternative ways of thinking about the situation.

Behavioural Self-management Training

In behavioural self-management training, adolescents are taught skills needed for reducing substance use to the levels that minimize the risk of physical illness and any other personal or social problems due to substance use (Jarvis *et al.*, 1995). Steps involved in behavioural self-management training include: (a) *Daily self-monitoring* that allows adolescents to keep a record of their substance use, and provides information as to when, where, and why they use it; (b) *Setting limits on substance use* helps minimize the risk of physical illness and other social problems due to substance use. Drinking can be set within limits using the "tapering off" approach (i.e., negotiating limits with adolescents each week until the final goal is reached). The second approach involves a period of abstinence after recommencing substance use within set limits. This "time out period" allows monitoring the situations in which the adolescents are tempted to use substances, and identify the strategies for coping with urges and temptations; (c) *Keeping to set limits* by teaching adolescents drink-refusal skills. The skills are especially useful for those who have difficulties in resisting social and/or peer pressures to drink or use drugs; (d) *Maintaining new drinking habits* by establishing self-rewards for cutting down drinking, and identifying alternatives to drinking to promote new drinking habits.

Drink-and Drug-refusal Skills

The main aim of the drink- and drug-refusal skills is to teach adolescents to refuse offers to drink or use drugs in an appropriate manner (Jarvis *et al.*, 1995). This training is best-suited for those who have little confidence in dealing with social pressure to use substances. The major components of a successful refusal include (Monti *et al.*, 1989): (a) *Body language*. The use of direct eye contact increase self-confidence and helps convey a convincing message that alcohol or drugs are refused to the person who offers the drink or drugs; (b) *Tone of voice*. An ability to say "no" in a firm and unhesitating manner to the offer to drink or use drugs will not give the other person the chance to question the refusal; (c) *What to say and do*. According to Monti *et al.* (1989), the best response to the offer to drink or use drugs is to firmly say "no thanks". Instead of consuming substances, adolescents should suggest other things to do and something else to drink. In order to avoid a long discussion about drinking or drug use it is advisable for the adolescents to change the topic of discussion. During the training session, it is important that the adolescents role-play this situation, as both a refuser and a pusher.

Communication Skills Training

The main goals of communication skills training are to teach adolescents to initiate and continue conversation appropriately, and to cope with silence, to develop sensitivity to social cues, to express their feelings and opinions to others, and to understand the feelings of others (Jarvis *et al.*, 1995). Appropriate communication could help reduce adolescents' feelings of embarassment and social tension that may lead to substance use (Jarvis *et al.*, 1995). The communication processes learnt during this training includes: (a) *Starting or entering a conversation*. Before entering a conversation, adolescents are told to listen to what the other people are interested in, and then to stay with a topics which is of mutual interest; (b) *Keeping the conversation going*. Use of appropriate non-verbal communication such as eye contact facial expression, and an interesting tone of voice which are important in maintaining conversations; and (c) *Active listening*. Telling adolescents to repeat what has been said to them helps verify that the message been heard accurately and show the speaker that they have been listening. Such approaches avoid misunderstanding from reading another people's mind.

Relapse.   Factors predictive of relapse include negative emotional state and interpersonal conflict (Brown *et al.*, 1989; Brown *et al.*, 1990). Adolescents with better treatment outcome reported using a greater number of behavioural coping strategies in high-risk situations (Myers and Brown, 1990). In a study by Friedman *et al.* (1986), successful treatment outcome was associated with long-term treatment, being White, and having few prior admissions. Since relapse rates are quite high, in the range of 35 to 70%, (Brown *et al.*, 1989), continued intervention efforts are needed.

Prevention

A number of prevention strategies for adolescents with substance use have been designed in recent years (Table 9.7, see also Hawkins *et al.*, 1992 for review). Prevention efforts can be divided into primary, secondary, and tertiary types. Primary prevention efforts aim to prevent substance use from occurring at all. To achieve this goal, the purpose of primary programs include (Milhorn, 1990): reducing social influences which promote substance use; increasing resistance to social influence by teaching adolescents refusal or communication skills; decreasing susceptibility to social influence by teaching adolescents skills to increase their social competence or sense of personal control; and finally by fostering the use of adaptive coping skills, thus making the use of substance as a coping strategy unnecessary.

If primary prevention effort fails, secondary prevention efforts need to be designed that involve reaching persons in the early stages (i.e., experimentation phase) of substance dependence providing treatment to prevent it from escalation. Tertiary prevention involves treating adolescents with substance use dependence and helping them lead a normal life in the community. Most prevention programs focus on one or more aspects of life (Schonberg, 1988) including: (a) individual (biological vulnerabilities, affective deficits, knowledge deficits, life skills deficits, invulnerability, sensation seeking); (b) family (family dynamics, socialization deficit, parental modelling, social control); (c) peer group (conformity, peer modelling, peer influence); (d) school and community (deterrence, availability, social climate, social bonding); and (e) larger social environment (advertising, portrayal of drug use).

Tobler (1986) differentiated between 5 types of preventive programs, which are aimed to reduce drug use. These approaches include: (i) affective enhancement to increase intrapersonal and social growth; (ii) alternative programs that focus on community and leisure activities; (iii) having knowledge or information regarding the use of drug; (iv) peer programs that focus on refusal skills and social life skills; and (v) a combination of knowledge and affective approaches.

Overall the results of these prevention studies suggest that changes are most often produced with regard to general knowledge and attitudes

Table 9.7   Preventive programs for substance use disorder

Preventive programs	Strategies/Target behavior
1. Early childhood and family support programs	Focus on the prenatal and early infancy periods. Interventions provided social support for mothers, health care, etc. The programs help buffer the effects of poverty by reducing the following risk factors for substance abuse: behaviour problems, family management problems, and academic failure.
2. Programs for parents of children and adolescents	Parenting skills training: Parents are taught to monitor their children's behavior, to use contingent discipline for undesired behavior, and to consistently reward prosocial behaviour. The training helps buffer the risk of substance use by decreasing family management problems.
3. Social competence skills training	Teaching adolescents behavioural skills to deal with interpersonal problems. Social competence promotion may affect adolescent's willingness to use nondrug or nonalcohol options when confronted with problem situation.
4. Academic achievement promotion	Substance use may be prevented by reducing risk factors of academic achievement and problem behaviour in school. The strategies to reduce these risk factors include early childhood education, changes in classroom teacher's instructional practices in school, academic tutoring of adolescents with low grades.
5. Organizational changes in school	Changes in school organization may reduce substance use risk factors through such activities as curriculum restructuring, greater school-faculty-community integration.
6. Youth involvement in alternative activities	Providing adolescents the opportunities to be involved in school activities to help reduce the likelihood of violating school rules such as proscription against substance use.
7. Comprehensive risk-focused programs	Consists of a combination of interventions that focus on different sources of social influence. Such interventions may include training parents in positive parent-child communication skills, training of community leader to organize drug abuse prevention task forces.

rather than reductions in actual substance use behaviours (Nathan, 1983). An exception is a study by Botvin *et al.* (1995) that assessed the long-term effects of a school-based prevention program consisting of drug related education classes and several maintenance sessions conducted with 7th-9th graders. At a six year follow-up assessment, significant reductions in drug use including alcohol, tobacco and marijuana were found in groups receiving the prevention program relative to controls. Unfortunately, many programs have not received the necessary evaluative efforts needed to establish their efficacy. This can be partially attributed to the low priority status that prevention research efforts have historically received.

CONCLUDING REMARKS

Substance use and abuse are major problems among adolescents, world wide. According to several surveys in the US, an average of about 30% of high school students have taken some types of drugs; the use of alcohol is more frequent, of about 60%. The prevalences for substance use disorders are much lower. The rates for alcohol abuse/dependence range from 1.9 to 32.4%, and for drug abuse/dependence from about 2 to 10%.

A large amount of research has been devoted to identifying factors which increase the adolescent's risk for substance use including genetic factors, individual vulnerability, psychopathology, familial vulnerability, siblings, family interaction, peers, school environment, and neighbourhood environment. However, little is known about their importance and interactions in the etiology of substance use disorders. Future research should therefore examine a broad range of risk factors through multidisciplinary approaches and considering the adolescents' developmental stages.

The age at which adolescents have first contact with the substance use on a regular basis is important, especially because childhood and adolescence are critical periods for developing personal and interpersonal competence, coping skills, and decision making. The use of substances may interfere with the development of skills which are requisite for successful functioning in adulthood, as well as other development that occurs during this life period. Consequently, these adolescents not only move into their adult roles prematurely, but also often fail in their adult roles. The fact that occasional substance use is more common than regular use suggests the need for prevention programs, although the efficacy of the existing prevention strategies has not yet been established.

This review also has important implications for the development of services for drug abuse. Treatment of drug abuse must provide a comprehensive assessment of psychopathology in both the individual and his/her family context, particularly among adolescents with substance abuse. The large gap between the philosophy of contemporary psychiatry and that which guides most current drug treatment programs which often discourage the use of all psychotropic medications may ironically lead to the exacerbation of the underlying psychopathology which may have been a major causative factor in the development of drug abuse in the first place. This is a particularly serious problem among adolescents with identified psychopathology who are often required to discontinue effective treatment regimens to participate in drug treatment programs. The widespread administrative distinction between substance abuse and mental illness also leads to overlapping services, and the lack of a comprehensive approach to treatment of the individual as the target rather than the specific disorders which may be manifest. The task for the future is clear: systematic research into all levels of prevention of substance abuse with children and adolescents.

REFERENCES

Abrams, D.B. and Niaura, R.S. (1987). Social learning theory. In H.T. Blane and K.E. Leonard (Eds.), *Psychological theories of drinking and alcoholism* (pp. 131–180). New York: Guilford.

Achenbach, T.M. and Edelbrock, C.S. (1983). *Manual for the Child Behavior Checklist and Revised Child Behavior Profile*. Burlington, VT: T.M. Achenbach.

Akers, R.L. and Cochran, J.E. (1985). Adolescent marijuana use: A test of three theories of deviant behavior. *Deviant Behavior*, **6**, 323–346.

Alexander, B.K. and Dibb, G.S. (1975). Opiate addicts and their parents. *Family Process*, **14**, 499–514.

Alterman, A.I. and Tarter, R.E. (1983). The transmission of psychological vunerability. *Journal of Nervous and Mental Disease*, **171**, 147–154.

American Psychiatric Association (1994). *Diagnostic and statistical manual of mental disorders* (4th ed.). Washington D.C.: American Psychiatric Association.

Anthony, J.C. and Helzer, J.E. (1991). Syndromes of drug abuse and dependence. In L.N. Robins and D.A. Regier (Eds.), *Psychiatric disorders in America*. New York, Free Press.

Bandura, A. (1986). *Social foundations of thought and action: A social cognitive theory*. Englewood Cliffs, NJ: Prentice Hall.

Barnes, G.M. and Windle, M. (1987). Family factors in adolescent alcohol and drug abuse. *Pediatrician*, **14**, 13–18.

Bean-Bayog, M. (1987). The adolescent drinker. In H.N. Barnes, M.D. Aronson, and T.L. Delbanco (Eds.), *Alcoholism: A guide for the primary care physician* (pp. 181–193). New York: Springer.

Block, J., Block, J.H., and Keyes, S. (1988). Longitudinally foretelling drug usage in adolescence: Early childhood personality and environmental precursors. *Child Development*, **59**, 336–355.

Botvin, G.J., Baker, E.B., Dusenbury, L., Botvin, E.M., and Diaz, T. (1995). Long-term follow-up results of a randomized drug abuse prevention trial in a white middle-class population. *JAMA*, **273**, 1106–1112.

Boyle, M.H., Offord, D.R., Racine, Y.A., Fleming, J.E., Szatmari, P., and Links, P.S. (1993). Predicting substance use in early adolescence based on parent and teacher assessments of childhood psychiatric disorders: Results from the Ontario Child Health Study follow-up. *Journal of Child Psychology and Psychiatry*, **34**, 535–544.

Brook, J.S., Whiteman, M., and Gordon, A.S. (1983). Stages of drug use in adolescence: Personality, peer, and family correlates. *Developmental Psychology*, **19**, 269–277.

Brook, J.S., Whiteman, M., Gordon, A.S., and Brook, D.W. (1988). Personality, family and ecological influence on adolescent drug use. *Journal of Chemical Dependence and Treatment*, **1**, 123–162.

Brown, S.A., Mott, M.A., and Myers, M.G. (1990). Adolescent alcohol and drug treatment outcome. In R.R. Watson (Ed.), *Drug and alcohol abuse prevention* (pp. 373–403). Clifton, NJ: Humana Press.

Brown, S.A., Vik, P.W., and Creamer, V.A. (1989). Characteristics of relapse following adolescent substance abuse treatment. *Addictive Behaviors*, **14**, 291–300.

Browne, A. and Finkelhor, D. (1986). Impact of child sexual abuse: A review of the research. *Psychological Bulletin*, **99**, 66–77.

Bukstein, O.G. (1995). *Adolescent substance abuse: Assessment, prevention, and treatment.* New York: John Wiley and Sons, Inc.

Bukstein, O.G., Brent, D.A., and Kamier, Y. (1989). Comorbidity of substance abuse and other psychiatric disorders in adolescents. *American Journal of Psychiatry*, **146**, 1131–1141.

Climent, C.E., De-Aradon, L.V., and Plutchik, R (1990). Prediction of risk for drug use in high school students. *International Journal of Addictions*, **25**, 545–556.

Cohen, P., Cohen, J., Kasen, S., Velez, C.N., Hartmark, C., Johnson, J., Rojas, M., Brook, J., and Streuning, E.L. (1993). An epidemiological study of disorders in late childhood and adolescence-I. Age-and gender-specific prevalence. *Journal of Child Psychology and Psychiatry*, **34**, 851–866.

Costello, A.J., Edelbrock, C., Dulcan, M., Kalas, R., and Klaric, S.H. (1984). *Development and testing of the NIMH Diagnostic Interview Schedule for Children in clinic populations.* Rockville, MD: National Institute for Mental Health.

Crowley, P. (1988). Family therapy approach to addiction. *Bulletin on Narcotics*, **40**, 57–62.

D'Agnone, O.A. and Basyk, D. (1989). Some familial dynamic aspects in drug abusers. *Medical and Law*, **8**, 431–432.

Dembo, R., Allan, N., Farrow, D., Schmeidler, J., and Burgos, W. (1985). A causal analysis of early drug involvement in three inner-city neighborhood settings. *International Journal of the Addictions*, **20**, 1213–1237.

Deykin, E.Y., Levy, J.C., and Wells, V. (1987). Adolescent depression, alcohol and drug abuse. *American Journal of Public Health*, **77**, 178–182.

Eccles, J. S., Midgley, C., Wigfield, A., Buchanan, C.M., Reuman, D., Flanagan, C., and Iver, D.M. (1993). Development during adolescence: The impact of stage-environment fit on young adolescents' experiences in schools and in families. *American Psychologist*, **48**, 90–101.

Feehan, M., McGee, R., Nada Raja, S., and Williams, S.M. (1994). DSM-III-R disorders in New Zealand 18-year-olds. *Australian and New Zealand Journal of Psychiatry*, **28**, 87–99.

Fergusson, D.M., Horwood, L.J., and Lynskey, M.T. (1993). Prevalence and comorbidity of DSM-III-R diagnoses in a birth cohort of 15 year olds. *Journal of American Academy of Child and Adolescent Psychiatry*, **32**, 1127–1134.

Friedman, A.S., Glickman, N.W., and Morrissey, M.R. (1986). Prediction of successful treatment outcome by client characteristics and retention in treatment in adolescent drug treatment programs: A large-scale cross-validation. *Journal of Drug Education,* **16,** 149–165.

Friedman, A.S. and Utada, A. (1989). A method for diagnosing and planning the treatment of adolescent drug abusers (The Adolescent Drug Abuse Diagnosis [ADAD] instrument). *Journal of Drug Education,* **19,** 285–312.

Garmezy (1985). Stress-resistant children: The search for protective factors. In J.E. Stevenson (Ed.), *Recent research in developmental psychopathology* (pp. 213–233). *Journal of Child Psychology and Psychiatry,* **4** (Book Supplement). Oxford: Pergamon Press.

Gelles, R.J. and Conte, J.R. (1990). Domestic violence and sexual abuse of children: A review of research in the eighties. *Journal of Marriage and Family,* **52,** 1045–1058.

Gittelman, R., Mannuzza, S., Shenker, R., and Bonagura, N. (1985). Hyperactive boys almost grown up. I: Psychiatric status. *Archives of General Psychiatry,* **42,** 937–947.

Hansen, W.B., Graham, J.W., Sobel, J.L., Shelton, D.R., Flay, B.P., and Johnson, C.A. (1987). The consistency of peer and parent influences on tobacco, alcohol and marijuana use among young adolescents. *Journal of Behavioral Medicine,* **10,** 559–579.

Hawkins, J.D., Catalano, R.F., and Miller, J.Y. (1992). Risk and protective factors for alcohol and other drug problems in adolescence and early adulthood: Implications for substance abuse prevention. *Psychological Bulletin,* **112,** 64–105.

Holden, G.W., Moncher, M.S., and Schinke, S.P. (1990). Substance abuse. In A.S. Bellack, M. Hersen, and A.E. Kazdin (Eds.), *International handbook of behavior modification and therapy* (pp. 869–880). New York: Plenum Press.

Holmberg, M.B. (1985). Longitudinal studies of drug abuse in a 15-year-old population, 2: Antecedents and consequences. *Acta Psychiatrica Scandinavica,* **71,** 80–91.

Huba, G.J. and Bentler, P.M. (1982). A developmental theory of drug use: Derivations and assessment of a causal modeling approach. In P.B. Baltes and O.G. Brim (Eds.), *Life span development and behavior* (Vol. 4, pp. 147–203). New York: Academic Press.

Huberty, D.J. (1975). Treating the adolescent drug abuser: A family affair. *Contemporary Drug Problems,* **4,** 179–194.

Jacob, T., Dunn, N.J., and Leonard, K. (1983). Patterns of alcohol use and family stability. *Alcoholism, Clinical and Experimental Research,* **7,** 382–385.

Jarvis, T.J., Tebbutt, J., and Mattick, R.P. (1995). *Treatment approaches for alcohol and drug dependence: An Introductory Guide.* Chichester: Wiley.

Jessor, R. (1973). A social psychology of marijuana use: Longitudinal studies of high school and college youth. *Journal of Personality and Social Psychology,* **26,** 1–15.

Jessor, R. (1993). Successful adolescent development among youth in high-risk settings. *American Psychologist,* **48,** 117–126.

Jessor, R., Donovan, J.E., and Costa, F.M. (1991). *Beyond adolescence: Problem behavior and young adult development.* Cambridge, England: Cambridge University Press.

Johnson, L.D., O'Malley, P.M., and Backman, J.G. (1994). *National survey results on drug use: The monitoring the future study, 1975–1993.* The University of Michigan Institute for Social Research.

Kaminer, Y., Wagner, E., Plummer, B., and Seifer, R. (1993). Validation of the teen addiction severity index (T-ASI). *American Journal on Addictions,* **2,** 250–254.

Kandel, D.B. (1980). Drug and drinking behavior among youth. *Annual Review Sociology* **6,** 235–285.

Kandel, D.B. and Logan, J.A. (1984). Patterns of drug use from adolescence to young adulthood: I. Periods of risk for initiation, continued use, and discontinuation. *American Journal of Public Health,* **74,** 660–668.

Kandel, D.B. (1985). On processes of peer influences in adolescent drug use: A development perspective. *Advances in Alcohol and Substance Abuse,* **4,** 139–163.

Kandel, D.B., Adler, I., and Sudit, M.S. (1981). The epidemiology of adolescent drug use in France and Israel. *American Journal of Public Health,* **71,** 256–265.

Kandel, D.B., Davies, M., Karus, D., and Yamaguchi, K. (1986). The consequences in young adulthood of adolescent drug involvement. *Archives of General Psychiatry,* **43**, 746–754

Kellam, S.G., Brown, C.H., Rubin, B.R., and Ensmiger, M.E. (1983). Paths leading to teenage psychiatric symptoms and substance use: Developmental epidemiologic studies in Woodlawn. In S.B. Guze, F.J. Earls, and J.E. Barrett (Eds.), *Childhood Psychopathology and Development* (pp. 17–47). New York: Raven.

Kiser, L. J., Ackerman, B.J., Brown, B.J., Edwards, N.B., McColgan, E., Pugh, R., and Pruit, D.B. (1988). Post-traumatic stress disorder in young children: A reaction to purported sexual abuse. *Journal of the American Academy of Child and Adolescent Psychiatry,* **27**, 645–649.

Knop, E.A. (1991). *A cohort study of young men at risk for alcoholism.* APA conference, New Orleans.

Kokkevi, A. and Stefanis, C. (1991). The epidemiology of licit and illicit substance use among high school students in Greece. *American Journal of Public Health,* **81**, 48–52.

Kumpfer, K. L. and Turner, C.W. (1990–1991). The social ecology model of adolescent substance abuse: Implications for prevention. *International Journal of Addictions,* **25**, 435–463.

Lewinsohn, P.M., Hops, H., Roberts, R.E., Seeley, J.R., and Andrews, J.A. (1993). Adolescent psychopathology: I. Prevalence and incidence of depression and other DSM-III-R disorders in high school students. *Journal of Abnormal Psychology,* **102**, 133–144.

Luthar, S.S. and Zigler, E. (1991). Vulnerability and competence: A review of research on resilience in childhood. *American Journal of Orthopsychiatry,* **61**, 6022.

MacDonald, D. (1984). *Drugs, drinking, and adolescents.* Chicago, Year Book.

Mayer, J.E. and Filstead, W.J. (1979). The Adolescent Alcohol Involvement Scale. *Journal of Studies on Alcohol,* **40**, 291–300.

McCord, J. (1988). Alcoholism: Toward understanding genetics and social factors. *Psychiatry,* **51**, 131–141.

Merikangas, K.R. (1990). The genetic epidemiology of alcoholism. *Psychological Medicine,* **20**, 11–22.

Merikangas, K.R., Rounsaville, B.J., and Prusoff, B.A. (1991). Familial factors vulnerability to substance abuse. In M. Glanz and R. Pickens (Eds.), *Vulnerability to drug abuse* (pp. 79–98). American Psychological Association Press.

Metzger, D.S., Kushner, H., and McLellan, A.T. (1991). *Adolescent Problem Severity Index. Administration manual.* Philadelphia: Biomedical Computer Research Institute.

Milhorn, H.T. (1990). *Chemical dependence: Diagnosis, treatment, and prevention.* New York: Springer.

Monti, P.M., Abrams, D.B., Kadden, R.M., and Cooney, N.L. (1989). *Treating alcohol dependence: A coping skills training guide.* New York: Guilford Press.

Myers, M.G. and Brown, S.A. (1990). Coping and appraisal in potential situations among adolescent substance abusers following treatment. *Journal of Adolescent Chemical Dependency,* **1**, 95–115.

Nathan, P.E. (1983). Failures in prevention: Why we can't prevent the devastating effect of alcoholism and drug use. *American Psychologist,* **April**, 456–467.

Needle, R., McCubbin, H., Wilson, M., Reineck, R., and Lazar, A. (1986). Interpersonal influence in adolescent drug use: The role of older siblings, parents and peers. *International Journal of the Addictions,* **21**, 739–766.

Newcomb, M.D. and Bentler, P.M. (1988). *Consequences of adolescent drug use: Impact on the lives of young adults.* Newbury Park, CA: Sage.

Newcomb, M.D. and Bentler, P.M. (1989). Substance use and abuse among children and teenagers. *American Psychologist,* **44**, 242–248.

Newcomb, M.D., Maddahian, E., and Bentler, P.M. (1986). Risk factors for drug use among adolescents: Concurrent and longitudinal analyses. *American Journal of Public Health,* **76**, 525–531.

Newcomb, M.D., Maddahian, E., Skager, R., and Bentler, P.M. (1987). Substance abuse and psychosocial risk factors among teenagers: Associations with sex, age, ethnicity, and type of school. *American Journal of Drug and Alcohol Abuse*, **13**, 413–433.

Nordlohne, E. (1992). *Die Kosten jugendlicher Problembewältigung. Alkohol, Zigaretten- und Arzeimittelkonsum im Jugendalter*. Weinheim: Juventa.

Oetting, E.R. and Beauvais, F. (1987). Peer cluster theory: Drugs and the adolescent. *Journal of Counseling and Development*, **65**, 17–22.

Perkonigg, A., Wittchen, H.-U., and Lachner, G. (in press). Wie häufig sind Substanzmißbrauch und-abhängigkeit? Ein methodenkritischer Überblick. *Zeitschrift für Klinische Psychologie*.

Pickens, R.W., Svikis, D.S., McGue, M., Lykken, D.T., Heston, L.L., and Clayton, P.J. (1991). Heterogeneity in the inheritance of alcoholism. *Archives of General Psychiatry*, **48**, 19–28.

Reich, W. and Welner, Z. (1988). *Revised version of the Diagnostic Interview for Children and Adolescents (DICA-R)*. St. Louis, MO: Department of Psychiatry, Washington University, School of Medicine.

Reuband, K.H. (1988). Drogenkonsum im Wandel. Eine retrospektive Prävelenzmessung der Drogenerfahrung Jugendlicher in den Jahren 1967–1987. *Zeitschrift für Sozialisationsforschung und Erziehungssoziologie*, **8**, 54–68.

Reilly, D.M. (1976). Family factors in the etiology and treatment of youthful drug abuse. *Family Therapy*, **2**, 149–171.

Reinherz, D.M., Giaconia, R.M., Pakiz, B., Silverman, A.B., Frost, A.K., and Lefkowitz, E.S. (1993). Prevalence of psychiatric disorders in a community population of older adolescents. *Journal of the American Academy of Child and Adolescent Psychiatry*, **32**, 369–377.

Robins, L. and McEvoy, L. (1990). Conduct problems as predictors of substance abuse. In L. Robins and M. Rutter (Eds.), *Straight and devious pathways from childhood to adulthood* (pp. 49–74). Cambridge: Cambridge University Press.

Rutter, M. (1979). Protective factors in children's response to stress and disadvantage. In M.W. Kent and J.E. Rolf (Eds.), *Primary Prevention of Psychopathology: Social Competence in Children* (pp. 49–74) Hanover: University Press of New England.

Rutter, M., Izard, C.E., and Read, P.B. (1986). *Depression in young people*. New York: Guilford Press.

Schinke, S.P. and Gilchrist, L.D. (1985). Preventing substance abuse with children and adolescents. *Journal of Counseling and Clinical Psychology*, **53**, 596–602.

Schonberg, S.K. (1988) (Ed.). Specific drugs. In *Substance Abuse: A guide for health professionals* (pp. 115–182). Illinois: American Academy of Pediatrics.

Schuckit, M.A. (1985). Genetics and the risk for alcoholism. *Journal of the American Medical Association*, **254**, 2614–2617.

Schuckit, M.A. and Russell, J.A. (1983). Clinical importance of the age at first drink in a group of young men. *American Journal of Psychiatry*, **140**, 1221–1223.

Schweitzer, R.D. and Lawton, P.A. (1989). Drug abusers' perceptions of their parents. *British Journal of the Addictions*, **84**, 309–314.

Selzer, M.L. (1971). The Michigan Alcoholism Screening Test: The quest for a new diagnostic instrument. *American Journal of Psychiatry*, **12**, 89–94.

Shedler, J. and Block, J. (1990). Adolescent drug use and psychological health. *American Psychologist*, **45**, 612–630.

Silbereisen, R.E., Robins, L., and Rutter, M. (1995). Secular trends in substance use: Concepts and data on the impact of social change on alcohol and drug abuse. In M. Rutter and D.J. Smith (Eds.), *Psychosocial disorders in young people: Time trends and their causes* (pp. 490–543). Chichester: John Wiley and Sons.

Simons, R.L., Conger, R.D., and Whitbeck, L.B. (1988). A multistage social learning model of the influences of family and peers upon adolescent substance abuse. *Journal of Drug Issues*, **16**, 7–28.

Skinner, H.A. (1982). The Drug Abuse Screening Test. *Addictive Behaviors, 7*, 363–371.

Spatz-Windom, C. (1989). The cycle of violence. *Science,* **244**, 117–264.

Stanton, M.D. (1985). The family and drug abuse. In T.E. Bratter and G.G. Forrest (Eds.), *Alcoholism and substance abuse: Strategies for clinical intervention* (pp. 398–430). New York: Free Press.

Stanton, M.D. and Todd, T.C. (1982). *The family therapy of drug abuse and addiction.* New York: Guilford.

Stoker, A. and Swadi, H. (1990). Perceived family relationships in drug abusing adolescents. *Drug and Alcohol Dependence, 25*, 293–297.

Swaim, R.C. (1991). Childhood risk factors and adolescent drug and alcohol abuse. *Educ. Psychol. Rev., 3*, 363–398.

Tarter, R.E. (1990). Evaluation and treatment of adolescent substance abuse: A decision tree method. *American Journal of Drug and Alcohol Abuse,* **16**, 1–46.

Tobler, N.S. (1986). Meta-analysis of 143 adolescent drug prevention programs: Quantitative outcome results of program participants compared to a control or comparison group. *Journal of Drug Issues,* **16**, 537–567.

Walter, H.J., Vaughan, R.D., and Cohall, A.T. (1991). Risk factors for substance use among high school students: Implications for prevention. *Journal of the American Academy of Child and Adolesence Psychiatry,* **30**, 556–562.

World Health Organization (1993). *The ICD-10 classification of mental and behavioural disorders.* Geneva: World Health Organization

CHAPTER 10
FEEDING AND EATING DISORDERS

Julie Hakim-Larson, Sylvia Voelker, Cheryl Thomas, and Linda Reinstein

Child psychologists have long understood that the self concept of the child and adolescent is closely linked to physical appearance (e.g., Hart and Damon, 1985) and developmental changes in the conceptual understanding of bodily functioning (e.g., Carey, 1985). Indeed, Lawrence and Thelen (1995) recently reported that as early as the third-grade some children are concerned about being overweight and that these concerns are negatively related to their feelings of self-worth. An adaptive task crucial to survival and related to this aspect of the physical and emotional self-concept involves feeding behaviours in infancy and eating behaviours in childhood and adolescence. When there is a severe disruption in such feeding or eating behaviours and medical etiological factors alone cannot account for the dysfunction, the need for psychological as well as medical intervention is critical to preventing irreversible physiological damage and maladaptive self development.

In this chapter, we will give an overview of the classification, diagnosis, and epidemiology of feeding disorder of infancy or early childhood, rumination disorder, pica, anorexia nervosa, bulimia nervosa, and disorders involving obesity. The remaining sections will emphasize the associated risks factors, course, outcome, and treatment of these feeding and eating disorders.

DEFINITION AND CLASSIFICATION

Disturbances in feeding or eating sufficiently severe to warrant clinical attention may occur from infancy through adulthood, but they are most likely to occur during two periods of life: infancy/early childhood and late childhood/adolescence. The type of disturbances manifested during these two developmental periods tend to be quite distinct, although some early eating problems may be precursors of later problems.

The Diagnostic and Statistical Manual, Fourth Edition (DSM-IV; American Psychiatric Association; APA, 1994) presents three categories of disorders likely to first manifest in infancy and early childhood: pica, rumination disorder, and feeding disorder of infancy or early childhood. The latter category is a new diagnosis in DSM-IV. Anorexia nervosa, bulimia nervosa, and eating disorders not otherwise specified comprise a separate eating disorders chapter in the general section of DSM-IV (1994), and they are distinguished from the infancy/early childhood disorders by affected individuals' preoccupation with body concerns and weight control. DSM-IV (APA, 1994) also contains a proposed new eating disorder category (binge-eating disorder, Appendix B, pp. 729–731) with research criteria recommended to facilitate further study.

Obesity is included as a general medical condition in the International Classification of Diseases (ICD-10; World Health Organization; WHO, 1993), but it is not recognized as a diagnostic category in DSM because research has not identified a specific psychopathology as characteristic of individuals who are obese. DSM-IV (APA, 1994) authors acknowledge that psychological factors may influence the etiology or course of obesity in some cases, for which "Psychological Factors Affecting Medical Condition" (p. 675) as the focus of treatment is appropriate.

DSM-IV (APA, 1994) is not inclusive of all juvenile eating and feeding disturbances. Bryant-Waugh and Lask (1995) have found that fully 25% of the children referred to their eating disorder clinic present with eating disturbances that do not fit the DSM-IV (APA, 1994) categories. These authors describe several additional categories of eating disorders in children. The present discussion will be limited to the DSM-IV (APA, 1994) diagnoses and obesity, but the reader should be aware that other manifestations of eating and feeding disturbances are being studied. As pointed out by Yates (1989), "The eating disorder diagnoses are somewhat arbitrary in definition and are likely to continue to evolve over the next several decades" (p. 814).

Feeding and Eating Disorders of Infancy or Early Childhood

Pica

Pica refers to the habitual, deliberate ingestion of non-nutritive substances, such as paint, plaster, or hair. Pica is usually associated with consumption of normal amounts of regular food as well. Epidemiological data on pica are quite limited. Historically and to the present day, the populations most likely to exhibit pica are young children, pregnant women, mentally retarded individuals, and geophagists (i.e., individuals who eat dirt or clay) in primitive cultures (Parry-Jones and Parry-Jones, 1994). Pica is reportedly rarer in the modern developed world, currently occurring predominately in infants and young children in lower socioeconomic groups. In less developed areas, culture-bound geophagy is still practised by both children and adults, especially in the lower classes in rural areas (Parry-Jones and Parry-Jones, 1992).

The DSM-IV (APA, 1994) criteria require that a diagnosis of pica be assigned if the behaviour is developmentally inappropriate, has persisted for at least a month, and is not culturally sanctioned. According to the Diagnostic and Statistical Manual of Mental Disorders, Third Edition, Revised (DSM-III-R; APA, 1987) criteria, a diagnosis of schizophrenia or pervasive developmental disorder precludes diagnosis of pica. The one change in DSM-IV (APA, 1994) is to permit dual diagnosis if the pica is sufficiently severe to warrant independent intervention.

Regarding pica as an independent disorder is unique to the 20th century. Parry-Jones and Parry-Jones (1992; 1994) suggest a return to the historical view of pica as a symptom complex associated with other conditions or disorders. These authors recommend that future classificatory efforts should at least expand the definition of pica to include excessive cravings for specific foods, such as the behaviour of restrained eaters who attempt to control their weight by restricting themselves to essentially non-nutritive, low-calorie food (e.g., spices, vinegar, and pickles). This change would facilitate studying subtypes of pica and the relationship between pica and other disorders, particularly anorexia and bulimia.

Rumination Disorder

Rumination, or merycism, involves deliberate regurgitation without nausea, followed by apparently pleasurable remastication of food. The re-chewed food is then either re-swallowed or spat out, the latter occurring most often in infants or mentally retarded individuals and sometimes resulting in significant nutritional deficits (Parry-Jones, 1994). As with pica, little is known about the incidence of rumination. It is apparently a rare disorder that occurs predominately in infants (typical onset between 3 and 12 months old) and mentally retarded individuals, and more often in males than females (DSM-IV; APA, 1994).

DSM-IV (APA, 1994) criteria require that the behaviour persist for at least a month, that it not be associated exclusively with anorexia or bulimia, and that medical causes be ruled out prior to assigning a diagnosis of rumination. The one change made in DSM-IV (APA, 1994) is to eliminate the criterion specifying weight loss or lack of gain. The rationale for this change is to distinguish rumination from feeding disorder of infancy or early childhood. In addition, research has demonstrated that clinically significant impairment may occur without the specified weight loss or failure to gain weight (APA, 1994).

In her extensive historical review of rumination, Parry-Jones (1994) found that prior to the 20th century, ruminators were predominately male juveniles or adults, both retarded and normally intelligent. Rumination in infants was not recognized until early in the 20th century when references to infants and mentally retarded populations began to dominate the rumination literature. Recently, rumination in non-retarded adults has been reported in connection with anorexia and bulimia (Fairburn and Cooper, 1984; Larocca, 1988). Parry-Jones (1994) indicated that obtaining accurate incidence estimates is difficult because of the secrecy of the behaviour. Based on her historical review and recent research, Parry-Jones (1994) concluded that rumination is not limited to infants and young children and that future nosologies should include retarded and normally intelligent adult ruminators and recognize the role of "covert rumination" in anorexia and bulimia.

Feeding Disorder of Infancy or Early Childhood

This new category has been included in DSM-IV (1994) for classifying infants and young children whose failure to eat sufficiently has had a significant impact on body mass (Table 10.1). This disorder resembles the medical syndrome of nonorganic failure-to-thrive (Kronenberger and Meyer, 1996) and is characterized by significant weight loss or failure to gain weight resulting from inadequate ingestion that is not attributable to a medical condition. DSM-IV (APA, 1994) criteria further specify that other sources of the eating disturbance be ruled out (e.g., rumination, lack of available food) and that the disturbance conform to specified onset (prior to six years old) and persistence (at least one month) parameters (APA, 1994). There has been little research to date that examines this new diagnosis, so it is necessary to incorporate existing knowledge about related disorders into discussion of Feeding Disorder of Infancy or Early Childhood (FDI). Two disorders that involve some aspects that overlap with this new diagnosis are nonorganic failure-to-thrive and Reactive Attachment Disorder (Kronenberger and Meyer, 1996).

FDI is most similar to nonorganic failure to thrive (NOFT), a well-established medical syndrome. NOFT is associated with low body mass, malnourished appearance, normal head circumference, abnormal social development, and delayed attainment of motor developmental milestones in the context of no organic causes. NOFT is attributed to psychological factors, most often thought to be caused by maladaptive parent/child relationships (Kronenberger and Meyer, 1996).

Feeding Disorder of Infancy or Early Childhood is distinct from Reactive Attachment Disorder, which involves no criterion addressing body mass and is defined by disturbed social relatedness associated with markedly pathogenic care (APA, 1994). Previously, the Diagnostic and Statistical Manual of Mental Disorders, Third edition (DSM-III; APA, 1980) classification included body mass in the definition of Reactive Attachment Disorder and referred to "failure to thrive" as a severe exemplar of the disorder (p. 57). In DSM-IV (APA, 1994), Reactive Attachment Disorder is presented as possibly associated with any of the three eating and feeding disorders of infancy and early childhood. Since mealtime is a likely venue for manifestation of parent/child relationship problems, the association between Reactive Attachment Disorder and eating and feeding disorders is not surprising.

The exact relationship between NOFT and Reactive Attachment Disorder has been a source of considerable confusion. Kronenberger and Meyer (1996) concluded that DSM-IV has taken a major step toward clarifying the area and encouraging more accurate classification by defining two distinct syndromes that may or may not co-occur.

Table 10.1 Diagnostic criteria for feeding disorder of infancy or early childhood

---

A. Feeding disturbance as manifested by persistent failure to eat adequately with significant failure to gain weight or significant loss of weight over at least 1 month

B. The disturbance is not due to an associated gastrointestinal or other general medical condition (e.g., esophageal reflux)

C. The disturbance is not better accounted for by another mental disorder (e.g., rumination disorder) or by lack of available food

D. The onset is before age 6 years

Reprinted with permission from the Diagnostic and Statistical Manual of Mental Disorders, Fourth Edition. Copyright 1994 American Psychiatric Association.

Late Childhood/Adolescent Eating Disorders and Obesity

Anorexia Nervosa

The most well-known of the eating disorders, anorexia nervosa, is characterized by self-starvation and failure to maintain minimally normal body weight (Table 10.2). DSM-IV (APA, 1994) criteria specify weight less than 85% of that expected, intense fear of becoming fat, disturbance in the way in which body weight or shape is experienced, and amenorrhea in postmenarchal females (APA, 1994; pp. 544–545). The major change from previous DSM versions is the inclusion of subtypes. When binge eating and purging occur exclusively during anorexia nervosa, the individual is diagnosed with anorexia nervosa, Binge-Eating/Purging Subtype (rather than being given a separate diagnosis of bulimia nervosa, as was true using DSM-III-R criteria). Individuals with anorexia nervosa who do not regularly binge and purge are diagnosed with anorexia nervosa, Restricting Subtype. As many as 50% of individuals with anorexia nervosa may show bulimic eating patterns (Kennedy and Garfinkel, 1992).

There are a number of potential biological sequelae of semistarvation and purging behaviours. Semistarvation can affect most major organ systems and produce a variety of physical abnormalities, such as anemia, bradycardia, hypotension, and growth of lanugo (fine body hair) on the trunk. Chronic purging behaviours are also linked to significant medical conditions, including impaired renal function, cardiovas-

Table 10.2   Diagnostic criteria for anorexia nervosa

A.   Refusal to maintain body weight at or above a minimally normal weight for age and height (e.g., weight loss leading to maintenance of body weight less than 85% of that expected; or failure to make expected weight gain during period of growth, leading to body weight less than 85% of that expected)

B.   Intense fear of gaining weight or becoming fat, even though underweight

C.   Disturbance in the way in which one´s body weight or shape is experienced, undue influence of body weight or shape on self-evaluation, or denial of the seriousness of the current low body weight

D.   In postmenarcheal females, amenorrhea, i.e., the absence of at least three consecutive menstrual cycles. (A woman is considered to have amenorrhea if her periods occur only following hormone, e.g., estrogen, administration)

Reprinted with permission from the Diagnostic and Statistical Manual of Mental Disorders, Fourth Edition. Copyright 1994 American Psychiatric Association.

cular abnormalities, dental problems (secondary to induced vomiting), and osteoporosis (resulting from reduced intake and absorption of calcium) (APA, 1994). Changing diagnostic criteria and differing study methodologies have led to striking variations in incidence and prevalence rates cited for anorexia nervosa. Whether eating disorders have recently increased at alarming rates or whether reports of increases are an artifact of methodologies used continues to be debated. In his comprehensive review of studies examining time trends in the incidence of eating disorders, Fombonne (1995) concluded that increased incidence of anorexia nervosa has not been compellingly demonstrated and that "there remains a need to demonstrate more firmly that an apparent increase does not merely reflect better recognition or different diagnostic and treatment practices or health-seeking behaviours" (p. 639).

There is also concern that rigorous diagnostic criteria exclude many individuals that present with clinically significant partial eating disorder syndromes and that this tendency toward under-diagnosing and under-reporting is a problem particularly for detecting eating disorders in prepubertal children. See Bryant-Waugh (1993) for a discussion of these issues and their impact on incidence estimates and treatment.

Bulimia Nervosa

Bulimia nervosa is defined by binge eating, or excessive intake of food, often high-calorie food, in a relatively brief period of time (Table 10.3). Like anorexia nervosa, bulimia nervosa is associated with morbid fear of becoming obese. The binge eating is often secretive, accompanied by feelings of shame and inability to control the eating behaviour, and interspersed with periods of restrained eating. Binges may be followed by purging through self-induced vomiting, laxatives, or diuretics (Husain and Cantwell, 1991).

For a diagnosis of bulimia nervosa, DSM-IV (APA, 1994) requires recurrent episodes of binge eating, recurrent maladaptive weight control behaviours, persistence of binge-eating and inappropriate compensatory behaviour (i.e., twice per week for 3 months), and preoccupation with body shape and weight. Changes in DSM-IV (APA, 1994) include adding an exclusion criterion to prevent diagnosis of bulimia nervosa during episodes of anorexia nervosa, and providing subtypes to distinguish between Purging Type for individuals who have regularly used vomiting, laxatives, or diuretics and Nonpurging Type for individuals whose attempts to compensate for binge eating include behaviours such as fasting or excessive exercise.

Table 10.3   Diagnostic criteria for bulimia nervosa

A.   Recurrent episodes of binge eating. An episode of binge eating is characterized by both the following:
   1)   eating, in a discrete period of time (e.g., within any 2-hour period), an amount of food that is definitely larger than most people would eat during a similar period of time and under similar circumstances
   2)   a sense of lack of control over eating during the episode (e.g., a feeling that one cannot stop eating or control what or how much one is eating)

B.   Recurrent inappropriate compensatory behavior in order to prevent weight gain, such as self-induced vomiting; misuse of laxatives, diuretics, enemas, or other medications; fasting; or excessive exercise

C.   The binge eating and inappropriate compensatory behaviors both occur, on average, at least twice a week for 3 months

D.   Self-evaluation is unduly influenced by body shape and weight

E.   The disturbance does not occur exclusively during episodes of anorexia nervosa

---

Reprinted with permission from the Diagnostic and Statistical Manual of Mental Disorders, Fourth Edition. Copyright 1994 American Psychiatric Association.

Obesity

Obesity in children and adolescents is conventionally defined as body weight that is 20% or more above the ideal based on gender, age, and height (Epstein and Wing, 1987). Dissatisfaction with the height-weight method of assessing obesity in children has led to experimenting with various methods of measuring adipose tissue directly, such as by measuring skin folds with calipers (see Foreyt and Cousins, 1989, pp. 407–409 for a review). The use of different criteria and methods has led to varying estimates of prevalence of juvenile obesity.

Obese children are at risk for a number of health problems, as well as psychological problems reactive to prejudicial attitudes (e.g., Siegel and Smith, 1991), and the research literature indicates that obesity is a common, chronic condition.

The experimental binge eating disorder category included in DSM-IV (APA, 1994) for further study is distinguished from bulimia nervosa by lack of the compensatory behaviours characteristic of bulimia nervosa. Field trials using this category have suggested that a substantial proportion of obese adults seeking treatment (about 30%) are struggling with binge eating, and that the bingers demonstrate more psychopathology than obese adults who do not binge (see Yanovski *et al.*, 1993 for a review). This relationship has not yet been investigated in adolescents.

EPIDEMIOLOGY

Feeding Disorder of Infancy or Early Childhood

The newness of the Feeding Disorder of Infancy or Early Childhood category, makes it difficult to obtain accurate epidemiological data. Approximately 1–5% of pediatric hospital admissions present with inadequate weight gain. Up to one half of these admissions may be secondary to feeding disturbances with no known medical cause. Feeding Disorder of Infancy or Early Childhood is apparently equally common in males and females. Age at onset is typically in the first year of life, but it may also occur in toddlers. Later onset (2–3 years) is associated with a better prognosis (APA, 1994).

Anorexia Nervosa

Anorexia nervosa primarily affects adolescent girls and women, but approximately 5 to 10% of cases across this age range are males (e.g., Barry and Lippmann, 1990). For females in the high-risk age group (12 to 18 years), incidence of anorexia nervosa may be as high as 1% (Yates, 1989). Higher incidences have been reported among groups that involve high achievement expectations and emphasize slimness, such as models, ballet dancers, and elite athletes (e.g., Garner *et al.*, 1987; Sundgot-Borgen, 1994). Once thought to be a Western disorder affecting primarily females of white racial origin (e.g., Russell, 1985), anorexia nervosa has since been documented in various cultures and ethnic groups, although it is still far more prevalent in middle and upper classes in industrialized societies with plentiful food (Wren and Lask, 1993). There are no epidemiological studies that examine eating disorders specifically in children under 14, but there have been several reports of early onset anorexia nervosa in children ages 8 to 13 (Fosson *et al.*, 1987; Hawley, 1985; Higgs *et al.*, 1989). These studies report a higher than expected proportion of the male cases (19 to 30%). Bryant-Waugh (1993) reviewed the sparse epidemiological data on early onset eating disorders and concluded that anorexia nervosa is likely less frequent in children than in older individuals.

Bryant-Waugh and Kaminski (1993) report that children with anorexia nervosa present with a clinical picture very similar to that of older individuals, but children also show some unique symptoms. Children are less likely to engage in binge-eating and use laxative abuse for weight control. Children are also more likely to restrict fluid intake and become dehydrated (Childress *et al.*, 1993). Because of differences in the way adipose tissue is distributed for children as compared to late adolescents or adults, children become more emaciated with a similar amount of weight loss and may develop depressive symptoms relatively early in the course of the disorder (Irwin, 1984). Bryant-Waugh and Lask (1995) recommend less stringent criteria for identification of anorexia nervosa in children to facilitate diagnosis earlier in the course when treatment is more likely to be effective.

Bulimia Nervosa

At least 90% of individuals who present with bulimia nervosa are females, predominately in the older adolescent and young adult age range (Foreyt and McGavin, 1989). Little is known about bulimia nervosa in children, but it is apparently rare before age 14 (Schmidt *et al.*, 1992; Bryant-Waugh and Lask, 1995). Rigorous criteria generally yield incidence rates of about 1–3% of females in the high-risk age range, with the rate in males about one-tenth of that for females (APA, 1994; p. 548.). However, given the secrecy and shame associated with bulimia nervosa, it is likely that it is underdiagnosed and underestimated by these prevalence rates (Husain and Cantwell, 1991).

Time trends in the incidence of bulimia nervosa are even more difficult to track than that of anorexia nervosa because of the recency of the formal description of bulimia nervosa as a distinct syndrome (APA, 1980) and because of the evolving nature of the diagnostic criteria used to identify bulimia nervosa. In his review of the limited data available, Fombonne (1995) concluded that no increase in incidence of bulimia nervosa has been demonstrated.

Obesity

Prevalence estimates of obesity in young children have ranged from 10–15%, and in adolescents from 15–30%. Obese children are not likely to outgrow the condition. If obesity persists through adolescence, it is highly unlikely that normal weight will be attained in adulthood (Foreyt and Cousins, 1989). There is evidence that the incidence of child and adolescent obesity is increasing (Siegel and Smith, 1991).

Wide cross-cultural variation in the incidence of childhood obesity has been reported. LeBow (1984) reported estimates of 10 to 40% in the United States (U.S.), 5 to 15% in Britain, 8% in West Germany, and 5% in Yugoslavia. Recent immigrants to the U.S. show elevated rates of obesity that decline to approximate typical U.S. rates by about the 3rd generation (Dietz, 1987). Prevalence estimates differ by gender, race, ethnicity, and socioeconomic status, but the relationships are complex and changing (Foreyt and Cousins, 1989). For example, obesity is typically found at higher rates in the lower classes, although the very poorest children tend to be the thinnest (LeBow, 1984).

RISK FACTORS

Despite burgeoning research on the feeding and eating disorders, no clear pathogenesis has emerged. The accumulated evidence regarding possible causes and associated risk factors suggests that these disorders are multidetermined syndromes produced and maintained through the interaction of a variety of factors — social, biological, psychological, and familial (Bryant-Waugh and Lask, 1995). The complex interplay of these factors has not yet been fully elucidated, but some compelling patterns have begun to take shape.

Feeding and Eating Disorders of Infancy or Early Childhood

Both pica and rumination disorder have multiple risks and etiological factors stemming from sociocultural conditions, biology, and psychological or familial influences. Pica has been associated with mental retardation, autism, developmental delays, conditions of poverty, neglect, and poor supervision, and possible nutritional deficiencies such as iron, calcium, and zinc (Benoit, 1993). Benoit (1993) also reviews evidence that rumination disorder or merycism is linked to mental retardation, or associated with parental psychopathology and disturbances in mother-infant interactions when it is not caused by a specific medical condition or complication.

Many risk factors having a possible association with feeding disorders and failure to thrive have been considered and studied. These include: *social* conditions involving poverty, stress, and limited parental resources and supports (Dubowitz *et al.*, 1989); *biological* factors affecting growth such as general medical condition, constitutional factors, amount of physical activity, and calories in diet (Benoit, 1993); and *psychological and familial* factors such as maternal depression (Singer *et al.*, 1990), infantile depression (Powell and Bettes, 1992), aversive or difficult infant temperament (Iwaniec *et al.*, 1985), and disturbances in mother-child interactions especially during feeding (Drotar *et al.*, 1990). Underfeeding by a caregiver may involve accidental errors in food preparation, deliberate underfeeding which is rare, or neglectful underfeeding due to maternal distress or pathology (Schmitt and Mauro, 1989). In addition, Chatoor and her colleagues (cited in Benoit, 1993) have proposed that some types of persistent and pervasive food refusal by the child may be caused by traumatic oral experiences as a result of medical procedures or ingestion of medications. Similarly, Wittenberg (1990) has described an iatrogenic form of failure to thrive whereby some children develop an aversion to eating due to various medical conditions or their treatment.

Anorexia Nervosa

Social Factors

Increasing societal pressures for thinness have been implicated as triggering the dissatisfaction that so many young women feel with their bodies. Beauty pageant participants and women photographed for popular magazines have become thinner on average over the last several decades while the number of articles devoted to dieting advice has dramatically increased. During the same time period, the average young woman has become heavier, making it increasingly difficult for her to attain the societal ideal (Agras and Kirkley, 1986). As Fombonne (1995) concluded, "secular changes in body weight, in conjunction with changing concepts of ideal body shape, may have increased vulnerability to eating disturbances" (p. 662).

Cross-cultural differences in incidence of eating disorders provides further evidence of the impact of sociocultural factors. Although the direction of causality has not yet been addressed, a correlation has been demonstrated between young girls' disturbed eating patterns and their reliance on fashion magazines as a source of information about ideal body shape and how to attain it (Levine *et al.*, 1994). Eating disorders are rare in cultures in which thinness is not highly valued. The fact that eating disorders are now being reported for children of immigrants from these cultures further supports the notion that cultural pressures trigger maladaptive eating patterns (Bryant-Waugh and Lask, 1995).

The relationship between dieting and eating disorders has not been clearly explicated. Hsu (1990) suggested that incidence of eating disorders and dieting behaviours are likely to be proportional within a given population. Dieting behaviour is often cited as a precursor of eating disorders, and some writers have proposed dieting as a precondition for the development of eating disorders (e.g., Bruch, 1974). Dieting behaviour is quite common among adolescents and older children and may be increasing (Hill *et al.*, 1989). Only a small proportion of dieters develop eating disorders, but the risk for dieters is much greater than that for non-dieters (Patton *et al.*, 1990). Hill and Robinson (1991) report that girls as young as nine years old are demonstrating dieting concerns and restricted eating at a rate similar to that of their older peers. In a prospective study of early adolescent girls, Killen *et al.* (1994) linked weight concerns with later onset of eating disorder symptoms. The literature suggests that dieting is a potential risk factor and implies that the risk for developing an eating disorder is increasing.

Individuals with anorexia may over-exercise as a means of weight control, but exercise *per se* does not cause eating disorders (Nash, 1987). There is, however, a connection between involvement in some competitive sports and pathogenic weight control (Biddle, 1993; Sundgot-Borgen, 1994). Sports and vocations that involve high achievement expectations and pressures for slimness, such as ballet and modelling, are associated with increased risk for eating disorders (e.g., Garner *et al.*, 1987).

Less is known about the relatively small number of males who develop eating disorders. Overall the symptoms, histories, and outcome measures for males and females with eating disorders are similar, but some differences have been reported. Eating disordered women are more likely to be married, whereas men with eating disorders are more likely to show unconventional psychosexual development and to report homosexual or bisexual preferences (Garfinkel *et al.*, 1987; Lowenstein, 1994; Yates, 1989). Sasson *et al.* (1995) suggest gender-linked developmental landmarks that precede the development of eating disorders. In both U.S. and Israeli samples (Maloney *et al.*, 1989; Sasson *et al.*, 1995), males and females showed similar eating attitudes and dieting behaviours until early adolescence (about age 12). Beginning at age 14 or 15, distinct gender differences emerged with boys aiming their efforts toward increasing upper body mass while girls increasingly tried to lose weight.

Biological Factors

There is now compelling evidence from family and twin studies that genetic factors contribute to vulnerability to anorexia. The risk for developing anorexia is significantly higher among first degree female relatives of anorexics than in the general population, while there is no increased risk for relatives of probands with other disorders (Strober *et al.*, 1990). Holland *et al.* (1988) studied 45 twin pairs and found substantially higher concordance for monozygotic (56%) than dizygotic pairs (5%). These studies and others implicate a genetic predisposition for the development of anorexia, but the exact mechanism is not known.

A number of other biological factors have been associated with anorexia. After reviewing research investigating the relationship between eating disorders, depression, and athleticism, Yates (1989) concluded that menstrual irregularities may be a biological marker for vulnerability to depression and eating disorders. Many of the abnormal laboratory findings typically obtained for individuals with anorexia, such as zinc deficiency, are secondary to semistarvation and dietary deficiencies and are *not* of etiological significance (Bryant-Waugh and Lask, 1995).

Other avenues of biological research may identify factors of causal significance. For example, Russell (1985) has proposed that endocrine abnormalities associated with anorexia may implicate hypothalamic dysfunction as a primary cause. Others have implicated brain serotonergic dysfunction (e.g., Weltzin *et al.*, 1993). It remains to be demonstrated whether these factors are primary or secondary (Bryant-Waugh and Lask, 1995).

Psychological and Familial Factors

Various theories regarding psychological characteristics have been suggested as contributing to the development of anorexia. For example, Husain and Cantwell (1991) report that Sigmund Freud first hypothesized fear of sexual maturity as the precipitant for anorexia. Others have emphasized premorbid history of perfectionism, feelings of ineffectiveness, distrust of others, and difficulty interpreting internal states (e.g., Bruch, 1977; Crisp, 1980; Strober, 1980). Bryant-Waugh and Lask (1995) point out that attempts to empirically validate these ideas have been sparse, and that none of the speculations proposed is sufficient "to explain the development of such a specific and idiosyncratic condition as anorexia nervosa" (p. 195).

Speculations regarding family dysfunction as a major contributing factor to the development and maintenance of anorexia have also been popular. Interactional patterns hypothesized as contributory include: overprotectiveness, enmeshment, poor conflict resolution, and lack of empathy and affection (Minuchin *et al.*, 1975; Strober and Humphrey,

1987). Recently, history of childhood sexual abuse has been associated with increased risk for eating disorders (e.g., Hall *et al.*, 1989). Again, empirical assessment of these ideas is lacking or inconclusive. Dysfunctional family interactions may be more common in families with an eating disordered member, but there is no evidence of a causal relationship (Lask and Bryant-Waugh, 1992; Fombonne, 1995).

Symptoms of depression are common among anorexics, but may be due, in part, to the effects of dietary restriction. It may be particularly difficult to rule out a primary affective disorder in children presenting with anorexia nervosa symptoms (Bryant-Waugh and Kaminski, 1993). There is evidence that adolescents with circumscribed eating problems are less likely to experience psychological and family problems, whereas those with concurrent eating and mood disturbances show aberrant psychological and family functioning (Steiger *et al.*, 1992). There is increased prevalence of affective disorders among first-degree relatives of anorexic probands (Weltzin *et al.*, 1993). High incidence of obsessive-compulsive symptoms has been reported for anorexics as well. Strober (1980) has described the obsessive thinking pattern as ingrained and not altered by changes in weight.

Marchi and Cohen (1990) investigated the prospective risks of eating and digestive problems in early childhood by tracing maladaptive eating patterns longitudinally. They reported that picky eating and digestive problems in early childhood are predictive of anorexia in adolescence. Greater vulnerability to eating disorders for children with chronic medical problems, such as diabetes and cystic fibrosis, has also been reported (e.g., Pollock *et al.*, 1995; Pumariega *et al.*, 1986).

Studies comparing binge-eating and restricting anorexics suggest that a premorbid personality characterized by overcontrol and reserve may be a risk factor for developing restricting anorexia (e.g., Casper *et al.*, 1992). Binge-eating anorexics have a higher incidence of premorbid and familial obesity, increased risk for depression, and higher incidence of childhood maladjustment and of impulsive behaviours, such as shoplifting, substance abuse, and sexual behaviour (Garfinkel *et al.*, 1980; Strober, 1986; Weltzin *et al.*, 1993).

Bulimia Nervosa

Social Factors

Young women who become bulimic may be particularly vulnerable to societal pressures for thinness because they tend to be slightly heavier than peers. Binge eating is paradoxically related to the persistent quest for thinness and consequent excessive dieting. A relationship between dieting and episodes of overeating has been well-established (e.g., Herman and Mack, 1975). Based primarily on the results of Herman and Polivy's (1975) classic study, Agras and Kirkley (1986) propose a model to explain bulimic binge eating as resulting from chronic dietary restraint and cognitive disinhibition. Eating behaviour of bulimics is generally restrained and under rigid cognitive control. There is evidence that when that control is disrupted, such as by a negative emotional state or the breaking of a rigid dietary intake rule, disinhibition and binge eating results (Agras and Kirkley, 1986). This cognitive disinhibition may be exaggerated by the effects of chronic restraint in eating, which may also paradoxically increase desire for sweets (Rodin *et al.*, 1977). Support for the model is found in Marchi and Cohen's (1990) report that dieting behaviours in early adolescence predicted increased risk for bulimia nervosa in late adolescence.

Since bulimic individuals have an intense fear of gaining weight, binge-eating increases anxiety. Purging behaviour is often conceptualized as an escape-avoidance response that is reinforced by anxiety reduction (Rosen and Leitenberg, 1982). An alternative interpretation consistent with the restrained eating and cognitive disinhibition model described above is that purging maintains bulimia by returning the body to a state of deprivation, thereby contributing to further binge eating (Agras and Kirkley, 1986).

Biological Factors

Bulimia nervosa as a distinct syndrome has a relatively short history, so less information regarding possible biological etiology specific to bulimia is available. Agras and Kirkley (1986) describe a biological theory, based on the work of Wurtman and Wurtman, that was developed to explain excessive carbohydrate intake and has particular relevance to bulimia. They suggest that some individuals have an abnormal craving for carbohydrates due to a faulty serotonergic carbohydrate feedback mechanism. Theoretically, such individuals would need to use extreme restraint in eating in order to stay thin, which would increase risk for onset of the binge eating and purging behaviour cycle. Other biological factors that have been implicated are increased plasma beta endorphin levels associated with vomiting, and diminished secretion of a peptide hormone, cholecystokinin, although the latter is more likely a perpetuating rather than a causative factor (Yates, 1989).

Psychological and Familial Factors

Bulimia nervosa has been associated with increased frequency of a number of disorders consistent with poor self-control of emotions and behaviour. The prevalence of depressed mood in bulimia nervosa, as well as the high incidence of affective disorders among relatives of individuals with bulimia has led to speculation that bulimia is a variant of affective disorder. Overall, this hypothesis has received only limited support (Weltzin *et al.*, 1993). Bulimia has also been associated with increased incidence of anxiety disorders and alcohol and substance abuse (e.g., Laessle *et al.*, 1989; Mitchell *et al.*,1985), as well as increased incidence of substance abuse among relatives (Hudson *et al.*, 1987). High incidence of personality disorders among individuals with bulimia nervosa has also been reported (Johnson *et al.*, 1989; Piran *et al.*, 1988). Perhaps because the age of onset is later than for anorexia nervosa, there has been less conjecturing about the role of family dysfunction in the development of bulimia. There is evidence that premorbid obesity or familial obesity may predispose one to the development of bulimia (Husain and Cantwell, 1991). In their longitudinal study, Marchi and Cohen (1990) found that pica in early childhood was associated with the development of bulimia in adolescence. The authors suggest that pica may be a symptom of a general lack of self-control of eating behaviour. This hypothesis is supported by their finding that picky eating in early childhood was a protective factor against developing bulimic symptoms in adolescence. History of sexual abuse has been implicated as a risk factor for bulimia; however, the evidence suggests that sexual abuse may be a risk for psychiatric disorder in general, but not specifically for bulimia (Pope *et al.*, 1994; Welch and Fairburn, 1994).

Studies comparing purging and nonpurging bulimics consistently suggest that purging defines a more serious form of the disorder. Purging bulimics eat less, report greater anxiety while eating, and show more pathological scores on eating attitudes scales and body image measures than do nonpurging bulimics (Prather and Williamson, 1988; Willmuth *et al.*, 1988).

Obesity

Biological Factors

The cause of obesity is deceptively simple: an energy imbalance due to consuming more calories than are used through exertion. Attempts to determine why this imbalance occurs for some children has led to no easy answers because of the complex interaction of various genetic and environmental influences (Siegel and Smith, 1991).

It has become increasingly clear that heritability is a substantial influence in the development of obesity. Children are more likely to be obese if a parent is obese, and the risk increases if both parents are obese (Epstein, 1986). Twin studies have indicated higher concordance of obesity in monozygotic twins (Foch and McClearn, 1980; Stunkard *et al.*, 1986). In an adoption study, the weight of children adopted as infants was found to be more similar to that of their biological parents than that of their adoptive parents (Stunkard *et al.*, 1986). As compelling as these data are, they do not explain similarities in fatness between unrelated spouses (Garn *et al.*, 1979) or between owners and their dogs (Mason, 1970). Clearly environmental factors also play a major role.

Psychological and Familial Factors

No specific psychopathology has been found to be regularly associated with obesity, so it is not recognized as a psychiatric disorder in DSM-IV (APA, 1994). Obese young people do face discrimination that may lead to psychological or behavioural problems, but these are likely to be the result, rather than a cause, of the obesity (Leon and Dinklage, 1989).

Family environment can potentially influence·the development of obesity in children and adolescents in a number of ways, including determining food availability and modelling attitudes toward food and eating behaviour (Foreyt and Cousins, 1989). Birch (1991) described infants as possibly the only "depletion-driven human eaters; they eat when they are hungry" (p. 265). Birch's research has demonstrated that by the end of the preschool period, children have learned through socialization and feeding practices to focus on external cues in addition to internal hunger states to control food intake. Parents influence their children's food preferences and the amount they consume using various techniques and at times producing paradoxical·results. For example, children learn to dislike foods that their parents reward them for eating (Birch *et al.*, 1984). The "reward" foods tend to be high in fat, salt, or sugar, and they become even more preferred after being used as rewards (Birch *et al.*, 1980). Birch (1991) suggests that feeding practices such as these may lead to development of maladaptive intake patterns.

Similarly, parents influence the level of physical activity in which their children engage (e.g., Klesges *et al.*, 1986). A number of studies have demonstrated that obese individuals engage in fewer physical activities and exert less energy in physical activities relative to peers of normal weight. This relationship between activity and obesity is less clear in children, but there is evidence that physical inactivity rather than excessive calorie intake may be the major determinant of obesity in some individuals (Leon and Dinklage, 1989). Consistent with this hypothesis is the fact that television viewing has been causally linked to obesity in children and adolescents (Dietz and Gortmaker, 1985).

COMORBIDITY

Anorexia Nervosa and Bulimia Nervosa

A variety of concomitant symptoms and comorbid disorders have been reported to occur with anorexia nervosa and bulimia nervosa. Herzog *et al.* (1988) reported that 27 of 33 outcome reports mentioned psychiatric disorders in anorexic patients at follow-up. Overlaps between eating disorders and depression, obsessive-compulsive disorder, substance abuse, and personality disorder have been most clearly documented (Kennedy and Garfinkel, 1992).

In examining the lifetime and current prevalence of psychiatric diagnoses in 62 women, Halmi *et al.* (1991) found significant comorbidity of both affective and anxiety disorders with the diagnosis of anorexia nervosa. Zerbe *et al.*, (1993) found that 73% of inpatients with anorexia nervosa, bulimia nervosa, and other eating disorders displayed Axis I or Axis II comorbidity, including a diagnosis of borderline personality for 46% of the sample and a diagnosis of depression for 45%. Their data suggests that patients presenting with eating disorders are often underdiagnosed, and therefore, undertreated. Similarly, in a study of 229 patients, Herzog *et al.* (1992) reported that 73% of anorexia nervosa, 60% of bulimia nervosa, and 82% of mixed anorexia nervosa/bulimia nervosa patients had a current comorbid DSM-III-R (1987) Axis I disorder, most commonly depression. Bossert-Zaudig and colleagues (1993) looked at psychiatric comorbidity in a sample of 24 women hospitalized with bulimia and found that more than 50% had two or three DSM-III-R (APA, 1987) Axis I disorders in addition to bulimia nervosa, and that almost 50% met criteria for at least one personality disorder.

It has been estimated that 21 to 91% of anorexia nervosa patients have depressive symptoms when they are underweight and malnourished (Eckert *et al.*, 1982; Hendren, 1983), and 15 to 58% of eating disorder patients continue to exhibit depressive symptoms after weight recovery over follow-up durations up to four years (Weltzin *et al.*, 1993).

Among the studies reviewed by Herzog *et al.* (1988) depression was the most common symptom in bulimic patients at follow-up, being reported in 15 to 36% of cases. However, none of the studies made diagnoses on the basis of standardized criteria. Antidepressants have been found to be partially effective in that they reduce binge-eating and purging behaviour and/or alleviate depression (e.g., Kennedy *et al.*, 1986; Lyles *et al.*, 1990), and family studies show a high prevalence of affective disorders in first-degree relatives of eating disorder patients (Biederman *et al.*, 1985; Strober *et al.*, 1990; Weltzin *et al.*, 1993). However, it remains controversial as to whether eating disorders and major depression share a common diathesis (Strober and Katz, 1987; Weltzin *et al.*, 1993).

Anxiety disorders have also been associated with eating disorders. For example, Laessle *et al.* (1989) found that 70% of bulimia nervosa patients had a lifetime diagnosis of anxiety disorders, a figure greater than the lifetime prevalence of depression (56%), whereas Hudson *et al.* (1987) found that bulimia nervosa patients had a 43% lifetime prevalence of anxiety disorders in comparison to a 67% prevalence of depression. Patients with anorexia nervosa have been found to show a high prevalence of obsessive-compulsive symptoms or disorders (e.g., Hudson *et al.*, 1983; Rothenberg, 1988). Conversely, adult women with obsessive-compulsive disorder appear to have an increased likelihood of a history of anorexia nervosa (Kasvikis *et al.*, 1986). In a recent review of research, Hsu *et al.* (1993) affirm the connection between eating disorders and obsessive-compulsive disorder, but note that without a clear understanding of the etiology of either category of disorders, it is difficult to determine whether anorexia nervosa is a variant of obsessive-compulsive disorder (OCD).

Studies of bulimia nervosa patients have shown a high incidence of alcohol abuse or dependency (Hudson *et al.*, 1987; Laessle *et al.*, 1989; Weltzin *et al.*, 1993). Mitchell and colleagues (1985) found that 23% of bulimic women acknowledged a history of alcohol abuse and 18% reported a prior history of treatment for chemical dependency. Moreover, between 33% and 83% of women with bulimia nervosa have at least one close relative with alcoholism (Bulik, 1987; Hudson *et al.*, 1987; Leon *et al.*, 1985; Mitchell *et al.*, 1988). The prevalence of eating disorders among substance abusers also appears to exceed general population norms (estimates range from 15 to 26%), although the basis for the comorbidity and the implications for treatment are uncertain (Hudson *et al.*, 1992; Peveler and Fairburn, 1990). The many clinical similarities that exist between these two groups of disorders do not and cannot prove a common addictive mechanism, but the high comorbidity of substance abuse with eating disorders means that clinicans should routinely screen for both disorders (Katz, 1990; Krahn, 1991).

Personality disorders appear to be quite common in patients with eating disorders. Herzog *et al.* (1992) found that 27% of 210 women seeking treatment for anorexia nervosa, bulimia nervosa, or mixed anorexia nervosa/bulimia nervosa had at least one personality disorder; the most commonly observed disorder was borderline personality disorder in 9% of subjects. The highest prevalence of personality disorders was found in the mixed anorexia nervosa/bulimia nervosa group (39%), followed by anorexia nervosa patients (22%) and bulimia nervosa patients (21%). The anorexia nervosa/bulimia nervosa group also had longer duration of eating disorder illness and much greater comorbid Axis I psychopathology compared with the rest of the sample. Skodol *et al.* (1993) found that bulimia nervosa was most frequently associated with borderline personality disorder and anorexia nervosa with avoidant personality disorder.

Obesity

Comorbidity of psychiatric disorders with obesity has not been a focus of much research and the studies that have been reported focus on obese adults. For example, Berman *et al.* (1992) found a comorbidity rate of 50% for DSM-III-R (APA, 1987) Axis I disorders among 37 moderately to severely obese patients seeking dietary treatment. Affective and personality disorders were most commonly identified. Similarly, Yanovski *et al.* (1993) found that more than 30% of obese women and 25% of obese men met criteria for binge-eating disorder. Moreover, compared to other obese subjects, those with binge-eating disorder also had significantly higher lifetime rates for Axis I and II disorders including depression, panic disorder, bulimia nervosa, borderline personality, and avoidant personality disorder.

COURSE AND OUTCOME

Course

Feeding and Eating Disorders of Infancy or Early Childhood

Pica may have an onset during infancy or the toddler years, remit after only a short duration, or persist sometimes into adulthood (APA, 1994; Kronenberger and Meyer, 1996). However, symptoms associated with pica may diminish over time in adults with mental retardation

(APA, 1994). For rumination disorder, the onset is often between 3 and 12 months of age, or later in individuals with mental retardation (APA, 1994; Kronenberger and Meyer, 1996). Although spontaneous remissions do occur with some infants and children merely outgrowing these disorders, medical complications can occur for each and can lead to variations in the outcome. For pica, negative outcomes may include choking from ingesting small objects (Kalfus *et al.*, 1988), lead poisoning, intestinal obstructions or perforations, infections, or death depending on the type and amount of substance ingested (Benoit, 1993). For rumination disorder, negative outcomes that can also result in death depending on problem severity include malnourishment with weight loss or a failure to gain weight (APA, 1994; Kronenberger and Meyer, 1996).

As for older age groups in which malnutrition occurs as a result of restricted food intake, NOFT can lead to a variety of medical complications or death. In their review of the literature, Powell and Bettes (1992) suggest that abnormal behaviours occur in NOFT infants and these include motor inactivity, lack of social smiles, abnormal gazes, poss- ible rumination, and a preoccupation with hand/finger activity and thumbsucking. These abnormal behaviours may persist even after some catch-up growth once proper nutrition has been restored. In a sample including both organic and nonorganic failure-to-thrive infants, Singer *et al.* (1990) found that these infants were likely to have feeding problems and to vomit, gag, or refuse food.

The long term negative outcome of NOFT appears to be pervasive. The available evidence suggests that as a group, infants and children with histories of organic or nonorganic forms of failure-to-thrive have poorer developmental outcomes and are delayed or impaired in terms of their physical, cognitive, emotional, and social development (e.g., Heffer and Kelley, 1994). Drotar and colleagues (1985) found that cognitive development at 18 months in infants with a history of failure-to-thrive was predicted by the interaction of biological factors, such as physical status at intake, and family resources (e.g., income and ratio of adults to children); thus, children with a better nutritional status and greater family resources had the potential for a better psychological outcome. Abramson (1991) and Polan *et al.* (1991) found evidence for disturbances in affect expression in infants and young children with histories of failure-to-thrive; in both studies, target infants were found to display more negative affect than control children. Abramson (1991) suggests that such negative affect displays may serve an adaptive function by signalling to others the infant's internal state.

Also of significance for the social and emotional functioning of children with NOFT are the disturbances in the parent-child relationship.
For example, one month post hospitalization, Drotar *et al.* (1990)
conducted home observations of mothers and their NOFT infants and
compared the observations to those for a matched group of control participants. They found more arbitrary termination of feeding and less
adaptive and less positive social-emotional interactions in the NOFT
participants as compared to the control participants.

Parental social cognition may be an additional contributing factor
related to outcome although further research is needed to substantiate
this possibility (Boddy and Skuse, 1994). Ayoub and Milner (1985) found
that parental awareness of the interactional nature of NOFT and their
cooperation in responding to instruction was related to a more positive
outcome resulting in increased infant weight. In contrast, parental denial
of the interactional nature of the disorder was related to more negative
infant outcomes. The course and outcome of NOFT may well depend
upon such parental attributions and social cognition, although the
potential processes leading to parental behaviours are as yet poorly
understood (Boddy and Skuse, 1994).

Anorexia Nervosa and Bulimia Nervosa

Onset of anorexia nervosa is typically in adolescence although it can
develop during adulthood (e.g., Bowler, 1992; Fornari *et al.*, 1994) or
before menarche (e.g., Bryant-Waugh and Lask, 1995). The age of risk
for onset of bulimia nervosa appears to be shorter than for anorexia
nervosa (Woodside and Garfinkel, 1992). Moreover, bulimia nervosa
tends to affect somewhat older individuals than anorexia nervosa
(Fairburn and Beglin, 1990) although onset of bulimia before menarche
has also been reported (Kent *et al.*, 1992). Anorexia nervosa and bulimia
nervosa are often unremitting, even after "successful" treatment. Husain
and Cantwell (1991) note that although milder cases may remit spontaneously without treatment or patients may recover completely after a
single episode, most patients require a variety of treatments for full
recovery, and more stubborn cases may follow a course of periodic
remission followed by relapse, or a gradually deteriorating course resulting in death.

Follow-up studies of both anorexia nervosa and bulimia nervosa
have shown that the disorders may cross over during the course of
illness (Kennedy and Garfinkel, 1992). However, the onset of anorexia

nervosa and bulimia nervosa symptoms appears to be independent, despite their frequent coexistence in the same person (Woodside and Garfinkel, 1992). Kennedy and Garfinkel (1992) estimate that 30 to 50% of anorexia nervosa patients have symptoms of bulimia nervosa; usually the bulimia symptoms occur within a year and a half after the onset of anorexia; sometimes the bulimic symptoms precede the onset of anorexia nervosa. Bulimia nervosa typically lasts for several years and the course of the illness is most often intermittent, with binges and fasting alternating with periods of normal eating; in extreme cases there may never be periods of normal eating.

Bulimia, unlike anorexia, is characterized by severe episodes of guilt and shame following binges, which are ego-dystonic and perceived as abnormal. For this reason, bulimics may be very secretive about their abnormal eating pattern and the illness may go undetected for years. Fairburn and Cooper (1982) suggest that the typical duration of bulimia nervosa prior to treatment is at least five years.

Outcome

Anorexia Nervosa and Bulimia Nervosa

Anorexia nervosa is one of the few psychiatric disorders of childhood and adolescence that shows an appreciable mortality rate. In their review of outcome studies, Herzog *et al.* (1988) found mortality rates ranging from 0 to 22% with over half of the studies they reviewed reporting rates of 4% or less over follow-up periods ranging from four months to 3 years. Of reported deaths, the cause was anorexia nervosa or its medical complications in 50% of cases, suicide in 24%, and other causes (diseases, accidents, unknown) in the remaining cases. Although bulimia is not typically viewed as life-threatening, deaths can occur. Indeed, Norring and Sohlberg (1993) suggest that the risk for premature death may be twice as high among bulimic patients as among restricting patients due to the severity of electrolyte imbalances that are associated with chronic purging. In general, the prognosis is better for restricting or non-binge-eating anorexics than it is for those anorexics who binge/purge (Foreyt and McGavin, 1989).

Over the long term, many eating disorder patients do poorly despite treatment. In a review of follow-up studies, Eckert (1985) noted that a high proportion of anorexic patients continued to have body weight below 75% of normal and to engage in abnormal eating practices, such as extensive dieting and avoidance of high-calorie food, often for many years after treatment. Vomiting, laxative abuse, and psychological diffi-culties, most notably depression and social phobias, were also common in treated anorexics. At six-year follow-up of 51 cases of anorexia nervosa, Gillberg *et al.* (1994) found a recovery rate of 47%. Although there were no deaths among the cases they followed, outcomes were poor to very poor in unrecovered patients. In a follow-up study of 50 German adolescents after a mean 58 months, Steinhausen and Seidel (1993) found that 68% had recovered, 10% still suffered from anorexia nervosa, 4% suffered from anorexia nervosa with bulimia, 14% still had partial syndromes of anorexia nervosa, and 4% had partial syndromes of bulimia nervosa. Herzog *et al.* (1993) assessed the course and outcome of anorexia nervosa and bulimia nervosa in 225 females with an eating disorder. They found that the recovery rate among bulimics was significantly better than the recovery rate of individuals with anorexia nervosa or mixed anorexia nervosa/bulimia nervosa diagnoses. Fallon and colleagues (1991) studied 46 women with bulimia nervosa 2–9 years after hospitalization; 39% had fully recovered, 20% had par-tially recovered, and 41% were currently bulimic.

Early outcome studies of anorexia nervosa suggested that younger age at onset was associated with a more favourable prognosis (e.g., Crisp *et al.*, 1977; Halmi *et al.*, 1975; Morgan and Russell, 1975). However more recent reports suggest that the long-term prognosis in early-onset eating disorders is poor (e.g., Bryant-Waugh *et al.*, 1988; Heebink *et al.*, 1995; Lask and Bryant-Waugh, 1992; Walford and McCune, 1991). Other variables that are consistently associated with poorer long-term outcome in anorexia nervosa are lower ideal body weight and mixed anorexia nervosa/bulimia nervosa symptoms (Herzog *et al.*, 1993). In bulimia, indicators of poor prognosis include duration of illness, positive family history of alcoholism and depression (Hsu and Holder, 1986), and higher frequency of binge eating and vomiting (Mitchell *et al.*, 1989). Root (1990) asked 21 women who had met criteria for bulimia nervosa to complete a variety of outcome measures and to endorse different defi-nitions of recovery. The majority of subjects endorsed the definition "I am recovered but still struggle with food, weight, and/or body image."

As Herzog *et al.* (1988) note, there are significant problems in assessing outcome across studies given the variability in research methodologies and study designs. Overly optimistic claims of success may be due to inadequate follow-up of patients (Vandereycken and Pierloot, 1983) or to the lack of standardisation in clinical definitions of recovery and relapse (Herzog *et al.*, 1991). Herzog *et al.* (1991) suggest that the persistent subclinical disturbances in attitudes toward food and body image following treatment may mean that alternative models for the course of eating disorders are needed. Specifically, they suggest that relapse should be defined as a resumption of symptoms during the vulnerable period immediately following remission, whereas recurrence should be defined as the appearance of a separate new episode subsequent to a low risk refractory period.

Obesity

Although empirical studies of forced infant feeding or overfeeding are sparse, such studies may be useful in better understanding the development of some forms of obesity (Benoit, 1993). The research literature suggests that children and adolescents are unlikely to "outgrow" obesity; the average obese child is likely to become an overweight adult (Foreyt and Cousins, 1989; Stark *et al.*, 1981). However, age at onset and the severity of childhood obesity are linked with the persistence of obesity into adulthood (Dietz, 1987). Interestingly, longitudinal studies suggest that infants who experience rapid weight gain during the first year of life do not necessarily experience later obesity (LeBow, 1984). However, when the obesity persists into middle and late childhood, it tends to persist into adolescence and adulthood (Foreyt and Cousins, 1989). Obese children and adolescents are thus at significant risk for physical problems, especially elevated levels of cholesterol, high blood pressure, and cardiovascular disease (Siegel and Smith, 1991; Stark *et al.*, 1981). Although there are positive reports concerning treatment efficacy and long-term outcome of childhood weight loss programs (Epstein *et al.*, 1994; Wilson, 1994), the question of whether treatment of childhood obesity contributes to later development of another eating disorder is unresolved (Wilson, 1994).

Relapse

Anorexia Nervosa and Bulimia Nervosa

Both anorexia nervosa and bulimia nervosa have a high rate of post-treatment relapse (Kennedy and Garfinkel, 1992). Norring and Sohlberg (1993) found a posttreatment relapse rate of 48% in a six-year follow-up study of 30 eating disorder patients with mixed diagnoses. Olmsted *et al.* (1994) reported a post-treatment relapse rate of 31% in a sample of 48 women with bulimia nervosa over a two year follow-up; most relapses occurred in the first six months following treatment. Variables predicting relapse have been assessed in a number of studies. For example, Fallon *et al.* (1991) found that likelihood of recovery increased with length of time since discharge from hospital. However, global functioning before hospitalization, lifetime DSM-III-R (APA, 1987) Axis I diagnoses and current Axis II diagnoses were not associated with outcome. Root (1990) found that elevated scores on the Eating Disorder Inventory were correlated with feeling an increased likelihood of relapse among 21 women recovering from bulimia nervosa. Olmsted *et al.* (1994) found that the strongest predictors of relapse were younger age, higher vomiting frequency, and a higher score on the bulimia sub-scale of the 26-item Eating Attitudes Test prior to treatment, and higher vomiting frequency and a higher score on the interpersonal distrust sub-scale of the Eating Disorder Inventory at the end of treatment.

Psychosocial Impairment

Anorexia Nervosa and Bulimia Nervosa

As Hsu (1990) and Husain and Cantwell (1991) note, follow-up studies show that weight loss and a persistent obsession with food dominate the clinical picture in chronic cases of anorexia nervosa and bulimia nervosa. Moreover, even in cases in which reasonable weight is achieved and maintained, long-term prognosis in terms of personality changes and social adjustment is often less promising. Although the normalization of weight is important in evaluating treatment outcome, it is also critical to assess a range of intra- and inter-personal variables since many patients exhibit significant depression, anxiety, poor sexual adjustment, academic underachievement, and impairment in self-image and social relationships at follow-up (Gillberg *et al.*, 1994; Phelps and Bajorek, 1991; Steiger *et al.*, 1992; Steinhausen and Vollrath, 1993). Ineffective coping strategies (e.g., avoidance, wishful thinking, self-blame, reluctance to seek social support) are common in patients with anorexia nervosa and bulimia nervosa (Soukup *et al.*, 1990; Troop *et al.*, 1994). Additionally, for individuals with bulimia nervosa, costly binge-purges can take up so many of their hours that social activities are restricted and financial resources squandered. In a study of 275 bulimics, Mitchell *et al.* (1985) found that 70% experienced difficulties with intimate or interpersonal relations, 53% reported family problems, and 50% had work impairment.

Obesity

Compared to their nonobese peers, obese children and adolescents worry significantly more about weight and body physique (Wadden *et al.*, 1991), are more vulnerable to disparagement and potential rejection by peers (DeJong, 1993; LeBow *et al.*, 1989; Sigelman, 1991), report more shyness (Page, 1991), and exhibit reduced academic achievement (e.g., Morrill *et al.*, 1991). Unfortunately, it appears that such psychosocial difficulties may also carry over into adulthood. Thus, individuals who are overweight as adolescents are likely to complete fewer years of school, less likely to marry, and more likely to have lower household incomes than individuals who are not obese during adolescence (Gortmaker *et al.*, 1993). Girls with high relative weights are more likely to be identified as overweight than boys with high relative weights (White *et al.*, 1991) and it appears that the long term consequences of early obesity may be more negative for girls (e.g., Gortmaker *et al.*, 1993).

Health Services Utilization

Anorexia Nervosa

Patients with anorexia nervosa tend to be more resistant to treatment than those with bulimia nervosa and the most important goal in treating such resistant patients is to keep them alive and relatively free from medical risk through the establishment of guidelines concerning weight, vital signs, and hospitalization (Hamburg *et al.*, 1989). This is especially crucial in children since self-starvation may affect growth (Hodes, 1993). Initially, in the treatment of anorexia nervosa, the goal is to restore the patient's nutritional state, since dehydration, starvation, and electrolyte imbalances can lead to serious health compromises, even death. The decision to hospitalize is based on the patient's medical condition and the degree of structure needed to ensure patient cooperation. According to Hamburg *et al.* (1989), anorexia nervosa patients who are 20% below their expected weight for height are typically recommended for inpatient programs, and patients who are 30% below expected weight require psychiatric hospitalization that ranges from two to six months. The short term response of patients to almost all hospital treatment programs is good.

Day hospital and other outpatient clinic treatment programs have become increasingly important in the treatment of eating disorders and there is some evidence suggesting that outpatients and inpatients may present for treatment with similar levels of psychopathology. Kennedy and Garfinkel (1989) compared psychopathologies of 85 female inpatients diagnosed with DSM-III-R (APA, 1987) eating disorders with those of 397 outpatients. Inpatients with anorexia nervosa who were admitted because of the severity of their symptoms did not differ significantly from anorexia nervosa outpatients on measures of eating disorder, age, duration of illness, or weight. However, bulimia nervosa inpatients showed more generalized psychopathology than bulimia nervosa outpatients with respect to those same variables.

Obesity

Parents with obese children or adolescents are most likely to consult their pediatricians about the problem. Unfortunately, although pediatricians are likely to inform parents of obese children about the health risks of obesity, they may not be the best resource for counselling and treatment. In a survey of pediatricians, Price *et al.* (1989) found that only 22% felt competent to prescribe weight-loss programs for children and even fewer found weight loss counselling to be professionally rewarding.

Assessment

Feeding and Eating Disorders of Infancy and Early Childhood

The following assessment recommendations are obtained from Kronenberger and Meyer's (1996) review of feeding disorders (pp. 302–319). Because cognitive impairment may either be the cause or the result of pica and rumination disorder and developmental delays may result from the malnutrition of NOFT, the assessment of these disorders should include standardized tests of intelligence (e.g., Bayley II or Wechsler scale) and adaptive behaviour (e.g., Vineland Adaptive Scales). In addition to parents' report of symptoms from the clinical interview or from a child behaviour checklist, a behavioural assessment is needed in which attention is given to the antecedents and consequences of the target behaviours. For rumination disorder, the observation of feeding interactions by a trained clinician may help to confirm that the diagnostic criteria are met and assist in determining whether or not an impaired mother–child interaction is contributing to the problem.

Egan *et al.* (1988) similarly recommend that assessment should include parental interviews as well as direct videotaped observations of the primary caregiver during meal time and play time with the infant; furthermore, such taped observations should be made repeatedly throughout treatment and used to monitor progress. Accurate assessment must also be conducted to determine the child's rate of weight gain, and weight and height relative to others of the same age (Schmitt and Mauro, 1989). Because certain personality characteristics (e.g., defensiveness, denial, depression) and a lack of marital or family social support have been found in mothers of NOFT infants, measures such as the MMPI-2 have been recommended as part of the assessment battery for this disorder (Kronenberger and Meyer, 1996). In addition, given that some children with Feeding Disorder of Infancy also develop Reactive Attachment Disorder, Kronenberger and Meyer (1996) recommend that children with Feeding Disorder of Infancy be routinely also evaluated for Reactive Attachment Disorder.

Anorexia Nervosa and Bulimia Nervosa

Weltzin *et al.* (1993) state that the assessment of eating disorders "… should include a complete history of weight, eating behavior, psychological functioning (including perceptions of weight and shape, depression, and anxiety), a complete medical history and examination, and family and developmental history" (p .220). Such a comprehensive assessment strategy also includes assessing: the person's weight at important intervals in the past (e.g., puberty, at onset of eating disordered behaviour), dieting behaviours, daily caloric intake, menstrual and sexual history, social and cognitive skills and history, prior efforts at medical or psychological treatment, family history in the form of a genogram, and a full physical and neurological examination (Weltzin *et al.*, 1993). Knibbs (1993) further suggests that the optimal form of behavioural assessment would involve direct videotaped observations of the target behaviours in the home setting.

While the clinical interview remains an important means of gathering much of the above information and structured interviews are available, there are also a number of psychological tests useful in the assessment of eating disorders. Some tests, such as the Eating Disorders Inventory (EDI; Garner *et al.*, 1983), Eating Attitudes Test (EAT; Garner and Garfinkel, 1979), or the Minnesota Multiphasic Personality Inventory (MMPI-2/MMPI-A) can be used in the assessment of either disorder

(Kronenberger and Meyer, 1996) (Table 10.4). While the EDI and EAT measures are typically used with adolescents and adults, The Kids' Eating Disorders Survey (KEDS) has been used to screen for anorexia nervosa and bulimia nervosa symptoms in children enrolled in grades 5 through 8 (Childress *et al.*, 1993). Childress *et al.* (1993) conducted follow-up interviews on children whose self-report on the KEDS suggested the possibility of an eating disorder; to further refine the diagnostic symptoms, they used DSM-III-R criteria for the interviews and the Eating Disorders module of the Diagnostic Interview Schedule for Children-Child Version (DISC-2.1C) developed by Shaffer *et al.* (1989; cited in Childress *et al.*, 1993) (Table 10.5).

Assessment of cognitive and achievement skills (e.g., WISC-III/ WIAT) affords an opportunity to observe for behavioural characteristics associated with anorexia nervosa, such as perfectionistic tendencies. There is evidence that individuals with anorexia nervosa tend to score in the High Average range, have higher Verbal than Performance scale scores, and to meet or exceed expected scores on achievement tests (Kronenberger and Meyer, 1996); however, there is disagreement as to whether such a pattern has been conclusively demonstrated (c.f., Fombonne, 1995). No specific pattern has been reported for the intellectual or achievement functioning of individuals with bulimia nervosa.

Corcoran and Fischer (1987) have reproduced the following measures for the assessment of eating disorders and have provided a review of the purpose and psychometric properties of these measures. The Bulimia Test (BULIT) was devised specifically to measure the various symptoms of bulimia using DSM-III criteria (Smith and Thelen, 1984). Other measures have been created to address efforts at controlling weight and diet. These include: the Restraint Scale (RS) to measure efforts made to control eating (Herman, 1978); the Compulsive Eating Scale (CES) and the Concern over Weight and Dieting Scale (COWD) to measure uncontrolled eating behaviours and compensatory dieting behaviours (Kagan and Squires, 1984); the Goldfarb Fear of Fat Scale (GFFS) to measure the fear of gaining weight (Goldfarb *et al.*, 1985); the Hunger-Satiety Scales (H-SS) to measure internal sensations of hunger and feeling full in individuals with anorexia nervosa (Garfinkel, 1974), and the Internal versus External Locus of Control of Weight Scale (IECW) to measure locus of control as applied to weight management efforts (Tobias and MacDonald, 1977).

Additional measures focus on body image. Knibbs (1993) cites Williamson (1990) as reviewing a number of body-image assessment

Table 10.4 Examples of questions to assess symptoms of eating disorders from selected self-report questionnaires

Instruments	Questions / Items	Rating Options		
Kids' Eating Disorders Survey (Childress *et al.*, 1993)	Have you ever thought that you looked fat to other people? Have you ever made yourself throw up (vomit) to lose weight? Have you ever taken laxatives to lose weight?	Yes	No	?
Compulsive Eating Scale (CES) (Kagan and Squires, 1984)	Feels completely out of control when it comes to food Eat so much food so fast that you don't know how much you ate or how it tasted Get out of bed at night, go into the kitchen, and finish the remains of some delicious food, because you knew it was there	"never" to "more than once a week"		
Eating Attitudes Test (EAT) (Garner and Garfinkel, 1979)	Find myself preoccupied with food Am preoccupied with the thought of having fat on my body Feel that food controls my life	"always" to "never"		
Bulimia Test (Smith and Thelen, 1984)	Do you ever eat to the point of feeling sick? How often do you intentionally vomit after eating? I have tried to lose weight by fasting or going on "crash"diets	varies for different questions		
Concern over Weight and Dieting Scale (Kagan and Squires, 1984)	How often do you skip one meal so you will lose weight? How often do you hate yourself or feel guilty because you cannot stop overeating? How often do you go without eating solid food for 24 hours or more so you will lose weight?	varies for different questions		

Table 10.5 Examples of questions to assess eating disorders from selected diagnostic interviews

Instruments	Examples of questions	Rating options			
		0	1	2	9
DISC (Costello *et al.*, 1984)	In the past 6 months, have you worried about being fat or becoming fat?	0	1	2	9
	IF YES, A. Would you say that you worry about this too much?	0	[1]	[2]	9
	B. How often have you worried about this? Would you say: Every day ... several times a week ... at least once a week ... or at least once a month?				
	Every day 5				
	4–6 days a week 4				
	1–3 days a week 3				
	1–3 days a month 2				
	Less than once a month 1				
	Don't know 9				
	Have you gone on eating binges, when you ate a whole lot of food in a very short time ... like a whole cake or two quarts of ice cream, or much more than you would usually eat?				
	IF YES, A. In the last 6 months, was there ever a period when you had an eating binge like that at least once a week?	0		[2]	9
	IF YES, B. How about twice a week?	0		2	9
	IF YES, C. Did you go on eating binges twice a week or more for as long as three months in a row?			2	9
	D. When you thought about bingeing, about a lot of food, was it something you couldn't stop thinking about, that you just couldn't put out of your head?	0	1	2	9

Note: DISC: 0 = no, 1 = sometimes/somewhat, 2 = yes, 9 = don't know

Table 10.5 *continued*

Instruments	Examples of questions	Rating options
K-SADS (Puig-Antich and Chambers, 1978)	Do you follow a diet in order to lose weight? How strict is it? What is your method of dieting? Do you use appetite suppressant pills? Which ones? Do you sometimes make yourself throw up? Have you had periods of at least 1 week during which you have eaten nothing but clear fluids (tea, coffee, water)? Or just diet drinks? Do you take laxatives to lose weight? Do you take water pills to lose weight (NOT JUST BEFORE MENSES) Do you exercise a lot to stay slim and in order to lose weight? How much? How many hours per day?	0 = no information; 1 = no; 2 = occasionally; 3 = sometimes; 4 = most of time *Manifestations include:* Use of specific appetite suppressants; Frequent, prolonged strict dietary restrictions; Absolute refusal to ingest other than clear, non-nutritive fluids; Self-induced vomiting; Abuse of laxatives; Extensive physical exercise
	Do you have "eating attacks" or binges? What happened? What triggers a binge? How does it end? What is the most food you have eaten during a binge? How often does it happen? Does your weight go up and down because of binges? By how much? Do you diet? What do you do? How do you feel after a binge? Happy, sad, sick, tired? Do you think this eating pattern is OK? Can you control it?	0 = no information; 1 = no; 2 = occasionally; 3 = sometimes; 4 = most of the time *Manifestations include:* Easily ingested, high caloric food; Hiding during binge; Binge ended by either abdominal pain, sleep, social interruption, induced vomiting; Weight fluctuates by 10 lbs. by binges and fasts; Feels lack of control over binging; Feels depressed following binging; Binges >/ 2 times/week for >/ 3 months

instruments. Two techniques that appear popular in the literature are attitudinal measures in which body size dissatisfaction is assessed, such as in the EDI; and the use of a series of silhouettes varying in size in which both actual and ideal body size and shape are assessed (e.g., Childress *et al.*, 1993).

TREATMENT PLANNING

In developing treatment plans for those with an identified eating disorder, a thorough assessment is an important first step to specify individual assets as well as specific problems psychologically, physically, socially, and systemically at the level of the family, neighbourhood/community, and society/culture (e.g., Looney, 1984). Assets in addition to problems are identified since personal assets, tangible resources, and areas of intact functioning can be utilized in treating the target problems. The problem common to the feeding and eating disorders addressed above is a disturbance in the child's ability to assimilate food and regulate physical activity in a manner that leads to adaptive, age-appropriate physical functioning (e.g., growth, menses). Thus, the common treatment goal underlying the disorders addressed in this chapter is to initiate or restore — and then most importantly maintain — appropriate food intake and regulation of physical functioning.

A comprehensive approach is considered necessary to manage the medical and psychological treatment and to prevent complications (e.g., Lask and Bryant-Waugh, 1993). Treatment approaches for anorexia nervosa, bulimia nervosa, and obesity include medical interventions, individual psychotherapy, family therapy, group therapy, or some combination of the above (e.g., Foreyt and Cousins, 1989; Foreyt and McGavin, 1989). Evidence for the efficacy of these approaches and various specific treatment techniques will be addressed separately below for anorexia nervosa, bulimia nervosa, and obesity.

Anorexia Nervosa and Bulimia Nervosa. Martin (1990) suggests that a systems model approach may be useful in conceptualizing case-specific interventions for anorexia nervosa, since it incorporates interactions between social, familial, intrapsychic, and physiological levels. Treatment of bulimia nervosa, like that of anorexia nervosa, involves a multicomponent, multidisciplinary approach consisting of medical as well as psychological interventions. A multidimensional assessment includes consideration of multiple biological factors (e.g., presence of a major affective disorder), family processes (e.g., communication, conflict), sociocultural demands (e.g., high achievement needs), and personality characteristics (e.g., low self-esteem); it is also important to conduct a macroanalysis of major life periods related to binge-purge behaviour, a microanalysis of daily binge-purging behaviour, and to note the contexts in which the bulimic behaviour occurs (Johnson and Pure, 1986).

Obesity. Epstein (1986) describes the goals of treating obese children as two-fold: to reduce weight until it is within 20% of what is average for the child's age and height, and to teach the child appropriate eating and exercise habits to maintain optimal growth and development. He proposes a four stage model based on the child's age: (i) for ages 1 to 5 years, parent management is the focus of treatment; (ii) for ages 5 to 8 years, parent management is still crucial since self-regulatory capabilities are still developing, but the child must also be taught ways to handle social situations involving food (e.g., at school); (iii) for ages 8 to 12 years, children can begin to take greater responsibility for their weight management by setting goals and self-monitoring although parental management is still important; and (iv) for adolescents 13 years and over who are motivated and possess the ability to manage their own program, parental support rather than management is an important treatment component.

Excess weight and body fat in childhood and adolescence, as reviewed earlier, may have an etiological basis involving genetic/biological factors and/or overeating due to environmental factors. Once a physical examination has ruled out a medical condition as the sole cause, weight management may become the focus of treatment. Foreyt and Cousins (1989) recommend utilizing multiple measures of body fat to increase measurement reliability and judgements as to whether or not the amount of body fat is excessive; such methods include densiometry (displacement when immersed in water), skinfold measurement, and measures of weight (absolute, relative, percent overweight, and the body mass index). In addition to targeting age-appropriate dietary changes involving both the quality and quantity of calories consumed, emphasis has also been placed on encouraging more exercise and physical activity in the daily lives of obese children (Foreyt and Cousins, 1989). Continued monitoring of excess weight and body fat and medical follow-up are important adjuncts to the weight management of obese children.

Pharmacotherapy

Anorexia Nervosa

The malnourishment associated with anorexia nervosa may lead to hormonal, neurotransmitter, and mood imbalances (Weltzin *et al.*, 1993). Restoring proper nutrition may thus require hospitalization where refeeding by oral, naso-gastric, or intravenous methods occurs to rehydrate, reverse electrolyte imbalance, remedy nutritional deficiencies, and promote weight gain (Lask and Fosson, 1993).

A variety of medications (antianxiety, antidepressants, appetite stimulants, neuroleptics) and vitamin/mineral supplements have been attempted in the treatment of anorexia nervosa. There is currently no firm evidence for the utility of these medications and supplements, with the possible exception of some antidepressants which are sometimes recommended if the adolescent also meets the criteria for major depression and has attained a normal weight after refeeding (see Andersen, 1986; Foreyt and McGavin, 1989; Lask and Fosson, 1993; Wells and Logan, 1987). The antidepressant fluoxetine may be particularly helpful in treating some individuals with the restricting subtype of anorexia nervosa; however, the currently available evidence is inconclusive and in need of double-blind placebo-controlled clinical research trials (Weltzin *et al.*, 1993). While zinc deficiency is a known concomitant of childhood-onset anorexia nervosa, zinc supplementation itself does not appear to be effective as a treatment. Furthermore, normal levels of zinc appear to be restored once the child's nutritional state has been improved (Lask *et al.*, 1993).

It is often recommended that the medical management of this disorder be accompanied by individual, family, and group treatments even though the relative efficacy of these approaches is yet to be determined as well (Foreyt and McGavin, 1989).

Bulimia Nervosa

To address dental and metabolic complications that may arise from repeated purgings (e.g., Mitchell, 1991), dental and medical assessment and follow-up are important adjuncts to psychotherapeutic and possible pharmacological treatment of bulimia nervosa.

Pharmacological treatments include anticonvulsants and antidepressants. Anticonvulsant medication may improve the functioning of those bulimics who are thought to have a neurological etiological basis for their disorder (e.g., McDaniel, 1986; Wells and Logan, 1987; Wilson, 1986). Some evidence now exists for the potential effectiveness of various antidepressants in reducing binge-eating, vomiting, and affective symptoms in some patients with bulimia nervosa (e.g., Ambrosini *et al.*, 1993; Wells and Logan, 1987; Weltzin *et al.*, 1993). In a study conducted by Goldbloom and Olmsted (1993), the antidepressant fluoxetine has been shown to be effective in producing clinically significant changes in behaviour and attitude in young adult women with bulimia nervosa; however, it is important to note that while no explicit form of psychotherapy was given to patients in this study, medical follow-up in the form of pharmacotherapy sessions was given, patients repeatedly completed self-report measures, and patients engaged in self-monitoring of their symptoms. This latter technique is a well-known specific component of the cognitive-behavioural therapy approach. The authors compared their results to intensive day treatment and brief psychoeducational group treatment and concluded nonetheless that their results were at least comparable in producing clinically significant change.

The comorbidity of depressive and bulimic symptoms have led some researchers to consider the potential seasonality of the disorder and the use of light therapy (Lam *et al.*, 1994). In the first reported controlled study of light therapy on patients with bulimia nervosa, Lam *et al.* (1994) found support for the efficacy of bright white light over baseline and over a dim red light condition for all mood and eating outcome measures; more improvement occurred for those participants with a seasonal bulimia than those with a nonseasonal bulimia pattern.

Psychological Interventions

Feeding and Eating Disorders of Infancy and Early Childhood

An important consideration in the treatment plan of pica is the correction of medical or surgical complications (Benoit, 1993). Since pica is often viewed as a learned behaviour, various behavioural modification programs have been devised for the treatment of individual cases. Kalfus *et al.* (1988) have successfully used such behavioural techniques as overcorrection, discrimination training, differential reinforcement, positive reinforcement, and time-outs in their treatment approach. Johnson *et al.* (1994) used face washing as a mild punishment for pica along with discrimination training to encourage the ability to distinquish appropriate from inappropriate edibles as generalized to several settings. To reduce pica behaviours, Duker and Nielen (1993) used negative prac-tice (repeated performances of pica behaviours such as biting and chewing of objects) as a punisher. In addition to medical evaluation or hospitalization and behavioural interventions such as those mentioned above, nutritional education, play therapy, and family therapy have been proposed as treatments (Kronenberger and Meyer, 1996).

For rumination disorder, attempted treatment methods have included the use of medication, mechanical devices, surgery, aversive behavioural techniques such as shocks or bitter tasting substances, or nonaversive techniques such as the use of attention or food (Benoit, 1993). Behavioural interventions include overcorrection, extinction, reinforcement of incompatible behaviours, and satiation techniques whereby the patient is fed large quantities of food. Family interventions to enhance parent-child interaction and the marital relationship have also been proposed (Kronenberger and Meyer, 1996).

Kronenberger and Meyer (1996) provide the following general overview of treatment options for feeding disorder of infancy. A medical evaluation to check for organic contributors to the problem must be con-ducted with possible hospitalization to restore weight gain. In some cases, home visits to monitor feeding behaviours are sufficient, but in other cases protective removal from the home is necessary. Therapies to alter feeding behaviours and the mother-infant interaction include both behavioural and family interventions. An interdisciplinary approach is important (Heffer and Kelley, 1994), and interventions must focus on addressing the needs of the infant, altering the behaviours of the primary caregiver(s), and altering certain stressful aspects of the environment (Powell and Bettes, 1992). Supportive services are an important adjunct if the mother lacks resources or is depressed; such services might also include parent education about normal child development and ways to structure healthy meal times (Egan *et al.*, 1988).

Some specific treatment approaches to NOFT have been attempted. Ayoub and Milner (1985) describe their three phase treatment program for infants hospitalized for NOFT. In Phase I, parents were interviewed to gather psychosocial and feeding history information and to begin parent counselling during regular hospital visits. Efforts were also made to substantiate the diagnosis based on the history, pediatric exams, infant weight gain during early hospitalization, and observations of feeding behaviours. During Phase II, parent and child were reunited during mealtimes with the focus of intervention on changing the nature of the feeding interaction. In Phase III, treatment continued on a long-term outpatient follow-up basis until catch-up growth occurred and feeding and eating patterns appeared stable; the average length of time for follow-up was two years. In their study of developmental outcome in infants with failure-to-thrive, Drotar *et al.* (1985) randomly assigned families post-hospitalization to outpatient family home interventions which varied in frequency of contact and approach (family-focussed or focussed on parent education).

Wittenberg (1990) suggests that although such early intervention for NOFT is costly due to its comprehensive and multidisciplinary nature, it is nonetheless less expensive than treatment later for the variety of problems that would persist or result otherwise. Some investigators have found it helpful to consider these various environmental and biological problems along a continuum (Benoit, 1993) or in the form of primary and secondary influences or effects (Wittenberg, 1990).

Anorexia Nervosa

Individual Psychotherapy

Early psychoanalytic approaches (1940s and 1950s) viewed anorexia nervosa as a form of conversion hysteria in which the patient symbolically expressed sexual conflict involving oral impregnation (Bruch, 1986). Bruch's (1986) own observations led her by the 1960s to conclude that developmental deficits — not sexual conflicts — were primary in this disorder. Body image distortion, disturbance in the ability to interpret hunger and appetite cues within the body, and a pervasive sense of ineffectiveness were seen as the main problems to be addressed in treatment. She considered the therapist's role as one of supportive, non-judgmental encouragement toward greater autonomy while simultaneously improving food intake and weight gain. To Bruch, the anorexic's control over her body gave her a "sense of identity or selfhood" and helped her to feel unique and special. The therapeutic task was to affirm the patient's abilities, bring them into awareness, and encourage more autonomous functioning. Although it is clear that Bruch's conceptualizations have had a wide impact on the study and treatment of anorexia nervosa, Gardner (1992) notes one possible limitation of the psychoanalytic approach; that is, gaining insight does not necessarily lead to behavioural change in food intake.

In contrast, some individual behavioural and cognitive behavioural techniques have been shown to be effective in producing weight gain and in changing eating behaviours. Siegel and Smith (1991) suggest that reinforcing food consumption immediately may be more appropriate for younger children than for adolescents (who may purge in some way at a later time); since reinforcement need not be immediate in adolescents, it is considered better to reinforce them for weight gain rather than for food consumption. They review studies using the following behavioural techniques to promote or maintain weight gain: (1) reinforcing lower frequency behaviours (weight gain as the result of increased caloric intake) with higher frequency behaviours (physical activity); (2) systematic desensitization to reduce fears of specific foods, weight gain, and social disapproval of appearance; and (3) self-monitoring of calories, number of mouthfuls of food eaten, and daily weight.

Family Therapy

Evidence has started to accumulate suggesting that family therapy or parent counselling are necessary adjuncts in treating anorexia nervosa (e.g., Lask, 1993) and in maintaining the gains made in behavioural treatments (see Siegel and Smith, 1991). In the first controlled study comparing individual and family treatment, Russell *et al.* (1987) found that female patients under the age of 19 whose illness was not chronic had markedly better outcomes with family therapy, while older patients had marginally better outcomes with individual supportive therapy. Thus, family therapy may be thought of as especially effective in the treatment of younger patients with anorexia nervosa (Dare *et al.*, 1990). LeGrange *et al.* (1992) compared family therapy to counselling of the parents plus individual counselling of the patient with anorexia nervosa; they found comparable changes in weight, eating attitudes, and self-esteem in both forms of treatment but no significant changes on the family measures they obtained.

To further address the issues raised by these studies, Robin *et al.* (1994) compared ego-oriented individual therapy (EOIT) to behavioural family systems therapy (BFST) in a study of 22 adolescent females with anorexia nervosa (no bulimic features). For the EOIT patients, ego strength, individuation, body image, and other identity and interpersonal issues were addressed individually and in separate parent counselling sessions. For the BFST patients, weekly family sessions were conducted with the patient, her parents, and sometimes with siblings. A behavioural weight control program was implemented with parents working as a team to promote the daughter's eating and weight gain. Cognitive, behavioural, and family systems techniques were used with parental monitoring in the initial phases gradually giving way to adolescent monitoring in the later phases. Both EOIT and BFST outpatient programs were found to be effective interventions for patients who were not in acute medical danger. It is important to note that parental involvement occurred in both cases, either collaterally or in family sessions.

With the aim of identifying the significant components of systemic family therapy in 15 adolescents with anorexia nervosa, Shugar and Krueger (1995) studied changes over time in eating attitudes, aggressiveness during family communication, and weight gain. They concluded that the therapeutic process led to a transition from covert to overt communication of aggression and that this was associated with improved eating attitudes. While all participants gained weight, those families with lower levels of covert aggression (e.g., sarcasm) or indirect aggression (e.g., body language), and higher levels of overt aggression (e.g, shouting) gained the most. Unfortunately, it appears that the category of overt aggression as defined in this study actually reflects a confounding of possibly adaptive conflict resolution initiation strategies (e.g., direct confrontation) with serious maladaptive overt aggression (e.g., actual physical aggression). To further explore such communication, future research will need to separate these definitions. It is the ability to openly resolve conflict via effective negotiation and problem solving that may be linked to efficacious changes as the result of family therapy (e.g., Foster and Robin, 1989).

Group Therapy

Group therapy approaches have also been utilized in the treatment of adolescents or their parents with treatment effectiveness obscured by the lack of well-controlled studies using valid and reliable measures. However, many clinicians have concluded that the group format nonetheless offers promise in providing a forum for enhancing the social functioning and skills of adolescents with anorexia nervosa (e.g., Andersen, 1986; Hendren *et al.* 1987; Trelfa and Britten, 1993). Group involvement for parents of an eating disordered adolescent may also be helpful. Parenting crisis support groups and multifamily treatment groups with parents of recovered eating disordered youths as cotherapists offer innovative approaches potentially worthy of further study for efficacy (e.g., Eliot, 1990).

Bulimia Nervosa

Individual Psychotherapy

In a study comparing 18 sessions of cognitive-behavioural treatment with supportive-expressive therapy in patients with bulimia nervosa, Garner *et al.* (1993) found that while both methods were effective in reducing binge-eating, the cognitive-behavioural approach was marginally more effective in reducing vomiting. Other differences as well in this study favoured the cognitive-behavioural approach; these differences included most of the measures involving concerns and attitudes about weight, shape, and eating, and measures of depression, self-esteem, personality, and general psychopathology.

Indeed, of the various psychotherapies, the cognitive-behavioural approach to the treatment of bulimia appears to be the most widely used and evaluated and seems to hold the most promise (Wilson, 1986). Among the cognitive-behavioural techniques used are: (1) self-monitoring of eating habits, bulimic behaviours, and thoughts and feelings including those involving body image, (2) cognitive restructuring of dysfunctional and distorted thoughts, (3) the introduction and use of more adaptive coping skills including methods of relaxation, and (4) a variety of other techniques such as coming up with adaptive alternative activities to binge-eating or purging as a means of response delay (e.g., Foreyt and McGavin, 1989; Wilson and Pike, 1993).

Family Therapy

As with anorexia nervosa, family therapy has been used at times as one component in the treatment of bulimia nervosa (e.g., Wooley and Kearney-Cooke, 1986). Little research appears to have been conducted on family therapy in young adult women with bulimia nervosa (Weltzin *et al.,* 1993); this may be because bulimia nervosa appears to affect primarily older adolescents and young adult women, some of whom no longer live with their families-of-origin. In addition, the efficacy of family treatment over other modalities for bulimia nervosa is yet to be determined. For example, Russell *et al.* (1987) found no differences in the effectiveness of individual supportive therapy and family therapy; in both cases, bulimic behaviours persisted in spite of the treatment.

However, research on family relationship variables suggests that bulimic women in treatment, but not those in a nonclinical college population, do report more conflict with their parents than normal women (Kent and Clopton, 1992). Kent and Clopton (1992) suggest that family conflict in those bulimics who are in treatment may not be unique to families with a bulimic member, but rather be similar to the family interaction patterns found in the general psychiatric population; furthermore, family conflict may arise once the secretive behaviour of the bulimic is uncovered and the need for treatment becomes apparent. When family therapy is conducted, in addition to altering the family interaction patterns, the focus of treatment will need to include the general goals of reestablishing and maintaining normal weight and eating patterns, and the empowerment of the family and patient through education about bulimia nervosa and its treatment (Weltzin *et al.*, 1993). Clearly, additional research is needed on these issues.

Group Therapy

Although they have also used their approach with individuals, Weiss *et al.* (1994) describe a cognitive-behavioural group treatment program for adolescents with bulimia nervosa. They address issues involving self-concept and body image, alternative means of coping, self-esteem, perfectionism, feelings of anger and/or depression, assertiveness, and countering the cultural expectations of thinness for women.

Obesity

Individual Therapy

Foreyt and Cousins (1989) review the following five components of behavioural treatment in obese preadolescents or adolescents. First, in the technique of *self-monitoring*, children note food intake, time, who shared the meal, where it occurred, and how they felt at the time, as well as their physical activity and sedentary behaviours. Second, *stimulus control* involves noting and modifying the cues that lead to inappropriate eating. Third, *eating management* includes slowing the rate of eating by chewing food throughly, laying down utensils frequently, and taking pauses during meals. Fourth, *contingency contracting* incorporates a system of rewards and punishments that are provided for *behaviours* associated with weight loss, but not for weight loss itself since this may encourage purging or fasting. And finally, various *cognitive behavioural strategies* can be implemented to alter maladaptive cognitions about food, self-image, and self-esteem, and to alter cognitions during eating and in social interactions.

Children and adolescents who are obese may also suffer a variety of psychosocial consequences such as peer rejection and teasing that may then become the focus of treatment to enhance their self-concept or social skills (Foreyt and Cousins, 1989). Little research has specifically addressed these issues and the findings are inconclusive (Siegel and Smith, 1991). Although Kimm *et al.* (1991) found that the overall self-concept of children who are obese fell within the norms on the Piers-Harris Self-Concept Scale, nonwhite obese children, particularly younger nonwhite females and nonwhite adolescent males, were found to score low in self-esteem. Thus, at least for some subgroups of obese children, self-esteem issues may need to be addressed. Kimm *et al.* (1991) conclude that there is variability in the self-concept of obese children and that both demographic factors and specific subscales of the self-concept are important considerations.

Parental Involvement in Therapy

When parents of obese children are also obese, they have often been encouraged to join in the weight loss program with their children. To ascertain the efficacy of a joint "weight loss" program in comparison to one in which the parental involvement was one of being a "helper", Israel *et al.* (1984) compared the two behaviourally-oriented procedures in a group of eight to twelve year old children with obesity. Separate parent and child treatment groups met and a four-prong treatment approach was used with emphasis on cue control rules, activity, intake, and rewards (CAIR). Israel *et al.* (1984) found that the two procedures were equally effective overall in producing weight loss in the children, although the results were suggestive of the weight loss condition being more effective for the younger children.

Indeed, many such programs include parents since it is well understood that parents regulate their children's food intake and activities, and provide models for their children; in addition, general child management skills and understanding of child development are important parental factors (Israel *et al.*, 1985). Israel *et al.* (1985) found that children with obesity whose parents received training in child management skills were better able to maintain their improved weight status than children who merely went through a weight loss program with their parents; they concluded that increasing parental knowledge may indeed be related to changes in parental behaviours.

Israel *et al.* (1986) note that studies involving the treatment of children who are obese will need to consider a variety of demographic characteristics (e.g., socioeconomic status, marital status, attending versus non-attending parent during treatment) and will need to include the entire family, since complex family patterns can emerge and may involve a variety of alliances involving the target child, one or both parents, and siblings. Israel *et al.* (1986) found that although none of the demographic factors they considered showed a statistically significant relationship to outcome, there was a tendency for some groups of children (i.e., only children, children with one or more overweight siblings, and children from an intact family with an attending overweight parent) to show greater decreases in percent overweight than other groups after participation in their CAIR treatment program. Israel *et al.* (1987) have also shown that whether or not a family adhered to the protocol for the collection of baseline data prior to participation in their treatment program was highly predictive of whether they continued with the program or dropped out. The authors conclude that such baseline information may be useful in identifying those families at risk for attrition.

Prevention

One promising way to prevent feeding disorder of infancy in those infants who are at risk is suggested by research that addresses the mother's internal working model of feeding and her understanding of infant feeding interactions (Pridham *et al.*, 1995). Pridham *et al.* (1995) have found that the mother's view of infant feeding changes throughout the first year, but it is as yet unclear what processes drive the changes. Future preventive efforts by pediatric staff may well be directed at helping parents with infants at risk for feeding disorders to have a more adaptive understanding of child development and parent-child interactions; of course, such preventive measures would need to supplement rather than replace the provision of more tangible resources and social supports.

Although childhood educators are aware of the possibility that school-based programs may assist in preventing eating disorders (e.g., Rhyne-Winkler and Hubbard, 1994), nutrition education researchers have found that knowledge about proper nutrition in adolescents does not necessarily coincide with eating a well-balanced diet (Wellington and Wellington, 1992). However, Sundgot-Borgen (1994) found that dieting athletes with an eating disorder were less likely to have been provided with guidance about how to go about weight reduction to improve their performance or appearance than those dieting athletes without an eating disorder. Thus, these latter data suggest that guidance or knowledge about nutrition and weight loss may indeed serve a preventative function.

In the first controlled longitudinal study with the aim of improving eating attitudes, encouraging healthful weight regulation, and preventing eating disorders in children, Killen and colleagues (1993) developed an 18 lesson prevention curriculum for nine hundred sixty-seven young adolescent girls. They found that while general knowledge showed a significant increase, the increase was not a meaningful one (i.e., test scores averaged less than 50% correct). They concluded that they were not able to achieve their objectives in that weight concerns and disordered eating behaviours remained relatively stable over time. They did however find that among those girls whose weight concerns put them "at risk", body mass index showed a slight increase. Killen *et al.* (1993) suggest that future prevention efforts need not be directed at all young adolescents but rather need to focus on those who particularly seem to be "at risk" for developing an eating disorder. In their attempt to identify those young adolescent girls most vulnerable to eating disorders, Killen *et al.* (1994) found that symptomatic girls in comparison to asymptomatic ones were more physically mature, heavier, more fearful of weight gain, more depressed, more dissatisfied with their bodies, and had greater feelings of inadequacy and worthlessness. The efficacy of prevention efforts directed at specific target groups is yet to be determined.

Planning Treatment Research on Feeding and Eating Disorders

Kazdin (1994) recommends the following series of steps that may be flexibly utilized in developing effective treatments for children and adolescents with developmental disorders. First, it is important to conceptualize the key causes and processes involved in the dysfunction. Then, research needs to be conducted on the processes thought to be involved to test the original theoretical model. According to Kazdin, attention also needs to be given to conceptualizing the treatment procedures and how they may be related to the processes involved in the disorder. The treatment procedures must be specified by operationalizing the concepts and processess involved, and by creating a treatment manual to codify and communicate the treatment techniques. Studies may then be conducted on the treatment process and treatment outcome. Finally, Kazdin (1994) discusses the need for studies of the boundaries or limits of treatment effectiveness by examining how the treatment interacts with other factors such as the context.

As reviewed in this chapter, conceptualizing the key causes and processes involved in eating disorders is a complex multidisciplinary effort and no comprehensive theoretical model exists as yet. As is true of other disorders of infancy, childhood, and adolescence, a developmental perspective is paramount. The relationship of feeding and eating behaviours to the various developmental tasks and challenges of each of these life periods needs to be addressed further in both theory and research (Attie *et al.*, 1990). Attie *et al.* (1990) point out that developmental psychopathology issues involving continuity and discontinuity, adaptive and maladaptive eating patterns, and socialization have rarely been explicitly addressed for eating problems and disorders.

The review provided in this chapter suggests that multiple processes — physiological, psychological, and familial/social — are involved in eating disordered behaviour. Some efforts thus far have been made to operationalize these processes (e.g., family conflict) and concepts (e.g., body image), and some treatment manuals currently exist (e.g., cognitive-behavioural treatment of bulimia by Weiss *et al.*, 1994). Additional research is needed on the various treatment processes, outcomes, and boundaries and limits. Because the long term course and outcome of eating disorders, in spite of treatment efforts, often remains intractable (e.g., Gillberg *et al.*, 1994), there is still a need for well-controlled treatment process and outcome research to identify those treatment components that are effective and the conditions under which they are efficacious. Prospective designs seem especially important in that individuals who are identified to be at risk and/or who begin to display eating problems earlier in childhood (e.g., food refusal, overeating) need to be followed as they face each succeeding developmental crisis and transition and need to be evaluated further at each developmental period for the possibility of eating disordered behaviours (Attie *et al.*, 1990). In addition to the family, other social and cultural contexts of the child and adolescent are worthy of further attention as well. For example, it is unknown to what extent eating behaviours are influenced by peers and by school-related experiences.

CONCLUDING REMARKS

Feeding and eating disorders are now recognized to be multidetermined syndromes necessitating multidisciplinary assessments and treatments. Current research is focused on identifying the interactive influence of various biological, sociocultural, psychological, and familial factors on predisposing individuals to the development of eating disorders. There is evidence that vulnerability to some of these disorders may be increasing and that eating disorders formerly associated with adolescence are being identified more often in younger children. A task remaining for researchers is to place the interactive causative factors as well as potential prevention and treatment components within a developmental framework and begin to build testable models.

REFERENCES

Abramson, L. (1991). Facial expressivity in failure to thrive and normal infants: Implications for their capacity to engage in the world. *Merrill-Palmer Quarterly*, **37**, 159–182.

Agras, W.S. and Kirkley, B.G. (1986). Bulimia: Theories of etiology. In K.D. Brownell and J.P. Foreyt (Eds.), *Handbook of eating disorders* (pp. 367–378). New York: Basic Books.

Ambrosini, P.J., Bianchi, M.D., Rabinovitch, H., and Elia, J. (1993). Antidepressant treatments in children and adolescents: II. Anxiety, physical, and behavioral disorders. *Journal of the American Academy of Child and Adolescent Psychiatry*, **32**, 483–493.

American Psychiatric Association (1980). *Diagnostic and statistical manual of mental disorders* (3rd ed.). Washington, DC: American Psychiatric Association.

American Psychiatric Association (1987). *Diagnostic and statistical manual of mental disorders* (3rd ed. rev.). Washington, DC: American Psychiatric Association.

American Psychiatric Association (1994). *Diagnostic and statistical manual of mental disorders* (4th ed.). Washington, DC: American Psychiatric Association.

Andersen, A.E. (1986). Inpatient and outpatient treatment of anorexia nervosa. In K.D. Brownell and J.P. Foreyt (Eds.), *Handbook of eating disorders* (pp. 333–350). New York: Basic Books.

Attie, I., Brooks-Gunn, J., and Petersen, A.C. (1990). A developmental perspective on eating disorders and eating problems. In M.Lewis and S.M. Miller (Eds.), *Handbook of developmental psychopathology* (pp. 409–420). New York: Plenum Press.

Ayoub, C.C., and Milner, J.S. (1985). Failure to thrive: Parental indicators, types, and outcomes. *Child Abuse and Neglect*, **9**, 491–499.

Barry, A. and Lippman, B.B. (1990). Anorexia in males. *Postgraduate Medicine*, **87**, 161–165.

Benoit, D. (1993). Failure to thrive and feeding disorders. In C.H. Zeanah, Jr. (Ed.), *Handbook of infant mental health* (pp. 317–331). New York: Guilford Press.

Berman, W.H., Berman, E.R., Heymsfield, S., and Fauci, M. (1992). The incidence and comorbidity of psychiatric disorders in obesity. *Journal of Personality Disorders*, **6**, 168–175.

Biddle, S. (1993). Children, exercise and mental health. *International Journal of Sport Psychology*, **24**, 200–216.

Biederman, J., Herzog, D.B., Rivinus, T.M., and Ferber, M.A. (1985). Amitryptyline in the treatment of anorexia nervosa: A double-blind, placebo-controlled study. *Journal of Clinical Psychopharmacology*, **5**, 10–15.

Birch, L.L. (1991). Obesity and eating disorders: A developmental perspective. *Bulletin of the Psychonomic Society*, **29**, 265–272.

Birch, L.L., Marlin, D., and Rotter, J. (1984). Eating as the "mean" activity in a contingency: Effects on young children's food preference. *Child Development*, **55**, 432–439.

Birch, L.L., Zimmerman, S., and Hind, H. (1980). The influence of social affective context on preschool children's food preferences. *Child Development*, **51**, 856–861.

Boddy, J.M., and Skuse, D.H. (1994). Annotation: The process of parenting in failure to thrive. *Journal of Child Psychology and Psychiatry*, **35**, 401–424.

Bossert-Zaudig, S., Zaudig, M., Junker, M., and Wiegand, M. (1993). Psychiatric comorbidity of bulimia nervosa inpatients: Relationship to clinical variables and treatment outcome. *European Psychiatry*, **8**, 15–23.

Bowler, C. (1992). Late-onset anorexia nervosa. *British Journal of Psychiatry*, **160**, 717.

Bruch, H. (1974). *Eating disorders: Obesity, anorexia nervosa and the person within.* London: Rutledge and Kegan Paul.

Bruch, H. (1977). Psychological antecedents of anorexia nervosa. In R.A. Vigersky (Ed.), *Anorexia nervosa* (pp. 1–10). New York: Raven Press.

Bruch, H. (1986). Anorexia nervosa: The therapeutic task. In K.D. Brownell and J.P. Foreyt (Eds.), *Handbook of eating disorders* (pp. 328–332). New York: Basic Books.

Bryant-Waugh, R. (1993). Epidemiology. In B. Lask and R. Bryant-Waugh (Eds.), *Childhood onset anorexia nervosa and related eating disorders* (pp. 55–67). Hove, UK: Lawrence Erlbaum.

Bryant-Waugh, R. and Kaminski, Z. (1993). Eating disorders in children: An overview. In B. Lask and R. Bryant-Waugh (Eds.), *Childhood onset anorexia nervosa and related eating disorders* (pp. 17–29). Hove, UK: Lawrence Erlbaum.

Bryant-Waugh, R., Knibbs, J., Fosson, A., Kaminski, Z., and Lask, B. (1988). Long term follow up of patients with early onset anorexia nervosa. *Archives of Disease in Childhood*, **63**, 5–9.

Bryant-Waugh, R. and Lask, B. (1995). Annotation: Eating disorders in children. *Journal of Child Psychology and Psychiatry*, **36**, 191–202.

Bulik, C.M. (1987). Drug and alcohol abuse by bulimic women and their families. *American Journal of Psychiatry*, **144**, 1604–1606.

Carey, S. (1985). *Conceptual change in childhood.* Cambridge, Mass.: The MIT Press.

Casper, R.C., Hedeker, D., and McClough, J.F. (1992). Personality dimensions in eating disorders and their relevance for subtyping. *Journal of the American Academy of Child and Adolescent Psychiatry*, **31**, 830–840.

Childress, A.C., Brewerton, T.D., Hodges, E., and Jarrell, M.P. (1993). The Kids' Eating Disorders Survey (KEDS): A study of middle school students. *Journal of the American Academy of Child and Adolescent Psychiatry*, **32**, 843–850.

Corcoran, K.J. and Fischer, J. (1987). *Measures for clinical practice.* New York: The Free Press.

Costello, A.J., Edelbrock, C., Dulcan, R.F., Kalas, R., and Klaric, S.H. (1984). *Development and testing of the NIMH Diagnostic Interview Schedule for Children in a clinic population.* Rockville, MD: National Institute of Mental Health.

Crisp, A. (1980). *Anorexia nervosa: Let me be.* New York: Grune and Stratton.

Crisp, A.H., Palmer, R.L., and Kalucy, R.S. (1977). How common is anorexia nervosa? A prevalence study. *British Journal of Psychiatry*, **128**, 549–554.

Dare, C., Eisler, I., Russell, G.F., and Szmukler, G.I. (1990). The clinical and theoretical impact of a controlled trial of family therapy in anorexia nervosa. *Journal of Marital and Family Therapy*, **16**, 39–57.

De Jong, W. (1993). Obesity as a characterological stigma: The issue of responsibility and judgments of task performance. *Psychological Reports*, **73**, 963–970.

Dietz, W.H., Jr. (1987). Childhood obesity. In R.J. Wurtman and J.J. Wurtman (Eds.), *Annals of the New York Academy of Sciences*, **499**, 47–54.

Dietz, W.H. and Gortmaker, S.L. (1985). Do we fatten our children at the TV set? Television viewing and obesity in children and adolescents. *Pediatrics*, **75**, 807–812.

Drotar, D., Eckerle, D., Satola, J., Pallota, J., and Wyatt, B. (1990). Maternal interactional behavior with nonorganic failure to thrive infants: A case comparison study. *Child Abuse and Neglect*, **14**, 41–51.

Drotar, D., Nowak, M., Malone, C.A., Eckerle, D., and Negray, J. (1985). Early psychological outcomes in failure to thrive: Predictions from an interactional model. *Journal of Clinical Child Psychology*, **14**, 105–111.

Dubowitz, H., Zuckerman, D.M., Bithoney, W.G., Newberger, E.H. (1989). Child abuse and failure to thrive: Individual, familial, and environmental characteristics. *Violence and Victims*, **4**, 191–201.

Duker, P. C., and Nielen, M. (1993). The use of negative practice for the control of pica behavior. *Journal of Behavior Therapy and Experimental Psychiatry*, **24**, 249–253.

Eckert, E.D. (1985). Characteristics of anorexia nervosa. In J.E. Mitchell (Ed.), *Anorexia nervosa and bulimia: Diagnosis and treatment* (pp. 3–28). Minneapolis, MN: University of Minnesota Press.

Eckert, E.D., Goldberg, S.C., Halmi, K.A., Casper, R.C., and Davis, J.M. (1982). Depression in anorexia nervosa. *Psychological Medicine*, **12**, 115–122.

Egan, J., Schaefer, S.S., and Chatoor, I. (1988). Clinical evaluation of nonorganic failure to thrive. In C.J. Kestenbaum and D.T. Williams (Eds.), *Handbook of clinical assessment of children and adolescents (Vol. II)* (pp. 831–841). New York: New York University Press.

Eliot, A.O. (1990). Group coleadership: A new role for parents of adolescents with anorexia and bulimia nervosa. *International Journal of Group Psychotherapy*, **40**, 339–351.

Epstein, L.H. (1986). Treatment of childhood obesity. In K.D. Brownell and J.P. Foreyt (Eds.), *Handbook of eating disorders* (pp. 159–179). New York: Basic Books.

Epstein, L.H., Valoski, A., Wing, R.R., and McCurley, J. (1994). Ten-year outcome of behavioral family-based treatment for childhood obesity. *Health Psychology*, **13**, 373–383.

Epstein, L.H. and Wing, R.R. (1987). Behavioral treatment of childhood obesity. *Psychological Bulletin*, **101**, 331–342.

Fairburn, C.G. and Beglin, S.J. (1990). Studies of epidemiology of bulimia nervosa. *American Journal of Psychiatry*, **147**, 401–408.

Fairburn, C.G. and Cooper, J.P. (1982). Self-induced vomiting and bulimia nervosa: An undetected problem. *British Medical Journal of Clinical Research*, **284**, 1153–1155.

Fairburn, C.G. and Cooper, P.J. (1984). Rumination in bulimia nervosa. *British Medical Journal*, **288**, 826–827.

Fallon, B.A., Walsh, B.T., Sadlik, C., Saoud, J.B., and Lukasik, V. (1991). Outcome and clinical course in inpatient bulimic women: A 2- to 9-year follow-up study. *Journal of Clinical Psychiatry*, **52**, 272–278.

Foch, R.R. and McClearn, G.E. (1980). Genetics, body weight, and obesity. In A.J. Stunkard (Ed.), *Obesity* (pp. 48–71). Philadelphia: W B Saunders.

Fombonne, E. (1995). Eating disorders: Time trends and possible explanatory mechanisms. In M. Rutter and D.J. Smith (Eds.), *Psychosocial disorders in young people: Time trends and their causes* (pp. 616–685). Chichester: John Wiley and Sons.

Foreyt, J.P. and Cousins, J.H. (1989). Obesity. In E.J. Mash and Barkley, R.A. (Eds.), *Treatment of childhood disorders* (pp. 405–422). New York: Guilford.

Foreyt, J.P. and McGavin, J.K. (1989). Anorexia nervosa and bulimia nervosa. In E.J. Mash and R.A. Barkley (Eds.), *Treatment of childhood disorders* (pp. 529–558). New York: The Guilford Press.

Fornari, V.M., Kent, J., Kabo, L., and Goodman, B. (1994). Anorexia nervosa: "Thirty something." *Journal of Substance Abuse Treatment*, **11**, 45–54.

Fosson, A., Knibbs, J., Bryant-Waugh, R., and Lask, B. (1987). Early onset anorexia nervosa. *Archives of Disease in Childhood*, **62**, 114–118.

Foster, S.L. and Robin, A.L. (1989). Parent-adolescent conflict. In E.J. Mash and R.A. Barkley (Eds.), *Treatment of childhood disorders* (pp. 493–528). New York: The Guilford Press.

Gardner, R.A. (1992). *The psychotherapeutic techniques of Richard A. Gardner* (Revised edition). Cresskill, New Jersey: Creative Therapeutics.

Garfinkel, P.E. (1974). Perception of hunger and satiety in anorexia nervosa. *Psychological Medicine*, **4**, 309–315.

Garfinkel, P.E., Garner, D.M., and Goldbloom, D.S. (1987). Eating disorders: Implications for the 1990's. *Canadian Journal of Psychiatry*, **32**, 624–630.

Garfinkel, P.E., Moldofsky, H., and Garner, D.M. (1980). The heterogeneity of anorexia nervosa. *Archives of General Psychiatry*, **37**, 1036–1040.

Garn, S.M., Bailey, S.M., and Cole, P.E. (1979). Synchronous fatness changes in husbands and wives. *American Journal of Clinical Nutrition*, **32**, 2375–2377.

Garner, D.M., and Garfinkel, P.E. (1979). The Eating Attitudes Test: An index of the symptoms of anorexia nervosa. *Psychological Medicine*, **9**, 273–279.

Garner, D.M., Garfinkel, P.E., Rockert, W., and Olmsted, M.P. (1987). A prospective study of eating disturbances in the ballet. *Psychotherapy and Psychosomatics*, **48**, 170–175.

Garner, D.M., Olmstead, M.P., and Polivy, J. (1983). Development and validation of a multidimensional eating disorder inventory for anorexia nervosa and bulimia. *International Journal of Eating Disorders*, **2**, 15–34.

Garner, D.M., Rockert, W., Davis, R., Garner, M.V., Olmsted, M.P., and Eagle, M. (1993). Comparison of cognitive-behavioral and supportive-expressive therapy for bulimia nervosa. *American Journal of Psychiatry*, **150**, 37–46.

Gillberg, I.C., Rastam, M., and Gillberg, C. (1994). Anorexia nervosa outcome: Six-year controlled longitudinal study of 51 cases including a population cohort. *Journal of the American Academy of Child and Adolescent Psychiatry*, **33**, 729–739.

Goldbloom, D.S. and Olmsted, M.P. (1993). Pharmacotherapy of bulimia nervosa with fluoxetine: Assessment of clinically significant attitudinal change. *American Journal of Psychiatry*, **150**, 770–774.

Goldfarb, L.A., Dykens, E.M., and Gerrard, M. (1985). The Goldfarb fear of fat scale. *Journal of Personality Assessment*, **49**, 329–332.

Gortmaker, S.L., Must, A., Perrin, J.M., and Sobol, A.M. (1993). Social and economic consequences of overweight in adolescence and young adulthood. *New England Journal of Medicine*, **329**, 1008–1012.

Hall, R., Tice, M., Beresford, T., Wooley, B., and Klassen, M. (1989). Sexual abuse in patients with anorexia and bulimia. *Psychosomatics*, **30**, 73–79.

Halmi, K.A., Brodland, G., and Rigas, C. (1975). A follow-up study of 79 patients with anorexia nervosa: An evaluation of prognostic factors and diagnostic criteria. In R.D. Wirt, G. Winokur, and M. Roff (Eds.), *Life history research in psychopathology* (Vol. 4, pp. 290–301). Minneapolis, MN: University of Minnesota Press.

Halmi, K.A., Eckert, E., Marchi, P., Sampugnaro, V., Apple, R., and Cohen, J. (1991). Comorbidity of psychiatric diagnoses in anorexia nervosa. *Archives of General Psychiatry*, **48**, 712–718.

Hart, D. and Damon, W. (1985). Contrasts between understanding self and understanding others. In R. L. Leahy (Ed.), *The development of the self* (pp. 151–178). Orlando, FL: Academic Press, Inc.

Hamburg, P., Herzog, D.B., Brotman, A.W., and Stasior, J.K. (1989). The treatment resistant eating disordered patient. *Psychiatric Annals*, **19**, 494–499.

Hawley, R.M. (1985). The outcome of anorexia nervosa in younger subjects. *British Journal of Psychiatry*, **146**, 657–660.

Heebink, D.M., Sunday, S.R., and Halmi, K.A. (1995). Anorexia nervosa and bulimia nervosa in adolescence: Effects of age and menstrual status on psychological variables. *Journal of the Academy of Child and Adolescent Psychiatry*, **34**, 378–382.

Heffer, R. W., and Kelley, M. L. (1994). Nonorganic failure to thrive: Developmental outcomes and psychosocial assessment and intervention issues. *Research in Developmental Disabilities*, **15**, 247–268.

Hendren, R. L. (1983). Bulimia in the adolescent. *American Journal of Disorders in Children*, **22**, 59–62.

Hendren, R.L., Atkins, D.M., Sumner, C.R., and Barber, J.K. (1987). Model for the group treatment of eating disorders. *International Journal of Group Psychotherapy*, **37**, 589–602.

Herman, C. P. (1978). Restrained eating. *Psychiatric Clinics of North America*, **1**, 593–607.

Herman, C.P. and Mack, D. (1975). Restrained and unrestrained eating. *Journal Personality*, **43**, 647–660.

Herman, C.P. and Polivy, J. (1975). Anxiety, restraint, and eating behavior. *Journal of Abnormal Psychology*, **84**, 666–672.

Herzog, D.B., Keller, M.B., and Lavori, P.W. (1988). Outcome in anorexia nervosa and bulimia nervosa: A review of the literature. *Journal of Nervous and Mental Disease*, **176**, 131–143.

Herzog, D.B., Keller, M.B., Lavori, P.W., and Sacks, N.R. (1991). The course and outcome of bulimia nervosa. *Journal of Clinical Psychiatry*, **52 (Suppl.)**, 4–8.

Herzog, D.B., Keller, M.B., Lavori, P.W., Kenny, G.M., and Sacks, N.R. (1992). The prevalence of personality disorders in 210 women with eating disorders. *Journal of Clinical Psychiatry*, **53**, 147–152.

Herzog, D.B., Keller, M.B., Sacks, N.R., Yeh, C.J., and Lavori, P.W. (1992). Psychiatric comorbidity in treatment-seeking anorexics and bulimics. *Journal of the American Academy of Child and Adolescent Psychiatry*, **31**, 810–818.

Herzog, D.B., Sacks, N.R., Keller, M.B., Lavori, P.W., von Ranson, A.B., and Gray, H.M. (1993). Patterns and predictors of recovery in anorexia nervosa and bulimia nervosa. *Journal of the American Academy of Child and Adolescent Psychiatry*, **32**, 835–842.

Higgs, J.F., Goodyer, I.M., and Birch, J. (1989). Anorexia nervosa and food avoidance emotional disorder. *Archives of Disease in Childhood*, **64**, 346–351.

Hill, A.J. and Robinson, A. (1991). Dieting concerns have a functional effect on the behaviour of nine-year-old girls. *British Journal of Clinical Psychology*, **30**, 265–267.

Hill, A.J., Rogers, P.J., and Blundell, J.E. (1989). Dietary restraint in young adolescent girls: A functional analysis. *British Journal of Clinical Psychology*, **28**, 165–176.

Hodes, M. (1993). Anorexia nervosa and bulimia nervosa in children. *International Review of Psychiatry*, **5**, 101–108.

Holland, A., Sicotte, N., and Treasure, J. (1988). Anorexia nervosa — evidence for a genetic basis. *Journal of Psychosomatic Research*, **32**, 561–571.

Hsu, L.K.G. (1990). *Eating disorders*. New York, NY: Guilford.

Hsu, L.K.G. and Holder, D. (1986). Bulimia nervosa: Treatment and long-term outcome. *Psychological Medicine*, **16**, 65–70.

Hsu, G.L., Kaye, W., and Weltzin, T. (1993). Are the eating disorders related to obsessive-compulsive disorder? *International Journal of Eating Disorders*, **14**, 305–318.

Hudson, J.I., Pope, H.C., Jonas, J.M., and Yurgelun-Todd, D. (1983). Family history study of anorexia nervosa and bulimia. *British Journal of Psychiatry*, **142**, 133–138.

Hudson, J.I., Pope, H.G., Jonas, J.M., Yurgelun-Todd, D., and Frankenburg, F.R. (1987). A controlled family history study of bulimia. *Psychological Medicine*, **17**, 883–890.

Hudson, J.I., Weiss, R.D., and Pope, H.G. (1992). Eating disorders in hospitalized substance abusers. *American Journal of Drug and Alcohol Abuse*, **18**, 75–85.

Husain, S.A. and Cantwell, D.P. (1991). *Fundamentals of child and adolescent psychopathology* (pp. 129). Washington, DC: American Psychiatric Press.

Irwin, M. (1984). Early onset anorexia nervosa. *Southern Medical Journal*, **77**, 611–614.

Israel, A.C., Silverman, W.K., and Solotar, L.C. (1986). An investigation of family influences on initial weight status, attrition, and treatment outcome in a childhood obesity program. *Behavior Therapy*, **17**, 131–143.

Israel, A.C., Silverman, W.K., and Solotar, L.C. (1987). Baseline adherence as a predictor of dropout in a children's weight-reduction program. *Journal of Consulting and Clinical Psychology, 5,* 791–793.

Israel, A.C., Stolmaker, L., and Andrian, C.A.G. (1985). The effects of training parents in general child management skills on a behavioral weight loss program for children. *Behavior Therapy, 16,* 169–180.

Israel, A.C., Stolmaker, L., Sharp, J.P., Silverman, W., and Simon, L.G. (1984). An evaluation of two methods of parental involvement in treating obese children. *Behavior Therapy, 15,* 266–272.

Iwaniec, D., Herbert, M., and McNeish, A.S. (1985). Social work with failure-to-thrive children and their families. *British Journal of Social Work, 15,* 243–259.

Johnson, C.R., Hunt, F.M., and Siebert, M. J. (1994). Discrimination training in the treatment of pica and food scavenging. *Behavior Modification, 18,* 214–229.

Johnson, C. and Pure, D.L. (1986). Assessment of bulimia: A multidimensional model. In K.D. Brownell and J.P. Foreyt (Eds.), *Handbook of eating disorders* (pp. 405–449). New York: Basic Books.

Johnson, C.L., Tobin, D., and Enright, A. (1989). Prevalence and clinical characteristics of borderline patient in an eating disorder population. *Journal of Clinical Psychiatry, 50,* 9–15.

Kagan, D.M. and Squires, R.L. (1984).Compulsive eating scale. Eating disorders among adolescents: Patterns and prevalence. *Adolescence, 19,* 15–29.

Kalfus, G.R., Fisher-Gross, S., Marvullo, M.A., and Nau, P.A. (1988). Outpatient treatment of pica in a developmentally delayed child. *Child and Family Behavior Therapy, 9,* 49–63.

Kasvikis, Y.G., Tasakiris, F., Marks, I.M., Basoglu, M., and Noshirvani, H.F. (1986). Past history of anorexia nervosa in women with obsessive-compulsive disorder. *International Journal of Eating Disorders, 37,* 1281–1285.

Katz, J.L. (1990). Eating disorders: A primer for the substance abuse specialist: II. Theories of etiology, treatment approaches, and consideration during comorbidity with substance abuse. *Journal of Substance Abuse Treatment, 7,* 211–217.

Kazdin, A. E. (1994). Psychotherapy for children and adolescents. In A.E. Bergin and S.L. Garfield (Eds.), *Handbook of psychotherapy and behavior change* (4th ed., pp. 543–594). New York: Wiley.

Kennedy, S.H. and Garfinkel, P.E. (1989). Patients admitted to hospital with anorexia nervosa and bulimia nervosa: Psychopathology, weight gain, and attitudes toward treatment. *International Journal of Eating Disorders, 8,* 181–190.

Kennedy, S.H. and Garfinkel, P.E. (1992). Advances in diagnosis and treatment of anorexia nervosa and bulimia nervosa. *Canadian Journal of Psychiatry, 37,* 309–315.

Kennedy, S.H., Piran, N., and Garfinkel, P.E. (1986). Isocarboxazide in the treatment of bulimia. *Journal of Psychology, 143,* 1495–1496.

Kent, J.S. and Clopton, J.R. (1992). Bulimic women's perceptions of their family relationships. *Journal of Clinical Psychology, 48,* 281–292.

Kent, A., Lacey, J.H., and McCluskey, S.E. (1992). Premenarcheal bulimia nervosa. *Journal of Psychosomatic Research, 36,* 205–210.

Killen, J.D., Hayward, C., Wilson, D.M., Taylor, C.B., Hammer, L.D., Litt, I., Simmonds, B., and Haydel, F. (1994). Factors associated with eating disorder symptoms in a community sample of 6th and 7th grade girls. *International Journal of Eating Disorders, 15,* 357–367.

Killen, J.D., Taylor, C.B., Hammer, L.D., Litt, I., Wilson, D.M., Rich, T., Hayward, C., Simmonds, B., Kraemer, H., and Varady, A. (1993). An attempt to modify unhealthful eating attitudes and weight regulation practices of young adolescent girls. *International Journal of Eating Disorders, 13,* 369–384.

Killen, J.D., Taylor, C.B., Hayward, C., Wilson, D.M., Haydel, K.F., Hammer, L.D., Simmonds, B., Robinson, T.N., Litt, I., Varady, A., and Kraemer, H. (1994). Pursuit of thinness and onset of eating disorder symptoms in a community sample of adolescent girls: A three-year prospective analysis. *International Journal of Eating Disorders*, **16**, 227–238.

Kimm, S.Y.S., Sweeney, C.G., Janosky, J.E., and MacMillan, J.P. (1991). Self-concept measures and childhood obesity: A descriptive analysis. *Developmental and Behavioral Pediatrics*, **12**, 19–24.

Klesges, R.C., Malott, J.M., Boschee, P.F., and Weber, J.M. (1986). Parental influences on children's food intake, physical activity and relative weight. *International Journal of Eating Disorders*, **5**, 335–345.

Knibbs, J. (1993). Behaviour therapy. In B. Lask and R. Bryant-Waugh (Eds.), *Childhood onset anorexia nervosa and related eating disorders* (pp. 163–176). Hove, UK: Lawrence Erlbaum.

Krahn, D.D. (1991). The relationship of eating disorders and substance abuse. *Journal of Substance Abuse*, **3**, 239–253.

Kronenberger, W. G., and Meyer, R. G. (1996). *The child clinician's handbook*. Boston, Mass.: Allyn and Bacon.

Laessle, R.G., Wittchen, H.U., Fichter, M.M., and Pirke, K.M. (1989). The significance of subgroups of bulimia and anorexia nervosa: Lifetime frequency of psychiatric disorders. *International Journal of Eating Disorders*, **8**, 569–574.

Lam, R.W., Goldner, E.M., Solyom, L., and Remick, R.A. (1994). A controlled study of light therapy for bulimia nervosa. *American Journal of Psychiatry*, **151**, 744–750.

Larocca, F.E. (1988). Rumination and its occurrence in conjunction with anorexia nervosa and bulimia nervosa. *American Journal of Psychiatry*, **145**, 1610.

Lask, B. (1993). Family therapy and parent counselling. In B. Lask and R. Bryant-Waugh (Eds.), *Childhood onset anorexia nervosa and related eating disorders* (pp. 211–219). Hove, UK: Lawrence Erlbaum.

Lask, B. and Bryant-Waugh, R. (1992). Early-onset anorexia nervosa and related eating disorders. *Journal of Child Psychology and Psychiatry*, **33**, 281–300.

Lask, B. and Bryant-Waugh, R. (1993). *Childhood onset anorexia nervosa and related eating disorders*. Hove, UK: Lawrence Erlbaum.

Lask, B. and Fosson, A. (1993). Physical treatments. In B. Lask and R. Bryant-Waugh (Eds.), *Childhood onset anorexia nervosa and related eating disorders* (pp. 157–161). Hove, UK: Lawrence Erlbaum.

Lask, B., Fosson, A., Rolfe, U., and Thomas, S. (1993). Zinc deficiency and childhood-onset anorexia nervosa. *Journal of Clinical Psychiatry*, **54**, 63–66.

Lawrence, C.M. and Thelen, M.H. (1995). Body image, dieting, and self-concept: Their relation in African-American and Caucasian children. *Journal of Clinical Child Psychology*, **24**, 41–48.

LeBow, M.D. (1984). *Child obesity: A new frontier of behavior therapy*. New York: Springer.

LeBow, M.D., Ness, D., Makarenko, P., and Lam, T. (1989). Attitudes, perceptions, and practices of Canadian teenagers towards obesity. *Journal of Obesity and Weight Regulation*, **8**, 53–65.

LeGrange, D., Eisler, I., Dare, C., and Russell, G.F.M. (1992). Evaluation of family treatments in adolescent anorexia nervosa: A pilot study. *International Journal of Eating Disorders*, **12**, 347–357.

Leon, G.R., Carroll, K., Chernyk, B., and Finn, S. (1985). Binge eating and associated habit patterns within college students and identified bulimic populations. *International Journal of Eating Disorders*, **4**, 43–57.

Leon, G.R. and Dinklage, D. (1989). Obesity and anorexia nervosa. In T.H. Ollendick and M. Hersen (Eds.), *Handbook of child psychopathology* (2nd ed., pp. 247–264). New York: Plenum Press.

Levine, M.P., Smolak, L., and Hayden, H. (1994). The relation of sociocultural factors to eating attitudes and behaviors among middle school girls. *Journal of Early Adolescence*, **14**, 471–490.

Looney, J.G. (1984). Treatment planning in child psychiatry. *Journal of the American Academy of Child Psychiatry*, **23**, 529–536.

Lyles, B., Sarkis, E., and Kemph, J.P. (1990). Fluoxetine and anorexia. *Journal of the American Academy of Child and Adolescent Psychiatry*, **29**, 984–985.

Lowenstein, L.F. (1994). Anorexia nervosa in boys: A review of the recent literature and a case treated in a therapeutic community. *Family Therapy*, **21**, 233–240.

Maloney, M.J., McGuine, J., Daniels, S.R., and Spector, B. (1989). Dieting behavior and eating attitudes in children. *Pediatrics*, **84**, 482–489.

Marchi, M. and Cohen, P. (1990). Early childhood eating behaviors and adolescent eating disorders. *Journal of the American Academy of Child and Adolescent Psychiatry*, **29**, 112–117.

Martin, F.E. (1990). The relevance of a systemic model for the study and treatment of anorexia nervosa in adolescents. *Canadian Journal of Psychiatry*, **35**, 496–500.

Mason, E. (1970). Obesity in pet dogs. *Veterinary Records*, **86**, 612–616.

McDaniel, K.D. (1986). Pharmacologic treatment of psychiatric and neurodevelopmental disorders in children and adolescents (Part 3). *Clinical Pediatrics*, **25**, 198–204.

Minuchin, S., Baker, L., Liebman, R., Milman, L., and Todd, T.C. (1975). A conceptual model of psychosomatic illness in children. *Archives of General Psychiatry*, **32**, 1031–1038.

Mitchell, J.E. (1991). Dental complications of bulimia nervosa. *Journal of the New Jersey Dental Association*, **14**, 73–76.

Mitchell, J.E., Hatsukami, D., Eckert, E.D., and Pyle, R.L. (1985). Characteristics of 275 patients with bulimia. *Journal of Clinical Psychopharmacology*, **142**, 482–485.

Mitchell, J.E., Hatsukami, D., Pyle, R.L., and Eckert, E.D. (1988). Bulimia with and without a family history of drug abuse. *Addictive Behaviors*, **13**, 245–251.

Mitchell, J.E., Soll, E., Eckert, E.D., Pyle, R.L., and Hatsukami, D. (1989). The changing population of bulimia nervosa patients in an eating disorders program. *Hospital and Community Psychiatry*, **40**, 1188–1189.

Morgan, H. and Russell, G.F.M. (1975). Value of family background and clinical features as predictors of long-term outcome in anorexia nervosa: Four-year follow-up study of 41 patients. *Psychological Medicine*, **5**, 355–371.

Morrill, C.M., Leach, J.N., Shreeve, W.C., and Radebaugh, M.R. (1991). Teenage obesity: An academic issue. *International Journal of Adolescence and Youth*, **2**, 245–250.

Nash, H.L. (1987). Do compulsive runners and anorectic patients share common bonds? *Physician in Sports Medicine*, **15**, 162–167.

Norring, C.E. and Sohlberg, S.S. (1993). Outcome, recovery, relapse, and mortality across six years in patients with clinical eating disorders. *Acta Psychiatrica Scandinavia*, **87**, 437–444.

Olmsted, M.P., Kaplan, A.S., and Rockert, W. (1994). Rate and prediction of relapse in bulimia nervosa. *American Journal of Psychiatry*, **151**, 738–743.

Page, R.M. (1991). Indicators of psychosocial distress among adolescent females who perceive themselves as fat. *Child Study Journal*, **21**, 203–212.

Parry-Jones, B. (1994). Merycism or rumination disorder: A historical investigation and current assessment. *British Journal of Psychiatry*, **165**, 303–314.

Parry-Jones, B. and Parry-Jones, W.Ll. (1992). Pica: Symptom or eating disorder? A historical assessment. *British Journal of Psychiatry*, **160**, 341–354.

Parry-Jones, W.Ll. and Parry-Jones, B. (1994). Implications of historical evidence for the classification of eating disorders. *British Journal of Psychiatry*, **165**, 287–292.

Patton, G.C., Johnson-Sabine, E., Wood, K., Mann, A.H., and Wakeling, A. (1990). Abnormal eating attitudes in London Schoolgirls — a prospective epidemiological study: Outcome at twelve month follow-up. *Psychological Medicine*, **20**, 383–394.

Peveler, R. and Fairburn, C. (1990). Eating disorders in women who abuse alcohol. *British Journal of Addiction*, **85**, 1633–1638.

Phelps, L. and Bajorek, E. (1991). Eating disorders of the adolescent: Current issues in etiology, assessment, and treatment. *School Psychology Review*, **20**, 9–22.

Piran, N., Lerner, P., Garfinkel, P.E., Kennedy, S.H., and Brouilette, C. (1988). Personality disorders in anorexia patients. *International Journal of Eating Disorders*, **5**, 589–599.

Polan, H.J., Leon, A., Kaplan, M.D., Kessler, D.B., Stern, D.N., and Ward, M.J. (1991). Disturbances of affect expression in failure-to-thrive. *American Academy of Child and Adolescent Psychiatry*, **30**, 897–903.

Pollock, M., Kovacs, M., and Charron-Prochownik, D. (1995). Eating disorders and maladaptive dietary/insulin management among youths with childhood-onset insulin-dependent diabetes mellitus. *Journal of the American Academy of Child and Adolescent Psychiatry*, **34**, 291–296.

Pope, H.G., Mangweth, B., Negrao, A.B., Hudson, J.I., and Cordas, R.A. (1994). Childhood sexual abuse and bulimia nervosa: A comparison of American, Austrian, and Brazilian women. *American Journal of Psychiatry*, **151**, 732–737.

Powell, G. F. and Bettes, B. B. (1992). Infantile depression, nonorganic failure to thrive, and DSM-III-R: A different perspective. *Child Psychiatry and Human Development*, **22**, 185–198.

Prather, R.C. and Williamson, D.A. (1988). Psychopathology associated with bulimia, binge eating, and obesity. *International Journal of Eating Disorders*, **7**, 177–184.

Price, J.H., Desmond, S.M., Ruppert, E.S., and Stelzer, C.M. (1989). Pediatricians perceptions' and practices regarding childhood obesity. *American Journal of Preventive Medicine*, **5**, 95–103.

Pridham, K.F., Van Riper, M., Schroeder, M., and Thoyre, S. (1995, March). *Mothers' working models of feeding: How stable are they through the first year?* Poster session presented at the Society for Research in Child Development, Indianapolis, IN.

Puig-Antich, J. and Chambers, W. (1978). *The Schedule for Affective Disorders and Schizophrenia for School-aged Children*. New York: State Psychiatric Institute.

Pumariega, A.J., Pursell, J., Spock, A., and Jones, J.D. (1986). Eating disorders in adolescents with cystic fibrosis. *Journal of the American Academy of Child Psychiatry*, **25**, 269–275.

Rhyne-Winkler, M.C. and Hubbard, G.T. (1994). Eating attitudes and behavior: A school counseling program. *The School Counselor*, **41**, 195–198.

Robin, A.L., Siegel, P.T., Koepke, T., Moye, A.W., and Tice, S. (1994). Family therapy versus individual therapy for adolescent females with anorexia nervosa. *Journal of Developmental and Behavioral Pediatrics*, **15**, 111–116.

Rodin, J., Slochower, J., and Fleming, B. (1977). The effects of degree of obesity, age of onset, and energy deficit on external responsiveness. *Journal of Comparative Physiology and Psychology*, **91**, 586–597.

Root, M.P. (1990). Recovery and relapse in former bulimics. *Psychotherapy*, **27**, 397–403.

Rosen, J.C. and Leitenberg, H. (1982). Bulimia nervosa: Treatment with exposure and response prevention. *Behavior Therapy*, **13**, 117–124.

Rothenberg, A. (1988). Differential diagnosis of anorexia nervosa and depressive illness: A review of 11 studies. *Comprehensive Psychiatry*, **29**, 427–432.

Russell, G. (1985). Anorexia and bulimia nervosa. In M. Rutter and L. Hersov (Eds.), *Child and adolescent psychiatry* (2nd ed., pp. 625–637). Oxford: Blackwell Scientific.

Russell, G.F.M., Szmukler, G.I., Dare, C., and Eisler, I. (1987). An evaluation of family therapy in anorexia nervosa and bulimia nervosa. *Archives of General Psychiatry*, **44**, 1047–1056.

Sasson, A., Lewin, C., and Roth, D. (1995). Dieting behavior and eating attitudes in Israeli children. *International Journal of Eating Disorders*, **17**, 67–72.

Schmidt, U., Hodes, M., and Treasure, J. (1992). Early onset bulimia nervosa — who is at risk? *Psychological Medicine*, **22**, 623–628.

Schmitt, B.D., and Mauro, R.D. (1989). Nonorganic failure to thrive: An outpatient approach. *Child Abuse and Neglect*, **13**, 235–248.

Shaffer, D., Fisher, P., Piacentini, J., Schwab-Stone, M., and Wicks, J. (1989). Diagnostic Interview Schedule for Children (DISC-2.1C) Child Version. New York: New York State Psychiatric Institute.

Shugar, G. and Krueger, S. (1995). Aggressive family communication, weight gain, and improved eating attitudes during systemic family therapy for anorexia nervosa. *International Journal of Eating Disorders,* **17**, 23–31.

Siegel, L.J. and Smith, K.E. (1991). Somatic disorders. In T.R. Kratochwill and R.J. Morris (Eds.), *The practice of child therapy* (2nd ed., pp. 222–256). New York: Pergamon.

Sigelman, C.K. (1991). The effect of causal information on peer perceptions of children with physical problems. *Journal of Applied Developmental Psychology,* **12**, 237–253.

Singer, L.T., Song, L., Hill, B.P., and Jaffe, A.C. (1990). Stress and depression in mothers of failure to thrive children. *Journal of pediatric psychology,* **15**, 711–720.

Skodol, A.E., Oldham, J.M., Hyler, S.E., Kellman, H.D., Doidge, N., and Davies, M. (1993). Comorbidity of DSM-III-R eating disorders and personality disorders. *International Journal of Eating Disorders,* **14**, 403–416.

Smith, M.C., and Thelen, M.N. (1984). Development and validation of a test for bulimia. *Journal of Consulting and Clinical Psychology,* **52**, 863–872.

Soukup, V.M., Beiler, M.E., and Terrell, F. (1990). Stress, coping style, and problem-solving ability among eating-disordered inpatients. *Journal of Clinical Psychology,* **46**, 592–599.

Stark, O., Atkins, E., Wolff, O.H., and Douglas, J.W.B. (1981). Longitudinal study of obesity in the National Survey of Health and Development. *British Medical Journal,* **283**, 13–17.

Steiger, H., Leung, F.Y.K., Puentes-Neuman, G., and Gottheil, N. (1992). Psychosocial profiles of adolescent girls with varying degrees of eating and mood disturbances. *International Journal of Eating Disorders,* **11**, 121–131.

Steinhausen, H.C. and Seidel, R. (1993). Outcome in adolescent eating disorders. *International Journal of Eating Disorders,* **14**, 487–496.

Steinhausen, H. C. and Vollrath, M. (1993). The self-image of adolescent patients with eating disorders. *International Journal of Eating Disorders,* **13**, 221–227.

Strober, M. (1980). A cross-sectional and longitudinal analysis of personality and symptomatological features in young, non-chronic anorexia nervosa patients. *Journal of Psychosomatic Research,* **24**, 353–359.

Strober, M. (1986). Anorexia nervosa: History of psychological concepts. In K.D. Brownell and J.P. Foreyt (Eds.), *Handbook of eating disorders* (pp. 231–246). New York: Basic Books.

Strober, M. and Humphrey, L.L. (1987). Familial contributions to the etiology and course of anorexia nervosa and bulimia. *Journal of Consulting and Clinical Psychology,* **55** 654–659.

Strober, M. and Katz, J.L. (1987). Do eating disorders and affective disorders share a common etiology? A dissenting opinion. *International Journal of Eating Disorders* **6**, 171–180.

Strober, M., Lampert, C., Morrell, W., Burroughs, J., and Jacobs, C. (1990). A controlled family study of anorexia nervosa: Evidence of familial aggregation and lack of shared transmission with affective disorders. *International Journal of Eating Disorders,* **9** 239–253.

Stunkard, A.J., Foch, R.R., and Hrubec, Z. (1986). A twin study of human obesity. *Journal of the American Medical Association,* **256**, 51–54.

Stunkard, A.J., Sorensen, T.I.A., Hanis, C., Teasdale, R.W., Chakraborty, R., Schull, W.J. and Schulsinger, F. (1986). An adoption study of human obesity. *New England Journal of Medicine,* **314**, 193–198.

Sundgot-Borgen, J. (1994). Risk and trigger factors for the development of eating disorders in female elite athletes. *Medicine and Science in Sports and Exercise,* **26** 414–419.

Tobias, L.L. and MacDonald, M.L. (1977). Internal locus of control and weight loss: A insufficient condition. *Journal of Consulting and Clinical Psychology,* **45**, 647–653.

Trelfa, J. and Britten, C. (1993). Group therapy. In B. Lask and R. Bryant-Waugh (Eds.), *Childhood onset anorexia nervosa and related eating disorders* (pp. 221–232). Hove, UK: Lawrence Erlbaum.

Troop, N.A., Holbrey, A., Trowler, R., and Treasure, J.L. (1994). Ways of coping in women with eating disorders. *Journal of Nervous and Mental Diseases,* **182**, 535–540.

Vandereycken, W. and Pierloot, R. (1983). Long-term outcome in anorexia nervosa: The problem of patient selection and follow-up duration. *International Journal of Eating Disorders,* **2**, 237–242.

Wadden, T.A., Brown, G., Foster, G.D., and Linowitz, J.R. (1991). Salience of weight-related worries in adolescent males and females. *International Journal of Eating Disorders,* **10**, 407–414.

Walford, G. and McCune, N. (1991). Long-term outcome in early-onset anorexia nervosa. *British Journal of Psychiatry,* **159**, 383–389.

Weiss, L., Wolchik, S., and Katzman, M. (1994). A treatment program for adolescent bulimics and binge eaters. In C.W. LeCroy (Ed.), *Handbook of child and adolescent treatment manuals* (pp. 278–306). New York: Lexington Books.

Welch, S.L. and Fairburn, D.M. (1994). Sexual abuse and bulimia nervosa: Three integrated case control comparisons. *American Journal of Psychiatry,* **151**, 402–407.

Wellington, C.M. and Wellington, W.J. (1992). A comparison of eating habits between Canadian male and female secondary school students. [Abstract] *Journal of the American Dietetic Association,* **(Suppl. Sept.),** A-15.

Wells, L.A. and Logan, K.M. (1987). Pharmacologic treatment of eating disorders. *Psychosomatics,* **28**, 470–479.

Weltzin, T.E., Starzynski, J., Santelli, R., and Kaye, W.H. (1993). Anorexia and bulimia nervosa. In R.T. Ammerman, C.G. Last, and M. Hersen (Eds.), *Handbook of prescriptive treatments for children and adolescents* (pp. 214–239). Needham Heights, MS: Allyn and Bacon.

White, D.R., Schliecker, E., and Dayan, J. (1991). Gender differences in categorizing adolescents' weight status. *Psychological Reports,* **68**, 978.

Williamson, D.A. (1990). *Assessment of eating disorders: Obesity, anorexia and bulimia nervosa.* New York: Pergamon Press.

Willmuth, M.E., Leitenberg, H., Rosen, J.C., and Cado, S. (1988). A comparison of purging and nonpurging normal weight bulimics. *International Journal of Eating Disorders,* **7**, 825–835.

Wilson, G.T. (1986). Cognitive-behavioral and pharmacological therapies for bulimia. In K.D. Brownell and J.P. Foreyt (Eds.), *Handbook of eating disorders* (pp. 450–475). New York: Basic Books.

Wilson, G.T. (1994). Behavioral treatment of childhood obesity: Theoretical and practical implications. *Health Psychology,* **13**, 371–372.

Wilson, G.T. and Pike, K.M. (1993). Eating disorders. In D.H. Barlow (Ed.), *Clinical handbook of psychological disorders* (2nd ed., pp. 278–317). New York: Guilford Press.

Wittenberg, J.V.P. (1990). Feeding disorders in infancy: Classification and treatment considerations. *Canadian Journal of Psychiatry,* **35**, 529–533.

Woodside, D.B. and Garfinkel, P.E. (1992). Age of onset in eating disorders. *International Journal of Eating Disorders,* **12**, 31–36.

Wooley, S.C. and Kearney-Cooke, A. (1986). Intensive treatment of bulimia and body-image disturbance. In K.D. Brownell and J.P. Foreyt (Eds.), *Handbook of eating disorders* (pp. 476–502). New York: Basic Books.

World Health Organization (1993). *The ICD-10 classification of mental and behavioural disorders.* Geneva: World Health Organization.

Wren, B. and Lask, B. (1993). Aetiology. In B. Lask and R. Bryant-Waugh (Ed.), *Childhood onset anorexia nervosa and related eating disorders* (pp. 69–89). Hove, UK: Lawrence Erlbaum.

Yanovski, S.Z., Nelson, J.E., Dubbert, B.K., and Spitzer, R.L. (1993). Association of binge eating disorder and psychiatric comorbidity in obese subjects. *American Journal of Psychiatry*, **150**, 1472–1479.

Yates, A. (1989). Current perspectives on the eating disorders: I. History, psychological and biological aspects. *Journal of the American Academy of Child and Adolescent Psychiatry*, **28**, 813–828.

Zerbe, K.J., Marsh, S.R., and Coyne, L. (1993). Comorbidity in an inpatient eating disordered population: Clinical characteristics and treatment implications. Psychiatric Hospital, 24, 3–8.

Acknowledgements. Support for this chapter was provided by the Child Study Centre, University of Windsor. The authors wish to thank Jody Levenbach for her assistance in the bibliographic research for this chapter.

CHAPTER 11
ELIMINATION DISORDERS

Richard J. Butler

The elimination disorders of childhood typically cover those problems arising from an inability to achieve appropriate control over bowel and bladder. From a developmental perspective most children (80% and above) will achieve bowel control by 2 years, bladder control during the day by 2 1/2–3 years, and bladder control at night between 3–4 years (Stein and Susser, 1967). Many children will naturally be delayed in their achievement of bowel and bladder control, yet some will continue to exhibit difficulties in young childhood and adolescence. The clinical description for such problems are "faecal soiling", "daytime wetting" and "nocturnal enuresis", each having a variety of aetiological models and requiring different treatment interventions. Children can be enormously distressed by their failure to stay clean and/or dry with widespread effect on parents' levels of tolerance and attachment relationships. Some children may threaten suicide (Butler, 1987) whilst parents can resort to nonaccidental injury (Jehu *et al.*, 1977) in their frustration with coping with the condition.

Historically the conditions have provoked separate medical and psychological theories of aetiology and methods of management. Whilst this chapter is inevitably psychologically focused, an attempt is made to investigate the more medical aspects. Hopefully this represents a more recent move to seek greater integration of psychological and medical models in the understanding and treatment of daytime wetting, nocturnal enuresis, and faecal soiling.

DEFINITION AND CLASSIFICATION

Day Wetting

The fourth edition of the Diagnostic and Statistical Manual of Mental Disorders (DSM-IV; American Psychiatric Association; APA, 1994) definition of enuresis includes both daytime wetting and nocturnal enuresis. It is described as repeated voiding of urine into the bed or clothes, and is

Table 11.1   Diagnostic criteria for enuresis

A.   Repeated voiding of urine into bed or clothes (whether involuntary or intentional)

B.   The behavior is clinically significant as manifested by either a frequency of twice a week for at least 3 consecutive months or the presence of clinically significant distress or impairment in social, academic (occupational), or other important areas of functioning

C.   Chronological age is at least 5 years (or equivalent developmental level)

D.   The behavior is not due exclusively to the direct physiological effects of a substance (e.g., a diuretic) or general medical condition (e.g., diabetes, spina bifida, a seizure disorder)

APA (1994), pp. 109–110

clinically manifested by either "a frequency of twice a week for 3 consecutive months or the presence of clinically significant distress or impairment in social academic or other area of functioning" (APA, p. 109) (Table 11.1). The definition also outlines a criteria of a chronological age of at least 5 years (or equivalent developmental level) and a cause not exclusively determined by direct physiological effect of a substance (e.g diuretics) or a general medical condition (e.g., diabetes, spina bifida, seizure, disorder) (APA, 1994). The ICD-10 definition (WHO, 1993) of enuresis differs only in severity — stating a frequency of twice a month (in contrast to twice a week under DSM-IV criteria) in children under 7 years and at least once a month in children older than 7 years. However, the ICD-10 criteria describe two further exclusion criteria — the lack of structural abnormality of the urinary tract, and the lack of any other psychiatric disorder.

Of particular interest is that both the DSM-IV and ICD-10 definitions include intentional voiding in the classification of enuresis. However, this remains a debatable point and indeed intentional or wilful micturition is not classified as enuresis in Great Britain (Forsythe and Butler, 1989) and interestingly the ICD-10 definition which excludes those who may have a "psychiatric disorder" would also tend to exclude such cases. In practice the two criteria — day wetting and nocturnal enuresis have quite distinct aetiologies and as such will be discussed separately.

Day wetting may be defined as "a lack of bladder control during waking hours in a child old enough to maintain bladder control" (Schmitt, 1982). As most children acquire daytime bladder control by the age of four years (Oppel *et al.*, 1968; Stein and Susser, 1967) this might be considered an appropriate age. However, Meadow (1990) takes the view that because of the natural variability of acquiring bladder control a considerable number of children are late in achieving dryness and the definition should therefore, reasonably, take 5 years as a minimal criteria.

There is some confusion over the terminology employed — day wetting or diurnal enuresis — to describe the problem. Enuresis (as with night time wetting) is traditionally used to describe lack of bladder control in the absence of organic causes at an age when control should be expected. However as more sophisticated methodology becomes available, Meadow (1990) suggests further physiological and functional causes surface, and for this reason he prefers the description of day wetting.

Schmitt (1982) has proposed a classification based on organic, physiological and psychological aetiology.

Organic Aetiology. According to Schmitt (1982) organic causes account for less than 5% of children with daytime wetting and clearly physical examination is required to screen for such abnormality. Consideration should be given to the following: (a) Ectopic ureter when dampness is present on a continual basis, and most usually in females Yue, 1974); (b) Neurogenic bladder which is rare and often associated with gait disturbance and inadequate bowel control (Schmitt, 1982); c) Lower urinary tract obstruction which may lead to bladder distension and the child having difficulty in starting to urinate, terminal dribbling or producing a weak urine stream on voiding (Redman and Seibert, 979); and (d) Stress incontinence where faecal masses which press on the bladder can lead to wetting with running, coughing or lifting Schmitt, 1982). Except in these rare cases, the child with day wetting rarely requires invasive urodynamic or radiographic investigations American Academy of Paediatrics, 1980; Lancet, 1987; Meadow, 1990).

Physiological Aetiology. Three types fall into this classification: a) Vaginal reflux (Butcher and Donnai, 1972) occurs following voiding, usually in overweight girls who find that on standing up and walking urine seeps out, an embarrassment which may continue for some minutes. Screening for this condition should seek to investigate whether the child hurriedly leaves the toilet after voiding (Schmitt, 1982). Managing this problem usually involves encouraging children to sit on the toilet after voiding for a few extra minutes; (b) Giggle micturition described as a sudden, involuntary, uncontrollable and complete emptying of the bladder when the child giggles or laughs (Cooper, 1973;

MacKeith, 1964). Other antecedents include excitement and being tickled, and at other times (including for some when sitting) the child achieves bladder control. Most sufferers are girls (Cooper, 1973) and encouragingly there is a good chance of "outgrowing" the problem in adolescence. There is a lack of any effective demonstrable technique in the literature (Brocklebank and Meadow, 1981), yet Schmitt (1982) advocates the use of stream interruption exercises; (c) Urge incontinence has been described as attacks of intense bladder spasms that lead to abrupt voiding and wetting (De Jonge, 1973a). It is the most common cause of daywetting in children (Meadow, 1990), adolescents and adults (Warwick and Whiteside, 1979), with 90% of sufferers being female (Hallgren, 1956). Van Gool and De Jonge (1989) report 1–3/1000 girls suffer with urge incontinence. Other terms for this problem are "bladder instability" or "detrusor instability" because overactivity of the detrusor and urethral muscles are thought to be responsible for the bladder sphincter dysfunction which causes the urge and wetting (Allen and Bright, 1978). Two patterns of bladder sphincter overactivity have been identified from urodynamic studies and summarised by Van Gool and De Jonge (1989). Firstly, strong, spontaneous and uninhibitable detrusor contractions give rise to urgency and frequency early in the filling phase while the child is attempting to inhibit micturition (Borzyskowski and Mundy, 1987; Whiteside and Arnold, 1975). Secondly, incomplete relaxation of the urethral and pelvic floor muscles interrupts voiding causing a staccato urinary flow. As Meadow (1990) points out, both patterns — detrusor contractions and incomplete relaxation of urethra and pelvic floor muscles — cause the bladder to "work" against resistance, generate high pressures and there needs to be concern about the transmission of such pressure to the kidneys. It is interesting that most children with nocturnal enuresis do not have bladder instability (Whiteside and Arnold, 1975). Urge incontinence is associated most markedly with urgency, frequency and urinary tract infection (Koff 1982; Lapides and Diokno, 1970; Van Gool and Tanagho, 1977).

Van Gool and De Jonge (1989) provide a cogent description of child's experience of the urge syndrome. Sudden and unexpected attacks of the urge to void tend to increase in number and severity during the day. The sensation is so acute that loss of urine can only be avoided by maximal compression of the urethra by contraction of the pelvic floor muscles and "external" mechanical compression. Children adopt all manner of postures to assist this compression, such as squatting on one foot with the heel of the foot against the perineum, known as the curtsey sign (Fielding *et al.*, 1978; Vincent, 1966). Often the compression is not completely successful and a small loss of urine occurs, but complete bladder emptying never arises. Van Gool and De Jonge (1989) note the symptoms of urge incontinence usually start around 4–5 years of age, with most cases referred for clinical intervention being 7–12 years of age, and a decrease in prevalence around puberty with a low incidence in adolescence.

The association between urge incontinence and urinary tract infection (UTI) is significant. Almost 50% of girls with urge syndrome have UTI (Berg *et al.*, 1977). As Van Gool and De Jonge (1989) suggest, UTI may not constitute the primary cause of the urge syndrome but it invariably occur in conjunction with it and have a key role in the persistence and severity of symptoms. Day wetting may facilitate the ascending infection (Savage *et al.*, 1969) and as Dodge *et al.* (1970) report, infected enuretic girls who continue to wet are more likely to become reinfected than enuretic girls who become dry. Effective antibiotic treatment for the UTI does not have an impact on reducing day wetting (Meadow, 1990). Other reported problems associated with urge incontinence include urgency and frequency (Lancet, 1987) and chronic constipation (Jarvelin *et al.*, 1990; Vincent, 1966) where the contraction of pelvic floor muscles in response to the urge is postulated as the cause mechanism. There is some evidence of emotional and behavioural disturbance in children with urge syndrome (Van Gool and De Jonge, 1989). It is noteworthy that whilst most studies of children with nocturnal enuresis tend to find little evidence of psychological distress or disturbance (Butler, 1994; Shaffer *et al.*, 1984), there is evidence of such disturbance with girls and particularly those wetting during the day (McGee *et al.*, 1984; Rutter *et al.*, 1973).

Psychological Aetiology. Types of day wetting which fall into this category include: (a) Transient or secondary wetting which may occur during illness, fear or stressful life events such as hospitalization, marital disharmony or loss of a parent (Meadow, 1990). Usually such wetting is restricted to the younger child and may be situation-specific as with an anxious child starting school and reluctant to use the school toilets or seek permission to leave the classroom during lessons (Shaffer, 1994). Schmitt (1982) notes that children with low functional bladder capacities are particularly vulnerable when restrictions on toilet use are made at school. He advocates support for children in coping with the stress, occasionally counselling for the families and where possible an improvement of facilities to reduce the child's anxieties about toilet use;

(b) Negligible wetting. Meadow (1990) suggests some parents, particularly those obsessed with cleanliness, are unwilling to accept any amount of tiny staining and such preoccupation may create undue tension in the child-parent relationship; (c) Resistive wetting. The tension between child and parent over toileting can escalate so that early toilet training becomes high pressured and the child resists toileting because it becomes associated with negative feelings (Schmitt, 1982). Parents may become punitive and coercive but more usually it is the endless reminding and prompting that children react against. Schmitt (1982) suggests most children with this form of wetting are boys, and about a third may have associated non-retentive soiling.

Nocturnal Enuresis

Nocturnal enuresis may be defined as an involuntary discharge of urine during sleep in the absence of congenital or acquired defects of the central nervous system or urinary tract in a child aged 5 or over (Forsythe and Butler, 1989). This divorces enuresis from incontinence and excludes acts of wilful micturition. The choice of 5 years is somewhat arbitrary but reflects the nocturnal course of bladder acquisition (Stein and Susser, 1967). Verhulst and colleagues (1985) argue for flexibility in age criteria due to different rates of acquisition for boys and girls. Brazelton (1973) and Butler (1987) suggest bed wetting becomes a problem, in the clinical context, at the point where parental concern and childhood distress surfaces.

Typically, children with nocturnal enuresis are separated into those with a primary type (who fail to demonstrate an extended period — usually 6 months — of dry nights) and those of a secondary type (where children resume bed wetting after a 6 month period of being dry). The risk of secondary enuresis is heightened where children acquire bladder control after 5 years of age (Fergusson *et al.*, 1990) and/or are exposed to stressful life events (Jarvelin *et al.*, 1990; Shaffer, 1980). Of perhaps more importance clinically is the division by sex. Girls with nocturnal enuresis, compared to boys, are more likely to have secondary enuresis (Rutter *et al.*, 1973), associated daytime wetting (Jarvelin *et al.*, 1988), daytime frequency (De Jonge, 1973a), associated emotional and behavioural problems (Rutter *et al.*, 1973) and more tolerant mothers (Butler *et al.*, 1986). There is also less evidence of a genetic aetiology (Bakwin, 1971) and girls therefore present a different picture in the clinical context (Butler, 1994).

Faecal Soiling

Functional encopresis may be defined as "the repeated passage of faeces into places not appropriate for that purpose (e.g., clothing) whether involuntary or intentional" (APA, 1994). Further elaboration of this statement is contained in three adjoiners which suggest there should be "at least one such event a month for at least three months, a chronological age of at least 4 years (or an equivalent developmental level) and "not due exclusively to the direct physiological effects of a substance (e.g., laxatives) or a general medical condition except through a mechanism involving constipation" (Table 11.2).

A variety of schemes of classification have been proposed. Because it is based on a description of the soiling behaviour and has clear implications for treatment intervention the classification developed by Rutter (1976) and Hersov (1994) has direct clinical relevance. Four types of faecal soiling have been described:

Psychological encopresis where a child can demonstrate adequate bowel control with motions of a normal consistency, but these are deposited in inappropriate places. This can take two forms: Secondary encopresis where control breaks down in circumstances where the child experiences emotional turmoil and stress such as the birth of a sibling, admission to hospital, separation from the family or sexual abuse (Boon, 1991; Buchanan, 1989). With relief from such circumstances, stress management counselling, and a supportive home background, bowel control is often regained (Hersov, 1994). Aggressive encopresis where the child, seemingly in response to family instability, parental disharmony and punitive attitude on behalf of the parents, deposits faeces in

Table 11.2   Diagnostic criteria for encopresis

A.   Repeated passage of feces into inappropriate places (e.g., clothing or floor) whether involuntary or intentional

B.   At least one such event a month for at least 3 months

C.   Chronological age is at least 4 years (or equivalent developmental level)

D.   The behavior is not due exclusively to the direct physiological effects of a substance (e.g., laxatives) or general medical condition except through a mechanism involving constipation inappropriate places such as cupboards, chairs and chests of drawers. Children may also smear their faeces, coupled with a denial of their encopresis, all of which appear designed to escalate parental annoyance and intolerance. Interventions with this form of soiling are primarily aimed at alleviating the disturbed family relationships and spiralling intolerance through family therapy.

Failure to learn bowel control where motions of a normal consistency are deposited randomly. Rutter (1976) argues that acquisition of bowel control requires maturation (both physical and intellectual) and the appropriate experience (toilet training), for the child to develop an awareness of bowel sensation, postponement of defecation until an appropriate place, and knowledge of an appropriate place. The absence of such conditions (e.g., where there are neurological problems as in spina bifida; delayed intellectual development; and/or inconsistent or inadequate toilet training) leaves children increasingly vulnerable to delayed bowel control. Appropriate toilet training coupled with a behavioural programme aimed at reinforcing appropriate toileting is usually advocated in these circumstances (Fielding and Doleys, 1988; Sluckin, 1975).

Stress *induced diarrhoea* where stools are abnormal in consistency and appearance. Hersov (1994) associates such soiling with children who react with fear and anxiety when confronted by unfamiliar and potentially stressful situations.

Retention with overflow is the most common type of functional encopresis with 80% of children classified in this way (Levine, 1975). It is identified by the presence of chronic constipation which arises because the child elects to hold and avoid defecating either to avoid the pain of passing motions, where there is an anal lesion, or for fear of passing motions where parents have established punitive or obsessive routines around toileting (Gleghorn *et al.*, 1991; Rutter, 1976; Woodmansey, 1967). Levine and Bakow (1976) present a system for classifying the degree of constipation. The hard compacted faeces lead to a dilation of the bowel with subsequent loss of normal anal reflex and the "overflow" or seepage of liquified motions. This will lead to multiple daily soiling (Levine, 1982).

Types of soiling which do not readily fit into this four way classification include children with a phobia or extreme fear of sitting on the toilet (Doleys, 1983) and anal masturbation where bedclothes are stained yet stools are only infrequently passed (Clark *et al.*, 1990).

EPIDEMIOLOGY

De Jonge (1973b) reports an incidence of 2–4% at 5–7 years of age, reducing to 1% in 7–12 year olds, which is not dissimilar to the rates reported by Bloomfield and Douglas (1956), although the degree of wetting was not defined very accurately. Meadow (1990) outlines the difficulty of acquiring accurate estimates because of the different types of day wetting, the different criteria employed to measure the presence of day wetting (e.g., once a month to every day) and the self selected nature of some of the populations surveyed.

Surveys suggest 13–19% of boys and 9–16% of girls at 5 years of age wet the bed at least once a month with a steady decline during the childhood years and adolescence but with 2–3% still regularly wetting during the late teens (Devlin, 1991; Feehan *et al.*, 1990; Rutter *et al.*, 1973; Verhulst *et al.*, 1985). The rate of spontaneous recovery is of the order of 14% a year for 5–9 years old and 16% for those 10–18 years old (Forsythe and Redmond, 1974). The rate of decline is less smooth and regular for girls (Devlin, 1991; Verhulst *et al.*, 1985) and is complicated by the influence of secondary enuresis, urinary tract infection, puberty and possibly sexual abuse.

There is broad agreement over the incidence of functional encopresis. Around 7 to 8 years the rate appears to be of the order of 1.5% (Bellman, 1966; Esser, 1993; Schaefer, 1979) with boys (2.3%) predominant over girls (0.7%). This incidence reduces to 1.2% for boys and 0.3% for girls at the 10–12 year range (Rutter *et al.*, 1970). Although many reports suggest that all children by late adolescence either spontaneously recover or respond to treatment, Rex and colleagues (1992) report on four cases of retention with overflow where this persisted beyond 15 years of age.

RISK FACTORS

Nocturnal Euresis

Physiological Factors

Organic pathology.   Schmitt (1990) suggests some 3% of bed wetting children seen in paediatric settings may have an organic basis for the condition, such as obstructive uropathy, neurogenic bladder and developmental anomalies of the urinary tract. Given the earlier defini-tion, such children should be excluded as cases of nocturnal enuresis.

Urinary tract infection (UTI). Children most susceptible are girls (Dodge *et al.*, 1970), those with frequency and mixed wetters (Jarvelin *et al.*, 1991). It is argued that UTI may be a consequence of bed wetting rather than a cause, as bed wetting is not reduced by clearing up the infection and it may also facilitate the ascent of pathogenic organisms to the bladder (Shaffer, 1980).

Nocturnal polyuria. Normally, the hormone arginine vasopressin (AVP) is released during sleep, causing the kidneys to concentrate urine by reabsorption of water and ensuring urine production during sleep does not exceed functional bladder capacity. It has been proposed that bed wetting children fail to produce AVP at night with consequent pro-duction of excess volume of urine with low osmolality (Norgaard *et al.*, 1985; Rittig *et al.*, 1989). However, it has yet to be demonstrated that a lack of AVP production accounts for all children's bed wetting and it remains unclear whether this mode of action is responsible for those children who become dry spontaneously.

Small functional bladder capacity. A popular formulation, elabo-rated initially by Starfield (1967) is that children with nocturnal enuresis have comparatively small functional bladder capacities which prevents them holding all the urine produced during night time. More recently the view being adopted focuses on the small functional bladder capacity being a correlate or a consequence rather than a cause of bed wetting (Fielding, 1980; Houts, 1991), because of the overlap in capacities between enuretic and non-enuretic children, the finding that an increase in functional bladder capacity is not a prerequisite for the attainment of dryness (Fielding, 1980), and that artificial filling of the bladder during sleep causes non-bed wetting children to wake yet enuretic children to wet, suggesting bladder capacity is less of a determinant than how bladder contractions are perceived and reacted to (Sorotzkin, 1984).

Unstable bladder. Houts (1991) suggests bed wetting results from spontaneous detrusor contractions during sleep, occurring at lower than normal pressure and leading to spontaneous voiding. He explains that avoidance of wetting occurs when children prevent detrusor contrac-tions by spontaneously contracting the pelvic floor muscles, but wetting occurs if the pelvic floor muscles fail to contract and respond as they do with daytime voiding, by relaxing.

Deep sleep. This is the most heavily endorsed view of children (Butler *et al.*, 1994) and parents (Butler *et al.*, 1986), yet a gathering body of evidence has accumulated to contradict the view. Enuretic episodes occur during all stages of sleep in proportion to the time spent in that stage (Mikkelsen *et al.*, 1980; Norgaard *et al.*, 1985), and further, there is no difference in sleep pattern of bed wetting children on dry nights compared with wet nights (Gillin *et al.*, 1982). In clinical practise, it may therefore prove important to emphasise not depth of sleep, but the child's difficulty in waking to an important signal (the full bladder) which logically leads to the employment of an enuresis alarm to assist the child to respond to an associated signal.

Maturational lag. Evidence of delayed maturation in enuretic children include lower birth weight (Jarvelin *et al.*, 1988), "soft signs" of neurological delay (Jarvelin, 1989), and delayed motor development (Fergusson *et al.*, 1986). Both Jarvelin (1989) and Fergusson *et al.* (1990) propose a model linking a delay in maturation of the physiological mechanism to primary enuresis, coupled with a view that such developmental "frailty" would leave a child more vulnerable to stressful situations and thus to a susceptibility for secondary enuresis. MacKeith *et al.* (1973) and Baller (1975) propose psychological variables may again be influential because delayed maturation generally leads to parental reactions (e.g., overprotection, anxiety) which possibly exacerbate vulnerability to delayed bladder control.

Genetic Factors

A history of nocturnal enuresis runs through many families (Devlin, 1991), with a risk of the order of 77% where both parents were enuretic as children (Bakwin, 1971; Jarvelin *et al.*, 1988). Further evidence of a link was found by Fergusson and colleagues (1986) where age of attaining bladder control was determined by family history of enuresis. The search for a genetic link was undertaken by Bakwin (1971) through twin study methodology. He found 70% concordance in monozygotic (MZ) male twins, compared with 31% concordance for dizygotic (DZ) males. Although the same trend was observed with girls (65% with MZ twins, 44% DZ twins) this difference was not statistically significant. An autosomal dominant gene with reduced penetrance is the model favoured by geneticists. However, questions remain over the mode of action (e.g., bladder vulnerability or release of AVP); the concept of vulnerability which suggests penetrance may be environmentally determined; and the mechanism of transfer, such as the different attitudes held by families with members who were formerly enuretic (Butler, 1994).

Psychological Factors

Social conditions.   Children from less advantageous environments such as those living in lower socio-economic groups (Devlin, 1991), large, overcrowded families (Foxman *et al.*, 1986; Miller, 1973) and institutional settings (Essen and Peckham, 1976) are more vulnerable to nocturnal enuresis. Such environments may increase stress, which disrupts acquisition of bladder control, or alternatively inhibit the production and release of AVP.

Interrupted learning.   This model proposes that enuresis is a consequence of disruptive and stressful events interfering with the acquisition of bladder control. It appears to necessitate three eventualities: (i) a vulnerability either genetically or maturationally determined (Fergusson *et al.*, 1986); (ii) the experience of stressful life events during a sensitive stage of bladder control acquisition, particularly separation from mother (Douglas, 1973); and (iii) a mechanism of action which assumes the anxiety resulting from distress either interferes with the process of learning bladder control, or exerts a detrimental effect on the acquisition of co-ordinated muscular responses leading to unstable detrusor activity (Houts, 1991).

Incomplete learning.   This hypothesis focuses on the child being inadvertently prevented from developing awareness of normal bladder sensation. Christmanson and Lisper (1982) found children with enuresis had parents who tended to regulate the frequency of urination through lifting at night and who adopted an attitude which emphasised a need to teach the child to be dry rather than respond to the child's needs. Such behaviour and attitude can prove counterproductive. Lifting, for example, prevents the child from developing an awareness of full bladder signals and often encourages the child to empty the bladder whilst asleep, both of which increase the chances of bed wetting persisting (Butler, 1994).

Behavioural/Attitudinal causes.   Exposition of the link between bed wetting and behavioural disturbance has been caught in a trap, because the search of an association between the two has subsequently led to a debate about the nature of the link (if it exists). Accumulating evidence lends weight to the notion that there is little evidence of an association between behavioural problems and nocturnal enuresis. Children assessed by parents on behavioural checklists tend to be placed within a normal range (Couchells *et al.*, 1981; Wagner *et al.*, 1982). However, a minority of mothers believe the child's bed wettting has behavioural causes such as laziness (Butler *et al.*, 1986; Wagner and Johnson, 1988) which leads to anger, intolerance and punitive reactions (Butler *et al.*,

1994), and whilst such families require immediate help, the indications are that such attitudes develop in response to coping with enuresis rather than act as a cause of enuresis.

Emotional causes. It seems axiomatic to suggest children with betwetting experience distress (Anon, 1987; Butler, 1994) yet evidence indicating emotional maladjustment is very sparse. Parental and teacher assessment suggest children with nocturnal enuresis fall within a normal range of emotional adjustment (Baker, 1969; Wagner *et al.*, 1982; Wagner and Matthews, 1985) and similarly self report measures indicate children generally construe themselves in similar ways to non-enuretic children (Butler *et al.*, 1994; Wagner and Geffken, 1986). Whilst most enuretic children appear emotionally well adjusted, it seems girls, those with associated daytime wetting (Fielding, 1980; Rutter *et al.*, 1973; Wagner *et al.*, 1982) and those with secondary enuresis (Shaffer, 1980) are more vulnerable to emotional disturbance. For this group, the causative link is difficult to determine because it can be argued the more public nature of daywetting and the stress associated with secondary enuresis, will create conditions whereby a child will exhibit more emotional disturbance. Thus, as Shaffer (1973) cogently argues, the association between enuresis and emotional disturbance may not be causal but linked as a result of the child's reaction to associated stress.

Faecal Soiling

Levine (1982) has proposed a multi-factorial three stage developmental model of risk where constitutional predisposition, environment and critical life events may interact to create functional encopresis. Levine (1982) suggests predisposing factors during the early years (0–2 years) include simple constipation, specific food intolerance, anal fissure and parental over-reaction resulting in bowel preoccupation on the part of the child. During pre-school years (2–5 years) accumulating risk factors include negative associations with defecation developing into fear of the toilet, and coercive and inappropriate toilet training. In the final stage during the early school years, Levine (1982) proposes new factors including avoidance of school toilets, prolonged medical illnesses such as gastroenteritis and a frenetic lifestyle where "tight schedules lead to tight sphincters" may increase the child's vulnerability to encopresis.

Given the influence of parental style and reactions in precipitating encopresis it is somewhat surprising to discover no relationship between family structure (size, age of parent and ordinal position of the child) and the development of faecal soiling (Anthony, 1957; Bemporad, 1978), although Wolters (1974) has shown some evidence of family disharmony being related to encopresis. The most common complaint from children is of abdominal pain, poor appetite and lethargy (Fielding and Doleys, 1988; Levine, 1975). It has been estimated that about 25% of children with encopresis also have enuresis (Fritz and Armbrust, 1982) most probably as a result of the rectal distension leading to urine dribbling during the day (Levine, 1982).

COURSE AND OUTCOME

Children experience nocturnal enuresis with perplexity, humiliation and fears of alienation (Anon, 1987; Butler, 1987) and have been subjected to a catalogue of misguided and harsh "treatments" (Schaefer, 1979). Most mothers attribute bed wetting to internal, stable and uncontrollable factors which leads them to feel helpless (Butler *et al.*, 1986). However, a minority of mothers attribute bed wetting to controllable factors, become angry, annoyed and intolerant and resort to punitive actions (Butler, 1994). Between 10–28% of bed wetting children have day-time bladder problems (Forsythe and Redmond, 1974) and are often described as "mixed" wetters. They are more resilient to treatment and more vulnerable to relapse (Fielding, 1980).

Meadow (1990) has postulated a model of parental reaction some-what similar to that described for nocturnal enuresis (Butler, 1994). Parents may construe the child as not trying, being lazy and unco-operative par-ticularly where they are continually prompting and urging the child to use the toilet. This may lead to intolerant attitudes developing with the threat of punitive reactions and physical abuse occurring.

Levine (1982) has comprehensively discussed the experience of encopresis. Children live with a constant fear of being discovered and anticipations of being bullied, ridiculed and ostracised. They often with-draw from others, avoid social engagements and suffer cruel nicknames when discovered. The shame and humiliation leads to low self esteem. Children sense, not unlike those with nocturnal enuresis, that they are alone with the problem and rarely know of any other child who suffers in a similar way.

Parents adopt a variety of strategies for dealing with the encopresis (Stark *et al.*, 1990), and perhaps more than with nocturnal enuresis they exhibit anger, annoyance, intolerance, punitive reactions and attribute the cause of the encopresis to controllable factors which means children are thought of as lazy and accused of being negligent (Levine, 1982). The encopresis may further incite conflict amongst family members who often advance contradicting theories about the cause, the child's responsibility and how the problem should be managed. Such disharmony typically leads to greater preoccupation with toileting, more hostility and blaming of the child with increased battles over the toilet, and hence further increasing the risk of toilet avoidance with consequent retention and overflow. A classic vicious circle of parental disharmony and soiling is promulgated.

ASSESSMENT

Enuresis

Medical screening is imperative along with a check of the urine for infection, but detailed radiological and invasive urodynamic investigations should be kept to a minimum (Lancet, 1987). Careful history taking as described by Meadow (1990) and Schmitt (1982) will reveal the type of day wetting and questionnaires developed by Butler (1993a) will reveal parental attitudes and concerns, particularly those relating to the development of intolerance. Baseline measures (Butler, 1993b; Meadow, 1990) are also important to build up a picture of frequency and severity of wetting. A number of diagnostic interview schedules have been developed to assess general psychopathology in children and adolescents, which also includes a section to measure enuresis. One such example is the Diagnostic Interview Schedule for Children (Costello *et al.*, 1984) (Table 11.3).

Nocturnal Enuresis

Butler (1993a) advocates a thorough joint parent-child assessment to elucidate factors which might influence the form of treatment intervention. Factors to cover include family structure, family disruption, wetting history, spontaneous waking, consequences of wetting, associated problems and the child's lifestyle. Additionally, parental and child attitude and beliefs are explored, because these can predict how well a child will respond to treatment (Butler, 1994). A baseline measure will additionally prove helpful, particularly if this is completed prior to a first appointment, as this may encourage families to "opt in" to treatment.

Table 11.3 Examples of question from a diagnostic interview schedule

Instruments	Examples of questions	Coding options			
DISC (Costello et al., 1984)	During this time, have you wet the bed at night?	0	1	2	9
	IF YES, A. Has this happened at least once a month?	0		2*	9
	IF YES, B. How about twice a month?	0		2*	9
	C. Since [NAME EVENT/MONTH], has this happened 6 or more times?	0		2*	9
	IF YES, D. How about 12 or more times?	0		2*	9
	IF YES (2*) TO A, B, C, OR D, ASK:				
	E. Does wetting the bed upset you a lot?	0	1	2	9
	F. Does wetting the bed get in the way of your doing things with others, such as spending the night away from home?	0	1	2	9
	G. Does it cause problems for you at home?	0	1	2	9
	H. Have other kids made fun of you for this?	0	1	2	9
	I. Does it cause problems for you at [school/work]	0		2	8	9

Note: 0 = no; 1 = sometimes/somewhat; 2 = yes; 8 = not applicable; don't know

TREATMENT

Enuresis

Psychological Intervention

Children with both nocturnal enuresis and daytime wetting should be helped at first to develop daytime bladder control. Schmitt (1982) provides written instructions for parents which can prove enormously beneficial. The aim must be to increase bladder sphincter awareness and control. The methods discussed below relate to the treatment of urge incontinence as this is the most familiar day wetting encompassed by clinicians. These include:

Reassurance, support, demystification. As with nocturnal enuresis and faecal soiling the best results occur when children feel relaxed, supported, praised for succeeding, understand the basis of treatment and expectation of success. Meadow (1990) recommends practical advice particularly with washing clothing and using fungicidal powder as it is stale, not fresh, urine, which causes an unpleasant odour. For children who show resistance wetting Schmitt (1982) advises the discontinuation of punishment, or overprompting and a structured way of delivering positive reinforcement for success.

Increase fluid. This provides the opportunity for the child to practise bladder control and reduce the frequency of UTI (Schmitt, 1982).

Encourage toileting regularly. Particularly for children with urge incontinence it seems imperative to encourage toilet use regularly or when the urge is felt. Bladder stretching (increasing interval between toileting) and retention control training (holding before voiding) should be avoided because they are counterproductive and prevent the child responding quickly to bladder sensations which is the required response (Meadow, 1990; Schmitt, 1982). Children should be encouraged to take responsibility for toileting regularly rather than become dependent upon parental prompts which may also be perceived by the child in an aversive way. For younger children, parents may prompt in a non-direct fashion to raise the child's awareness of bodily cues (e.g., postures) as an indication of the need to toilet (Fielding *et al.*, 1978). Meadow (1990) recommends toileting every 90 minutes to begin with and suggests the use of a kitchen timer or wrist watch alarm to alert the child when it is time to go. Such a programme is supported by the work of Halliday *et al.* (1987) where in a controlled trial, a contingent alarm (sounding when the child wet) was found to be no more effective than a non-contingent alarm (sounding at intermittent intervals). Meadow (1990) suggests regular toileting in this way enables children to achieve bladder awareness and reliable dryness 4–8 weeks.

Stream interruption.   Schmitt (1982) suggests this exercise suppresses the bladder spasm and improves control over the bladder sphincter. It involves the child attempting to stop the stream of urination whilst voiding, counting to ten and then resuming voiding. This might be used on each toilet visit and, with boys, a ping pong ball in the toilet can add some interest.

Positive reinforcement.   This might include social reinforcers (e.g., praise) or stars for a younger child when success is achieved. Success might be defined as those behaviours which the child performs which increase the chances of being dry (e.g., regular toileting) or the achievement of dryness itself.

Responding to accidents.   Parental responses should be non punitive and based on encouraging the child to take some responsibility for changing him/herself (Schmitt, 1982).

Cognitive bladder training (biofeedback).   For children who fail to respond to the more straightforward management programmes described, Van Gool and De Jonge (1989) propose intense training in bladder awareness. They argue that children with urge incontinence need to recognise the first sensations of urge, develop means of central inhibition, and learn to void with a relaxed pelvic floor, and they can achieve this through biofeedback using signals of urine flow rate and pelvic floor electromyogram. Their results are impressive, with 60% of 93 children overcoming the detrusor overacting and wetting and a further 22% finding an improvement in the symptoms. The findings suggest both detrusor over activity and urethral overactivity are to some extent results of inappropriate learning processes, triggered or aggravated by UTI. Such intensive training must remain with professionals specialising in this field (Meadow, 1990).

Pharmacotherapy

Meadow (1990) maintains there is no convincing evidence for the effectiveness of any medication for day wetting. However, Oxybutinin is widely used and recommended by Borzyskowski and Mundy (1987), and double blind studies by Thompson and Lauvetz (1976) and Baigrie *et al.* (1988) show it to be effective in reducing day wetting. Van Gool and De Jonge (1989) suggest the anticholinergic drugs offer little advantage in the long term, as relapse tends to occur with withdrawal of medication, but indicate they may have a use in short term trial or as an adjunct to other behaviourly based treatment programmes.

Predictors of Outcome

Many aspects of service delivery can adversely affect treatment outcome of nocturnal enuresis (Butler, 1994) yet the most obvious is lack of supervision during treatment and follow up, which has been demonstrated to lead to drop out (Dische, 1973), failure (Houts *et al.*, 1994) and relapse (Bollard and Nettelbeck, 1981). A model of supervision proposed by Morgan (1993) in his influential "Guidelines on Minimum Standards" is regular 2–3 weekly contact during treatment and an arrangement whereby assistance can be provided between appointments, when necessary.

Butler (1993b) outlines an approach to improving clinical practice. This includes the *abandonment of lifting and fluid restriction* which is practised by some 97% and 88% of families, respectively (Butler *et al.*, 1986), yet which enhance the continuation of bed wetting; the encouragement of reassuring, supportive and patient *parental involvement* with removal of intolerant attitudes; *the involvement of the child* through explanation of bladder functioning, demystification of the deep sleep theory, building on the attempts and efforts already tried to achieve dryness, taking responsibility for wetting episodes, and encouraging the child's choice over treatment inventions; development of *positive reinforcement* for behaviours which improve the child's chances of achieving bladder control (e.g., Van Londen *et al.*, 1993); establishing good *record keeping*; developing *child focused* assessment and treatment interventions; and *tailoring treatment* to the child's needs.

Houts *et al.* (1994) highlights how differences in outcome criteria between medication where management of enuresis is the aim and reduction in bed wetting frequency the measure, and alarm based treatment where cessation of wetting is the aim and achievement of bladder control the measure, has made comparison between the two treatment methods difficult to interpret. Butler (1991) has proposed a set of working definitions for initial success, failure, drop out, continued success and complete success, which should lead to standardarised and comparable means of measuring treatment effectiveness.

Nocturnal Enuresis

A vast array of treatment interventions have been advocated. Under rigorous scrutiny, only the enuresis alarm and pharmacological measures have proved consistently effective. Other interventions may be recommended as adjuncts to the enuresis alarms, and some programmes, such as dry bed training (Azrin *et al.*, 1974) and full spectrum home training (Houts *et al.*, 1986) have incorporated such interventions into training packages. Dry bed training is an intensive programme involving waking schedules, positive practice following a wetting episode, social reinforcement, increased fluid intake and cleanliness training (Azrin *et al.*, 1974). Full-spectrum home training is a manual guided package involving retention control training, cleanliness training and overlearning (Houts *et al.*, 1986). Both programmes employ the enuresis alarm, and component analysis reveals the alarm to be by far the most effective component of such packages (Houts *et al.*, 1986).

Psychological Intervention

The Enuresis Alarm. The essential principle is to alert and sensitise the body to respond quickly and appropriately to a full bladder during sleep, to convert the signal from one of urination to the exact opposite response — that of inhibition of urination and waking (Baller, 1975). Theoretical interest resides in the learning paradigm which was originally considered to be classical conditioning (Mowrer and Mowrer, 1938). Other principles are now thought to be involved, including avoidance conditioning (Lovibond, 1972), the development of an increased functional bladder capacity (Houts, 1991), increased production of anti-diuretic hormone (Houts, 1991), alteration of social and motivational factors (Azrin *et al.*, 1974), and increased expectancy (Butler, 1987).

Johnson (1980) reviewed early uncontrolled studies of the enuresis alarm and found a good rate of initial success (35–100%), but with reports of up to 40% drop out and 56% relapse. Reviews of controlled studies suggest the alarm is the most effective intervention compared with other treatment methods. It can be expected to enable 65–70% of children to achieve nocturnal bladder control, the duration of treatment averages around 5–12 weeks, and relapse following treatment may be of the order of 30% (Doley, 1977; Forsythe and Butler, 1989; Johnson, 1980).

The standard pad and bell alarm with mat(s) placed on the child's bed, has recently received competition from the body worn alarm, which consist of a lightweight alarm box worn by the child and connected to a small sensor. There are a few varieties of such alarm (Butler, 1994). Whilst they remain as effective as the pad and bell (Butler *et al.*,1990a; Fordham and Meadow, 1989), they appear to enable children to respond quicker. They also have advantages over the pad and bell in terms of face validity (the child is often woken before the bed becomes wet), preventing sabotage, and have consumer acceptability (Butler, 1994).

Pharmacotherapy

Only three types survive as effective interventions following vigorous evaluative trials — the tricyclic antidepressants (imipramine) which acts on the brain and bladder, the synthetic analogue of vasopressin (desmopressin) which influence kidney functioning and the anticholinergics (oxybutinin) which affect bladder functioning.

The most favoured in clinical practice, because of reduced side effects, is desmopressin (Houts *et al.*, 1994). Norgaard *et al.* (1989) found evidence of a lack of circadian vasopressin release in older enuretic children which resulted in an inability to reduce urine volume at night and thus the child's bladder capacity is exceeded. What Moffatt *et al.* (1993) point out, however is that for a child to be enuretic, not only must the bladder's capacity be exceeded, but the child must also fail to arouse from sleep at that point. Thus, whilst desmopressin may reduce urine volume, and enable children to stay dry, there is no evidence it helps children become aware of bladder sensations. The effect of administration of desmopressin is immediate (Terho, 1993), wetting frequency is reduced, cessation of wetting for 2 weeks whilst taking medication is around 25% (Moffatt *et al.*, 1993), prolonged use of desmospray does not increase effectiveness (Evans and Meadow, 1992) and removal of medication provokes relapse in most children (Moffatt *et al.*, 1993; Rittig *et al.*, 1989; Terho, 1991). In a comparison with the alarm, Wille (1986) found desmopressin had a superior initial response rate, inferior long term success rate and greater chance of relapse following treatment termination.

Because of these results, it has been suggested that desmopressin has a place in the treatment of childhood nocturnal enuresis where a rapid response is required, for example, under adverse social circumstances and developing maternal intolerance (Butler, 1994), to enhance the child's confidence when sleeping away from home, with the older child who has failed with alarm treatment and in combination with the alarm treatment (Sukhai *et al.*, 1989).

Other Interventions

These may be considered as adjuncts to the alarm, to be employed where appropriately indicated. Butler (1992) has described a range of such interventions and how they might be most effectively employed. They include: (i) *Customary routines* such as cleanliness training to enhance the child's responsibility (Azrin *et al.*, 1974), active responsibility to encourage active participation and a feeling of being instrumental in change (Marshall *et al.*, 1973) and counselling and support to reassure, educate, demystify and avoid blame (White, 1971). (ii) *Bladder training*, which involves retention control training to increase functional bladder capacity (Fielding, 1980), sphincter control to strengthen the bladder sphincter and pelvic floor muscles (Bennett *et al.*, 1985) and bladder stretching to prolong the duration between voiding (Starfield, 1967). Retention control training involves increased fluid intake, a request of the child to resist toileting for as long as possible and at the point of voiding are encouraged to postpone voiding for as long as possible (Fielding, 1980). Although often recommended, particularly for children with both daytime and nocturnal wetting, and an indication that it increases functional bladder capacity (Doleys *et al.*, 1977), there is little evidence that it increases the child's ability to stay dry at night (Fielding, 1980). (iii) *Arousal techniques.* Such as positive practice which aims to strengthen the desired response of waking and toileting (Azrin *et al.*, 1974), waking schedules to encourage arousability from sleep (e.g., Young, 1964) and self awakening which seeks to internalise the waking response (Schmitt, 1990). (iv) *Increased cognitive* awareness involving auto suggestion which aims to develop a preparedness to respond to bladder signals (Butler and Parkin, 1989), development of internal attributes for success (Butler, 1987) and visualisation, which employs imagery as a vehicle for establishing bladder control (Butler, 1993b); and (v) *Overlearning* to strengthen the detrusor muscles with increased fluid intake in order to prevent relapse (Morgan, 1978).

Decisions regarding treatment intervention should be made in light of the child's needs and wishes but also in cognizance of the principles of an expectation of a spontaneous recovery rate of approximately 15% a year (Forsythe and Redmond, 1974), the need for minimal side effects (Fitzwater and Macknin, 1992) and selection of interventions with proven effectiveness rates (Butler, 1994).

Predictors of Outcome

An understanding of pre-treatment factors which influence outcome can assist greatly in selecting the type of treatment intervention. With the enuresis alarm, a range of variables have proved important. Drop out is significantly increased where there is maternal intolerance (Butler *et al.*, 1988; Morgan and Young, 1975; Wagner *et al.*, 1982), behavioural problems (Wagner and Johnson, 1988) and a negative self image on the child's part (Butler *et al.*, 1994; Geffken *et al.*, 1986). Butler (1994) has suggested medication might be most appropriately employed initially in such circumstances in order to promote the child's confidence, reduce maternal intolerance and encourage attendance at clinics. *Failure* is increased where there is unsatisfactory housing (Dische *et al.*, 1983), family discord and stress (Devlin and O'Cathain, 1990), daytime wetting (Fielding, 1982; Houts *et al.*, 1994) and where the child construes the enuresis as having positive implications (Butler *et al.*, 1990b). *Relapse* is more likely in cases of secondary enuresis (Butler *et al.*, 1990c; Butler *et al.*, 1990b), multiple wetting (Finley *et al.*, 1982), and associated daytime wetting (Bollard, 1982; Fielding, 1980).

With desmospray, the chances of success are increased with the older child (Rittig *et al.*, 1989), where there is high morning osmolality (Dimson, 1986), with children already achieving some dry nights (Pederson *et al.*, 1985), where there is a family history of enuresis (Hogg and Husmann, 1993) and in cases of primary rather than secondary enuresis (Moffatt *et al.*, 1993).

Faecal Soiling

Levine (1982) has outlined the aims of treatment: independent regular toileting; reduced stool retention; optimal neuromuscular bowel function; and alleviation of the emotional scars. Most clinicians advocate a comprehensive assessment to delineate the type of soiling and thus develop treatment programmes tailored to the child and family's needs (Boon and Singh, 1991). Given that the most common form of faecal soiling is of the retention with overflow type, treatment methods will be discussed with this as a frame of reference.

An interesting claim made by Swanwick (1991) is that many children with encopresis can be managed within General Practice and there is good reason to support this contention. It appears however that General Practitioners may be put off by the psychoanalytical theories proposed to account for the aetiology. These suggest that encopresis is a symptom representing some underlying unconscious conflict. The power struggles between child and parent that often develop during toilet training have been well described by Anthony (1957), Levine (1982) and Hersov (1994), yet Fielding and Doleys (1988) coherently

argue against the view that such "battles" become the source of unconscious conflicts. Most children tend to be seen clinically in out-patient
settings, although more severe and resistant cases tend to be admitted
for in-patient treatment. Levine (1982) identifies the criteria for hospitalization as severe stool retention, disturbed or punitive parent-child
relationships where treatment interventions might be adopted in a coercive manner, and where there are questions about the parents' ability to
manage the treatment programme.

The predominant view regarding effective intervention for children
with faecal soiling supports a collaborative medical-psychological
approach. Components of effective programmes can be summarized as
follows:

Reassurance.   A positive and non accusatory approach needs fostering throughout (Levine, 1982). Some of the major themes to emphasize are that the child is not alone with the problem, and that it is highly
likely other children in the child's school will have similar difficulties;
that the child should not feel on trial when discussing the problem; that
the child and parents are not to blame for what has happened; that it is
usually the case that most children will develop a pattern of appropriate defecation with help.

Demystification.   Levine (1982) has raised awareness of the need
to help children understand their problem, advocating the use of draw-
ings to portray the mechanism of stretched out bowels which have lost
sensation and muscle tone. Explanations of the function of the bowel is
also stressed by Blackwell (1989). Levine (1982) further emphasizes the
need to provide a plausible explanation for the child's retention, utilizing a metaphor of accumulating "rocks" or waste which become
impacted, forcing the muscles to stretch and weaken to the point of
being unable to push the "rocks" out. The stretching also causes the
nerves to stretch, preventing them responding properly and thus the
child fails to get a warning of a need to visit the toilet.

Parental support.   This means both offering parents support and
advice, plus encouraging their supportive involvement with the child.
As Levine (1982) again illustrates, parents are likely to require a considerable amount of support to co-exist with a child who soils. They
require advice and help in terminating all coercive measures and punitive reactions and support in refraining from anger and frustration. As
Blackwell (1989) points out these will only service to exacerbate the
soiling. Accidents should be handled as far as possible in a matter of
fact way (Houts *et al.*, 1988). Parental concerns that the child has diarrhoea because of evidence of "seepage" need to be addressed otherwise

they may encourage a "binding" diet which will exacerbate the constipation (Blackwell, 1989). A noticeable source of frustration for parents is their difficulty in understanding how their child can "live" with the smell, which can evoke parental beliefs that the child is not bothered, or lazy. Levine (1982) invites parents to consider that children get accustomed to the smell in the way that people have difficulty in detecting their own bodily odours, because of the way the olfactory sensory apparatus accommodates to odours that are present incessantly. Finally parents may be encouraged to develop patience because relief from soiling, even with the most effective treatment interventions, may take some months (Blackwell, 1989).

Child responsibility. Most authors suggest that the child should be encouraged to take some responsibility for washing themselves and placing soiled clothing in the laundry following an accident but that the child should not be expected to launder the clothing (Houts *et al.*, 1988; Levine, 1982). Additionally children should have the opportunity to discuss with the clinician all aspects of a proposed treatment programme. Their involvement and understanding is vital to the success. Involvement in choices regarding treatment options (such as reinforcement programmes) and understanding of the relevance of each aspect of treatment and the details of how the child is expected to participate.

Co-operation of school. Levine (1982) has highlighted the need for children to have access to toilets with a degree of privacy. This may involve practical issues such as having a change of clothing available and access to a staff toilet, plus fostering a sensitive attitude towards the child's needs whereby requests to use the toilet during lessons are guaranteed.

Clearing the blockage. The aim in clearing the bowel of faeces is to remove the pain and fear of the younger child and prevent gross impaction of faeces (Hersov, 1994). Levine (1982) suggests this is particularly required where children have a functional megacolon, and claims that many treatment failures stem from an incomplete initial clean out. Some clinicians favour enemas to remove the blockage followed by senna laxatives coupled with stool softeners such as docusate or lactuloze to ensure the passage of soft painless stools (Hersov, 1994). Fielding and Doleys (1988) make the point well that normal muscle tone, bowel control and toileting behaviour are unlikely to return by simply removing the impaction. They argue that toileting skills and muscle control may need retraining and it may take some months for the muscle tone to return to normal. There is criticism in the literature about the use of enemas, laxatives and suppositories in the treatment of faecal soiling, except in severe cases of psychogenic megacolon: (i) prolonged use of purgatives may lead to "passive defecation" where the child fails to learn how to initiate appropriate bowel movements, and instead relies on the artificially induced urge to defecate (Doleys *et al.*, 1977); (ii) an emphasis on purgatives may neglect the struggles and disharmony in the child-parent relationship (Hersov, 1994); and (iii) a retrospective account by Gleghorn *et al.* (1991) suggested 94% of children with retention and overflow were successfully treated without the use of enemas.

In a randomized trial comparing behaviour modification with and without laxatives Nolan *et al.* (1991) found the addition of laxatives enabled children to achieve bowel control quicker and success rates at 12 months favoured those who had a combination of laxative plus behaviour modification. Of interest was the high number of children (1 in 8) who failed to comply with the toileting programme and when analysis was performed on the two groups, with the non compliers excluded, there was no statistical difference between those treated with and without laxatives. This study suggests that laxatives may have a place in the treatment of those children who might object to a regular toileting programme.

Diet.   Increases in dietary fibre increase bowel movement in normal and constipated adults (e.g., Graham *et al.* 1982) and many programmes therefore now advocate an increased intake of dietary fibre, such as fruit and cereals containing bran. However Levine (1982) warns of possible increases in parent-child conflict if the child dislikes such additions as bran. Some clinicians also advocate the reduction of milk products (Wright and Walker, 1976), with increased fluid, regular mealtimes and regular exercise to promote regular bowel movements (Blackwell, 1989). Houts *et al.* (1988) subjected a programme of increased dietary intake plus regular toileting to some scrutiny and found it to be very effective for children with retention plus overflow, although they suggest children with functional megacolon would still require initial artificial evacuation before benefitting from the programme.

Regular toileting.   This is almost invariably combined with clearing the blockage and alterations in diet (Levine, 1982). Blackwell (1989) outlines common clinical practice: a warm drink at breakfast; attempt sitting on the toilet after 20 minutes; sit and attempt to defecate (no longer than 10 minutes); ensure toileting is made as pleasant as possible for the child; reduce parental prompting and encourage self-initiated toileting, producing a "handing over" of responsibility.

Reinforcement of appropriate response.   The arrangement of environmental consequences (from praise to reward systems) to initiate and establish appropriate behaviour is the cornerstone of a behavioural approach to the problem (Fielding and Doleys, 1988). The target behaviour may differ for individual children. Houts *et al.* (1988) reinforced dietary fibre intake through arranging a points system for increased fibre consumption plus feedback on a publicly displayed graph. Most clinicians favour a reward system (e.g., points, stars) for appropriate toileting (Neals, 1963) although some advocate rewards for clean pants (e.g., Logan and Garner, 1971) and some a combination of both these (e.g., Doleys *et al.*, 1977).

Most programmes which employ a combination of these methods (with appropriate enemas, softeners, increased fibre diet, regular toileting and reinforcement of appropriate responses) have proved to be generally effective in treating constipation with overflow type soiling (Berg and Jones, 1964; Houts *et al.*, 1988; Levin and Bakow, 1976; McClung *et al.*, 1993). Stark *et al.* (1990) found such programmes could also be effectively conducted within small groups which has cost-effective implications, and Dawson *et al.* (1990) demonstrated the effectiveness of a combined programme in an in-patient setting with severely emotionally disturbed youngsters.

Other interventions. Success has been claimed for paradoxical intention when a child expresses denial of the soiling and takes to hiding the soiled clothing in "embarrassing" places (Knights, 1993). This involves skilled clinical interviewing with a paradox in which the clinician sets up a situation which encourages the child to take control over the bowel by "defeating" the clinician's expectations. Feldman and colleagues (1993) used play with modelling clay as a metaphor for faeces in treating 6 children, 4 of which responded during the session and went 12 months free of soiling. Biofeedback involves a balloon being inserted in the anus which transmits pressure changes to an oscilloscope, visible to the child who attempts to use this information to alter their sphincter responses voluntarily and has been employed by Olness *et al.* (1980) and Benninga *et al.* (1993) with some success. As Hersov (1994) notes, the employment of paradoxical intention, play therapy or biofeedback requires specialist training and does not form the basis of an initial treatment programme.

Predictors of Outcome

The question of identifying which pre-treatment variables might predict successful outcome and/or increase the risk of failure in treatment has received only minimal attention. There appears to be no difference between treatment successes and failures in terms of demographic variables (Landman *et al.* 1983), a result not dissimilar to that with nocturnal enuresis, or with parenting style (Stark *et al.*, 1990). However, two variables have emerged as important predictors: (i) children who fail treatment are more likely to be perceived by their parents as having behavioural problems (Levine and Bakow, 1976; Stark *et al.*, 1990) and thus such children would presumably tend to adopt non co-operative attitudes towards treatment regimes; (ii) children who respond to treatment tend to have a more internal locus of control (Rappaport *et al.*, 1986) which suggests they adopt a belief that the problem and solution is within their control.

CONCLUDING REMARKS

Given the incidence of faecal soiling, day wetting and nocturnal enuresis these conditions might accurately be regarded as amongst the most prevalent of childhood problems, and coupled with the low spontaneous recovery rate, nocturnal enuresis might also be regarded as one of the most chronic. All three problems deserve an integrated medical and psychological approach. Organic causes require screening and classification of most children that remain appear divided between those with a predominant physiological or medical aetiology and those where psychological factors play a major contributory role.

The most common forms — retention with overflow, urge incontinence and monosymptomatic nocturnal enuresis — all require a combined medical and psychological input. Common management themes include reassurance, demystification, encouraging parental support, developing the child's responsibility and reinforcing appropriate responses. The treatment of choice for retention with overflow is clearance of the blockage, consideration of diet and regular toileting; for day wetting it is increased fluid intake, stream interruption and regular toileting; and for nocturnal enuresis the employment of an enuresis alarm coupled with regular monitoring.

Exploration of the impact of soiling, day wetting and bed wetting has interestingly led to similar conclusions. The child fears discovery, tends to feel alone with the problem, sometimes withdraws socially and may suffer low self esteem. Researchers from different perspectives have found the development of parental intolerance with a minority of families in all three conditions, leading to attributions of laziness and lack of effort. The model of intolerance developed within the field of nocturnal enuresis has clear treatment implications — the need to intervene quickly and possibly with medication to avoid the development of increasingly punitive attitudes and drop out from treatment.

This raises the importance of developing accurate pre-treatment predictors of outcome, which will influence the type of treatment intervention prescribed. So far most of the work in this area has been undertaken with nocturnal enuresis, with particularly exciting results in assessing parental and child attitudes. To a large extent drop out from treatment, failure, success and relapse with alarm treatment can be predicted with sensitive pre-treatment measures. The indications are that similar parent and child focused measures are leading to predictors of treatment outcome with faecal soiling. Such findings highlight the importance of discovering and employing sensitive measures to meet the needs of children with elimination problems, but also they recognize the importance of involving both children and parents in both the process of assessment and decision making regarding treatment interventions.

REFERENCES

Allen, T.D. and Bright, T.L. (1978). Urodynamic patterns in children with dysfunctional voiding problems. *Journal of Urology*, **119**, 247–249.

American Academy of Paediatrics. (1980). Excretory urography for evaluation of enuresis. *Paediatrics*, **65**, 644–645.

American Psychiatric Association (1994). *Diagnostic and statistical manual of mental disorders* (4th ed.). Washington, DC: American Psychiatric Association.

Anon (1987). My enuresis. *Archives of Disease in Childhood*, **62**, 866–868.

Anthony, E.J. (1957). An experimental approach to the psychopathology of childhood encopresis. *British Journal of Medical Psychology*, **30**, 146–175.

Azrin, N.H., Sneed, T.J., and Foxx R.M. (1974). Dry-bed training: Rapid elimination of childhood enuresis. *Behaviour Research and Therapy*, **12**, 147–156.

Baigrie, R.J., Kellehaer, J.P., Fawcett, D.P., and Pengelly, A.W. (1988). Oxybutin: Is it safe? *British Journal of Urology*, **62**, 319–322.

Baker, B.L. (1969). Symptom treatment and symptom substitution in enuresis. *Journal of Abnormal Psychology*, **74**, 42–49.

Bakwin, H. (1971). Enuresis in twins. *American Journal of Disease in Childhood*, **121**, 222–225.

Baller, W.R. (1975). *Bed-wetting: Origins and treatment.* New York: Pergaman Press.

Bellman, M. (1966). Studies in encopresis. *Acta Paediatrica Scandinavica*, **170**, 1.

Bemporad, J.R. (1978). Encopresis. In B. Wolman, J. Egon, and A. Ross, (Eds.), *Handbook of treatment of mental disorders in childhood and adolescence* (pp. 143–161). New Jersey: Prentice Hall.

Bennett, G.A., Walkden, V.J., Curtis, R.H., Burns, L.E., Rees, J., Gosling, J.A., and McQuire, N.L. (1985). Pad-and buzzer training, dry-bed training, and stop-start training in the treatment of primary nocturnal enuresis. *Behavioural Psychotherapy*, **13**, 309–319.

Benninga, M.A., Buller, H.A., and Timinau, J.A. (1993). Biofeedback training in chronic constipation. *Archives of Disease in Childhood*, **68**, 126–129.

Berg, I., Fielding, D., and Meadow, S.R. (1977). Psychiatric disturbance, urgency and bacteriuria in children with day and night wetting. *Archives of Disease in Childhood*, **52**, 651–657.

Berg, I. and Jones, K.V. (1964). Functional faecal incontinence in children. *Archives of Disease in Childhood*, **39**, 465–472.

Blackwell, C. (1989). A guide to encopresis. Northumberland Health Authority.

Bloomfield, J.M. and Douglas, J.M.B. (1956). Bedwetting: Prevalence among children aged 4–7 years. *Lancet*, **1**, 850–852.

Bollard, J. (1982). A 2-year follow up of bedwetters treated by dry bed training and standard conditioning. *Behaviour Research and Therapy*, **20**, 571–580.

Bollard, J. and Nettelbeck, T. (1981). A comparison of D.B.T. and standard urine-alarm conditioning treatment of childhood bedwetting. *Behaviour Research and Therapy*, **19**, 215–226.

Boon, F. (1991). Encopresis and sexual assault (letter). *American Journal of Academic Child and Adolescent Psychiatry*, **30**, 509–510.

Boon, F.F. and Singh, N.N. (1991). A model for the treatment of encopresis. *Behaviour Modification*, **15**, 355–371.

Borzyskowski, M. and Mundy, A.R. (1987). Videourodynamic assessment of diurnal urinary incontinence. *Archives of Disease in Childhood*, **62**, 128–131.

Brazelton, T.B. (1973). Is enuresis preventable? In I. Kolvin, R. MacKeith, and S.R. Meadow (Eds.), *Bladder control and enuresis*. London: Heinemann.

Brocklebank, J.T. and Meadow, S.R. (1981). Cure of giggle micturation. *Archives of Disease in Childhood*, **56**, 232–234.

Buchanan, A. (1989). Soiling and sexual abuse. The danger of mis-diagnosis. *Association for Child Psychoanalysis Newsletter*, **11**, 3–8.

Butcher, C. and Donnai, D. (1972). Vaginal reflex and enuresis. *British Journal of Radiology*, **45**, 501–502.

Butler, R.J. (1987). *Nocturnal enuresis: Psychological perspectives*. Bristol: John Wright and Son.

Butler, R.J. (1991). Establishment of working definitions in nocturnal enuresis. *Archives of Disease in Childhood*, **66**, 267–271.

Butler, R.J. (1992). *Nocturnal enuresis: A manual of treatment methods*. Leeds: CMH Services.

Butler, R.J. (1993a). *Enuresis resource pack*. Bristol: E.R.I.C.

Butler, R.J. (1993b). Establishing a dry run: A case study in securing bladder control *British Journal Clinical of Psychology*, **32**, 215–217.

Butler, R.J. (1994). *Nocturnal enuresis: The child's experience*. Oxford: Butterworth Heinman.

Butler, R.J., Brewin, C.R., and Forsythe, W.I. (1986). Maternal attributions and tolerance for nocturnal enuresis. *Behaviour Research and Therapy*, **24**, 3, 307–312.

Butler, R.J., Brewin, C.R., and Forsythe, W.I. (1988). A comparison of two approaches to the treatment of nocturnal enuresis and the prediction of effectiveness using pre treatment variables. *Journal of Child Psychology and Psychiatry*, **29**, 501–509.

Butler, R.J., Brewin, C.R., and Forsythe, W.I. (1990c). Relapse in children treated for nocturnal enuresis: Prediction of response using pre-treatment variables. *Behavioura Psychotherapy*, **18**, 65–72.

Butler, R.J., Forsythe, W.I., and Robertson. (1990a). The body worn alarm in the treatment of nocturnal enuresis. *British Journal of Clinical Practice*, **44**, 237–241.

Butler, R.J. and Parkin, G. (1989). *Eric's wet to dry bedtime book*. Nottingham: Nottingham Rehab.

Butler, R.J., Redfern, E.J., and Forsythe, W.I. (1990b). The child's construing of nocturnal enuresis: A method of enquiry and prediction of outcome. *Journal of Child Psychology and Psychiatry*, **31**, 447–454.

Butler, R.J., Redfern, E.J., and Holland, P. (1994). Children's notions about enuresis and the implication for treatment. *Scandinavian Journal of Urology and Nephrology*.

Christmanson, L. and Lisper, H.O. (1982). Parent behaviour related to bed-wetting and toilet-training as etiological factors in primary enuresis. *Scandinavian Journal of Behaviour Therapy*, **11**, 29–37.

Clark, A.F., Taylor, P.J., and Bhate, S.R. (1990). Nocturnal faecal soiling and anal masturbation. *Archives of Disease in Childhood*, **65**, 1367–1368.

Cooper, C.E. (1973). Giggle micturation. In I. Kolvin, R.C. MacKeith, and S.R. Meadow (Eds.), *Bladder control and enuresis* (pp. 61–65). London: Heinemann.

Costello, A.J., Edelbrock, C., Dulcan, R.K., Kalas, R., and Klaric, S.H. (1984). *Development and testing of the NIMH Diagnostic Interview Schedule for Children.* Rockville, MD: National Institute of Mental Health.

Couchells, S.M., Johnson, S.B., Carter, R., and Walker, D. (1981). Behavioural and environmental characteristics of treated and untreated enuretic children and matched nonenuretic controls. *Journal of Paediatrics*, **99**, 812–816.

Dawson, P.M., Griffith, K., and Boeke, K.M. (1990). Combined medical and psychological treatment of hospitalised children with encopresis. *Child Psychiatry and Human Development*, **20**, 181–190.

De Jonge, G.A. (1973a). The urge syndrome. In I. Kolvin, R.C. MacKeith and S.R. Meadow (Eds.), *Bladder control and enuresis* (pp. 66–69). London: Heinemann.

De Jonge, G.A. (1973b). Epidemiology of enuresis: A survey of the literature. In I. Kolvin, R.C. MacKeith, and S.R. Meadow (Eds.), *Bladder control and enuresis* (pp. 22–29). London: Heinemann.

Devlin, J.B. (1991). Prevalence and risk factors for childhood nocturnal enuresis. *Irish Medical Journal*, **84**, 118–120.

Devlin, J.B. and O'Cathain, C. (1990). Predicting treatment outcome in nocturnal enuresis. *Archives of Disease in Childhood*, **65**, 1158–1161.

Dimson, S.B. (1986). DDAVP and urine osmolality in refractory enuresis. *Archives of Disease in Childhood*, **61**, 1104–1107.

Dische, S. (1973). Treatment of enuresis with an enuresis alarm. In I. Kolvin, R. MacKeith, and S.R. Meadow (Eds.), *Bladder control and enuresis* (pp. 211–230). London: Heinemann.

Dische, S., Yule, W., Corbett, J., and Hand, D. (1983). Childhood nocturnal enuresis: Factors associated with outcome of treatment with an enuresis alarm. *Developmental Medicine and Child Neurology*, **25**, 67–80.

Dodge, W.F., West, F.F., Bridgforth, E.B., and Travis, L.B. (1970). Nocturnal enuresis in 6–10 year old children: Correlation with bacteriuria, proteinuria and dysuria. *American Journal of Diseases of Children*, **120**, 32–35.

Doleys, D.M. (1977). Behavioural treatments for nocturnal enuresis in children: A review of the recent literature. *Psychological Bulletin*, **84**, 30–54.

Doleys, D.M. (1983). Enuresis and encopresis. In T.H. Ollendick and M. Hersen (Eds.), *Handbook of child psychopathology* (pp. 201–226). New York: Plenum Press.

Doleys, D.M., Ciminero, A.R., Tollison, J.W., Williams, C.L., and Wells, K.C. (1977). Dry bed training and retention control training: A comparison. *Behaviour Therapy*, **8**, 541–548.

Doleys, D.M., McWhorter, A.Q., Williams, S.C., and Gentry, W.R. (1977). Encopresis: Its treatment and relation to nocturnal enuresis. *Behaviour Research and Therapy*, **8**, 77–82.

Douglas, J.W.B. (1973). Early disturbing events and later enuresis. In I. Kolvin, R. MacKeith, and S.R. Meadow (Eds.), *Bladder control and enuresis* (pp. 109–117). London: Heinemann.

Essen, J. and Peckham, C. (1976). Nocturnal enuresis in childhood. *Developmental Medicine and Child Neurology*, **18**, 577–589.

Esser, G. (1993). Diagnosis and therapy of functional encopresis. *Kinderärztliche Praxis*, **61**, 104–107.

Evans, J.H.C. and Meadow, S.R. (1992). Desmopressin in bedwetting: Length of treatment, vasopressin secretion and response. *Archives of Disease in Childhood*, **67**, 184–188.

Feehan, M., McGee, R., Stanton, W., and Silva, P.A. (1990). A 6 year follow up of childhood enuresis: Prevalence in adolescence and consequences for mental health. *Journal of Paediatric Child Health*, **26**, 75–79.

Feldman, P.C., Villanueva, S., Lanne, V., and Devroede, G. (1993). Use of play with clay to treat children with intractable encopresis. *Journal of Paediatrics*, **122**, 483–488.

Fergusson, D.M., Horwood, L.J., and Shannon, F.T. (1986). Factors related to the age of attainment of nocturnal bladder control: An 8 year longitudinal study. *Paediatrics*, **78**, 884–890.

Fergusson, D.M., Horwood, L.J. and Shannon, F.T. (1990). Secondary enuresis in a birth cohort of New Zealand children. *Paediatric and Perinatal Epidemiology*, **4**, 53–63.

Fielding, D. (1980). The response of day and night wetting children and children who wet only at night to retention control training and the enuresis alarm. *Behaviour, Research and Therapy*, **18**, 305–317.

Fielding, D. (1982). An analysis of the behaviour of day and night wetting children: Towards a model of micturition control. *Behaviour Research and Therapy*, **20**, 49–60.

Fielding, D., Berg, I., and Bell, S. (1978). An observational study of posture and limb movements of children who wet by day and night. *Developmental Medicine and Child Neurology*, **20**, 453–461.

Fielding, D.M. and Doleys, D.M. (1988). Elimination problems: Enuresis and encopresis. In E.J. Mash and L.G. Terdal (Eds.), *Behavioural assessment of childhood disorders* (pp. 586–623). New York: Guilford Press.

Finley, W.W., Rainwater, A.J., and Johnson, G. (1982). Effect of varying alarm schedules on aquisition and relapse parameters in the conditioning treatment of enuresis. *Behaviour Research and Therapy*, **20**, 69–80.

Fitzwater, D. and Macknin, M.L. (1992). Risk/benefit ratio in enuresis therapy. *Clinical Paediatrics*, **May**, 308–310.

Fordham, K.E. and Meadow, S.R. (1989). Controlled trial of standard pad and bell alarm against mini alarm for nocturnal enuresis. *Archives of Disease in Childhood*, **64**, 651–656.

Forsythe, W.I. and Butler, R.J. (1989). Fifty years of enuretic alarms. *Archives of Disease in Childhood*, **64**, 879–885.

Forsythe, W.I. and Redmond, A. (1974). Enuresis and spontaneous cure rate: Study of 1129 enuretics. *Archives of Disease in Childhood*, **49**, 259–263.

Foxman, B., Burciaga Valdez, R.B., and Brook, R.J. (1986). Childhood enuresis: Prevalence, perceived impact and prescribed treatments. *Paediatrics*, **77**, 482–487.

Fritz, G.K. and Armbrust, J. (1982). Enuresis and encopresis. *Psychiatric Clinics of North America*, **5**, 283–296.

Geffken, G., Johnson, S.B., and Walker, D. (1986). Behavioural interventions for childhood nocturnal enuresis: The differential effect of bladder capacity on treatment progress and outcome. *Health Psychology*, **5**, 261–272.

Gillin, J.C., Rapoport, J.L., Mikkelsen, E.J., Langer, D., Vanskiver, C., and Mendelson, W. (1982). EEG sleep patterns in enuresis: A further analysis and comparison with nocturnal enuresis. *Biological Psychiatry*, **17**, 947–953.

Gleghorn, E.E., Heyman, M.B., and Rudolph, C.D. (1991). No-enema therapy for idiopathic constipation and encopresis. *Clinical Paediatrics*, **30**, 669–672.

Graham, D.Y., Moser, S.E., and Esters, M.K. (1982). The effect of bran on bowel function in constipation. *American Journal of Gastroenterology*, **77**, 599–603.

Hallgren, B. (1956). Enuresis: A study with reference to the morbidity risk and symptomatology. *Acta Psychiatrica et Neurologica Scandinavica*, **31**, 379–403.

Halliday, S., Meadow, S.R., and Berg, I. (1987). Successful management of daytime enuresis using alarm procedures: A randomly controlled trial. *Archives of Disease in Childhood*, **67**, 132–137.

Hersov, L. (1994). Faecal Soiling. In M. Rutter, E. Taylor, and L. Hersov (Eds.), *Child and adolescent psychiatry: Modern approaches* (pp. 520–528). Oxford: Blackwell Scientific Publishers.

Hogg, R.J. and Husmann, D. (1993). The role of family history in predicting response to desmopressin in nocturnal enuresis. *Journal of Urology, 150,* 444–445.

Houts, A.C. (1991). Nocturnal enuresis as a biobehavioural problem. *Behaviour Therapy, 22,* 133–151.

Houts, A.C., Berman, J.S., and Abramson, H. (1994). The effectiveness of psychological and pharmacological treatments for nocturnal enuresis. *Journal of Consulting and Clinical Psychology, 62,* 737–745.

Houts, A.C., Mellon, M.W., and Whelan, J.P. (1988). Use of dietary fibre and stimulus control to treat retentive encopresis: A multiple baseline investigation. *Journal of Paediatric Psychology, 13,* 435–445.

Houts, A.C., Peterson, J.K., and Whelan, J.P. (1986). Prevention of relapse in full-spectrum home training for primary enuresis: A component analysis. *Behaviour Therapy, 17,* 462–469.

Jarvelin, M.R. (1989). Developmental history and neurological findings in enuretic children. *Developmental Medicine and Child Neurology, 31,* 728–736.

Jarvelin, M.R., Huttunen, N.P., Seppanen, J., Seppanen, U., and Moilanen, U. (1990). Screening of urinary tract abnormalities among day and night wetting children. *Scandinavian Journal of Urology and Nephrology, 24,* 181–189.

Jarvelin, M.R., Moilanen, I., Kangas, P., Moring, K., Vikevainen-Tervonen, L., Huttunen, N.P., and Seppanen, J. (1991). Aetiological and precipitating factors for childhood enuresis. *Acta Paediatrica Scandinavica, 80,* 361–369.

Jarvelin, M.R., Moilanen, I., Vikevainen-Tervonen, L., and Huttunen, N.P. (1990). Life changes and protective capacities in enuretic and non-enuretic children. *Journal of Child Psychology and Psychiatry, 31,* 763–774.

Jarvelin, M.R., Vikevainen-Tervonen, L., Moilanen, I., and Huttunen, N.P. (1988). Enuresis in seven year old children. *Acta Paediatrica Scandinavica, 77,* 148–153.

Jehu, D., Morgan, R.T.T., Turner, R.K., and Jones, A. (1977). A controlled trial of the treatment of nocturnal enuresis in residential homes for children. *Behaviour, Research and Therapy, 15,* 1–16.

Johnson, S.B. (1980). Enuresis. In R.D. Daitman (Ed.), *Clinical behaviour therapy and behaviour modification* (Vol. 1, pp. 81–142). London: Garland STPM Press.

Knights, B.W. (1993). *Welcome to poo land: A paradoxical approach to encopresis.* Paper presented at Encopresis study day, North Tyneside.

Koff, S.A. (1982). Bladder sphincter dysfunction in childhood. *Urology, 19,* 457–461.

Lancet (1987) Diurnal enuresis (editorial). *Lancet,* **August,** 314–315.

Landman, G.B., Levine, M.D., and Rappaport, L. (1983). A study of treatment resistance among children referred for encopresis. *Clinical Paediatrics, 23,* 449–452.

Lapides, J. and Diokno, A.C. (1970). Persistence of the infant bladder as a cause for urinary tract infection in girls. *Journal of Urology, 103,* 243–248.

Levine, M.D. (1975). Children with encopresis: A descriptive analysis. *Paediatrics, 56,* 412–416.

Levine, M.D. (1982). Encopresis: Its potentiation, evaluation and alleviation. *Paediatric Clinics of North America, 29,* 315–330.

Levine, M.D. and Bakow, H. (1976). Children with encopresis: A study of treatment outcome. *Paediatrics, 50,* 845–852.

Logan, D.C. and Garner, D.G. (1971). Effective behaviour modification for reducing chronic soiling. *American Annals of the Deaf, 116,* 382–384.

Lovibond, S.H. (1972). Critique of Turner, Young, and Rachman's conditioning treatment of enuresis. *Behaviour Research and Therapy, 10,* 287–289.

MacKeith, R.C. (1964). Micturation induced by giggling. *Guy's Hospital Report, 1113,* 250–260.

MacKeith, R.C., Meadow, S.R., and Turner, R.K. (1973). How children become dry. In I. Kolvin, R. MacKeith, and S.R. Meadow (Eds.), *Bladder control and enuresis* (pp. 3–21). London: Heinemann.

Marshall, S., Marshall, H.H., and Lyon, R.P. (1973). Enuresis: An analysis of various therapeutic approaches. *Paediatrics*, **52**, 813–817.

McClung, H.J., Boyne, L.J., Linshied, T., Heitlinger, L.A., Murry, R.D., Fyda, J., and Li, B.U. (1993). Is combination therapy for encopresis nutritionally safe? *Paediatrics*, **91**, 591–594.

McGee, R., Makinson, T., Williams, S., Simpson, A., and Silva, P. (1984). A longitudinal study of enuresis from five to nine years. *Australian Paediatric Journal*, **20**, 39–42.

Meadow, S.R. (1990). Day wetting. *Paediatric Nephrology*, **4**, 178–184.

Mikkelsen, E.J., Rapoport, J.L., Nee, L., Gruenau, C., Mendelson, W., and Gillin, J.C. (1980). Childhood Enuresis 1. Sleep Patterns and Psychopathology. *Archives of General Psychaitry*, **37**, 1139–1144.

Miller, F.J.W. (1973). Children who wet the bed. In I. Kolvin, R. MacKeith, and S.R. Meadow (Eds.), *Bladder control and enuresis* (pp. 231–245). London: Heinemann.

Moffatt, M.E.K., Harlos, S., Kirshen, A.J., and Burd, L. (1993). Desmopressin acetate and nocturnal enuresis: How much do we know? *Paediatrics*, **92**, 420–425.

Morgan, R.T.T. (1978). Relapse and therapeutic response in the conditioning treatment of enuresis: A review of recent findings on intermittent reinforcement, overlearning and stimulus intensity. *Behaviour Research and Therapy*, **16**, 273–279.

Morgan, R.T.T. (1993). *Guidelines on minimum standards of practice in the treatment of enuresis*. Bristol: ERIC.

Morgan, R.T.T. and Young, G.C. (1975). Parental attitudes and the conditioning treatment of childhood enuresis. *Behaviour Research and Therapy*, **13**, 197–199.

Mowrer, O.H. and Mowrer, W.M. (1938). Enuresis — a method for it's study and treatment. *American Journal of Orthopsychiatry*, **8**, 436–459.

Neals, D.H. (1963). Behaviour therapy and encopresis in children. *Behaviour Research and Therapy*, **1**, 139–149.

Nolan, T., Debelle, G., Oberklaid, F., and Coffey, C. (1991). Randomised trial of laxatives in treatment of childhood encopresis. *Lancet*, **338**, 523–527.

Norgaard, J.P., Pedersen, E.B., and Djurhuus, J.C. (1985). Diurnal antidiuretic hormone levels in enuretics. *Journal of Urology*, **134**, 1029–1031.

Norgaard, J.P., Rittig, S., and Djurhuus, J.C. (1989). Nocturnal enuresis: An approach to treatment based on pathogenesis. *Journal of Paediatrics*, **114**, 705–710.

Olness, K., McParland, F.A., and Piper, J. (1980). Biofeedback: A new modality in the management of children with faecal soiling. *Journal of Paediatrics*, **96**, 505–509.

Oppel, W.C., Harper, P.A., and Rider, R.V. (1968). The age of attaining bladder control. *Paediatrics*, **42**, 614–626.

Pederson, P.S., Hejl, M., and Kjoller, S.S. (1985). Desamino-d-arginine vasopressin in childhood nocturnal enuresis. *Journal of Urology*, **133**, 65–66.

Rappaport, L., Landman, G., Fenton, T., and Levine, M.D. (1986). Locus of control as predictor of compliance and outcome in treatment of encopresis. *Journal of Paediatrics*, **109**, 1061–1064

Redman, J.F. and Seibert, J.J. (1979). The uroadiographic evaluation of the enuretic child. *Journal of Urology*, **122**, 799–801.

Rex, D.K., Fitzgerald, J.F., and Goulet, R.J. (1992). Chronic constipation with encopresis persisting beyond fifteen years of age. *Diseases of the Colon and Rectum*, **35**, 242–244.

Rittig, S., Knudsen, U.B., Norgaard, J.P., Pedersen, E.B., and Djurhuus, J.C. (1989). Abnormal diurnal rhythm of plasma vasopressin and urinary output in patients with enuresis. *American Journal of Physiology*, **256**, 664–667.

Rutter, M. (1976). *Helping troubled children*. Hammonsworth: Penguin.

Rutter, M., Tizard, J., and Whitmore, K. (1970). *Education, health and behaviour*. London: Longman.

Rutter, M.L., Yule, W., and Graham, P.J. (1973). Enuresis and behavioural deviance: Some epidemiological considerations. In I. Kolvin, R. MacKeith, and S.R. Meadow (Eds.), *Bladder control and enuresis* (pp. 137–147). London: Heinemann.

Savage, D.C.L., Wilson, M.I., Ross, E.M., and Fee, W.M. (1969). Asymptomatic bacteriuria in girl entrants to Dundee primary schools. *British Medical Journal*, **3**, 75–80.

Schaeffer, C.E. (1979). *Childhood encopresis: Causes and therapy*. New York: Van Nostrand Reinhold.

Schaffer, D., Gardner, A., and Hedge, B. (1984). Behaviour and bladder disturbance in enuretic children: A rational classification of a common disorder. *Developmental Medicine and Child Neurology*, **26**, 781–792.

Schmitt, B.D. (1982). Day wetting (diurnal enuresis). *Paediatric Clinics of North America*, **29**, 9–20.

Schmitt, B.D. (1990). Efficacy and safety of drugs available for the treatment of nocturnal enuresis. *Drug Investigation*, **2**, 9–16.

Shaffer, D. (1973). The association between enuresis and emotional disorder: A review of the literature. In I. Kolvin, R. MacKeith, and S.R. Meadow (Eds.), *Bladder control and enuresis* (pp. 118–136). London: Heinemann.

Shaffer, D. (1980). The development of bladder control. In M. Rutter (Ed.), *Scientific foundations of developmental psychiatry* (pp. 129–137). London: Heinemann.

Shaffer, D. (1994). Enuresis. In M. Rutter, E. Taylor, and L. Hersof (Eds.), *Child and adolescent psychiatry: Modern approaches* (pp. 505–519). Oxford: Blackwell Scientific Publications.

Sluckin, A. (1975). Encopresis: A behavioural approach described. *Social Work Today*, **5**, 643–646.

Sorotzkin, B. (1984). Nocturnal enuresis: Current perspectives. *Clinical Psychology Review*, **4**, 293–316.

Starfield, B. (1967). Functional bladder capacity in enuretic and non-enuretic children. *Journal of Paediatrics*, **70**, 777–781.

Stark, L.J., Spirito, A., Lewis, A.V., and Hart, K.J. (1990). Encopresis: Behavioural parameters associated with children who fail medical management. *Child Psychiatry and Human Development*, **20**, 169–179.

Stein, Z.A. and Susser, M.W. (1967). Social factors in the development of sphincter control. *Developmental Medicine and Child Neurology*, **9**, 692–706.

Sukhai, R.N., Mol, J., and Harris, A.S. (1989). Combined therapy of enuresis alarm and desmopressin in the treatment of nocturnal enuresis. *European Journal of Paediatrics*, **148**, 465–467.

Swanwick, T. (1991). Encopresis in children: A cyclical modal of constipation and faecal retention. *British Journal of General Practice*, **41**, 514–516.

Terho, P. (1993). Desmopressin in the treatment of nocturnal enuresis in children. *Ferring Literature Service*, **2**, 2–4.

Terho, P. (1991). Desmopressin in nocturnal enuresis. *Journal of Urology*, **145**, 818–820.

Thompson, I.M. and Lauvetz, R. (1976). Oxybutynin in bladder spasm, neurogenic bladder and enuresis. *Urology*, **8**, 452–454.

Van Gool, J.D. and De Jonge, G.A. (1989). Urge syndrome and urge incontinence. *Archives of Disease in Childhood*, **64**, 1629–1634.

Van Gool, J.D. and Tanagho, E.A. (1977). External sphincter activity and recurrent urinary tract infection in girls. *Urology*, **10**, 348–353.

Van Londen, A., Van Londen-Barentsen, M.W.M., Van Son, M.J.M., and Mulder, G.A.L.A (1993). Arousal training for children suffering from nocturnal enuresis: A 2 1/2 year follow up. *Behaviour Research and Therapy*, **31**, 613–615.

Verhulst, F.C., Vander Lee, J.H., Akkerhuis, G.W., Saunders-Woudstra, J.A.R., Timmer, F.C., and Donkhorst, I.D. (1985). The prevalence of nocturnal enuresis: Do DSM-III criteria need to be changed? *Journal of Child Psychology and Psychiatry*, **26**, 989–993.

Vincent, S.A. (1966). Postural control of incontinence: The curtsey sign. *Lancet*, **ii**, 631–632.

Wagner, W.G. and Geffken, G. (1986). Enuretic children: How they view their wetting behaviour. *Child Study Journal*, **16**, 13–18.

Wagner, W.G. and Johnson, J.T. (1988). Childhood nocturnal enuresis: The prediction of premature withdrawal from behavioural conditioning. *Journal Abnormal Child Psychology*, **16**, 687–692.

Wagner, W., Johnson, S.B., Walker, D., Carter, R., and Wittner, J. (1982). A controlled comparison of two treatments for nocturnal enuresis. *Journal of Paediatrics*, **101**, 302–307.

Wagner, W.G. and Matthews, R. (1985). The treatment of nocturnal enuresis: A controlled comparison of two models of urine alarm. *Developmental and Behavioural Paediatrics*, **6**, 22–26.

Warwick, R.T. and Whiteside, G. (1979). Nocturnal enuresis. *Urologic Clinics of North America*, **6**, 255–258.

White, M. (1971). A thousand consecutive cases of enuresis: Results of treatment. *Child and Family*, **10**, 198–209.

Whiteside, C.G. and Arnold, E.P. (1975). Persistent primary enuresis: A urodynamic assessment. *British Medical Journal*, **1**, 364–367.

Wille, S. (1986). Comparison of desmopressin and enuresis alarm for nocturnal enuresis. *Archives of Disease in Childhood*, **61**, 30–33.

Wolters, W.H.G. (1974). *Kindred mid Encopresis*. Utrecht: Elinkivijk.

Woodmansey, A.C. (1967). Emotion and the motions: An inquiry into the causes and prevention of functional disorders of defecation. *British Journal of Medical Psychology*, **40**, 207–223.

Wright, L. and Walker, C.E. (1976). Behavioural treatment of encopresis. *Journal of Paediatric Psychology*, **4**, 35–37.

Young, G.C. (1964). A "staggered-wakening" procedure in the treatment of enuresis. *The Medical Officer*, **111**, 142–143.

Yue, P.C. (1974). Ectopic ureter in girls as a cause of wetting. *Journal of Paediatric Surgery*, **9**, 485–489.

ACKNOWLEDGEMENTS

I am grateful to Amanda Pullan, Julie Kemp, Emma Hiley and Shirley Robinson for their assistance in the writing of this chapter.

CHAPTER **12**

PROGRESS AND UNRESOLVED ISSUES IN DEVELOPMENTAL PSYCHOPATHOLOGY

Joseph A. Sergeant and Pier J.M. Prins

This chapter reviews a number of basic issues in developmental psychopathology. These include the definition of abnormality, the association between disorders, the role of age, maturation and developmental processes in the manifestation, recognition and assessment of childhood disorders. This is not an exhaustive list, but certain key issues which require resolution are addressed.

In the last 25 years, child and developmental psychopathology has come to be considerably more placed upon an empirical basis than hitherto (see the three journals: Development and Psychopathology, Journal of Abnormal Child Psychology, Journal of Child Psychology and Psychiatry). This is partly due to divergent research strategies which include: epidemiological studies, prospective longitudinal studies, the improved methodology in behavioural genetics and psychometrics, the influence of cognitive psychology and behavioural psychopharmacology. We will restrict ourselves in this chapter to primarily the life-span approach to child psychopathology and in passing refer to some of the main issues generated by these other approaches. It is evident, however, that the last 25 years has been a period of data-driven research. For further progress to be made, we believe that a more theoretically oriented type of research will be needed to explain existing data bases and to make testable predictions in future studies. In this sense the primary issue of child psychopathology is how to initiate research based on a theory (or mini-theory) of childhood disorders, which will account for their developmental transitions and for their relation with one another. From longitudinal and genetic research it has become evident that behavioural disorders in children are not random processes but have predictable associations. How can we account for this? Why do some children share and others not share common developmental pathways? The answer to these questions cannot be given here. We raise them, fully aware that it is easier to state a question than to answer it, but in the hope that by asking them, we will be able to suggest what needs to be answered as the building blocks of a future model of child psychopathology. We begin by reflecting upon the first model of psychopathology, namely the definition of abnormality.

DEFINITION OF ABNORMALITY

One of the major unresolved issues in psychopathology (both child and adult) is the definition of abnormality. Current classifications of mental disease (Diagnostic and Statistical Manual of Mental Disorders, fourth edition; DSM-IV, American Psychiatric Association, 1994; p. xxi) define mental disease as a "clinically significant behavioral or psychological syndrome or pattern that occurs in an individual and that is associated with present distress (e.g., a painful symptom) or disability (i.e., impairment in one or more important areas of functioning) or with a significantly increased risk of suffering death, pain, disability, or an important loss of freedom." This definition has sufficient undetermined degrees of freedom that a wide variety of symptoms and disorders can fall under it. For example, crucial terms and qualifications such as "clinically significant" and "distress" are undefined and can result in wide differences in diagnostic practice between clinicians. A restriction in the definition is that the response pattern not be a culturally acceptable response to an event such as bereavement.

Over sixty years ago, the role of culture upon the expression and interpretation of behaviour along a dimension "deviant-normal" was pointed out by Benedict (1934; edition 1959). Progress has been made in the quantification of cultural influences, especially using the dimensional approach to psychopathology. The dimensional approach to abnormality has treated abnormality as a deviation from a statistical average. This contrasts with the inexact nature of mental disorder as conceived from a categorical approach. Here abnormality is conceived of as a cluster of behaviours. For both approaches, the role of cultural factors remains an important issue in psychopathology. Nevertheless, some progress in this area has been made. Using a dimensional approach to quantifying child psychopathology with the Child Behavior Checklist (CBCL), Verhulst (1995) reviewed studies comparing Dutch with American children. He concluded that American and Dutch parents rated children in a rather similar manner on problem behaviours, but not on their competencies. Why problem behaviours and competencies should differ in this manner is not self-evident.

Cultural differences with using the CBCL have, nevertheless, emerged. Higher T-scores on the CBCL, for example, have been reported for Thai compared with American and Dutch children (Weisz *et al.*, 1987). Thai children were rated higher on internalizing problems, particularly somatic complaints. Similarly, Puerto Rican and Australian children were rated higher on some of the scales of the CBCL than both American and Dutch children (Achenbach, 1991a, 1991b). Differences between American samples rated on the CBCL seem to be minor with some Northern European countries (Doepfner *et al.*, 1995; Vermeersch and Fombone, 1995) but are distinctly different in some southern European countries (Fonseca *et al.*, 1995). These results suggest that the psychometric (dimensional) approach has something to offer in terms of cultural comparisons of child psychopathology (see also Fonseca *et al.*, 1994).

Heredity

DSM-IV (APA, 1994; p. xxi) in its definition of mental disorder indicates that whatever the cause, mental disorders are a "manifestation of a behavioral, psychological or biological dysfunction in the individual." While the first two manifestations seem intuitively correct, a biological manifestation does not seem to be a self-evident one. Nevertheless, biological differences associated with development appear a key issue. Heredity has long been an issue in abnormality varying between pure determinism to probabilistic relations. The developmental perspective concerns itself with the intergenerational expression of similar disorders, either through environmental or genetic (heredity) modes of transmission. While not extensively considered in this chapter, it is clear from current behavioural genetics research that the message today is "that widely used environmental measures show significant genetic influence" (Plomin, 1995). The issue is not do genes influence behaviour, nor that genetic factors imply untreatability. Rather the issue concerns expression and variation of disorders within a framework of genetic stability. Plomin (1995) further noted that in the genetic environmental interaction genes may have operation at given points in the developmental process and not at all points. For example, genes do not influence scores on the Bayley Mental Development Index at one year but do so at two years old. Further, some items such as verbal and lexical items show greater genetic influence. A similar issue is, why do two disorders have different levels of intergenerational expression? A recent family study of the relatives of anxiety disordered children indicate an increased rate of anxiety disorders compared with the relatives of psychopathological (Attention-Deficit/Hyperactivity Disorder; ADHD) and "normal" comparison groups.

Even within the general classification "anxiety disorder" there appear to be differences in expression. Panic disorder and obsessive-compulsive disorder appear to have a specific relationship for parents and their children. Psychosocial influences leading to increases in anxiety do not preclude the influence of genetic factors, as individuals may inherit a predisposition to develop anxiety disorders which become evident during different developmental stages. Anxiety disorders may be more likely to occur in individuals with behavioural inhibition, an early temperamental characteristic which may have a significant heritable component (Biederman *et al.*, 1990; Rosenbaum *et al.*, 1992). Recently, a molecular genetic study has been reported in which the D4 transporter gene has been found to have in 40% of hyperactive children significantly longer allele repetitions than in controls (LaHoste *et al.*, 1996). This suggests that at least a subgroup of these children have a high genetic loading. Although studies to date have generated intriguing data, more definitive results await longitudinal studies examining the relationship among multiple anxiety dimensions, temperament, sex-hormone levels, cognitive development, social demands, and self-perception.

Rutter (1994), in this respect, notes that a matter of concern for developmental psychopathologists is the causes of variations in level. Given the same genes, what causes the variation in expression? Similarly, genetic factors play a major role in individual differences in height and the timing of puberty. However, they are not responsible for the very substantial increase in the average height of the population, and the parallel fall in the age of menarche, that has taken place in industrialised countries over the last century. Thus, while genes are given, their behavioural expression is not and the nature of the mechanisms of expression remains an issue for developmental psychopathologists. A difficulty here is in finding environmental and developmental measures which are sufficiently strong to permit the required genetic analysis (Plomin, 1995).

Age, Maturation, and Developmental Appropriateness

For developmental psychopathologists the distinction between normal and abnormal is complicated by developmentally appropriate deviations from the normal average development. Social anxiety for example, may be particularly problematic in adolescent populations. Development of social anxiety is to some extent normal in adolescents. The interpretations of its severity defined in the diagnostic criteria including such qualifications as "almost invariably", "intense anxiety", and "marked distress", become particularly important. More explicit definitions for these elements would be useful. Furthermore, the functional significance of anxiety at particular phases in life may be different. ·

In assessing age-appropriateness versus clinical relevance of children's behaviour the age-appropriateness of the behaviour is normative. Sometimes this means that certain behaviour should disappear with increasing age. As children grow older other behaviours should become evident. Two examples are given: First, children who are younger than three years are accepted to be boisterous. It is only later towards four and five years old that motoric unrest becomes an issue. Even then, motoric unrest in itself only gives rise to problems in particular contexts, such as the classroom or in the neat living room. Hyperactive children can be shown to have motoric unrest even in sleep (Porrino *et al.*, 1984). In this context, the behaviour is not considered problematic. The issue of situational specificity will be addressed later.

The question of developmental appropriateness is also of central importance when assessing possible phobias in children and adolescents, because research indicates that certain fears are age-appropriate (i.e., it is thought "normal" to have certain fears at a young age). Fear of the dark might be considered nonclinically significant in a 4-year-old child, but developmentally inappropriate (and clinically significant) in a 13-year-old. Thus persistence of a fear evident at a younger age into adolescence is considered "inappropriate" and potentially clinically significant. What is clear is that the seriousness of a disorder is partially dependent upon clinical opinion of whether the behaviour in question commenced before a particular age (see DSM-IV, ADHD) or manifests itself at an early age and rather than disappearing, as in normal development, is maintained. For example, many young children have fear of dogs which mitigates with age.

The difficulty in defining and operationalizing "age appropriate" is a considerable one. As noted above, since the development of social anxiety is to some extent normal in adolescents, the interpretation of its severity is defined in the diagnostic criteria by such phrases as "almost invariably", "intense anxiety", and "marked distress", all of which are correct clinical terms but with very poor operationalization. Milestones of normal development might be here more useful, but for these to be useful, researchers and clinicians will need to account for the relative heterogeneity in development of children. Cross-sectional, large scale epidemiological investigations of anxiety symptoms and disorders need to be undertaken to further our understanding of normal versus psychopathological anxiety at different stages across the life span. There are indications that particular stages in the lifespan may have differing "pathological profiles". For example, adolescents with separation anxiety disorder tend to have a different symptom profile than preadolescent children. Preadolescent children tended to present with more symptoms, with an emphasis on unrealistic fears and nightmares about harm to attachment figures, while adolescents meeting criteria tended to do so with minimal symptoms, with school refusal and somatic complaints predominating (Francis *et al.*, 1987; Last, 1991).

An issue which is often overlooked is behavioural transience. Anxiety symptoms which occur during adolescence may be transient responses to developmental challenges. Thus developmental pathologists insist upon a period such as six months or two years before the child's behaviour is considered "diagnostic". However, there are actually no norms which indicate for a particular age, how long behaviour should be expressed to say that it is "diagnostic" at that particular age. The other approach to define abnormality on the basis of norms for particular disorders has also not produced a "golden" standard by which to define deviant behaviour. Added to this is the fact that certain periods of life, such as puberty, are recognised to be turbulent for all children. In a retrospective epidemiological study with adults, the median age of onset of anxiety disorders was shown to be 15 years (Christie *et al.*, 1988). Discrimination of which adolescents cases are truly at risk for adult anxiety disorders versus those with a transient response at this turbulent age will remain a task for future research.

Pervasive versus Situational Features of Disorder

For some time, it has been recognised that some disorders are by their very definition situational in character, for example, dental phobia. Among the externalizing disorders, particularly hyperactivity, strong claims have been made concerning the differential effects of situational versus pervasive hyperactivity. Schachar (1991) argued that it was primarily the pervasive disorder which deemed to be considered the equivalent of European hyperkinesis. He marshalled evidence showing that these children were subject to greater deficits. Differences have been shown in the degree of attention deficit (van der Meere *et al.*, 1991) lower intelligence and poorer psychopathological prognosis (Taylor, 1995) between pervasive and situational hyperactive children. Consequently, the distinction is not merely an academic one. Clearly, situationality versus pervasiveness is an operationalization of severity. The issue is not "Are children pervasive or situationally disordered, but what determines specific versus generalised dysfunction?" The answer to this issue is more relevant than the current practice of selecting children on a dimension of situationality-pervasiveness.

Until this point we have treated disorders as though they are independent and uncorrrelated. We now proceed to consider the relation between disorders and the development of disorders in the context of the Kraepelinian taxonomy and the concept of comorbidity.

KRAEPELIN'S HIERARCHICAL MODEL AND THE CONCEPT OF COMORBIDITY

Historically, psychodiagnostics developed out of medical practice (Kraepelin, 1899). The medical model assumed that psychological dysfunctioning reflected a structural condition, that is to say, a relatively permanent state characterised by a cluster of symptoms. This is referred to as the "categorical model" of psychopathology. When the signs of the disorder were absent, recovery or health was assumed to be present or imminent. The original hierarchical model of psychiatric disorders proposed by Kraepelin and later emphasised by Foulds (1976) suggested that disorders high in the hierarchy were relatively permanent conditions and more serious than those lower in the hierarchy. In addition, disorders high in the hierarchy could contain the symptoms of disorders lower in the hierarchy. On the basis of a single diagnosis such as schizophrenia, it was possible that the patient had not only psychotic symptoms but also depression and/or anxiety symptoms. Symptoms lower in the hierarchy were not given a separate diagnosis but were "explained" by the primary diagnosis, in this example, schizophrenia. In the development of the third edition of the Diagnostic and Statistical Manual of Mental Disorders (DSM-III, APA, 1980) and the subsequent field studies in preparation for DSM-IV, it became evident that the co-occurrence of two disorders was not a matter of chance: some disorders are highly correlated with one another, such as anxiety and depression (Boyd *et al.*, 1984; Brady and Kendall, 1992). The simultaneous association in time of two independent disorders is known as "comorbidity" (Caron and Rutter, 1991). At first, this was conceived in the hierarchical model as a special case. In childhood disorders, epidemiological and field studies showed that two conditions: ADHD and conduct disorder were highly correlated (Loeber *et al.*, 1991). Comorbidity in clinic samples tends to be higher than in community-based samples (children with both depressive and anxiety symptoms may be more likely to present for treatment), leading research based on clinical populations to show higher rates of comorbidity.

The general level of the correlation between ADHD and conduct disorder using exploratory analytic methods has been about 0.6 (Loney *et al.*, 1981; Quay, 1986). More recently, Fergusson *et al.* (1991) using confirmatory factor analysis and data from the Christchurch study (a longitudinal follow-up study of an epidemiologically derived sample of New Zealand children), showed that the correlation between ADHD and conduct disorder was in fact much higher, around 0.9. Despite this, Fergusson *et al.* (1991) concluded that both ADHD and conduct disorder are independent disorders but share overlap in symptoms (see also Abikoff and Klein, 1992). Loeber *et al.* (1991) developed a model in which they argued that ADHD was a general early childhood condition, which changed its form to oppositional defiant disorder and, in some cases, went on to become conduct disorder. From this perspective, the overlap in symptoms (comorbidity) is dependent upon the pathological trajectory of the child and must necessarily show overlap. These empirical facts suggest that a simple hierarchical model of psychopathology is untenable, since the disorders at different levels of the hierarchy are too highly correlated with one another. Further, a more dynamic model of developmental psychopathology is required which reflects the transitions and links along a lifespan pathway of risk and dysfunction. This can be illustrated by the recent report by Loeber's group that ADHD symptoms are predictive of conduct disorder which develops prior to puberty but not of conduct disorder which develops after age 16 (Keenan *et al.*, 1995).

Longitudinal follow-up studies have confronted developmental psychopathologists with the fact that children not only could have comorbid diagnoses, but that they could move from one diagnostic group to another (Anderson *et al.*, 1987). Anderson *et al.* (1987) found that 55% of their sample met criteria for more than one diagnosis and Schmidt and Moll (1995) report changes from one diagnosis to another and back to a former diagnosis. As Ollendick and King (1994, p. 923) put it: "Does comorbidity imply a blurring of boundaries between presumably "distinct" disorders or that disorders are indistinct and part of a more general, "broad" internalizing disorder? Might it be the case that disorders truly coexist in some children and adolescents and that their coexistence carries important implications for recovery and treatment?"

Children often report a heterogeneous rather than a specific anxiety disorder. An explanation for this is that the presence of one anxiety disorder acts as a risk factor for other, different anxiety disorders. These disorders are hypothesised as having the same aetiology, or overlapping symptoms of anxiety disorders resulting in subjects meeting criteria for multiple diagnoses (Kashani and Orvaschel, 1990). Another, more parsimonious explanation, may be that "there is considerable overlap in symptoms among the various DSM anxiety disorders (e.g., avoidant disorder and social phobia, overanxious disorder and generalised disorder); as a result, two or more of the disorders can be diagnosed in a particular child or adolescent at the same time." (Ollendick and King, 1994, p. 918).

Several explanations for the comorbidity between anxiety and depression have been posited. The "unitary model" suggests that anxiety and depression exist on a continuum, with depression at one end and anxiety at the other, and are variants of the same disorder. Brady and Kendall (1992) conclude that, while there is considerable symptom overlap, anxiety and depression syndromes are in fact distinguishable and should be considered separate entities. Anxiety disorders are apparently not simply a consequence of depressive disorders, as anxiety disorders typically predate depression (Kovacs *et al.*, 1989). However, the frequent association between these syndromes suggest a fundamental relationship which has not been fully explicated.

Before closing this section, it might be worth emphasising that comorbidity is not just a theoretical issue. Caron and Rutter (1991) pointed out that the co-occurrence of two childhood disorders may be the precursors of more severe adult disorders. For example, childhood conduct disorder is predictive of adult anti-social personality disorder. Moreover, to illustrate the practical implications of comorbidity, we note that it is well established that methylphenidate can achieve short term modification of hyperactivity (Pelham and Hinshaw, 1992). Taylor and colleagues (1987) found that in boys with disruptive behaviour disorder methylphenidate did not improve behaviour when anxiety was also present. Pliszka (1989) reported that ADHD children who were also comorbid for anxiety did not have a significant benefit from methylphenidate. Consequently, assessment of associated psychopathology (comorbidity) is important for predicting treatment outcome and argues against use of diagnostic procedures which are restricted to a specific disorder rather than a global assessment.

CONTINUITY (PHENOTYPE VERSUS PSYCHOPATHOLOGICAL DIMENSION)

A concern for child psychopathologists is the validity of diagnostic categories developed to classify adult symptomatology for children. We give here two examples of this issue. The manifestation of aggression in children, for example, differs from that of adults in a variety of ways. A mild form of aggression is childhood temper tantrums, which is a symptom of oppositional defiant disorder. This may involve behaviour which occurs frequently in the average child, but because of its high frequency or intensity is considered to have passed a "clinical" threshold. Developmental norms for anger and aggression are currently unavailable. Therefore, the presence of the "phenotype" is defined by a clinical judgement as opposed to a score on a psychopathological dimension. In order to replace assessment of phenotype by clinical judgement, it will be necessary for developmental psychopathology to give more attention to a theory of emotions (Frijda, 1989) which can explain the (dys)functional significance of emotions. Whether the same degree of behaviours observed in adults may be applicable to the expression of an emotion in children is unclear. It will necessarily involve the study of emotions in children (Harris, 1989).

A second example concerning the generation of a developmentally appropriate classification scheme for children comes from the role of somatic complaints in anxiety disorders. Research on somatic complaints in anxiety-disordered children suggests that stomach aches and headaches are the two most frequently offered symptoms. Recent research indicates that many of the somatic complaints described in the DSM-diagnosis "generalised anxiety disorder" hardly occur with young children or adolescents! This diagnosis is seldom given to large groups of children referred for anxiety disorder.

These two examples raise the issue of the validity of many (in particular) adult diagnostic categories of various subtypes of anxiety disorders for children. Somatic equivalents of anxiety disorders in paediatric clinics, such as gastro-intestinal symptoms and headaches should be identified and studied. "Worrying about future events" appears to be the hallmark of the disorder in both children and adolescents, whereas wor-rying about past events (another criterion of the disorder) is frequently seen among adolescents, but not in young children. The importance of temporal perception in young children (their ability to deal with the concept of "past" as opposed to "future") has received little attention in the design of instruments and diagnostic procedures. This is obviously a matter requiring urgent diagnostic research, aside from its implications for the formulation of diagnostic criteria.

Continuity/Discontinuity

In the discussion of the significance of comorbidity above, we noted that an underlying assumption of many developmental psychopathologists is that there may be (and there is evidence to support this position) conti-nuity rather than the discontinuity of disorders from childhood to adult-hood. Where previously the continuity versus discontinuity issue was polarised, it is currently recognised that this dimension has validity and that there are differences between anxiety which emerges in childhood and progresses into adulthood versus anxiety which is peculiar to child-hood. Similarly, several investigations have demonstrated that obsessive-compulsive disorder begins in childhood in one third to one half of adult cases (Berg *et al.*, 1989). The clinical picture for obsessive-compulsive disorder in adolescents has been found to be similar to that of adults (Last and Strauss, 1989). In other words, there is for obsessive-compulsive dis-order, at least in some cases, continuity between childhood and adult dis-orders. The developmental or longitudinal approach to understanding psychopathology, in contrast to early psychometric models of psy-chopathology, does not presume constancy or similarities in the presen-tation of mental disorders throughout the life span. Rather, as individuals continue to grow and change (physically, socially, and cognitively), the manifestations of psychopathology are expected to vary (Last, 1993).

There is some degree of continuity between childhood, adoles-cence, and adulthood psychopathology. Some anxiety symptoms increase from childhood to adolescence, including panic attacks and obsessive-compulsive disorder. Anxiety symptomatology occurring during adolescence, like other developmental phases, may be transient responses to developmental challenges (Achenbach, 1990). There may be a relationship between separation anxiety disorder during childhood or adolescence and the later emergence of adult panic disorder with agoraphobia. The characteristics of these disorders do overlap in some ways, including avoidance of being alone and less anxiety when with an attachment figure. There may be a latent period or a period of transition between the manifestations these two disorders, with symptoms of agoraphobia emerging in these same individuals in late adolescence or early childhood. Controlled longitudinal studies of children with sep- .aration anxiety through adolescence and into adulthood are needed to empirically determine whether or not separation anxiety predicts agoraphobia (Thyer, 1993).

The developmental approach to psychopathology does not presume constancy or similarities in the presentation of mental disorders throughout the life span. The life span approach concerns itself with predictive links between different developmental stages. Do childhood disorders predict disorders in adolescence or adulthood? We will discuss this issue in terms of both the life-span approach to psychopathology, and the issue of stability.

Questions addressed by this approach are for example: Does ADHD with conduct disorder have a poorer prognosis than ADHD without conduct disorder? Recently, Taylor (1995) indicated that the answer to this question is dependent upon whether one uses data derived from clinical or epidemiological research and upon the age at which a cohort is studied. There seem to be two contrasting positions on the developmental significance of ADHD. One position, Taylor points out, is that attention deficit disorder symptoms in themselves are the key to outcome (Gittelman *et al.*, 1985). Only those children with the clinical diagnosis are at risk, while subthreshold levels of disturbance are not associated with the same kinds of adverse outcome. The contrasting position, Taylor suggests, stems from epidemiological studies. Risk appears in these studies to be associated with quite minor degrees of elevation of rated ADHD (e.g., Fergusson *et al.*, 1991; McGee *et al.*, 1987). Taylor (1995) argued that children with ADHD who had been identified from clinical records as hyperactive were even more at risk than a group of children referred at the same time for psychiatric help — usually because of conduct disorder. Despite this, many children grow out of ADHD, although the proportion of children who do so is still a matter of some controversy (see Barkley, 1990). Those who persist are likely to show an explosive or an immature kind of personality, rather than a formal psychiatric illness. More information concerning which child develops in a more normalised fashion as opposed to a disordered one is required.

Several reviewers have pointed to the developmental significance of ADHD, conduct disorder and their correlation (Hinshaw, 1987;

Schachar, 1991). Taylor (1995) argued that it is not yet clear whether ADHD is still a risk factor when one allows for comorbidity with oppositional/defiant symptomatology. An epidemiological study of 7 year-old boys by Taylor *et al.* (1991) suggested that children rated as hyperactive but not defiant were at risk for both hyperactivity and defiance aggression nine months later; while children who were defiant but not hyperactive were at risk for defiant aggressive symptoms later but not for hyperactivity. This finding contrasts with that of Fergusson and Horwood (1993). These New Zealand researchers used latent dimension analysis of the Christchurch epidemiologically defined cohort. They found that children with aggression/ defiance were at risk for antisocial behaviours and criminality later in adolescence. However, children with attention deficit symptomatology were not. Children with ADHD were, unlike the defiant aggressive child, more often at risk for poor educational outcomes. Taylor (1995) suggests that one possible resolution of these discrepant findings is to suppose that the risk factors interact in different ways at different points in the life span. In earlier childhood, ADHD is a risk for later conduct disorder; but the risk is completely expressed by the age of about 8 or 9 years. Thereafter — during the period studied by Fergusson and Horwood (1993) — the two types of disorder pursue different developmental pathways. Some support for this argument may be found in the recently reported finding that hyperactive-attention symptoms predict the onset of conduct disorder before but not after puberty (Keenan, *et al.*, 1995).

Prospective, longitudinal studies are the most empirically rigorous means for assessing pathways and "predictive links", i.e. the course and outcome of disorders. Such studies are costly and time-consuming and therefore rarely done. However, follow-up studies of children are essential for most of the issues discussed here. Last and colleagues (1992) recently completed a blind, controlled, follow-up study of clinically referred anxiety-disordered children. Children were reassessed every 12 months for 3 to 5 years to determine clinical course and prognosis (outcome) as the children entered adolescence and young adulthood. Analyses indicate that most of the anxiety disordered youngsters were free from their initial anxiety disorders at follow-up. The findings did not support, in contrast to adult research (Lechman *et al.*, 1984), the notion that anxiety disordered children are at increased risk for depressive disorders. The risk was equally low among the anxiety disordered probands, a psychopathological control group of ADHD children, and a "normal" control group who were never psychiatrically ill children.

A related finding concerns the relation between separation anxiety disorder and generalised anxiety disorder. The hypothesis that childhood separation anxiety disorder is a risk factor for the development of adult-onset panic disorder has appeared in the clinical literature for decades. Current empirical data on the whole do not support such a relationship (Last, 1993). This is also true for childhood and adolescent overanxious disorder and adult-onset generalised anxiety disorder.

Another line of enquiry has been to assess the relative risk of a disordered child for developing other forms of anxiety disorder. Recent prospective follow-up study of DSM-III-R (APA, 1987) diagnosed anxiety-disordered children indicated that these children were at increased risk for developing additional (new) anxiety disorders relative to normal (never psychiatrically disturbed) children, but that they did not significantly differ from psychopathological control (ADHD) children in risk rates. Thus, it is possible that anxiety disorders are equally likely to develop in adolescents and adults with a childhood history of any type of psychiatric disorder, not specifically those with a childhood history of anxiety disorder. Given the relatively young ages of the children, further extended follow-up may reveal a different pattern of results as the children enter late adolescence and early adulthood. Consequently, the picture which is emerging may be one of stability and continuity between childhood and adult psychopathology, but not a specific continuity between a particular childhood and adult disorder.

We discuss in the following sections the issue of stability followed by the issue of risk and protective factors.

Stability

Using the CBCL Achenbach (1991a) reported respectable stability coefficients for symptoms. One may note that around 50% of the internalizing and externalizing disorders (see below) have been reported to be stable over time (Ollendick and King, 1994). Clearly, this stability coefficient is indicative of a considerable fluctuation either in individuals and/or disorders and could possibly be related to age. Ollendick and King (1994, p. 921) remark: "For a significant number of children, early behavior problems portended negative future outcomes; yet the pathways were not always direct, as some children left but then re-entered the deviant score range. For a significant minority, the problems desisted". The factors generating persistence as opposed to termination are presently poorly known and are an unresolved issue. Nevertheless, the literature does contain some suggestions. For example, it has been found that family dysfunction and poor peer relations were related to persistence of disorders four years later. This was independent of the type of disorder. In contrast, low income, but not family dysfunction or peer relationship difficulties at the first measurement point were related to onset of new disorders during this interval, independent of the type of disorder (Offord *et al.*, 1992).

Cantwell and Baker (1989) showed that internalizing disorders were characterised by lower rates of stability than externalizing disorders (66% compared with 87%). Nevertheless, considerable persistence within the broad range of internalizing disorders was evident in that study. Offord *et al.* (1992) found that the persistence of emotional disorders in 26.2% of the children could be found over a period of four years. This proportion is lower than that reported by Cantwell and Baker (1989) and may be due to sampling differences between the two studies.

Ollendick and King (1994, p. 923) suggest further that "internalizing disorders are malleable — a significant number of youths escape their risk status in the absence of active treatment and do not show persistent symptoms of internalizing disorders; for a significant minority of children and adolescents, however, internalizing disorders are persistent — stability is evident although the expression of the disorder may change over time." This position is similar to that taken by Taylor (1995), which we noted above. With respect to externalizing disorders, Campbell (1995) in a review of preschool children concluded that serious externalizing disorders identified early in prospective longitudinal research often persist. It may be the case that current data reflect differences in the time point at which studies have sampled or reflect differences in severity, as suggested by Taylor, or that there may be specific risk-protective factors working which expose/protect the one and not the other child. This point is taken up in the section below.

RISKS, PROTECTIVE FACTORS, AND MEDIATING MECHANISMS

Here the unresolved issue is that it is absolutely crucial in the testing of causal hypotheses to go beyond the indexing of risk variables to some postulated mechanism by which risk factors might operate. Rutter (1994) illustrates this point with the broken home. For an understanding of the mixed picture of findings in the literature, it is necessary to go beyond broken homes to the postulated mechanism of marital discord. It is necessary to go on to consider whether, for example, the individual differences in response to discord reflect the extent to which different children are scapegoated or drawn into the family conflict or whether the differences reflect individual differences in vulnerability as a result of some other mechanism. Albeit that no single mechanism of abnormality has as yet been identified, there do appear several hypothetical mechanisms such as sexual abuse, parental rearing, temperament, and interactions (in particular attachment theory). Before addressing these issues we note that in recent years greater attention has been given to the resilience or ability to recover from adverse experiences. This concerns the protective mechanisms which serve as a buffering function. So far, understanding of these mechanisms is distinctly limited, mainly because of the lack of adequate conceptualisation of measurement of which features might operate in this fashion (i.e., modifying the impact of a risk factor rather than having a directly positive effect). Thus we do not treat this area here, although it is clearly an issue for future research and related to the many hypothetical mechanisms of abnormal behaviour.

Considerable attention has been devoted recently to the impact of childhood sexual abuse and its effect upon the psychological health of the victim. Kendall-Tackett *et al.* (1993) reviewed 45 published studies on the subsequent symptomatology of sexually abused children. Analysis indicated that sexually abused children exhibited more sexualized behaviour as well as a range of more global symptoms such as depression, aggression and withdrawal. Compared with other clinically referred children they did not appear to be more symptomatic except for the diagnosis of post-traumatic stress disorder and sexualized behaviour. On the other hand, the absence of symptoms in abused children is significant. The literature suggests that absence of symptoms in abused children may range between 21% (Conte and Schuerman, 1987) and 49% (Caffaro-Rouget *et al.*, 1989). Child sexual abuse appears to be a non-specific risk factor for psychopathology and of equal severity to other childhood conditions.

Another risk factor is the child's temperament. Temperament is the characteristic style of emotional and behavioural response of an individual in a variety of situations (Prior, 1992). In her review, Prior points out that there are a variety of factors associated with temperament: activity, mood, intensity and threshold of response, persistence, approach-withdrawal, adaptability, distractibility, and rhythmicity. Stability of temperament has been shown to vary considerably varying from 0.25 across the first five years of life to 0.82 at ages 5–7 years (Freiberg-Golvan and Prior, 1991). Clusters such as difficult temperament appear to be more stable than specific dimensions. Furthermore, the stability is greater in those who score at extreme ends of a dimension.

Temperament has been used to predict behaviour disorders of various kinds (see for review Prior, 1992). Relationships are generally found to be moderate and indirect (Kyrios and Prior, 1990). Temperament, and this suggests a mechanism that mediates psychopathology, seems to have its effect via interaction with the care-giver. In a study of maternal perception of childhood temperament, Bates (1987) found that difficulties in the first year of life predicted later externalizing disorders in boys (Bates and Bayles, 1988; Bates *et al.*, 1985). Sanson *et al.* (1991) found that maternal ratings of temperamental problems and ratings of the child as being more difficult than the average were weakly associated with later maternal ratings of behaviour problems. Temperament in combination with other risk factors such as perinatal stress, low birth weight, and being a boy have been found to be good predictors of hyperactivity (Sameroff, 1975). The role of biological risk factors in combination with temperament do not appear strong predictors of a specific type of problem behaviour. For example, in a very low birth weight group (biological factor), it was found that the low weight babies differed from controls only on the rating of depression (temperament factor) (Weisglas-Kuperus *et al.*, 1993). Similarly, Sanson *et al.* (1991) retrospectively examined data on temperament and perinatal functioning in ADHD children, while able to make predictions based on temperament, biological data did not differentiate ADHD, aggressive and control children. This seems to suggest firstly that biological risk factors *may be* aspecific for later diagnoses. On the other hand, biological measures such as Magnetic Resonance Imagining has been able to suggest brain loci in which subgroups of ADHD children can be differentiated. For example, it has been recently reported that the attention-impulsivity items of ADHD may be related to the parietal attenton circuit (Filipek *et al.*, 1997) Secondly, the role of environment may be an important explanatory variable in producing differences between studies (Werner and Smith, 1982). Thus biological and temperamental factors may be associated with the probability of risk for developing deviant behaviour but they are neither necessary nor sufficient for doing so.

Another risk factor, noted by Campbell (1995), is negative, inconsistent parental interactional behaviour combined with high levels of family adversity, which are associated with the emergence of problems in early childhood and which persist into school age. However, the severity of the initial problems and family context are related to different developmental outcomes.

Using observational measures, Egeland *et al.* (1990) and Renken *et al.* (1989) found that children of 3 years old with negative affect in interaction with maternal hostility predicted later teacher ratings of child aggression for both boys and girls. Anderson *et al.* (1986) showed that mothers of conduct disordered boys were more negatively interacting with their sons than with boys of similar behaviour. It has been argued by attachment theorists that infants who experience inconsistent, unresponsive or rejecting care develop a sense of worthlessness and regard their caregivers as unreliable and untrustworthy.

The quality of early caregiving will influence the attachment relationship, which, in turn, will have an impact on perception of control and efficacy. Attachment theory (Bowlby, 1973) proposed that parental relationship with the child was crucial in the development of experience and psychological adjustment. Rutter (1995) concluded that attachment theory has had a seminal effect in developmental psychopathology but it remains unclear how distortions in parent-child relationships are a mechanism in the development of psychopathology. The data in support of attachment theory is, according to Campbell (1995), equivocal. Five studies support this notion but only in the context of current family stress. Parenting style: harsh-warm, interested-uninvolved in combination with family adversity such as maternal depression, marital discord, and stressful life events which have been suggested to be aspecific with respect to their effect upon the child (Cowan *et al.*, 1993; Patterson *et al.*, 1989). Nevertheless, it is clear that marital discord is consistently associated with externalizing problems such as conduct disorder, delinquency and aggression (Emery, 1982). As pointed by Grych and Fincham (1992), marital discord is also associated with internalizing symptomatology of children whose mothers are depressed. It would seem, therefore, that both discord and maternal depression may be interactive factors working upon the temperament of the child to produce symptomatology.

Other possible reasons for diversity in outcome include the existence of individual differences in susceptibility to the stress experiences. Study of individual differences in stress responsivity requires conceptualisation of the possible mechanism (or mechanisms) involved, together with a focus on the subsamples in which the process might operate. It is not sufficient to rely solely on the detection of statistical interaction effects. However, with respect to longitudinal studies, a key consideration is that the vulnerability or resistance to stress may sometimes derive from earlier experiences rather than from any constitutional given (Rutter, 1994).

Concluding Remarks

The unresolved issues in developmental psychopathology may be attributed to the lack of a theoretical model which has sufficient parsimony and comprehensiveness to explain the phenomena. In this chapter we have emphasised the definition of abnormality, the association between disorders, the role of age, maturation and developmental processes in the manifestation of psychopathology. In this discussion we offer some concluding remarks.

We have emphasised, firstly, that the definition and the expression of abnormality, a problem shared by both adult and childhood psychopathology, is complicated in clinical developmental research by the complex interaction between biological development and child-parent interaction, which may lead to behavioural transience, stability and either predisposition or protection from life stressors. It is evident that mixed rather than specific disorders are the rule and comorbidity is a critical feature of childhood psychopathology, which has both conceptual and methodological repercussions. Developmental norms are not available for both the majority of disorders as single entities and for the transitions between comorbid disorders. The mundane task of collecting developmental norms for both of these is a primary goal for the area.

Secondly, there is seldom a single cause or a single ultimate outcome or even a single causal pathway (Rutter, 1994). With most types of psychopathology multifactorial causation is operative at most points in the causal chain. In many instances, it is necessary to consider the causes of individual differences in susceptibility to some risk-factor (person-environment interactions), as well as the processes involved in risk mediation. An adequate model of developmental psychopathology should contain a number of characteristics: it should explain the causes, manifestation, development, and therap(y)ies for a disorder. Currently, no single model meets these requirements. What is available is a set of mini-models which tackle specific issues. The absence of a general theory is not particular to developmental psychopathology and can be found in a variety of psychological domains.

Thirdly, we note that, while longitudinal follow-up of a cohort is the best methodological approach to developmental psychopathology, it is the most difficult research strategy in assessing continuity and discontinuity. We have noted that the point at which it is sampled may produce differences between studies. Clear differences exist between studies using clinic versus epidemiologically derived samples. Thus longitudinal follow-up needs to account for both temporal and phenotypic differences, which currently are present in the studies reviewed above. An alternative strategy is cross-sectional research for a specific disorder (McGee *et al.*, 1990). Critics of this strategy note that: "Unfortunately, McGee *et al.* did not track the DSM disorders in those 15 year-old youths who were found to have the same disorders as 11 year-olds. Consequently, we do not know the extent of continuity of specific disorders over time in an individual youth." (Ollendick and King, 1994, p. 920). In reply to this, one can argue that individual patterns will give individual patterns and what, at this stage of the research, would seem necessary, is discovery of relatively stable pathways. However, identification of reasonably stable pathways has not proven an easy matter and follow-up of a German clinical sample of ADHD children has shown wide fluctuation of diagnoses, even in severe cases (Schmidt and Moll, 1995). Thus a key issue at present is whether some (evidently not all) childhood disorders predict specific adult disorders. It is evident that childhood disorders do predict risk for future deviance.

The combination of longitudinal research with behavioural genetic methodology is clearly a powerful research strategy for future developments in psychopathology research. It goes beyond the scope of this chapter to give a detailed description of behavioural genetics. Nevertheless, in the recently published review by Plomin (1995) of this approach, it is clear that one may expect from this approach not only an improvement in our understanding of the role of genetic factors but also how genetics influences the apparent environmental factors.

Fourthly, cross-cultural factors in developmental psychopathology are receiving increasing attention. Comparisons between American and European samples suggest that there are differences but that they are subtle. In contrast, the differences between American and Asian samples seem greater. This may provide the basis for a natural experiment to show the role of rearing practices upon the expression of deviance and should be researched in the future.

Unresolved is, fifthly, the issue of pathological mechanisms. Part of the difficulty here maybe that the models which have been proposed appear to be univariate models but are in fact multi-variate models. That is, at first sight, for example, attachment theory suggests a relatively evident fact but, when investigated, findings are dependent upon a host of variables. A multivariate approach brings with it a considerable logistic problem to say nothing of its conceptual ramifications. As argued at several points in this chapter, fundamental research into the nature of dynamic processes such as the emotions seem a necessary prerequisite in order to solve some of the unresolved issues. It may be expected that the behavioural genetics and modern brain imaging techniques in combination with cognitive paradigms will in the coming decennium resolve some of the riddles of current developmental psychopathology.

REFERENCES

Abikoff, H. and Klein, R. G. (1992). Attention-deficit-hyperactivity and conduct disorder: Comorbidity and implications for treatment. *Journal of Consulting and Clinical Psychology*, **60**, 881–892.

Achenbach, T.M. (1990). Conceptualization of developmental psychopathology. In L. Michael and S.M. Miller (Eds.), *Handbook of developmental psychopathology* (pp. 3–14). New York: Plenum Press.

Achenbach, T.M. (1991a). *Integrative guide for the 1991 CBCL/4-18, YSR, and TRF profiles*. Burlington, VT: University of Vermont, Department of Psychiatry.

Achenbach, T.M. (1991b). *Manual for the Child Behavior Checklist/4-18 and 1991 profile*. Burlington, VT: University of Vermont, Department of Psychiatry.

American Psychiatric Association (1980). *Diagnostic and statistical manual of mental disorders* (3rd ed.). Washington, DC: American Psychiatric Association.

American Psychiatric Association (1987). *Diagnostic and statistical manual of mental disorders* (3rd ed. rev.). Washington, DC: American Psychiatric Association.

American Psychiatric Association (1994). *Diagnostic and statistical manual of mental disorders* (4th ed.). Washington, DC: American Psychiatric Association.

Anderson, K.E., Lytton, H., and Romney, D.M. (1986). Mothers' interactions with normal and conduct-disordered boys: Who affects whom? *Developmental Psychology*, **22**, 604–609.

Anderson, J.C., Williams, S., McGee, R., and Silva, P.A. (1987). DSM-III disorders in preadolescent children: Prevalence in a large sample from the general population. *Archives of General Psychiatry*, **44**, 69–76.

Barkley, R.A. (1990). *Attention deficit hyperactivity disorder. A handbook for diagnosis and treatment*. New York: Guilford Press.

Bates, J.E. (1987). Temperament in infancy. In J. Osofsky (Ed.), *Handbook of infant development* (2nd ed., pp. 1101–1149). New York: Wiley

Bates, J. E. and Bayles, K. (1988). Attachment and the development of behavior problems. In J. Belsky and T. Nezworski (Eds.), *Clinical implications of attachment* (pp. 253–299). Hillsdale, NJ: Lawrence Erlbaum Associates.

Bates, J., Maslin, C., and Frankel, K. (1985). Attachment security, mother-child interaction, and temperament as predictors of behavior problem ratings at age 3 years. *Monographs of the society for research in child development* (Serial No. 209), 167–193.

Benedict, R. (1934). *Patterns of culture. Edition 1959*. Boston: Houghton Mifflin Company.

Berg, C.Z., Rapoport, J.L., Whitaker, A., Davies, M., Leonard, H., Swedo, S.E., Braiman, S., and Lenane, M. (1989). Childhood obsessive-compulsive disorder: A two-year prospective follow-up of a community sample. *Journal of the American Academy of Child and Adolescent Psychiatry*, **28**, 528–533.

Biederman, J., Rosenbaum, J.F., Hirschfeld, D.R., Faraone, S.V., Bolduc, E.A., Gersten, M., Meminger, S.R. , Kagan, J., Snidman, S., and Reznick,, J.S. (1990). Psychiatric correlates of behavioral inhibition in young children of parents with and without psychiatric disorders. *Archives of General Psychiatry*, **47**, 21–26.

Boyd, J.H., Burke, J.D., Grünberg, E., Holzer, C.E., Rae, D.S., George, L.K., Karno, M., Stoltzman, R., McEvoy, L., and Nestadt, G. (1984). Exclusion criteria of DSM-III. *Archives of General Psychiatry*, **41**, 983–989.

Bowlby, J. (1973). *Attachment and loss, vol 2. Separation, anxiety and anger.* London: Hogarth Press.

Brady, E.U. and Kendall, P.C. (1992). Comorbidity of anxiety and depression in children and adolescents. *Psychological Bulletin*, **111**, 244–255.

Caffaro-Rouget, A., Lang, R.A., and VanSanten, V. (1989). The impact of child sexual abuse. *Annals of Sexual Research*, **2**, 29–47.

Campbell, S.B. (1995). Behavior problems in preschool children a review of recent research. *Journal of child Psychology and Psychiatry*, **36**, 113–150.

Cantwell, D.P. and Baker, L. (1989). Stability and natural history of DSM-III childhood diagnoses. *Journal of American Academy of Child and Adolescent Psychiatry*, **28**, 691–700.

Caron, C. and Rutter, M. (1991). Comorbidity in childhood psychopathology: Concepts, issues and research strategies. *Journal of Child Psychology and Psychiatry*, **32**, 1063–1080.

Christie, K.A., Burke, J., Regier, D.A., Rae, D.S., Boyd, J.H., and Locke, B.Z. (1988). Epidemiologic evidence for early onset of mental disorders and higher risk of drug abuse in young adults. *American Journal of Psychiatry*, **145**, 971–975.

Conte, J. and Schuerman, J. (1987). The effects of sexual abuse on children: A multi-dimensional view. *Journal of interpersonal Violence*, **2**, 380–390.

Cowan, P.A., Cowan, C.P., Schulz, M., and Heming, G. (1993). Prebirth to preschool family factors predicting children's adaptation to kindergarten. In R. Parke and S. Kellam (Eds.), *Advances in family research* (Vol. 4, pp. 75–114). Hillsdale, NJ: Lawrence Erlbaum Associates.

Doepfner, M., Berner, W., Schmeck, K., Lehmkuhl, G., and Poustka, F. (1995). Internal consistency and validity of the CBCL and TRF in a German sample: A cross-cultural comparison. In J. Sergeant (Ed.), *Eunethydis: European approaches to hyperkinetic disorder* (pp. 47–76). Trumpi: Zürich.

Egeland, B., Kalkoske, M., Gottesman, N., and Erickson, M.F. (1990). Preschool behavior problems' stability and factors accounting for change. *Journal of Child Psychology and Psychiatry*, **31**, 891–909.

Emery, R.E. (1982). Interparental conflict and the children of discord and divorce. *Psychological Bulletin*, **92**, 310–330.

Fergusson, D.M., Horwood, L.J., and Lloyd, M. (1991). Confirmatory factor models of attention deficit and conduct disorder. *Journal of Child Psychology and Psychiatry*, **32**, 257–274.

Fergusson D.M. and Horwood L.J. (1993). The structure, stability and correlations of the trait components of conduct disorder, attention deficit and anxiety/withdrawal reports. *Journal of Child Psychology and Psychiatry*, **34**, 749–766.

Filipek, P.A., Semrud-Clikeman, M., Steingard, R.J., Renshaw, M.D., Kennedy, D.N., and Biederman, J. (1997). Volumetyric MRI analysis comparing attention-defcit hyper-activity disorder and normal control. *Neurology*, in press.

Fonseca, A.C., Simoes, A., Rebelo, J.A., Cardoso, F., and Temudo, P. (1995). Hyperactivity and conduct disorder among Portugese children and adolescents: Data from parents' and teachers' reports. In J. Sergeant (Ed.), *Eunethydis: European approaches to hyper-kinetic disorder* (pp. 115–129). Trumpi: Zürich.

Fonseca, A.C., Yule, W., and Erol, N. (1994). Cross-cultural issues. In T.H. Ollendick, N.J. King, and W. Yule (Eds.), *International handbook of phobic and anxiety disorders in children and adolescents* (pp. 67–87). New York: Plenum Press.

Foulds, G. A. (1976). *The hierarchical nature of personal illness.* London: Academic press.

Francis, G., Last, C.G., and Strauss, C.C. (1987). Expression of separation anxiety disorder: The roles of age and gender. *Child Psychiatry and Human Development*, **87**, 82–89.

Freiberg-Golvan, D. and Prior, M. (1991). *Continuity, stability and change in temperament: A review of research.* (unpublished manuscript).

Frijda, N. H. (1989). *The emotions.* Cambridge: Cambridge University press.

Gittelman R., Mannuzza S., Shenker R., and Bongura N. (1985) Hyperactive boys almost grown up. I. Psychiatric status. *Archives of General Psychiatry,* **42**, 937–947.

Grych, J.H. and Fincham, F.D. (1992). Intervention for children of divorce: Toward greater integration of research and action. *Psychological Bulletin,* **111**, 434–454.

Harris, P. (1989). *Children and Emotion.* Oxford: Basil Blackwell Ltd.

Hinshaw, S.P. (1987). On the distinction between attentional deficits/hyperactivity and conduct problems/aggression in child psychopathology. *Psychological Bulletin,* **101**, 443–463.

Kashani, J.H. and Orvaschel, H. (1990). A community study of anxiety in children and adolescents. *American Journal of Psychiatry,* **147**, 313–318.

Keenan, K., Loeber, R., Zhang, Q, Stouthamer-Loeber, M., and Van Kammen, W.B. (1995). The influence of deviant peers on the development of boys' disruptive and delinquent behavior: A temporal analysis. *Development and Psychopathology,* **7**, 715–726.

Kendall-Tackett, K.A., Meyer-Williams L., and Finkelhor, D. (1993). Impact of sexual abuse on children: A review and synthesis of recent empirical studies. *Psychological Bulletin,* **113**, 164–180.

Kovacs, M., Gatsonis, C., Paulaskas, S.L., and Richards, C. (1989). Depressive disorders in childhood. *Archives of General Psychiatry,* **46**, 776–782.

Kraepelin, E. (1899). *Psychiatrie: Ein lehrbuch für Studierende und Aertzte.* Leipzig: Verlag von J.A. Barth.

Kyrios, M. and Prior, M. (1990). Temperament, stress and family factors in behavioural adjustment of 3–5 year old children. *International Journal of Behavioural Developmental,* **13**, 67–93.

LaHoste, G.J., Swanson, J.M., Wigal, S.B., King, N., and Kennedy , J.L.(1996). Dopamine D4 receptor gene polymorphism is associated with attention deficit hyperactivity disorder. *Molecular Psychiatry,* in press.

Last, C.G. (1991). Somatic complaints in anxiety disordered children. *Journal of Anxiety Disorders,* **5**, 125–138.

Last, C.G. (1993). *Anxiety across the life-span: A developmental perspective.* New York: Springer Publishing Company.

Last, C.G., Hersen, M., Kazdin, A.E., and Perrin, S. (1992). *Prospective study of anxiety disordered children.* Unpublished manuscript.

Last, C.G. and Strauss, C. C. (1989). Obsessive-compulsive disorder in childhood. *Journal of Anxiety Disorders,* **3**, 295–302.

Lechman, J.F., Weissman, M.M., Prussoff, B.A., Caruso, K.A., Merikangas, K.R., Pauls, D.L., Kidd, and K.K. (1984). Subtypes of depression: Family study perspective. *Archives of General Psychiatry,* **41**, 833–838.

Loeber, R., Lahey, B.B., and Thomas, C. (1991). Diagnostic conundrums of oppositional defiant disorder and conduct disorder. *Journal of Abnormal Psychology,* **100**, 379–390.

Loney, J., Kramer, J., and Milich, R.S. (1981). The hyperactive child grows up: Predictions of symptoms, delinquency, and achievement at follow-up. In K.D. Gadow and J. Loney (Eds.), *Psychosocial aspects of drug treatment for hyperactivity* (pp. 381–415). Boulder, CO: Westview Press.

McGee R., Williams S., and Silva, P.A. (1987). A comparison of girls and boys with teacher-identified problems of attention. *Journal of the American Academy of Child and Adolescent Psychiatry,* **26**, 711–717.

McGee, R., Feehan, M., Williams, S., Partridge, F., Silva, P.A., and Kelly, J. (1990). DSM-III disorders in a large sample of adolescents. *Journal of the American Academy of Child and Adolescent Psychiatry,* **29**, 611–619.

Offord, D.R., Boyle, M.H., Racine, Y. A., Fleming, J.E., Cadman, D.T., Blum, H.M., Byrne, C., Linds, P.S., Lipman, E.L., MacMillan, H.L., Grant, N.I.R., Sanford, M.N., Szatmari, P., Thomas, H., and Woodward, C.A. (1992). Outcome, prognosis, and risk in a longitudinal follow-up study. *Journal of American Academy of Child and Adolescent Psychiatry*, **31**, 916–923.

Ollendick, T. H. and King, N.J. (1994). Diagnosis, Assessment, and treatment of internalizing problems in children: The role of longitudinal data. *Journal of Consulting and Clinical Psychology*, **62**, 918–927.

Patterson, G.R., DeBaryshe, B.D., and Ramsey, E. (1989). A developmental perspective on antisocial behavior. *American Psychologist*, **44**, 329–335.

Pelham, W.E. and Hinshaw, S.O. (1992). Behavioural intervention for Attention Deficit-Hyperactivity Disorder. In Turner, Calhoun, and Adams (Eds.), *Handbook of clinical behavior therapy* (pp. 259–285). New York: Wiley.

Pliszka, S. (1989). Effect of anxiety on cognition, behavior and stimulant response in ADHD. *Journal of the American Academy of Child and Adolescent Psychiatry*, *28*, 882–887.

Plomin, R. (1995). Genetics and children's experiences in the family. *Journal of Child Psychology and Psychiatry*, **36**, 69–112.

Porrino, L.J., Rapoport, J.L., Behar, D., Sceery, W., Ismond, D.R., and Bunney, W.E. (1984). A naturalistic assessment of the motor activity of hyperactive boys. *Archives of General Psychiatry*, **40**, 681–687.

Prior, M. (1992). Childhood Temperament. *Journal of Child Psychology and Psychiatry and Allied Disciplines*, **33**, 249–279.

Quay, H.C. (1986). Classification. In H.C. Quay and J.S. Werry (Eds.), *Psychopathological disorders in childhood* (3rd ed., pp. 1–34). New York: Wiley.

Renken, B., Egeland, B., Marvinney, D., Mangelsdorf, S., and Sroufe, L.A. (1989). Early childhood antecedents of aggression and passive-withdrawl in early elementary school. *Journal of Personality*, **57**, 257–281.

Rosenbaum, J. F., Biederman, J., Bolduc, E.A., Hirschfeld, D.R., Faraone, S.V., and Kagan, J. (1992). Comorbidity of parental anxiety disorders as risk for childhood-onset anxiety in inhibited children. *American Journal of Psychiatry*, **149**, 475–481.

Rutter, M. (1994). Beyond longitudinal data: Causes, consequences, changes and continuity. *Journal of Consulting and Clinical Psychology*, **62**, 928–940.

Rutter, M. (1995). Clinical implications of attachment concepts. *Journal of Child Psychology and Psychiatry*, **36**, 1549–571.

Sameroff, A.J. (1975). Early influences on development: Fact or fancy? *Merrill-Palmer Quarterly*, **21**, 265–294.

Sanson, A., Oberklaid, F., Pedlow, R., and Prior, M.(1991). Risk indicators: Assessment of infancy predictors of pre-school behavioural maladjustment. *Journal of Child Psychology and Psychiatry*, **32**, 609–626.

Schachar R.J. (1991) Childhood hyperactivity. *Journal of Child Psychology and Psychiatry*, **32**, 155–191.

Schmidt, M.H. and Moll, G.H. (1995). The course of Hyperkinetic Disorders and symptoms: A ten year prospective longitudinal study. In J.A. Sergeant (Ed.), *Eunethydis: European approaches to hyperkinetic disorder* (pp. 189–205). Zurich: Trumpi.

Taylor, E. (1995). Developmental psychopathology of Hyperactivity. In J.A. Sergeant (Ed.), *Eunethydis: European approaches to hyperkinetic disorder* (pp. 171–187). Zurich: Trumpi.

Taylor E., Sandberg S., Thorley G., and Giles S. (1991). *The epidemiology of childhood hyperactivity*. Maudsley monographs No. 33. Oxford: Oxford University Press.

Taylor, E., Schachar, R., Thorley, G., Wieselberg, H.M., Everitt, B., and Rutter, M. (1987). Which boys respond to stimulant medication? A controlled trial of methylphenidate in boys with disruptive behavior. *Psychological Medicine*, **17**, 121–143.

Thyer, B.A. (1993). Childhood separation anxiety disorder and adult-onset agoraphobia: Review of the evidence. In C.G. Last (Ed.), *Anxiety across the life-span: A developmental perspective* (pp. 128–147). New York: Springer Publishing Company.

Van der Meere, J.J., Wekking, E., and Sergeant, J.A. (1991). Sustained attention and pervasive hyperactivity. *Journal of Child Psychology and Psychiatry*, **32**, 275–284.

Verhulst, F.C. (1995). The cross-cultural generalizability of the CBCL. In J.A. Sergeant (Ed.), *Eunethydis: European approaches to hyperkinetic disorder* (pp. 15–31). Zurich: Trumpi.

Vermersch, S. and Fombone,E. (1995). Attention and aggressive problems among French school-aged children. In J.A. Sergeant (Ed.), *Eunethydis: European approaches to hyperkinetic disorder* (pp. 33–45). Zurich: Trumpi.

Weisglas-Kuperus, N., Koot, H.M., Baerts, W., Fetter, W.P., and Sauer, P.J. (1993). Behaviour problems of very low birthweight children. *Developmental Medicine and Child Neurology*, **35**, 406–416.

Weisz, J.R., Suwanlert, S., Chaiyasit, W., Weiss, B., Achenbach, T.M., and Walter, B.A. (1987). Epidemiology of behavioral and emotional problems among Thai and American children. Parent reports from ages 6 to 11. *Journal of the American Academy of Child and Adolescent Psychiatry*, **26**, 890–897.

Werner, E.E. and Smith, R.S. (1982). *Vulnerable but invincible: A longitudinal study of resilient children and youth.* New York: Adams, Bannister, Cox.

INDEX